E-Health and Telemedicine:

Concepts, Methodologies, Tools, and Applications

Information Resources Management Association
USA

Volume III

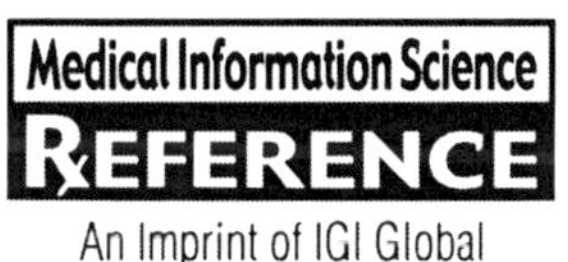

Managing Director:	Lindsay Johnston
Managing Editor:	Keith Greenberg
Director of Intellectual Propery & Contracts:	Jan Travers
Acquisitions Editor:	Kayla Wolfe
Production Editor:	Christina Henning
Multi-Volume Book Production Specialist:	Deanna Jo Zombro
Cover Design:	Samantha Barnhart

Published in the United States of America by
Medical Information Science Reference (an imprint of IGI Global)
701 E. Chocolate Avenue
Hershey PA, USA 17033
Tel: 717-533-8845
Fax: 717-533-8661
E-mail: cust@igi-global.com
Web site: http://www.igi-global.com

Library of Congress Cataloging-in-Publication Data

E-Health and telemedicine : concepts, methodologies, tools, and applications / Information Resources Management Association, editor.
     pages cm
  Includes bibliographical references and index.
  Summary: "This reference explores recent advances in mobile medicine and how this technology impacts modern medical care"-- Provided by publisher.
  ISBN 978-1-4666-8756-1 (hardcover) -- ISBN 978-1-4666-8757-8 (ebook) 1. Medical care--Technological innovation. 2. Medical informatics. 3. Telecommunication in medicine. I. Information Resources Management Association.
  R858.E223 2016
  610.285--dc23
                                   2015019904

British Cataloguing in Publication Data
A Cataloguing in Publication record for this book is available from the British Library.

For electronic access to this publication, please contact: eresources@igi-global.com.

List of Contributors

Table of Contents

Volume I

Section 1
Fundamental Concepts and Theories

This section serves as a foundation for this exhaustive reference tool by addressing underlying principles essential to the understanding of E-Health and Telemedicine. Chapters found within these pages provide an excellent framework in which to position E-Health and Telemedicine within the field of information science and technology. Insight regarding the critical incorporation of global measures into E-Health and Telemedicine is addressed, while crucial stumbling blocks of this field are explored. With 15 chapters comprising this foundational section, the reader can learn and chose from a compendium of expert research on the elemental theories underscoring the E-Health and Telemedicine discipline.

Cynthia M. LeRouge, Saint Louis University, USA
Bengisu Tulu, Worchester Polytechnic Institute, USA
Suzanne Wood, Saint Louis University, USA

Jasmine Tehrani, University of Reading, UK

Randike Gajanayake, Queensland University of Technology, Australia
Tony Sahama, Queensland University of Technology, Australia
Renato Iannella, Queensland University of Technology, Australia

Andrew Georgiou, University of New South Wales, Australia

Section 2
Frameworks and Methodologies

This section provides in-depth coverage of conceptual architecture frameworks to provide the reader with a comprehensive understanding of the emerging developments within the field of E-Health and Telemedicine. Research fundamentals imperative to the understanding of developmental processes within E-Health and Telemedicine are offered. From broad examinations to specific discussions on methodology, the research found within this section spans the discipline while offering detailed, specific discussions. From basic designs to abstract development, these chapters serve to expand the reaches of development and design technologies within the E-Health and Telemedicine community. This section includes 11 contributions from researchers throughout the world on the topic of E-Health and Telemedicine.

Section 3
Tools and Technologies

This section presents an extensive coverage of various tools and technologies available in the field of E-Health and Telemedicine that practitioners and academicians alike can utilize to develop different techniques. These chapters enlighten readers about fundamental research on the many tools facilitating the burgeoning field of E-Health and Telemedicine. It is through these rigorously researched chapters that the reader is provided with countless examples of the up-and-coming tools and technologies emerging from the field of E-Health and Telemedicine. With 21 chapters, this section offers a broad treatment of some of the many tools and technologies within the E-Health and Telemedicine field.

Volume II

**Section 4
Cases and Applications**

*This section discusses a variety of applications and opportunities available that can be considered by
practitioners in developing viable and effective E-Health and Telemedicine programs and processes. This
section includes 13 chapters that review topics from case studies to best practices and ongoing research.
Further chapters discuss E-Health and Telemedicine in a variety of settings. Contributions included in
this section provide excellent coverage of today's IT community and how research into E-Health and
Telemedicine is impacting the social fabric of our present-day global village.*

Volume III

Section 5
Issues and Challenges

This section contains 17 chapters, giving a wide variety of perspectives on E-Health and Telemedicine and its implications. Within the chapters, the reader is presented with an in-depth analysis of the most current and relevant issues within this growing field of study. Crucial questions are addressed and alternatives offered along with theoretical approaches discussed.

Section 6
Emerging Trends

This section highlights research potential within the field of E-Health and Telemedicine while exploring uncharted areas of study for the advancement of the discipline. Introducing this section are chapters that set the stage for future research directions and topical suggestions for continued debate, centering on the new venues and forums for discussion. A pair of chapters on space-time makes up the middle of the

Preface

The constantly changing landscape of E-Health and Telemedicine makes it challenging for experts and practitioners to stay informed of the field's most up-to-date research. That is why Medical Information Science Reference is pleased to offer this three-volume reference collection that will empower students, researchers, and academicians with a strong understanding of critical issues within E-Health and Telemedicine by providing both broad and detailed perspectives on cutting-edge theories and developments. This reference is designed to act as a single reference source on conceptual, methodological, technical, and managerial issues, as well as provide insight into emerging trends and future opportunities within the discipline.

E-Health and Telemedicine: Concepts, Methodologies, Tools and Applications is organized into six distinct sections that provide comprehensive coverage of important topics. The sections are:

1. Fundamental Concepts and Theories;
2. Frameworks and Methodologies;
3. Tools and Technologies;
4. Cases and Applications;
5. Issues and Challenges; and
6. Emerging Trends.

The following paragraphs provide a summary of what to expect from this invaluable reference tool.

Section 1, "Fundamental Concepts and Theories," serves as a foundation for this extensive reference tool by addressing crucial theories essential to the understanding of E-Health and Telemedicine. Introducing the book is *Project Initiation for Telemedicine Services* by Cynthia M. LeRouge, Bengisu Tulu, and Suzanne Wood; a great foundation laying the groundwork for the basic concepts and theories that will be discussed throughout the rest of the book. Another chapter of note in Section 1 is titled *Principles of Information Accountability: An eHealth Perspective* by Randike Gajanayake, Tony Sahama, and Renato Iannella. Section 1 concludes, and leads into the following portion of the book with a nice segue chapter, *Telemedicine Program for Management and Treatment of Stress Urinary Incontinence in Women: Design and Pilot Test* by Anna Abelló Pla, Anna Andreu Povar, Jordi Esquirol Caussa, Vanessa Bayo Tallón, Dolores Rexachs, and Emilio Luque.

Section 2, "Frameworks and Methodologies," presents in-depth coverage of the conceptual design and architecture of E-Health and Telemedicine. Opening the section is *Information Architecture for Pervasive Healthcare Information Provision with Technological Implementation* by Chekfoung Tan and Shixiong Liu. Through case studies, this section lays excellent groundwork for later sections that will get into present and future applications for E-Health and Telemedicine. The section concludes with an excellent work by Sabah Al-Fedaghi, titled *Design Principles in Health Information Technology: An Alternative to UML Use Case Methodology.*

Section 3, "Tools and Technologies," presents extensive coverage of the various tools and technologies used in the implementation of E-Health and Telemedicine. Section 3 begins where Section 2 left off, though this section describes more concrete tools at place in the modeling, planning, and applications of E-Health and Telemedicine. The first chapter, *Healthinfo Engineering: Technology Perspectives from Evidence-Based mHealth Study in WE-CARE Project* by Anpeng Huang and Linzhen Xie, lays a framework for the types of works that can be found in this section. Section 3 is full of excellent chapters like this one, including such titles as *A System for the Semi-Automatic Evaluation of Clinical Practice Guideline Indicators* by Alexandra Pomares Quimbaya, María Patricia Amórtegui, Rafael A. González, Oscar Muñoz, Wilson Ricardo Bohórquez, Olga Milena García, and Melany Montagut Ascanio; and *Ambulance Dispatching System with Integrated Information and Communication Technologies on Cloud Environment* by Jian-Wei Li, Chia-Chi Chang, Yi-Chun Chang, and Yung-Fa Huang. The section concludes with *Using a Smartphone as a Track and Fall Detector: An Intelligent Support System for People with Dementia* by Chia-Yin Ko, Fang-Yie Leu, and I-Tsen Lin. Where Section 3 described specific tools and technologies at the disposal of practitioners, Section 4 describes the use and applications of the tools and frameworks discussed in previous sections.

Section 4, "Cases and Applications," describes how the broad range of E-Health and Telemedicine efforts has been utilized and offers insight on and important lessons for their applications and impact. The first chapter in the section is titled *The Role and Use of Telemedicine by Physicians in Developing Countries: A Case Report from Saudi Arabia* written by Dana Alajmi, Mohamed Khalifa, Amr Jamal, Nasria Zakaria, Suleiman Alomran, Ashraf El-Metwally, Majed Al-Salamah, and Mowafa Househ. This section includes the widest range of topics because it describes case studies, research, methodologies, frameworks, architectures, theory, analysis, and guides for implementation. The breadth of topics covered in the chapter is also reflected in the diversity of its authors, from countries all over the globe, such as: *A Case for Enterprise Interoperability in Healthcare IT: Personal Health Record Systems* by Mustafa Yuksel, Asuman Dogac, Cebrail Taskin, and Anil Yalcinkaya. The section concludes with *Political Attitudes on the Dutch Electronic Patient Record* by Evert Mouw, a great transition chapter into the next section.

Section 5, "Issues and Challenges," presents coverage of academic and research perspectives on E-Health and Telemedicine tools and applications. The section begins with *Detection of Pre-Analytical Laboratory Testing Errors: Leads and Lessons for Patient Safety* by Wafa Al-Zahrani and Mohamud Sheikh. Chapters in this section will look into theoretical approaches and offer alternatives to crucial questions on the subject of E-Health and Telemedicine. For example, *Operative Role Management in Information Systems* written by Taina Kurki and Hanna-Miina Sihvonen. The section concludes with *Approaches to Evidence-Based Management and Decision-Making in Healthcare Organizations: Lessons for Developing Nations* by Nouf Al Saleem and Mohamud Sheikh.

Section 6, "Emerging Trends," highlights areas for future research within the field of E-Health and Telemedicine, opening with *Mobile Health Services: A New Paradigm for Health Care Systems* by Nabila Nisha, Mehree Iqbal, Afrin Rifat, and Sherina Idrish. This section contains chapters that look at what might happen in the coming years that can extend the already staggering amount of applications for E-Health and Telemedicine. The final chapter of the book looks at an emerging field within E-Health and Telemedicine, in the excellent contribution, *Coalitions: The Future of Healthcare in Public Private Partnerships* by Erinn N. Harris.

Although the primary organization of the contents in this multi-volume work is based on its six sections, offering a progression of coverage of the important concepts, methodologies, technologies, applications, social issues, and emerging trends, the reader can also identify specific contents by utilizing the extensive indexing system listed at the end of each volume. As a comprehensive collection of research on the latest findings related to using technology to providing various services, *E-Health and Telemedicine: Concepts, Methodologies, Tools and Applications*, provides researchers, administrators and all audiences with a complete understanding of the development of applications and concepts in E-Health and Telemedicine. Given the vast number of issues concerning usage, failure, success, policies, strategies, and applications of E-Health and Telemedicine in countries around the world, *E-Health and Telemedicine: Concepts, Methodologies, Tools and Applications* addresses the demand for a resource that encompasses the most pertinent research in technologies being employed to globally bolster the knowledge and applications of E-Health and Telemedicine.

Chapter 59
Factors Enabling Communication–Based Collaboration in Interprofessional Healthcare Practice:
A Case Study

Ramaraj Palanisamy
St. Francis Xavier University, Canada

Jacques Verville
SKEMA Business School, USA

ABSTRACT

The healthcare system has moved from autonomous practice to a cross-disciplinary interprofessional team-based approach in which communication for collaborative care is vital. Ineffective communication contributes to the team's inability to work collaboratively and significantly increases the possibilities of mistakes occurring in the delivery of patient care. So, effective communication for collaborative care becomes necessary for ensuring patient safety. This paper aims to advance our understandings of current communication-based collaborative healthcare practices. Specifically, it explores the factors enabling communication-based inter-professional practice. A qualitative study was selected for obtaining real life experiences of healthcare professionals. Twenty-five participants participated in the study, and the descriptive interview method was used to obtain qualitative data. The enabling factors were grouped into five main themes: communication, coordination, cooperation, trust, and collaboration. Quotes from the participants are presented to augment the interpretation and enhanced description of the enabling factors. Managerial implications, areas for future research, and limitations are given besides the conclusions of the study.

DOI: 10.4018/978-1-4666-8756-1.ch059

1. INTRODUCTION

In the modern healthcare system, healthcare provision has shifted from that of autonomous practice to interprofessional team based approach which involves multiple professionals with different educational background, training and expertise, working on behalf of patients, sharing a common goal (Woods et al., 2011). In providing high-quality care to patients, professionals have to interact with a number of other healthcare professionals cultivating relationships using best communication practices ensuring better patient outcomes. Patients receive safer and higher-quality care when healthcare professionals work as a team and communicate effectively while they practice. Effective interprofessional communication is not only important for patient care, but it is an essential element of healthcare environment. Ineffective communication contributes to the professional team's inability to collaboratively work together (Thomas et al., 2004). Healthcare professionals cannot provide safer care for patients without correct information and so communication has life-and-death implications (Haeuser & Preston, 2005).

The past research has found the communication of healthcare professionals as highly variable and often ineffective due to individual differences in culture and environment (McKinney, Barker, Davis, & Smith 2005; Pearce, 2003; Shorter, 1995). In the complex healthcare environment, poor communication and collaboration among health professionals significantly increases the possibilities of mistakes occurring in the delivery of patient-care, medication-error-related deaths, wrong-site surgeries and increased staff turnover (Woods et al., 2011; Spath, 2005; Anonymous, 2005). So, clear and precise communication among professionals becomes necessary for ensuring patient safety and safe patient environment (Joint Commission on the Accreditation of Healthcare Organizations, 2004).

The objective of this paper is to advance our understandings of current practices by examining the communication processes used in inter-professional collaborative practice in healthcare settings. Specifically, the paper explores the ways in which health professionals can communicate more effectively and identify the factors enabling communication-based inter-professional collaborative practice in complex environment. The remaining part of the paper is organized as follows. Section 2 documents the research methodology followed for this study; Section 3 shows the qualitative findings; Section 4 discusses the managerial implications of this study followed by the areas of future research; and Section 5 gives the limitations and the concluding remarks.

2. RESEARCH METHODOLOGY

The purpose of this study is to improve our understandings of current communication based collaboration used in inter-professional practice in healthcare settings. In other words, the research study is intended to deepen the understandings of communication based collaboration by obtaining real life experiences of healthcare professionals. Since the study aimed for straight descriptions of the phenomena of communication-based inter-professional practice and collaboration, the qualitative descriptive study method was chosen for the research design (Sandelowski, 2000). The qualitative study was selected as it is a process used to examine the lived experiences of healthcare professionals in the field; and it provides a comprehensive summary of real life experiences in terms of events. To know and understand a phenomenon, facts about that phenomenon is required. The facts could be in the form of events or experiences which are descriptive in nature. These descriptions depend on the describer's perceptions and sensitiveness of the described events (Emerson, Fretz, & Shaw, 1995). Based on the descriptive findings the theory development was done which is common in qualitative research studies (Neuman, 2003).

A descriptive interviewing method was applied for collecting qualitative data as the concepts and theories were not fully developed. The shift to the qualitative study enabled the researchers to examine the current practices and based on the findings a valid theory was evolved. Qualitative interviewing process helps to find what others feel, think, and perceive about their own worlds by collecting several types of information including narratives, stories and myths (Rubin & Rubin, 1995). These information types determine the completeness, accuracy and important facts about the targeted event or experience. The problems and solutions described in the events and the narrated practices are useful to predict the future performance in similar circumstances. A notable outcome of the qualitative research is the emergence of themes and subthemes out of the descriptive data. The participants in the study were healthcare professionals in North America including nurses, physicians, pharmacists, technologists, and nonclinical personnel. The opinion of healthcare professionals whose positions require ongoing skill development and experience may yield more appropriate data for accomplishing the study objectives. Furthermore, the emergence of themes and subthemes cannot be arrived by statistical methods and are notable outcome of qualitative research (Glaser and Strauss, 1967).

Having understood the difficulties of scheduling interviews with busy healthcare professionals, a sample size of 70 potential contacts was targeted. Out of which 25 respondents including both male and female professionals participated in the study. The average length of each interview was about 75 minutes. The participants selected for this study were possessing minimum of five years professional experience and actively participated in interprofessional communication for collaboration. Besides the purpose of the study,

the key words and their meaningful definitions were given to the participants beforehand. The interviews were administered with the objective of describing and understanding the occurrences of various events from the respondents' point of view (Leedy & Ormrod, 2001). The interviews were taped and transcribed for better understanding. In addition to the main questions, a set of supplemental questions were asked for deeper understanding.

3. FINDINGS

Several recurring sub-themes emerged as enabling factors for communication-based interprofessional practice. These sub-themes were grouped into five main themes: communication, coordination, cooperation, trust, and collaboration. All these themes were considered to be equally important. Quotes from the participants are presented to augment the interpretation and enhanced description of the enabling factors.

3.1. Communication

The sub-themes related to communication for inter-professional practice are: methods for communication, openness, social structure and impediments for effective communication.

3.1.1. Methods for Communication

There is no single way for communication. Most common methods for communication are face-to-face, telephone, computer (e-mail, or specific software), etc.

… I think we are all very open in our meetings and whether we use a phone or whether we use the computer or whether we just stop in the hall or chat or whether we actually have formal meeting set up with our Manager,…

... is all meet and sort of brainstorm around how the weeks have gone and how we are going to do next week in the various areas that you in... Having positive conflict resolution skills, so that the issues don't go on and on and build...

There is no consensus/agreement regarding the choice of media about communication. Employees sometimes feel more comfortable with specific ways to communicate each other. While several employees see face-to-face communication as the best way to communicate sensitive issues (i.e., patient related, business related, etc.), several other employees prefer technology to communicate sensitive information.

...we have to respect the fact that – of course we never do it if somebody is in there, if a client is in the room for confidentiality.

Promise is open to the whole team.

Where as Meditec which is another system...

Email is not an appropriate medium we believe for medical emergencies management.

Employees have various options to communicate. While they prefer face-to-face communication for sensitive and complex information, location and attitude or familiarity with technology may impact the choice of communication media for daily conversation. In those cases, technology may be a substitute for face-to-face communication. Even employees may feel more comfortable using technology under specific conditions (i.e., sensitivity).

...a lot of information that not shared because this is really sensitive and so we would only share that as it was needed in either verbally or in writing.

Sometimes face-to-face communication is preferred since it allows more effective communication and richer information.

the conversation might elaborate into something much, much bigger and I will learn, I think, personal learn a lot more talking face to face rather than email. I am just too slow at typing, most of us are.

we are learning how to be a little bit more careful with emails and learning how they can be misinterpreted and how there is no body language or context around the email.

Sometimes, technology is preferred as a reliable way to communicate among team members and also in whole department or hospital.

..they have their information posted on it so while it might not be personal as speaking face to face at least we are sure that the information is there and available for everyone and then at some point the onus is on them to make sure that you know that they are looking at it, that their up to date...a bulletin board...

Education and providing several toolkits may enhance communication among team members from different disciplines.

... institution here has offered us communication workshop and they have a communication tool kit that is actually available to the portal so for anyone that wants that education or that support in communication it's there.

3.1.2. Openness

Team members are encouraged joining the meetings and also members feel comfortable to discuss any issue (i.e., roles) about the agenda in meetings. During meetings, each participant feels free to share their opinions openly, and also without fear of being misunderstood.

Staff meetings for sure and we all have access to the staff meeting agenda so anybody can put anything on the agenda at a staff meeting.

…there is a really good comfort level here I think just being able to say what is on your mind.

Those (everybody has a voice that they can speak up in terms of your meetings) that attend on a regular basis do.

These meetings allow people from different groups or people from different areas but in the same group to gain knowledge about up-to-date news about field or even about issues in their work place.

…the leaders or all the professional groups in the building come together to communicate any issues that come up from their individual areas.

The Doctors bringing issues forward, whoever has an issue to be informed. Keeping each other informed what each of us is doing in our various programs.

In addition, employees feel very comfortable about going to see anyone including the management and talking about any issue: work related, information sharing, etc.

…very much more open door policy and I mean that it really is an open door policy that you can come and feel much more comfortable talking to someone or talking to the management here compared to when we initially opened here.

… Here it is more or less open door approach. You wander down the hallway and if someone is in their office then you go in and have your chat so there you go your issues over and done with…

Feedback makes communication more effective.

Feedback is another thing like people are very quick to be critical…. I think we would like to encourage people to provide us with some good feedback as well, constructive feedback as well as…

3.1.3. Social Structure

The relationships are considered mainly based on "trust, honesty, respect, and openness" and employees prefer a social structure based on these values.

Employees also find guidance and support from more experienced employees.

While employees have the opportunity to speak during meetings as they wished, in some cases where members do not feel comfortable with speaking, they are encouraged and a friendly environment is created so that everyone will be able to join the discussion comfortably. The social structure inhibits the interaction among team members.

… we have the opportunity to speak and sometimes I, just because of me I wouldn't necessarily open up at a meeting but maybe ask the manager afterwards if she had a few minutes just to chat because I am not always comfortable talking in large groups."

And our interviews reveal that this type of informal conversations, friendly talks encourages members to talk and share their opinions freely.

..we started to collaborate on a couple of things or once we were starting to have some successes in working through some of our planning groups all of a sudden we've shared a few laughs and you've agreed with what I've had to say on these things or I've seen your point of view and I agreed with what you've had to say and all of a sudden yeah I am more willing to kind of share what my weaknesses are or what I'm curious about.

Employees feel comfortable when they have an environment that they can say what they want. And they believe that this environment helps them to improve collaboration and fix the things that need to be handled.

... So having a safe environment where we can say what it is that we need to say and it might not be perfect but we can repair if there is something that didn't work out well.

Based on the interviews, employees who find their environment more encouraging communicating also state that their organization does not have strict rules and less hierarchy.

... it is a much more flat hierarchy in ... than many other organizations involved in health care.

..I think that we are all on the same level. I do not think, oh well, you are better than me so I will just....we are all here to work and do a good job.

3.1.4. Impediments for Effective Communication

The impediments to effective communication or even collaboration do exist in health-care industry. These impediments can be in several ways: location, social image, lack of trust, lack of feedback, timeliness, attitude to technology, etc. For example, while working in the same floor or even sometimes the same building, the opposite is considered as an impediment in order to communicate effectively, share knowledge, and even developing interpersonal relationships.

...we did have a lot of interaction with the three of us because we were all in the same floor for most of the time.

...how the building was designed I guess...

Physical surrounding or location of the offices that team members work may affect the communication as well as the medium of communication among the members.

All of their offices are on the second floor and they very rarely go to the actual treatment units any more they used to have to go there to do a certain function but they don't anymore so I do think that we are losing touch with them a bit on a daily basis because just...

Impediments regarding social image, how people think about him/her sometimes become an impediment to communicate. This fact is more obvious during group/team meetings. Members sometimes prefer not to ask questions or speak because of being misunderstood or judged.

... sometimes it is really hard to communicate stuff that is uncomfortable, it is always easy to say 'Hey you're doing a great job' 'Hey that's really neat' but some of us were less willing to expose what we didn't know, right, because we weren't trusting and 'everybody is going to think I'm stupid so I'm not going to ask', 'how do I do a blood pressure again' ...

Trust plays an important role in communication and collaboration. Lack of trust causes several problems. For example, support is one of these problems that may take place between team members.

There has been a falling out between the Nurses and Doctors lately because the Doctors have felt unsupported by the Nurses...

On the other hand, friendly conversations before the meetings can eliminate this impediment.

...sudden we've shared a few laughs and you've agreed with what I've had to say on these things or I've seen your point of view and I agreed with what you've had to say and all of a sudden yeah I am more willing to kind of share what my weaknesses are or what I'm curious about.

Lack of feedback is another impediment for effective communication.

... the thing that I find most difficult with is the two way communication like I communicate to them but I don't always get communication back.

Not all employees can attend the meetings and exchange information. This may happen because of various reasons (i.e., timing, announcement, etc.). This may create problem and unpleasant feeling among employees.

It is just that I feel sometimes that I do not know everything that is going on because they have their separate meeting.

The biggest challenge is trying to get their managers here to meet with us as a group.

Technology is supposed to help individuals to have an easier and probably better life (personal and business life). However, in some cases, people have a negative attitude for technology and claim that technology is not making their lives easier, on the contrary making their lives more complicated.

...whatever and these are like schedules, Oncologists, Nurses schedules. All our policies and procedures all kinds of things that has really been the best way that we have found of communicating on a non-verbal level at least you know for us it is a way... much, much, much better than email.

3.2. Coordination

The two sub-factors related to coordination that enabled the interprofessional practice were: leadership and power.

3.2.1. Leadership

Leadership is important in teams. Members feel more comfortable when they feel like they can discuss any concerns with the team leaders. They have an effect on the style of communication among the team members. Generally, team members prefer an open door policy where they can discuss any concerns with the leaders.

The listening to what your concerns are. If you have a concern, we feel able to communicate a concern.

Our interview results show that employees can feel the difference in management when the hospital was new and more established. As the organization has become more established, employees felt the leadership more. And they were comfortable to have a collaborative environment, good communication opportunities, and open door policy with the management.

...we have gone through a lot of ups and downs and trials and tribulations with the way they... Leadership, yes. Very much more open door policy and I mean that it really is an open door policy that you can come and feel much more comfortable talking to someone or talking to the management here compared to when we initially opened here.

Leaders also dedicated themselves to help team members to perform better. They find helping employees on their performance issues one-to-one, setting goals and measuring their position and level, as well as giving feedback to enhance the performance of team members.

… from performance evaluation and helping people work on goals and assessing where their level andhow their practicing. I'll sit in and observe classes periodically and give feedback afterwards or I'll sit in and join people individually and observe.

The most effective way to enhance the team members' performance is the communication and feedback.

…The only way that ….and the clinicians agree to that…. they said absolutely come in and give me feedback on what I am doing well and where I could improve. So it was with permission doing some observations but also if I was doing some observation as part of an annual performance and appraisal I would get permission and say yeah well I'll come and watch and see what's going on.

The characteristics of a good leader are described as:

…be somebody who listens, somebody who plans ahead, who is data driven, somebody who is transparent, somebody who is punctual and somebody who communicates regularly so that all the players on the team are aware of the things going on around.

…It is much better to be able to arrive at a consensus for the group that you are leading and have them feel that they made the decision and as often as possible.

Collaboration and performance improve when the team members are following the meetings and aware of latest improvements and conditions in the hospital. Therefore, not participating in meetings, or not following the agenda of the meeting are the impediments for an effective collaboration. An effective leadership can increase the aware-ness and interest to meetings and also increase collaboration.

They (Physicians) have a clinical meeting and I am wondering if sometimes they may not realize what they are discussing may impact the rest of the people in the building.

It is just that I feel sometimes that I do not know everything that is going on because they have their separate meeting.

3.2.2. Power

When the power and hierarchy of the leader is less, the employees or team members feel more involved in decision making and this perception leads to a better collaboration according to our interview results.

in BCCA the answers probably yes but it's a much more flat hierarchy in BCCA than many other organizations involved in health care.

…one of the most valuable things to do is to make as few decisions as you can on an island. It is much better to be able to arrive at a consensus for the group that you are leading and have them feel that they made the decision and as often as possible.

Hierarchy was….That was one of the things we did have to kind of break down and say 'no this is not how it's going to work'.

3.3. Cooperation

In an effort to cooperate during interprofessional practice, the teams have to organize meetings for knowledge sharing, have to make use of technology for effective communication. The impediments in organizing meetings and using technology were also identified and given below.

3.3.1. Knowledge Sharing

Knowledge sharing and discussing the responsibilities are encouraged during meetings and for this purpose, there are established regular meetings.

There are staff meetings here usually every second Thursday, ...

We do every week we come together and do case consults and we also come together and have a staff meeting...

...also have smaller meetings maybe every six weeks...

...they are encouraged to go there because that is where a lot of information is shared but there is no sort of rules or policies or circumstances...

Meetings, exchanging opinions are crucial and they are more crucial especially when the organization is new and there is an intense need to put things in order.

... when we first opened we would meet daily and we did a check in for about a half an hour every morning.

Meetings create an ideal environment for exchanging information, discussing concerns, decision making, and sharing responsibilities.

... who meet to look at some policy development... about something to do with in the center we might be involved in making decisions about that...

The more time passes and the routines are established, there may be less need to meet but it does not mean that there will be no meetings. Therefore, even if works are in flow, there must be meetings so that people can decide their responsibilities and share information. In addition, there

is more than one way for exchanging information such as hallway conversations, lunch meetings, etc.

And then we started to meet you know once a week for about an hour to go through things and then it became you know twice a month more or less. So we have staff meetings regularly, hallway conversations, chit chatting over lunch hours, planning meetings, yeah.

Team members use different methods and environment to communicate and share their opinion for several issues as well as decision making.

At the end of the clinic we all get together and go through all the patients that we've seen and each person has equal opportunity to speak up and voice their opinion and state what they think the medical management should be...

Main goal of meetings among team members from other disciplines was to share information and expertise.

It was made very clear right from Management, high up level Management, that the expectation was that we would learn each other's disciplines because the patient comes in and if they have got Diabetes, Heart Disease and Kidney Disease it is not good enough for me to know just about Kidney Disease.

Sharing information leads to enhanced collaboration.

And as we were sharing more things would come up and more pieces would come together and we would begin to build.

3.3.2. Impediments for Meetings

Although meetings are required and perceived as crucial, some conditions make the meetings and sharing information more difficult. Location, time concerns, announcements of the meetings and fear of misunderstanding are among the highly mentioned impediments for gathering together to exchange information.

... we never meet as a team... Except tonight and a couple of times prior to that.

... We do have staff meetings probably not as regularly as you...

... because they are seeing patients to get everybody away from their work place for an hour to have a meeting...

Not so much with attendance, if we let everybody know when the meetings are going to be with enough advanced notice all the staff that are here will clear their calendar for that.

... five or six different buildings. So if you wanted to meet with someone you would actually have to pick up the phone and make an appointment basically to meet with them because not only were they not in your building but you had to go a few blocks down the street in order to meet with them so.

Information can be shared through several methods.

... what information gets spread via email, what information gets spread via bulletin boards, what information gets shared in some of the smaller program meetings so we have a Diabetes Meeting, we've got a Renal Meeting, a Cardiovascular Meeting where we tend to bring those issue.

When information sharing is done through informal ways, such as mouth-to-mouth, there is a danger of losing or modifying the information. If this information is critical, this situation may cause harm for an organization.

... especially with changes in policies and procedures of things, it is sometimes difficult because I find you know the first couple of people that you communicate with is great but as it gets filtered down either people are not here and they don't hear it or the rest of (022) switch changed along the way.

Impediments to sharing or exchanging information include fear of misunderstanding, image on others' eyes.

Sometimes it's really hard to communicate stuff that is uncomfortable.

... some of us were less willing to expose what we didn't know, right, because we weren't trusting and 'everybody is going to think I'm stupid so I'm not going to ask'...

3.3.3. Technology enabled Communication

Usually hospitals have the entire technological infrastructure but the matter is how much employees want to use it.

... we found most valuable lately actually is a web site that we have, a portal on the PH (033) website and I can show it to you if you'd like but it's a portal where we post information. We post announcements, we post schedules for the therapists, all our policies and procedures any information that anybody might need to know that we can think of to put on there is on the portal and it's the very easy it's the desktop on the computer.

Sometimes people may be less willing to communicate face-to-face and choose technology as a medium to communicate. In addition, they may prefer one type of communication to another based on the case. In that case employees usually find technology as an easier and more efficient way of communication.

So you don't want to actually phone them because you are a little bit scared or anxious so you email them. You never actually bridge that gap because you don't have to.

Hospitals usually provide the current communication technologies for their employees in work environment. Wiki, portal, e-mail, phone, blackberry, bulletin board, and specific software systems are among the most highly used technologies in hospitals.

Although technology is supposed to make life easier and better, it is not always the case. Sometimes technology can be scary for employees and be an obstacle for collaboration. Therefore there is no consensus about the attitude towards using technology for communication.

I need that reassurance and the biggest fear with technology from other people is 'oh my god I am going to screw up and press the wrong button, right.

Sometimes technology may not be perceived as the appropriate media for communication. Usually this is the case when members are talking about "sensitive" information. Another reason may be lack of interest or knowledge about technology.

I would suggest that we use email as a last resort rather than a first resort for one thing.

Impediments regarding acceptance and use of technology include bureaucracy, fear of being hacked, and perception of less richness of communication.

It {website} is very bureaucratic...

...make sure that we can't be hacked or somebody can get into our...

... we kind of steered away from email a bit more was because you don't get that richness of the dialog and you don't get that clarification automatically...

One of the main reasons that employees are not willing to use technology is the richness of communication. Employees state that face-to-face communication provides richer information than any technology does. This is also what media richness theory says.

the conversation might elaborate into something much, much bigger and I will learn, I think, personal learn a lot more talking face to face rather than email. I am just too slow at typing, most of us are.

we are learning how to be a little bit more careful with emails and learning how they can be misinterpreted and how there is no body language or context around the email.

'I am a nurse I am not here to work on the computer you want to pay me to be spending all this time working on the computer'.

Sometimes technology is not preferred as an optimum way of communication because of the accessibility of the technology by team members.

...it would be verbally and again we use email outside of the meetings which again are not an ideal way to communicate because I know that some of the front line people don't have access to email on a routine basis.

Some of them are so patient care driven that email the last thing on their mind. And I know that some of the therapists actually don't even read their emails so email is not the best way of communicating.

3.4. Trust

Our results reveal that trust has an impact on communication (effectiveness, openness, medium choice, etc.).

... I think if you are not getting to know somebody on a more personal level it is really difficult not only to communicate with them but you know you don't build the same trust in them and I think that goes both ways that they'll be...

Trust also can be critical for communication. If team members do not trust each other, they may be less willing to communicate and share information. This may affect the decision making process.

... because we weren't trusting and 'everybody is going to think I'm stupid so I'm not going to ask', 'how do I do a blood pressure again' ...

3.5. Collaboration

Other impediments to collaboration include gathering the team members together as well as their attention during (or priority to) team meetings.

... it is very difficult to bring the team together to work on...

... they jump up and answer their blackberry you know it's like that to no end just drives me crazy like you are either committed to a...and fully focused on being at the meeting and participating or to me if someone flipping you know flipping through their blackberry or running out of the room to me that is sending a message that the meeting is not top priority so...

...I try to hold a meeting that is no longer than an hour because I find that I mean because I have attended two and three hour meetings and it's just you reach a point in time where you start to think about all the other stuff... so you start to get

distracted so I try and hold meetings that are no longer than an hour because I just find that you loose your attention...

Having a conversation with someone who has their Blackberry down there and they're trying to read their email. Completely disrespectful you know it's just horrific actually you know.

4. DISCUSSION

This study examined the factors enabling communication-based collaborative interprofessional practice in healthcare settings and organized the factors into five main themes and several subthemes. In particular, the study identified the practical communication barriers among the healthcare professionals in team meetings. Besides identification of the themes, the study found huge potential in using new communication technologies for healthcare interactions and practice. Using the communication/collaboration tools and technologies for meetings are beneficial for achieving the goal of delivering quality healthcare. In particular, growing popularity and usage of mobile technologies are important enablers for healthcare communication and collaboration. The communication/ collaboration environment- technology fit needs to be based on the comparison of technology requirements of the healthcare groups and the features offered by available communication technologies (Sarker et al., 2010). Nonetheless, choosing technology for communication is not always the best choice especially when team members are of different nationalities with diverse cultural background (Duranti & de Almeida, 2012). As the communication cannot be limited to only two actors, there is a need to consider all possible multi-party interactions among healthcare professionals in order to understand how they work, particularly before using new communication technologies. As the same technologies are to be used by professionals, the usage has a practical impact on all of them and bound by practical constraints. The interactions among healthcare professionals are considered to be delicate ones because of their key contents such as patients' health and illness, symptoms and diagnoses, diseases and therapies (Pilnick et al., 2010). The research finds that the healthcare professionals choose several media for communication such as face-to-face, telephone, computer (e-mail, or specific software), etc. The complexity of the healthcare situation, importance and urgency of the message are the factors influencing the selection of media for communication (Bok et al., 2012). Therefore, the healthcare professionals must be able to balance the face-to-face meetings and technology enabled communications in the context of communicating sensitive and complex information.

This study identified the following impediments for effective communication: location of healthcare professionals, fear of social image, lack of trust, lack of feedback, hierarchical structure of organization, timeliness, and attitude towards technology. Generating a favorable communicative environment by addressing these barriers is important as they have a significant impact on patient safety and care. Having healthcare professionals in the same building premises increases the possibilities for having more face-to-face interactions. For overcoming the fear of being misunderstood and concerns for social image, the team members should be encouraged to ask questions or speak out in meetings. Having one-on-one conversations with members and providing guidance from experienced team members may also create a friendly environment so that everyone can discuss comfortably and can say what they want. Communication is an important enabler for building trust and it facilitates to understand the contributions of professionals aiming quality care (Henneman et al., 1995). Trust keeps the professionals' mind open to ideas and secures more dialogue and communication. The professionals consider the trust beliefs based on their

past communication with others and develop a good or bad attitude towards multi-disciplinary team work. Building trust through effective communication is so important for lessening the impact of negative attitude and continuance interactions among professionals. The professionals get more confidence in interactions when the communicative experience is positive. Winning trust at the beginning is important as initial trust could be a starting point for continuance participation in interactive decision making aiming quality care of patients. So an open and positive communicative environment facilitates more trust among professionals.

Daiski (2004) found non-supportive relationships between nurses and physicians in a specific context. The existence of mutual non-supportiveness was because of nurses' oppression caused by hierarchical relationships and dis-empowering. As lack of autonomy and assertiveness suppress initiatives and creativeness, the voices of the nurses are to be heard as they are the forefront care delivery professionals. Having frequent friendly conversations create support and trust among the professionals. The communicative breakdowns occur when there is a lack of feedback due to absence of closure in the communication loop while making patient care decisions (Roberts & Kuo, 2006; Behara et al., 2005). A hierarchical relationship can alter one's ability to close the communication loop as the boundaries of a relationship suppress the interaction from occurring (Roberts, 2003). So team performance could be enhanced by providing feedback in a flat hierarchical environment.

Besides the existence of traditional subordinate-superior relationship between nurses and physicians, there are other hierarchies within the healthcare profession. For instance, hierarchies exist among technological specialists/ nonclinical professionals; nurses based on their professional education; physicians based on qualification, skill and specialty; and these multiple overlapping hierarchy does not support an openly communicative environment due to domination and subordination

(Forsythe, 2007). Furthermore, hierarchical communication can be a significant barrier to safe care and can influence the way professionals communicate with each other (Miller, 2005; Thomas et al., 2004). So the professionals need to understand their communication boundaries by encouraging open communication and better to have less or flat hierarchy to serve the best interests of the patients. The diverse educational experiences, backgrounds, skills, personalities of the healthcare teams may create barriers to inter-professional communication as they have different philosophies of practice. Showing mutual recognition to each other's contribution to patient care can overcome these barriers. In the remainder of this section, the main enabling factors and recommendations for fostering them are discussed.

Consensus is the level of agreement of team members' views on the communication process (Rittgen, 2013). Though consensus is a key measure for the success of the communication process, conflict between healthcare professionals may be detrimental to the patient care and eventually may destroy the lines of communication. Conflicts and ineffective communication among healthcare professionals may occur due to professional, cultural, individual and environmental differences (Mckinney et al., 2005; Pearce, 2003). Though the variability can develop rich interactions (Pearce, 2005), conflicts are unavoidable as each team member brings his or her own unique frame of reference, knowledge and understanding to the communication space (Shorter, 2005a, 2005b). So, the team members have to keep this in mind while communicating and should be capable of handling conflicts if any.

Energy-draining conflicts are frequently the result of communication breakdowns. In healthcare settings, conflicts could be resolved and minimized by establishing a standard that keeping other professionals informed about key issues, making them to understand each other's priorities, encouraging face-to-face communication throughout the process, creating opportunities for

informal meetings, and conducting routine audits of communication processes to ensure the receiver understands the intent of the sender (Haeuser & Preston, 2005). For instance, to avoid a conflict or offence, a healthcare recommendation needs to be communicated in a more assertive way without offending the opinion of the team members. Similarly, how a discussion or communication ends is just as essential as how it begins. Inappropriate end may spoil the discussion and all the efforts in starting the communication may go in vain.

Healthcare decisions and communication are influenced by cognitive abilities of professionals (Croskerry, 2005) and the safe patient environment depends on clear and precise communication. The decisions can be influenced by an individual to group or group to individual in a collaborative setting (Papanikolaou & Gouli, 2013). So, educating healthcare professionals to enhance their communication skills is essential for providing safe-care for patients. Thereby, precautions could be taken to avoid any harmful events happen for patient. Organizing (online) communication workshops are recommended in this regard. For efficiency reasons, the communication toolkit has to be made available in the portal site for facilitating the download by the team members anywhere and at any time. The communicative environment in healthcare and inter-professional relationships need to be free from intimidation and avoidance, where communication of information flows openly and the team members should be given equal opportunity to express their voices (Forsythe, 2007). Thereby, the team members feel free to share their opinion in an atmosphere of equality in healthcare meetings.

Leaders of healthcare teams need to establish team goals and motivate team members toward achieving the goals (Spears & Lawrence, 2002). Lack of leadership competencies in healthcare settings could negatively affect patient care and safety (Smith, 2004). Leadership competencies refer to knowledge, key capabilities, skills, and abilities that team leaders have to motivate the team members to achieve goals and thereby enhancing performance (Tubbs & Schulz, 2006; Thompson, Repko & Staggers, 2003). Possessing skills such as forward thinking, planning ahead, producing vision, data-driven, transparency and regular communication are important for team-leaders as they greatly influence the healthcare delivery system (Wheatley, 2010; Hartley & Benington, 2010; Sultz & Young, 2009). Besides regular communication, listening is also an important characteristic of leadership for encouraging team members to express their thoughts freely. Traditionally physicians are the team leaders mediating between healthcare teams and management for enhancing agreement and understanding (Guthrie, 1999). As physicians are the key people in motivating the team members to produce the required changes for the common goal of patient care (Zaleznik, 1992), reasonable steps are to be taken to improve the quality of physician leadership. This makes the physicians to see themselves as leaders, physicians, and managers.

The modern healthcare services system moves from traditional hierarchical structure to cooperative multidisciplinary healthcare team structures for delivering safe and complex healthcare services (Carley, 2008; Krause et al., 2006; McCallin, 2003; Webster & Anderson, 2002). The teams are expected to have deeper levels of collaborative interactions and mentoring approach result in a shifting of leadership roles from the traditional hierarchy. The multidisciplinary configuration enables the teams to interact, intellectually stimulate, obtain professional inputs from different disciplines and operate in a flexible way responding to healthcare needs (Carley, 2008; Caramanica et al. 2003). So a leader must be able to influence, inspire, motivate and intellectually challenge the team members in a rewarding way and to achieve the goals. The team leader has to understand the constantly changing healthcare environment to refocus the team's efforts by providing regular feedbacks for improving the team's performance (Estep, 2005). The leadership communication in

workplaces needs to be open and mutual among the interdisciplinary teams by encouraging flexible flow of ideas as healthcare is constantly searching for excellence in patient care (Stuart-Kregor, 2005). The new and prospective leaders are to be developed by training them to improve their decision-making skills and successfully attaining the goals. Power in healthcare organizations especially with inter-professionals needs to be distributed evenly among multiple teams where members are involved in decision making.

As the majority of medical errors are caused by issues in interpersonal communication and a lack of shared understandings (''Silence Kills'', 2005), conducting regular meetings would enable the team members for sharing knowledge, information, responsibilities and discussing concerns. To develop shared understandings, healthcare professionals have to exchange their stories in an open communicative environment (Shorter, 2005a; Roberts, 2003). When a healthcare professional discusses a patient's case with other team members, it is in the best interest of the patient for sharing information in a cooperative and collegial manner. The more a team member knows about a patient's diagnosis, the more effectively the member can interact and contribute for the betterment of the patient.

In inter-professional communication, more opportunities are to be created for having regular meetings so as to learn each other's discipline for enhancing collaboration. Furthermore, the capability to function as a communicator in one's professional role is a learned behavior. So, healthcare professionals need to increase their capabilities to partner, trust each other and develop collaborative decision-making skills for delivering safety care to the patients (Forsythe, 2007). When a professional is consulted in the context of patient's course of treatment, the professional should demonstrate professional decision making skills. The more information a healthcare professional has, more the quality of the decisions that can be made on patient care.

The continuous changes in healthcare communication, ongoing pressure to reduce healthcare costs and demand for new communication skills force the healthcare institutions to evaluate and implement innovative technologies for transforming and advancing professional practices (Leach, 2005; Christensen, Bohmer, & Kenagy, 2000; Sachdeva, 2001). Often, new technologies are implemented ignoring users' knowledge level to use those technologies (Amendola, 2008). Often, professionals are offered little or no training after implementing the technology. Lack of skills to use the technology may result in communication gaps that could harm patients (Anonymous, 2005). So user training is the key to implementation success of new (communication) technologies as it increases user confidence, nurtures the skill development and thereby removes the fear over using the new technology (Glenzer & Middleberg, 2006). The team leaders should realize the benefits of communication technologies and should incorporate training for the team members in order to move from a low-technology to a high-technology environment for enhancing the quality of patient care (Parker, 2005). Creating knowledge about current communication technologies generate positive attitude towards using them.

Collaboration in healthcare is defined as a teamwork of individual healthcare experts in diverse fields working together agreeably, sharing responsibilities in solving problems assuming complementary roles (Woods et al., 2011). The collaborative practice increases the awareness of each team member's professional knowledge and skill set so as to enable effective decision making in patient care related decisions. Collaborative communication has to occur among healthcare professionals by creating a greater understanding of meaning by knowledge transfers for patient care (Nieva et al., 2005). For this, an open communicative environment in which all the professionals are encouraged to speak and to be heard is to be created. For ensuring effective collaboration, an evaluative process has to be established focusing on the team interaction (Forsythe, 2007). The teams are to be trained to work collaboratively. This process ensures whether healthcare professionals do have consistent understandings of each other's meanings. The major challenges for collaborative communication are gathering the team members together as well as getting their attention during team meetings.

Our overall findings reveal that communication-based healthcare professional practice is enabled by five mechanisms: communication, coordination, cooperation, trust, and collaboration. The future research can focus on empirically examining the relationships between these factors to develop evidence-based theory for improving the patient care. Exploring the role of technology especially the social media for communication-based healthcare practice is another significant research issue. The areas of conflict resolution in healthcare communicative environment, leadership strategies for creating favorable climate for effective communication, role of gender and culture in inter-professional communication may also of interest to the future researchers.

5. LIMITATIONS

The recommendations given in this study are to be used as guidelines for improving communication-based collaborative practices in healthcare settings. As sampling in this qualitative research is purposive rather than random, the experiences of the study-participants may not represent and generalize the experiences of all the healthcare professionals. As the study relies on a smaller sample size with the aim of studying communication-based collaborative practices in depth and detail, a large group of participants with different experience may outline additional (or different) themes/ sub-themes with added characteristics. So results and recommendations might have been different with large or another sample of respondents. It is important to acknowledge that the factors presented in this paper do not represent an exhaustive list. The recommendations given in this study for practice are mostly based on the personal experiences of the study-participants. The context-specific experience may not be valid in all circumstances and hence may prevent generalizability of the findings. Although, qualitative studies are not usually generalizable in the statistical sense, lack of empirical validation of the findings (e.g, trust has an impact on communication) is another limitation of the recommendations given in the study. Furthermore, limitation in the number of case studies restricts the ability to generalize the findings across the population of all the healthcare organizations. The variations in the competence, experience, and other skills of the study-participants have an impact on the reliability of the findings. In other words, subjectivity plays a role on the participants' reflections on the issues considered during the interview.

6. CONCLUSION

The study findings can guide professionals, managers and decision-makers toward a better understanding of the factors for communication based collaboration in interprofessional healthcare practice. The ineffective communication is a key barrier for the professionals to collaborate in a multi-disciplinary environment (Haeuser & Preston, 2005). Based on the study, the factors enabling communication-based collaborative practices are: coordination, cooperation, and trust. The key elements of communication are openness, and methods (media) of communication. Open communication enables the professionals to understand each other's perspective, boundary, discipline and the value of mutual contributions in a team-based approach for delivering care. Thereby, conflicts are resolved and collegial relationships are developed. As open communication is a key enabler for effective team collaboration, the implication for management is to implement

various methods of communication in interprofessional team work. The study finds various methods of communication in interprofessional healthcare practice. Based on the study, most of the information sharing takes place through face-to-face interactions, email communications, messaging, team meetings, interprofessional committees, team retreats, hallway conversations, and mini-conferences. In emergency situations, email may not be the preferred way of communicating health professionals. At the same time, physically divided office locations may impede opportunities for more face-to-face interactions.

Communication based collaboration can benefit, in particular, by providing good leadership so that members feel comfortable in discussing with the team leaders in sessions, group discussions, forums or formal meetings involving all team professionals. The team leader exhibits leadership roles by constantly communicating with the team members, encouraging an open door policy for obtaining inputs and providing feedback for care-related decisions by serving as the communicative hub of their healthcare teams. Although healthcare industry demands for new competencies for healthcare professionals, the care delivery must remain more patient focused rather than technology focused. Of course, the healthcare leaders must respond to the technological changes. At the same time, the presence of sophisticated communication technology alone cannot solve care related problems. On the other hand, the usage skills and leadership competencies are to be nurtured for enhancing patient care. Educating the healthcare team for effectively using the communication technology will get rid of the fear over the technology. Thereby, knowledge about the technology creates a positive attitude for using it. So exploring the alternative ways of technology-enabled communication is important for enhancing the patient-care. The organizations can use the guidelines for handling the impediments for effective communication in their own organizational context. In general, flattening the hierarchical structure and moving to team based health care creates a friendly environment for open and effective communication.

Communication brings the professionals working together as a team in a collaborative way. Communication-based cooperation enables information and knowledge sharing for enhanced decisions and optimal care of patients. In the inter-disciplinary team work, lack of knowledge about other professional's area of competence may hinder opportunities for collaboration. Creating opportunities for knowledge sharing and clarifying the professionals' positions, roles and responsibilities to team objectives lead to effective collaboration. The common methods of information sharing are: dissemination thru' emails, bulletin boards, smaller program meetings and informal ways such as hallway conversations, lunch meetings, chitchatting etc. Besides, trust has an impact on communication-based collaborative practice. Having competent, skilled and experienced professionals in the healthcare team enhances the level of trust which enhances collaborative working relationships.

The study findings have implications for the intervention of government policies. For the implementation of effective communication-based collaboration projects, government interventions are required in the areas of budget allocations, professional practice regulations and compensating professionals for their services (Rodriguez et al., 2005). It is hard to draw boundary for the roles and responsibilities of a professional in a multi-disciplinary team environment. So, regulations on professionals' jurisdiction need to be reviewed for permitting more flexible roles in the teamwork. The government funding for communication-based collaboration projects in healthcare are to be more objective-driven rather than traditional resource-driven. The compensation for professionals especially for physicians has to be based on time, service, competition and clientele. Besides, medico-legal considerations,

clear policies are to be laid out for governing professional practice.

Overall, for the safety care of the patients, acquiring skills to communicate effectively and efficiently with the team members is critical. It is vital that the whole team takes the responsibility for patient care. Team leaders must initiate and cultivate mutually beneficial relationships with team members. Opportunities to nurture these relationships should be created through effective collaborative communication among the inter-professionals. Furthermore, failing to properly manage the conflicts or disrupted communication may progress to adverse events. Healthcare professionals should prevent communication related problems for protecting the best interests of the patients. Conflicts in communication could be resolved by providing effective leadership. As automation becomes a critical part of healthcare, using the technological advancements for developing a solid collaborative leadership between healthcare professional will be the future trend of this profession.

REFERENCES

Amendola, M. L. (2008). *An examination of the leadership competency requirements of nurse leaders in healthcare information technology*. (Ph.D. Dissertation). University of Phoenix, Faculty of Management in Organizational Leadership, Phoenix, AZ.

Anonymous,. (2005). Hospitals must improve workplace communication to help reduce medical errors. *Hospitals & Health Networks*, 79(3), 66. PMID:15828545

Behara, R., Wears, R. L., Perry, S. J., Eisenberg, E., Murphy, L., Vanderhoef, M., et al. (2005). A conceptual framework for studying safety transitions in emergency care. In *Advances in patient safety: From research to implementation*. Retrieved from www.ahrg.gov/qual/advances/

Bok, H. S., Kankanhalli, A., Raman, K. S., & Sambamurthy, V. (2012). Revisiting media choice: A behavioral decision-making perspective. *International Journal of e-Collaboration, 8*(3), 19–35. doi:10.4018/jec.2012070102

Caramanica, L., Cousino, J. A., & Petersen, S. (2003). Four elements of a successful quality program: Alignment, collaboration, evidence-based practice, and excellence. *Nursing Administration Quarterly, 27*(4), 336–343. doi:10.1097/00006216-200310000-00012 PMID:14649026

Carley, P. J. (2008). *Generational perceptions of leadership behaviors and job satisfaction among healthcare professionals in western New England.* (Ph.D. Dissertation). University of Phoenix, Faculty of Health Administration, Phoenix, AZ.

Christensen, C. M., Bohmer, R., & Kenagy, J. (2000). Will disruptive innovations cure health care? *Harvard Business Review, 78*(5), 102–112. PMID:11143147

Croskerry, P. (2005). Diagnostic failure: A cognitive approach. In *Advances in patient safety: From research to implementation.* Retrieved from www.ahrg. gov/qual/advances/

Daiski, I. (2004). Changing nurses'dis-empowering relationship patterns. *Journal of Advanced Nursing, 45*(1), 43–50. doi:10.1111/j.1365-2648.2004.03167.x PMID:15347409

Duranti, C. M., & de Almeida, F. C. (2012). Is more technology better for communication in international virtual teams? *International Journal of e-Collaboration, 8*(1), 36–52. doi:10.4018/jec.2012010103

Emerson, R. M., Fretz, R. I., & Shaw, L. L. (1995). *Writing ethnographic ®endnotes.* Chicago: University of Chicago Press. doi:10.7208/chicago/9780226206851.001.0001

Estep, T. (2005). Vikings who don't work together don't plunder together. *T&D, 59*(8), 71-72.

Forsythe, L. L. (2007). *Healthcare communication and the creation of a culture of safety.* (Ph.D. Dissertation). The Fielding Graduate University, Faculty of Human And Organizational Systems, Santa Barbara, CA.

Glaser, J. A., & Strauss, A. L. (1967). *The discovery of grounded theory: Strategies for qualitative research.* New York: Arline de Gruyter.

Glenzer, K., & Middleberg, M. I. (2006). *Preparing for the global health transition.* San Francisco, CA: Wiley & Sons.

Guthrie, M. B. (1999). Challenges in developing physician leadership and management. *Frontiers of Health Services Management, 15*(4), 3–26. PMID:10387764

Haeuser, J. L., & Preston, P. (2005, January/February). Communication strategies for getting the results you want. *Healthcare Executive, 20*(1), 16. PMID:15656222

Hartley, J., & Benington, J. (2010). *Leadership for healthcare.* Bristol, UK: Policy Press. doi:10.1332/policypress/9781847424877.001.0001

Henneman, E. A., Lee, J. L., & Cohen, J. I. (1995). Collaboration: A concept analyses. *Journal of Advanced Nursing, 21*(1), 103–109. doi:10.1046/j.1365-2648.1995.21010103.x PMID:7897060

Krause, C. M., Joyce, S., Curtin, K., Jones, C. S., & Kuhn, M. E. (2006). The impact of a multidisciplinary, integrated approach on improving the health and quality of care for individuals dealing with multiple chronic conditions. *The American Journal of Orthopsychiatry, 76*(1), 109–114. doi:10.1037/0002-9432.76.1.109 PMID:16569134

Leach, L. S. (2005). Nurse executive transformational leadership and organizational commitment. *JONA, 35*(5), 228–237. doi:10.1097/00005110-200505000-00006 PMID:15891486

Leedy, P. D., & Ormrod, J. E. (2001). *Practical research planning and design* (7th ed.). Upper Saddle River, NJ: Merrill Prentice Hall.

McCallin, A. (2003). Interdisciplinary team leadership: A revisionist approach for an old problem? *Journal of Nursing Management, 11*(6), 364–370. doi:10.1046/j.1365-2834.2003.00425.x PMID:14641717

Mckinney, E. H., Barker, J. R., Davis, K. J., & Smith, D. (2005). How swift starting action teams get off the ground. *Management Communication Quarterly, 19*(2), 198–237. doi:10.1177/0893318905278539

Miller, L. A. (2005). Patient safety and teamwork in perinatal care. *The Journal of Perinatal & Neonatal Nursing, 19*(1), 46–51. doi:10.1097/00005237-200501000-00011 PMID:15796424

Neuman, W. L. (2003). *Social research methods: A simple guide* (5th ed.). Boston: Allyn & Bacon.

Nieva, V. F., Murphy, R., Ridley, N., Donaldson, N., Combes, J., & Mitchell, P. et al. (2005). *From science to service: A framework for the transfer of patient safety research into practice. In Advances in patient safety: From research to implementation.* Agency for Healthcare.

Papanikolaou, K. A., & Gouli, E. (2013). Investigating influences among individuals and groups in a collaborative learning setting. *International Journal of e-Collaboration, 9*(1), 9-25.

Parker, P. J. (2005). One nurse informatics specialists views the future: Technology in the crystal ball. *Nursing Administration Quarterly, 29*(2), 123–124.

Pearce, W. B. (2003). *The coordinated management of meaning (CMM): Theorizing about communication and culture.* Thousand Oaks, CA: Sage.

Pearce, W. B. (2005). The coordinated management of meaning (CMM). In W. B. Gudykunst (Ed.), Theorizing about intercultural communication. Thousand Oaks, CA: Sage.

Pilnick, A., Hindmarsh, J., & Gill, V. (Eds.). Communication in healthcare settings: Policy, participation and new technologies. Chichester, UK: Wiley-Blackwell. doi:10.1002/9781444324020

Rittgen, P. (2013). Group consensus in business process modeling: A measure and its application. *International Journal of e-Collaboration, 9*(4), 17–31. doi:10.4018/ijec.2013100102

Roberts, K., & Kuo, Y. (2006). *Patient safety is an organizational system issue: Lessons from a variety of industries. In Handbook in patient safety.* Berkley, CA: Aspen.

Roberts, K. H. (2003). HRO has prominent history. *HRO Has Long, Credible History.* Retrieved from http://apsf.org/resourcecenter/newletter/2003/spring/hrohistorv.htm

Rodriguez, L. S., Beaulieu, M., D'Amour, D., & Ferrada-Videla, M. (2005). The determinants of successful collaboration: A review of theoretical and empirical studies. *Journal of Interprofessional Care, 19*(s1), 132–147. doi:10.1080/13561820500082677 PMID:16096151

Rubin, H., & Rubin, I. (1995). *Qualitative interviewing: The art of hearing data.* Thousand Oaks, CA: Sage.

Sachdeva, R. M. (2001). Measuring the impact of new technology: An outcomes-based approach. *Critical Care Medicine, 29*(8), 190-195.

Sandelowski, M. (2000). Focus on research methods: Whatever happened to qualitative description? *Research in Nursing & Health, 23*(3), 334–340. doi:10.1002/1098-240X(200008)23:4<334::AID-NUR9>3.0.CO;2-G PMID:10871540

Sarker, S., Campbell, D.E., Ondrus, J., & Valacich, J.S. (2010). Mapping the need for mobile collaboration technologies: A fit perspective. *International Journal of e-Collaboration, 6*(4), 32–53.

Shorter, J. (2005a). *Talk of showing, gesturing, and feeling in Wittgenstein and Vygotsky*. Retrieved at w.massev.ac.nz/~alock/virtual/wittwg.htm

Shorter, J. (2005b). Inside processes: Withness-thinking and action-guiding anticipations. *International Journal of Action Research*.

Silence Kills. (2005). *Nursing, 55*(4), 33-33.

Smith, C. (2004). New technology continues to invade healthcare: What are the strategic implications/outcomes? *Nursing Administration Quarterly, 28*(2), 92–98. doi:10.1097/00006216-200404000-00004 PMID:15181674

Spears, L., & Lawrence, M. (Eds.). (2002). *Focus on leadership: Servant leadership for the 21st century*. New York: John Wiley & Sons.

Stuart-Kregor, P. (2005). Having the guts to be different. *Journal of Medical Marketing, 5*(1), 74–76. doi:10.1057/palgrave.jmm.5040204

Sultz, H. A., & Young, K. M. (2009). *Health care USA: Understanding its organization and delivery* (6th ed.). Sudbury, MA: Jones and Bartlett.

Thomas, E. J., Sherwood, G. D., Mulhollem, J. L., Sexton, J. B., & Helmreich, R. L. (2004). Working together in the neonatal intensive care unit: Provider perspective. *Journal of Perinatology, 24*(5), 552–559. doi:10.1038/sj.jp.7211136 PMID:15141266

Thompson, C., Repko, K., & Staggers, N. (2003). A Delphi study to validate competencies required of Air Force medical surgical (46N3) nurses in mobilized environments. *Military Medicine, 168*(8), 618–625. PMID:12943036

Tubbs, S. L., & Schulz, E. (2006). Exploring a taxonomy of global leadership competencies and meta-competencies. *The Journal of American Academy of Business, 8*(2), 29–35.

Webster, C. S., & Anderson, D. J. (2002). A practical guide to the implementation of an effective incident reporting scheme to reduce medication error on the hospital ward. *International Journal of Nursing Practice, 8*(4), 176–183. doi:10.1046/j.1440-172X.2002.00368.x PMID:12100674

Wheatley. (2010). *Leadership styles of healthcare executives: Comparisons of transformational, transactional, and passive-avoidant styles.* (Ph.D. Dissertation). Northcentral University, Faculty of Business and Technology Management.

Woods, J. A., Jackson, D. J., Ziglar, S., & Alston, G. L. (2011). Interprofessional communication. *Drug Topics, 155*(8), 42–53.

Zaleznik, A. (1992). Managers and leaders: Are they different? *Harvard Business Review, 70*(2), 126–137. PMID:10119712

This work was previously published in the International Journal of e-Collaboration (IJeC), 11(2); edited by Ned Kock, pages 8-27 copyright year 2015 by IGI Publishing (an imprint of IGI Global).

Chapter 60
Political Attitudes on the Dutch Electronic Patient Record

Evert Mouw
Independent Researcher, The Netherlands

ABSTRACT

In the Netherlands, the introduction of a nationwide electronic patient record (EPR) infrastructure was rejected in 2011 after a heated political debate. Such debate is influenced by the political attitudes of politicians and voters, such as their trust in governments. The objective is to explore the relation between political attitudes of individuals and the priority they give to health privacy. The method is from a new survey that was developed; the Health Privacy and Political Attitudes Survey. The survey is as compatible as possible with a few well-known surveys. With 218 respondents enough data was collected for a first explorative study. Little correlations were found between political attitudes and the individual's priorisation of health privacy or their trust in a nationwide EPR. In general, most respondents valued their health privacy highly and trust in a nationwide EPR was low, irrespective of their political affiliation or their political attitudes. One exception were respondents with authoritarian attitudes. Such individuals had, on average, more trust in (government regulated) electronic records. More trust in the law correlates with less fear for problems with the EPR. Interestingly, higher educated and older respondents have, on average, the same level of trust in the EPR as others but are more apt to act when they distrust the system (opt-out). In general, political attitudes and one's trust in electronic patient records (EPRs) are not strongly related, but individuals who score high on authoritarian attitudes and trust in the law are more likely to also trust EPRs. Still, nearly everybody places a high value on health privacy, so EPR providers should be careful in this regard.

1. INTRODUCTION

In April 2011, the plan to introduce legislation for a nationwide Electronic Patient Record (EPR) communications system in the Netherlands failed. It was a close call – the letters informing civilians about the new EPR were already sent. The Lower Chamber of Dutch Parliament had passed the legislation. The Senate (Upper Chamber) usually agrees with the Lower Chamber, although sometimes minor adjustments are required. But this time, the minister of health, Schippers (VVD[1], a

DOI: 10.4018/978-1-4666-8756-1.ch060

conservative-liberal party), saw her law proposal unanimously rejected, mainly over concerns over data security and privacy[2]. One of the leading Senate senators vocally rejecting the proposal was Dupuis, also member of the VVD. This disagreement within one political party already hints at the unconventional political cleavages separating people on this issue.

The unanimous rejection of the EPR law does not reflect the finding of most opinion reseach surveys that hint to a strong public support for digitalised health records – see table 1. As much of the political debate was over privacy concerns, a better understanding of health pricacy might help to understand why the Dutch Senate rejected the proposal.

This study explores the relation between the importance given by voters to a nationwide EPR (enforced by law) and the voters' political attitudes. How voters appreciate a nationwide EPR is related to their attitudes on health privacy and their trust in the rule of law. Attitudes predict behaviour and opinions and are thus important for understanding the political debate about EPRs.

Little is known about a possible relation between political attitudes of individuals and the valuation of health privacy by the same individuals. This study explores such a possible relation by measuring both political attitudes and health privacy preferences in a sample of the Dutch population. For measurement, the survey as described in the "Methods" section is used.

First, the Dutch EPR, health privacy and political attitudes will be introduced. Second, previous work and the relevance of this study will be discussed. Thereafter the survey and its results will be presented and discussed. The paper will be concluded with a reflection on policy implications and suggestions for future research.

1.1 The Dutch EPR

The Dutch EPR is not a centralised medical records database, but more of a decentralised storage structure with a centralised communications infrastructure for medical records, so that medical care providers can easily access patient records from each other. In practice, most medical data stored by participating parties such as hospitals, pharmacies, and general practitioners can be accessed by all other participating parties. Access logs provide after-the-fact security.

The proposed opt-out system ensured that people would take part in the system by default. In an opt-out system, one has to actively object to be excluded from the system. An opt-in system is harder to introduce because all participants must actively give permission beforehand.

A number of medical specialists, politicians, and computer scientist did raise objections to the legal proposal to make participation in the EPR compulsory for health care providers. One of them, van 't Noordende (2010), wrote a paper on the security of the proposed EPR and showed important shortcomings and vulnerabilities.

Table 1. Public popularity of health databases by country

Country	Year	Perc.	Support in favour of	Source
Canada	2003	78%	genetic research database	Pollara and Earnscliffe, 2003
Sweden	2005	80%	shared, national HER	Rynning, 2007
USA	2005	72%	health information network	Public Opinion Strategies, 2005
USA	2008	79%	electronic PHR	Westin, 2008
Australia	2008	82%	individual HER	UMR Research, 2008
Netherlands	2009	63%	electronic EPR	de Hond, 2009
Netherlands	2009	85%	electronic EPR	TNS NIPO, 2009

Currently, the EPR infrastructure is no longer maintained by the Dutch government because the law did not pass the Senate. Still, many health care providers recognize the advantages and have decided to support the central communications infrastructure for the EPR.

2. PREVIOUS WORK

2.1. Health privacy

Privacy can mean a lot of different things in the literature. Solove (2002) mentions six general headings:

1. The right to be let alone (from Samuel Warren and Louis Brandeis, 1891).
2. Limited access to the self – the ability to shield oneself from unwanted access by others.
3. Secrecy – the concealment of certain matters from others.
4. Control over personal information – the ability to exercise control over information about oneself.
5. Personhood – the protection of one's personality, individuality, and dignity.
6. Intimacy – control over one's intimate relationships or aspects of life.

With the rise of information technology, new challenges arise. To cite Holvast (2009): "History of privacy makes clear that there is a strong relationship between privacy and the development of technology. The modern discussion started with the use of cameras and went on to include the development and use of computers in an information society in which personal data on every individual is collected and stored. Not only is it a great concern that privacy is eroding but also that we are entering a surveillance society."

Apart from the political risk of a technology-driven surveillance society, there is also another privacy risk in the digital realm: weak technical security, which can result in the access, modification or deletion of data by non-authorised persons.

An important subclass of privacy is *health privacy*. This is sometimes recognised in law: the USA federal government has issued the Model State Public Health Privacy Act. Gostin et al. (2001) stress the importance of health privacy for the quality of public health. But what makes health privacy so special?

Medical records and genetic data contain very personal information. Both are related to health and life expectancy. A breach of confidentiality would infringe one's privacy – often quite personal things such as sexually transmittable diseases, mental illness, and genetic disorders. Health privacy is a special category, on which people often have other feelings and opinions than on "normal" privacy or other privacy matters. One example of a group that advocates health privacy is the American based Health Privacy Project[3].

Health privacy mostly concerns medical records and genetic information. It is a very general term, not only including medical records and genetic information but also (medical) images and public information about one's health status. Especially when the data is stored in electronic databases, health privacy becomes an issue because data security could be compromised.

Castle and DeBusk (2008) write about nutritional genomics and the ethical difficulties which face registered dieticians. Electronic health records often contain genetic information. Health privacy concerns not only affect isolated individuals. Genomic disorders often affect whole families. Medical records can reveal family implications, like "increased risk of Alzheimer's disease to other family members." Another problem noted by Castle and DeBusk (2008) is the problem of unsolicited information: after a genetic test for some problem x, the doctor might see test results for some other illnesses y. The patient might profit from pro-active treatment for y, but maybe he/she does not want to know about that problem y. Patients who can read their own medical records might face such unsolicited information.

Hustead and Goldman (2002) discern four components of medical information privacy protection: *1)* access (who has access to one's data, and when), *2)* use (how should the data be used), *3)* disclosure (to whom can the data be disclosed), and *4)* storage and security (safety precautions). They also stress the importance of non-discriminatory use, for example meaning that health insurers are not allowed to use such health information to deny clients or set prices. Goldman and Hudson (2000) recommend both self-regulatory policies and better legislation "to engender public trust and confidence in both traditional health care as well as e-health activities."

Margulis (2003) discusses "genetic privacy" in the US. He calls the "genetic/medical privacy" a "major policy battleground." Hustead and Goldman (2002), Solove (2002), Cross (2006), Tanne (2008), and others stress the importance of new legislation. The emerging technological possibilities must be covered by law. Castle and DeBusk (2008) advise "strict controls around electronic health records to ensure that registered dietitians can make the most of the benefits of electronic record management, while gaining the client's trust that private health records will remain private." These calls for new legislation are reflected in the proposal for a new privacy and data protection Regulation of the European Union, which contains specific saveguards for genetic privacy (Mouw, 2012).

Indeed, technological advances in the Information Age give health privacy a new dimension with new problems and new insights. That is why this new term, "health privacy", is being used in this paper.

2.2. Political Attitudes

The politicians in the Netherlands that proposed the national EPR wanted to regulate medical records and health privacy. This implies that party politics and political attitudes come into play. Political attitudes can determine the weight given to privacy *vis-à-vis* central regularisation of medical patient information.

Many authors have written about political attitudes. One of the first was Allport (1929). He described an attitude as a "disposition to act", a generic and broad neural "set" leading to some behaviour or some ad-hoc opinion. In this way, political attitudes can be a predictor of voting behaviour. This study tries to link political attitudes to public opinions on the Dutch EPR.

One's political attitudes are related to one's position in the political space. Political space or the political spectrum can be represented by a simple left-right divide, but many social scientists find this unsatisfactory. Most models are two-axial models, although models with more axes are also used [4].

In the Netherlands, a model well known by the public is the two-axial model used by the Electoral Compass (Dutch: "Kieskompas"). The academic director is Krouwel, a political scientist. The two axes are the conservative – progressive axis and the left – right axis (Kieskompas, 2010). The first axis is about someone's cultural values, while the latter axis is about one's economic views. The model is very useful because the resulting map is often updated to reflect actual party positions.

The well-known British Social Attitudes Survey (BSAS)[5] lists four different dimensions under its topic "attitude and values scales". These dimensions show some similarity to the other multi-axial models mentioned. The dimensions or scales are: left – right, libertarian – authoritarian, postmaterialist – materialist, and welfarist – individualist. Note that some of these dimensions show some overlap or at least are suspected of intercorrelation, which is why simpler two-axis models are often preferred.

Another way to divide the political space is to identify political (or social) cleavages (Lipset and Rokkan, 1967). Manza and Brooks (1999), for example, identified four major social cleavages in the US: class, religion, gender, and race.

2.3. Earlier Surveys

Data on health privacy related to political attitudes is scarce because electronic medical records are so very recent. Only very few nations have implemented EPRs. So, the subject is too recent to be subjected to much social research, and the number of countries is too small to have attracted many researchers and their surveys. This has lowered the number of datasets that contain data on both political attitudes and health privacy. The next two paragraphs will serve to illustrate this by mentioning data sources that do *not* contain both data types.

Surveys designed by medical researchers, information scientists and public opinion experts only measure the popularity of medical records and how people feel about a number of practical issues; they do not care about political attitudes. Examples of such surveys are reported by Pollara and Earnscliffe (2003), Public Opinion Strategies (2005), Rynning (2007), UMR Research (2008), Westin (2008), de Hond (2009), and TNS NIPO, 2009. A survey to measure the opinions of persons working in the medical field was held by Katzenbauer (2009). Although all these surveys give indications about the public support for an EPR, none of them contains questions or data on political attitudes.

Most surveys and theories designed by social scientists do not recognize health privacy as a separate concept. Examples are Margulis (2003), Westin (2003), and NKO Stichting Nationaal Kiezersonderzoek (2006). Those that do mention health privacy as a separate concept, such as Hustead and Goldman (2002), Solove (2002), Cross (2006), Castle and DeBusk (2008), and Tanne (2008), do not explore the relation with political attitudes.

The British Social Attitudes Survey (BSAS) is an exception. The inclusion of health privacy questions might be inspired by the fact that the UK is one of the first countries to use electronic health databases. Still, while a lot of questions related to political attitudes are available, the number of questions related to health privacy is very low. In fact, no questions on medical records are included, only just one question on genetic databases can be found. Also, the number of years in which health privacy questions were included is only three.

One reason why there is not much research being published on the relation between political attitudes and health privacy issues might be that most discussions on the EPR and genetic databases have been done by medical researchers and computer scientists. Another reason might be that the introduction of the EPR is such a recent development. But now that the EPR is part of the political debate, that might change. The Dutch Senate asked the Rathenau Instituut to do research.

The Rathenau Instituut (2009) conducted a qualitative research using focus groups to explore the public opinion on the EPR. The total number of participants was 38, and they were divided over five focus groups, based on factors such as level of education and frequency of contact with the medical world. The research concluded that lower educated persons tend to have more trust in the EPR than higher educated persons. Because of the qualitative nature of the research and the limited size of the focus groups, Rathenau Instituut (2009) warned that their results could *not* be extrapolated to the Dutch population at large.

3. METHODS

How to find a possible relationship between political attitudes and the subjects' opinions on the Dutch EPR and health privacy? Using earlier work or datasets is not a feasable option, as explained in the "Earlier surveys" subsection. One method is to do qualitative interviews, as did

Rathenau Instituut (2009). But instead we wanted a method that actually could be "extrapolated to the population at large". Also, having the option to compare parts of the survey results (e.g. the privacy subset) to other, earlier or later surveys would be attractive because it increases the value of the data collection. So, a quantitative method is preferred, but we had to design our own survey.

3.1. Survey Design

Furthermore, because of limited funding, we aimed for a small but just big enough sample, between 200 and 300 respondents. That allows to do explorative research and to find relationships, which we intended to do in any case, but it does not allow to give much precision of the strenght of relationships, if any. Ideally, the respondents would come from all trades, age groups, educational levels and so on, to reflect the diversity of the Dutch population. We intended to test the diversity in the sample to validate the results (see "Demographics" in "Results").

To increase the participation rate and to avoid selection bias (busy people do not fill in long surveys), it was a requirement to keep the survey short, ideally between 10 and 20 questions, including the questions on basic demographics.

Survey design is hard, so we decided to copy survey questions from well-known surveys if possible. That also satisfied our wish to make it possible to compare subsets of the survey to other surveys. These subsets or categories include, among others, health privacy and political attitudes. A disadvantage of such "cherry picking" is that the range of possible answers sometimes differ. For example, some questions score on a five-point scale, others on a seven-point scale. One then has to transform one scale to another for calculations. Luckily, that is well possible because both scale systems are Likert-style questions using equally spaced intervals.

Questions were borrowed from the BSAS, the NKO ("Nationaal Kiezersonderzoek", which is Dutch for National Parliamentary Election Studies), and from Katzenbauer (2009). We also included questions on gender, age, occupation, religion, education, political attitudes, and privacy attitudes. See table 2 for a detailed overview.

The survey was held at the end of 2009 using a self-developed online tool under the name "Health Privacy and Political Attitudes Survey". The survey was located at www.epd-enquete.nl. Approximately 2000 email invites were sent to people using the circles of contacts surrounding the author. The invited persons could invite other people (a kind of viral marketing to exploit the idea of the principle of six degrees of separation (Milgram, 1967)). Also, small-scale limited use of online advertisement was used. Other data collection methods, such as normally used by public opinion polling organizations, have not been used due to severe time and budget constraints. Full results (survey data) are available on the same website.

Religion: **0.** not religious **1.** believer, but not a member of a church or religious association **2.** Roman Catholic **3.** Reformed **4.** Presbyterian / Calvinist **5.** Protestant **6.** Islam **7.** other church or religious association.

Origins: **BSAS** British Social Attitudes Survey. **EM** Evert Mouw. **MC** Medisch Contact (Katzenbauer, 2009). **NKO** Nationaal KiezersOnderzoek (NKO, 2006).

The *party* variable of the survey is not a direct measurement of one's political attitudes, so a mapping is still needed to the derived variables *leftright* and *conservative*. Each political party is given an score (integer) from 1 to 10 on two political axes based on a two-axis model from Kieskompas (2010). A Boolean score is assigned based on a party being self-proclaimed Christian or secular.

Table 2. Overview of the survey questions

Category	Variable	Question wording (abbreviated)	Range	Value assignment	Origin
health privacy	principle	in principle I... the introduction of the EPR	-1 ~ 1	1 = favour	MC
	objection	have objected to the EPR	-1 ~ 1	1 = objected	MC
	longterm	EPRs are on long term useful	-1 ~ 1	1 = yes	EM
other privacy	idcard	every adult should carry an ID card	-2 ~ 2	2 = strongly agree	BSAS
DNA privacy	- - -	likelyhood of genetic data being used for...	- - -	- - -	- - -
	gen-insurance	... health or life insurance	-2 ~ 2	2 = very likely	BSAS
	gen-job	... a job	-2 ~ 2	2 = very likely	BSAS
	gen-load	... credit (loan)	-2 ~ 2	2 = very likely	BSAS
left-right	levelling	more income difference or less?	1 ~ 7	0	7 = more	NKO
	management	management tries to profit from employees	-2 ~ 2	2 = very likely	BSAS
authoritarian	criminality	government should be harder on crime	1 ~ 7	0	7 = strongly agree	NKO
	law	law should always be respected	-2 ~ 2	2 = strongly agree	BSAS
	euthanasia	euthanasia should be possible	1 ~ 7	0	7 = strongly agree	NKO
party	party	which party did you vote	MC	*see table 2*	EM NKO
personal	age	year of birth	0 ~ 100	2009 - integer	NKO
	gender	male or female	f | m	f = female m = male	NKO
	religion	which religious denomination /... ?	1 ~ 7	0	*see below*	NKO
	education	highest education followed	1 ~ 7	≥ 6 = higher educated	NKO
comments	comments	- - -	- - -	- - -	- - -

Table 3. Party mapping. How one's party preference maps to political attitudes

party	leftright	conservative	christian
cda	8	7	1
cu	5	8	1
d66	6	3	0
gl	1	1	0
pvda	3	5	0
pvdd	4	2	0
pvv	10	9	0
sgp	7	10	1
sp	2	4	0
vvd	9	6	0
other	0	0	-1

3.2. Method of Statistical Analysis

Because this is an explorative study, aiming at finding correlations between political attitudes and opinions on health privacy, the main instrument of analysis is testing for correlations between variables using a cross table. Three variables measure the attitude to the Dutch EPR directly: *principle*, *objection*, and *longterm*. These three variables will be tested for correlation with all other variables.

Not Pearson but Spearman correlation was used because ordinal data is being analysed and varying Likert scales were used. The Spearman method makes less assumptions on the data. According to Gauthier (2001), no normality is assumed, outliers have little impact, and no large sample size is required, although the power of the test is slightly lower that Pearson's. The correlation strength will be in the range $[-1,1]$, with zero being no correlation.

We aim for a confidence level of 95% ($p < 0.5$). A relatively small sample size suffices because we only want to prove correlation itself, not the strength of the correlation. Power calculations for the Spearman non-parametric correlation test are not straighforward, but one method is described by Bonett and Wright (2000). Using their formula, and given $\alpha = 0.05$, desired width of the confidence interval $\omega = 0.3$, and estimated correlation $\theta = 0.3$, a sample size $n = 150$ is needed. Note that this is just an indication for the *minimum* number of respondents needed to detect correlations given these requirements.

How well the sample represents the Dutch population at large depends on the demographics of the sample. In the "Demographics" subsection of "Methods", a comparison between the survey sample and the Dutch population will be made based on educational level, gender, age, and political preferences.

4. RESULTS

In total, 218 respondents filled in the survey. The survey started on 2009-11-17 and ended on 2009-12-17, so the running time was exactly one month. Most responses were recorded during the first two weeks of the survey.

4.1. Demographics

Does the sample offer a good representation if the population? In this subsection, the sample is compared with the Dutch population at large.

In the Dutch general population of 2008, 25% has a higher degree[6]. In my sample, it is 63%. Of the 218 respondents, 57% are male and 43% are female. The average age of the respondents was 36. That is only slightly below the average age of the Dutch population, which was 38 years in 2003 (NIDI, 2003). In the sample, people aged 30 to 50 are somewhat underrepresented, while older people and especially young adults are somewhat overrepresented.

The female respondents (*mean*=32,3; *sd*=13,0) are, on average, younger than the males (*mean*=39,5; *sd*=15,9) but the standard deviations have a big overlap. Still, the gender difference in age is of statistical significance (Wilcoxon Mann-Whitney test p=0,0007 < 0,05).

The attempt at viral marketing did not result in a very diverse pool of respondents. Many respondents were close to me, studying at Leiden University (causing the high educational level of the sample) or close to my family or former work circles (IT and graphical industry).

Overall, the political attitudes seem to be well distributed in the sample – see figure 1 and figure 2. Figure 1 shows on the *x*-axis the *conservative* score, as derived from the political party preference (see table 2 and Kieskompas (2010)), and on the *y*-axis the number of respondents. It is easy to see that all political flavours on the scale are represented in the sample, although very progressive voters are better represented than very conservative voters. Figure 2 shows the same, but now with the right-left score on the *x*-axis, again showing much variation in the sample. The high variability of political attitudes in the sample is important, because it makes an extrapolation of the findings of this study more justified.

4.2. Correlations

The correlations of the health privacy variables *principle*, *objection*, and *longterm* with other variables can be found in table 4. The survey questions associated with these variables can be looked up in table 2.

The correlations between the health privacy variables *principle*, *objection*, and *longterm* are expected because they fall in the same category. The strong correlation between these variables

Figure 1. Political party preferences in the sample, measured against conservatism. This histograms show how the respondents are divided between progressive and conservative parties

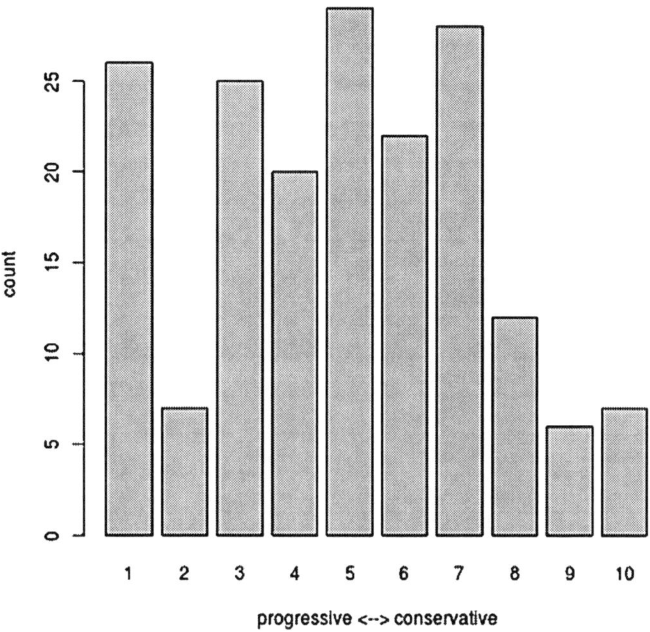

Figure 2. Political party preferences in the sample, measured against left vs. right. This histograms show how the respondents are divided between left-wing and right-wing parties

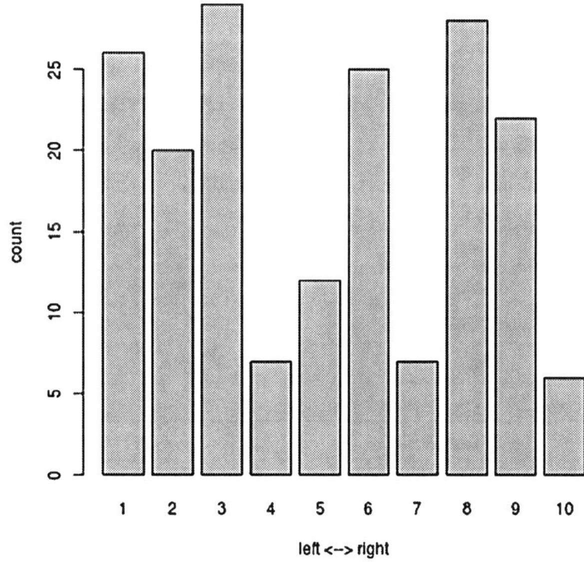

confirms the validity of placing them in the same category. The same holds for the correlations with *idcard* (other privacy) and *gen_** (DNA privacy).

Correlations that are noteworthy because they do include variables from different categories will now be discussed.

Table 4. Correlations (Sprearman's rho, with p ~ sig. (2-tailed)). Please refer to table 2 for the meaning of the variables

	N		principle	objection	longterm
principle	218	corr. coeff.	1,000		
		sig. (2-tailed)	.		
objection	218	corr. coeff.	-,591**	1,000	
		sig. (2-tailed)	,000	.	
longterm	218	corr. coeff.	,755**	-,652**	1,000
		sig. (2-tailed)	,000	,000	.
control	218	corr. coeff.	,237**	-,253**	,260**
		sig. (2-tailed)	,000	,000	,000
idcard	218	corr. coeff.	,277**	-,269**	,268**
		sig. (2-tailed)	,000	,000	,000
gen_insurance	218	corr. coeff.	-,295**	,288**	-,315**
		sig. (2-tailed)	,000	,000	,000
gen_job	218	corr. coeff.	-,358**	,301**	-,367**
		sig. (2-tailed)	,000	,000	,000
gen_loan	218	corr. coeff.	-,274**	,301**	-,340**
		sig. (2-tailed)	,000	,000	,000
levelling	208	corr. coeff.	-,068	,071	-,095
		sig. (2-tailed)	,328	,310	,174
management	218	corr. coeff.	-,120	,069	-,121
		sig. (2-tailed)	,076	,309	,075
criminality	216	corr. coeff.	,094	-,121	,044
		sig. (2-tailed)	,169	,076	,517
law	218	corr. coeff.	,203**	-,185**	,143*
		sig. (2-tailed)	,003	,006	,035
priority	203	corr. coeff.	-,187**	,102	-,116
		sig. (2-tailed)	,008	,149	,098
euthanasia	217	corr. coeff.	,128	-,102	,152*
		sig. (2-tailed)	,060	,133	,025
party_leftright	182	corr. coeff.	-,065	,020	-,057
		sig. (2-tailed)	,386	,791	,442
party_conservative	182	corr. coeff.	,012	,054	-,069
		sig. (2-tailed)	,873	,467	,358
party_christian	182	corr. coeff.	,128	-,112	,018
		sig. (2-tailed)	,086	,131	,813
age	218	corr. coeff.	-,059	,188**	-,160*
		sig. (2-tailed)	,382	,005	,018
gender	218	corr. coeff.	-,122	-,017	-,123
		sig. (2-tailed)	,072	,804	,070

continued on following page

Table 4. Continued

	N		principle	objection	longterm
religion	218	corr. coeff.	-,017	,027	-,094
		sig. (2-tailed)	,801	,695	,165
occupation	218	corr. coeff.	,014	-,042	,021
		sig. (2-tailed)	,835	,536	,761
education	218	corr. coeff.	-,112	,210**	-,137*
		sig. (2-tailed)	,098	,002	,043

- Respondents who agree with the statement that "the law should always be obeyed" (an authoritarian political attitude) are more likely to have a positive stand towards the EPR. The correlation is clear; all three EPR related variables show correlation with *law*.
- The correlation with *euthanasia* is less clear, only with *longterm*.
- People of higher *age* and with a higher *education* seem to have actively objected against the EPR more often, but they are in *principle* not more against an EPR than others.

Other correlations could not be found.

Apart from these correlations, we noticed that respondents opposing the Dutch EPR were more active to add free text comments or to send emails expressing their concerns. Many of those comments were well-informed, raising the suspicion that many of the opponents had taken the trouble to learn more about the subject.

5. DISCUSSION

5.1. Respect for the Law Comes With Trust in the EPR

A correlation between trust in the EPR and trust in authoritarian government was found. A possible explanation of this correlation is that respect for the law, and for authority and regulation in general, is based on the assumption that rules and regulations will be valued and followed. Much fear and some real risks surrounding the EPR are based on the breach of rules and security. More trust in the application of the law decreases the fear for such risks, and thus makes the EPR appear less risky. Note that our sample allows to find correlations, but might be too small to make definite statements about the strength of the correlation.

5.2. Political Debate

What can we learn from the unanimous rejection by the Senate, and the cleavages *within* political parties on this issue? Maybe Dutch political parties have not "politicised" the EPR topic. This might explain why no relation between the individual preference for the EPR and one's political party preference could be found, not even using multiple groupings (left vs. right, conservative vs. progressive, Christian vs. secular). Or it might be the other way round: the EPR preference divides all parties. Whatever the case, in the Netherlands, party preferences are not measurably connected to individual EPR preferences. This was well illustrated by the fact that the legislative proposal of the minister of health, Schippers, was met by strong resistance in the Senate with senator Dupuis as the leading critic. Both are member of the same political party, the conservative-liberal VVD.

5.3. Reasons for a Lack of Correlation

This study could not prove a correlation between religion and health privacy. Assumptions about a supposed "Christian" trust in authority (and thus, government) might be mistaken, at least on the subject of EPRs. A possible explanation for the lack of correlation could be that "religion" is a big umbrella term, under which many worldviews and attitudes manifest themselves.

The correlation between health privacy and other privacy comes as no surprise, as both concepts are related. But at the same time they differ enough to have a weakening effect on the correlation: the correlation between *idcard* with the health privacy variables is half of the value of the correlation between *principle*, *objection*, and *longterm*. That supports our notion that health privacy is different from "general" privacy.

5.4. The Role of Education

Higher educated respondents were more likely to fill in an objection form against the EPR, which is understandable because better educated individuals and older people have more experience with filling in forms, and maybe they also have a better understanding of technological risks and political pressures. This finding is also consistent with earlier work from the Rathenau Instituut (2009). Also respondents of older age are more likely to fill in an objection form, possibly for the same reasons. But in relation to their "in *principle*" preference for the EPR, no difference could be found with the lower educated or the younger respondents. This contrasts with the suggestion from the Rathenau Instituut (2009) that higher educated persons are less likely to support the EPR. This study is quantitative, while the Rathenau research is qualitative – they already mentioned that their results could not be extrapolated to the Dutch population at large. This survey based research finds that the level of education has little

to do with one's preference (attitude) for the EPR, although one is more likely to take active actions when one is higher educated (or of higher age).

5.5. Bias and Reliability

The short running time of the survey is likely to reduce the chance that new political developments or media coverage during the survey had much influence on the outcomes.

In the results section, the problems with the viral marketing method and the bias towards the author's study, work and family circles was noted. The sample is still quite diverse, but the conclusions from this study are thus primarily applicable to the groups that were preferred by the selection method (selection bias). The sample is heavily biased towards people with a higher education. So, the study results are more reliable for the higher educated parts of the population.

5.6. Policy Recommendations

The message of this study is clear: health privacy issues in the Netherlands transcend political attitudes. One's position in the political space is not a good predictor for one's opinion on the electronic patient record (EPR). Based on that finding and based on various talks during the study, a few policy recommendations are given below. These recommendations are not necessarily supported by our data, but they do reflect the views obtained during the study.

Political leaders should handle EPRs carefully because it is likely that their own parties – and voters – are divided on the topic. Also, discussions on privacy and health evoke much emotion, especially when electronic networks are involved. For leaders of parties that are libertarian and focused on privacy, this study adds even more incentive for such caution. Such parties value privacy even more, and likely their voters do the same. In this respect, it is remarkable that people from the study sample that voted Green-Left (GL) do not take a more critical stance towards the EPR. GL is one of the best scoring parties on the privacy ranking from Privacy Barometer (2010), a website measuring a privacy score for political parties based on their law proposals.

Possibly, opinions about the EPR and attitudes regarding health privacy do not follow traditional political cleavages and are not much related to political attitudes. In that case, feelings about the balance between privacy and health are very personal and varying. So an opt-in system will likely provoke less resistance, although that will probably necessitate a slower and more gradual approach.

The fact that critics of the EPR were more motivated to add free text comments or to send emails and that those critics were often quite knowledgeable is another warning that resistance to eHealth initiatives can be strong and well-informed.

A suggestion for policy makers is to create a more patient-oriented EPR. Trust in a computerised system (or any system) comes more easily when you can control (or at least view) and access that system, especially when it's about personal and private health data. A system designed only for medical personnel, hospitals, and insurance companies will not be trusted by voters. In the age of the Internet, online access to one's own (medical) data is a requirement (Mandl et al., 2001; Jacobs, 2010).

Programs for technological advancement should be accompanied with a deep understanding of the technology itself and the possible consequences of a bad design. In other words, such programs should be subject to the highest standards. Technical or security incidents can cause lots of distrust.

6. CONCLUSION

The Dutch EPR proposal met much political resistance, with views on the subject cleaving all groups, even dividing political parties. This study could not prove political attitudes to be a predicting factor for one's view on the Dutch EPR, with one exception: trust in the law is weakly linked with trust in the EPR. Higher educated persons are more likely to fill in an objection form against the EPR, but their average trust in the EPR is the same as for lower educated persons.

This study was explorative in the sense that it was the first study that tried to link health privacy to political attitudes using multiple variables. The weak correlation found between one's preferences for the EPR and for authoritative government seem worth further investigation.

ACKNOWLEDGMENT

I am grateful for the following people: Prof. Dr. Joyce Outshoorn, Leiden University, department of Political Science, for advising during the project. Dr. Frits G.J. Meijerink, Leiden University, department of Political Science, for reviewing the statistical analysis. Drs. Mireille Schaap, Leiden University Medical Centre, department of Human Genetics, for her support.

REFERENCES

Allport, G. W. (1929). The composition of political attitudes. *American Journal of Sociology*, *35*(2), 220–238. doi:10.1086/214980

Bonett, D. G., & Wright, T. A. (2000). Sample size requirements for estimating Pearson, Kendall and Spearman correlations. *Psychometrika*, *65*(1), 23–28. doi:10.1007/BF02294183

Castle, D., & DeBusk, R. (2008). The electronic health record, genetic information, and patient privacy. *Journal of the American Dietetic Association*, *108*(8), 1372–1374. doi:10.1016/j. jada.2008.06.369 PMID:18714474

Cross, M. (2006). GPs' leader sets conditions for electronic care records. *British Medical Journal, 332*(7542), 627. doi:10.1136/bmj.332.7542.627-b PMID:16543319

de Hond, M. (2009). Veel Nederlanders negatief over elektronisch patiënten dossier. Retrieved 2009-11-10 from www.radio1.nl. Dutch.

Gauthier, T. D. (2001). Detecting trends using Spearman's rank correlation coefficient. *Environmental Forensics, 2*(4), 359–362. doi:10.1006/enfo.2001.0061

Goldman, J., & Hudson, Z. (2000). Virtually exposed: Privacy and e-health. *Health Affairs, 19*(6), 140–148. doi:10.1377/hlthaff.19.6.140 PMID:11192397

Gostin, L. O., Hodge, J. G. Jr, & Valdiserri, R. O. (2001). Informational privacy and the public's health: The model state public health privacy act. *American Journal of Public Health, 91*(9), 1388–1392. doi:10.2105/AJPH.91.9.1388 PMID:11527765

Holvast, J. (2009). *The Future of Identity in the Information Society, chapter History of Privacy* (pp. 13–42). Boston: Springer. doi:10.1007/978-3-642-03315-5_2

Hustead, J., & Goldman, J. (2002). Genetics and privacy. *American Journal of Law & Medicine, 28*(2), 285–307. PMID:12197466

Jacobs, B. (2010). The electronic patient record from the perspective of data protection. In *Databases – The promises of ICT, the hunger for information, and digital autonomy* (pp. 42–51). Rathenau Instituut.

Katzenbauer, M. (2009). Te vroeg voor landelijk EPD. [Dutch.]. *Medisch Contact, 64*(20), 880–883.

Kieskompas (2010). Electoral compass at www.kieskompas.nl. Note: The academic director is André Krouwel.

Lipset, S. M., & Rokkan, S. (1967). *Party Systems and Voter Alignments: Cross-National Perspectives*. Free Press.

Mandl, K. D., Szolovits, P., & Kohane, I. S. (2001). Public standards and patients' control: How to keep electronic medical records accessible but private. *British Medical Journal, 322*(7281), 283–287. doi:10.1136/bmj.322.7281.283 PMID:11157533

Manza, J., & Brooks, C. (1999). *Social cleavages and political change: voter alignments and U.S. party coalitions*. Oxford University Press.

Margulis, S. T. (2003). Privacy as a social issue and behavioral concept. *The Journal of Social Issues, 59*(2), 243–261. doi:10.1111/1540-4560.00063

Milgram, S. (1967). The small world problem. [On the six degrees of separation principle.]. *Psychology Today, 2*, 60–67.

Mouw, E. (2012). Legal constraints on genetic data processing in European grids. In Studies in Health Technology and Informatics: Vol. 175. Healthgrid. IOS Press. PMID: 22941987.

NIDI. (2003). *De bevolkingsontwikkeling in een notendop. Demos*. Dutch.

Pollara and Earnscliffe (2003). *Public opinion research into genetic privacy issues* (Tech. Rep.).

Privacy Barometer. (2010). De actuele stand van de politiek over privacy, at www.privacybarometer.nl. Dutch.

Public Opinion Strategies. (2005). *Attitudes of Americans regarding personal health records and nationwide electronic health information exchange (Tech. Rep.)*. The Markle Foundation.

Rathenau Instituut (2009). *Presentatie focusgroepen EPD* (Tech. Rep.). Dutch. Expertmeeting EPD - Eerste Kamer op 2009-12-09.

Research, U. M. R. (2008). *National e-health transition authority quantitative survey report* (Tech. Rep.). eGovernment Resource Centre at www.egov.vic.gov.au

Rynning, E. (2007). Public trust and privacy in shared electronic health records. [Editorial]. *European Journal of Health Law*, *14*(2), 105–112. doi:10.1163/092902707X211668 PMID:17847827

Solove, D. J. (2002). Conceptualizing privacy. *California Law Review*, *90*(4), 1088–1155. doi:10.2307/3481326

Stichting Nationaal Kiezersonderzoek, N. K. O. (2006). Dutch parliamentary electoral studies website at www.dpes.nl

Tanne, J. H. (2008). Fears over security as Google launches free electronic health records service for patients. *British Medical Journal*, *336*(7655), 1207. doi:10.1136/bmj.a208 PMID:18511778

TNS NIPO. (2009). *Meerderheid Nederlanders heeft vertrouwen in elektronisch patiënten dossier* (Tech. Rep.). TNS NIPO and NPCF.Retrieved 2009-11-10 from http://www.npcf.nl/images/stories/Actueel/eindrapport_epd_tns_nipo_npcf.pdf. Dutch.

van 't Noordende, G. (2010). Security in the Dutch electronic patient record system. In *2nd ACM Workshop on Security and Privacy in Medical and Home-Care Systems (SPIMACS)* (pp. 21–31). Chicago, Illinois, USA. doi:10.1145/1866914.1866918

Westin, A. (2008). *Americans overwhelmingly believe electronic personal health records could improve their health (Tech. Rep.).* The Markle Foundation.

Westin, A. F. (2003). Social and political dimensions of privacy. *The Journal of Social Issues*, *59*(2), 431–453. doi:10.1111/1540-4560.00072

ENDNOTES

[1] VVD: (Dutch) *Volkspartij voor Vrijheid en Democratie*, (English) *People's Party for Freedom and Democracy*. The VVD is one of the largest political parties in the Netherlands. It is considered a conservative-liberal party.

[2] Dutch source: Eerste Kamer, "Wetsvoorstel EPD verworpen", 2011-04-05, URL: http://www.eerstekamer.nl/nieuws/20110405/wetsvoorstel_epd_verworpen_en

[3] www.healthprivacy.org

[4] A non-academic but nice introductory overview can be found at https://en.wikipedia.org/wiki/Political_spectrum

[5] See www.britsocat.com

[6] CBS, Statistics Netherlands, 2007

This work was previously published in the International Journal of Privacy and Health Information Management (IJPHIM), 2(1); edited by Muaz A. Niazi, pages 34-50 copyright year 2014 by IGI Publishing (an imprint of IGI Global).

Section 5
Issues and Challenges

This section contains 17 chapters, giving a wide variety of perspectives on E-Health and Telemedicine and its implications. Within the chapters, the reader is presented with an in-depth analysis of the most current and relevant issues within this growing field of study. Crucial questions are addressed and alternatives offered along with theoretical approaches discussed.

Chapter 61
Detection of Pre-Analytical Laboratory Testing Errors:
Leads and Lessons for Patient Safety

Wafa Al-Zahrani
Saudi Health Council, Saudi Arabia

Mohamud Sheikh
University of New South Wales, Australia

ABSTRACT

A Few years later, after the publication of 'To Err is Human: building a Safer Health System', patient safety became the major concern of the medical services and for the public. The clinical laboratory is not completely empty of errors, and these errors may affect the patient's health and the health care service. Evidence from studies indicate that a large percentage of laboratory errors occur in the pre-analytical and post-analytical phases. Based on reliable data, laboratories that established ongoing quality monitoring system have low percentage of errors. Most of laboratory errors are attributed to ineffective systems and less attributed to the individual malpractice, thus the laboratory quality improvement programs should focus more on the system in a holistic manner. This chapter aims to explore the critical issues that underpin laboratory errors and in particular the pre-analytical errors and provides some recommendations of ways to overcome such critical domains.

INTRODUCTION

The Institute of Medicine's report (IOM's) 1999, *To Err is Human: Building a Safer Health System*, about medical errors in the United States (U.S), was a driver for the creation of a national agenda to address massive costs in terms of life lost, injury, and the financial burden of medical care required as the result of clinical mistakes, and ultimately the ever increasing burden of medical indemnity. Widespread curiosity about the consequences of medical errors emerged in 1999 when the Institute of Medicine unexpectedly reported that medical errors accounted for up to 98,000 deaths in US hospitals each year. One of the outcomes of the magnitude of these deaths was that they exceeded the annual deaths as the results of car accidents, breast cancer, or Acquired Immunodeficiency Syn-

DOI: 10.4018/978-1-4666-8756-1.ch061

drome (AIDS), although preventative measures had been highlighted for several years. The IOM report estimated that medical errors cost the U.S. $17-$29 billion a year, and called for huge changes to the health-care system to improve patient safety (Kohn, Corrigan & Donaldson, 1999). The IOM followed their 1999 report with several other reports, including a 2001 report titled, *Crossing the Quality Chasm: A New Health System for the 21st Century*. This report was prepared by the IOM committee on quality of the health care in the United States. As the result of rapid changes, the country's health care delivery system has developed better ability to translate knowledge into practice and applies new technology for patient safety. Crossing the *Quality Chasm* concentrates more extensively on how the health system care can be transformed and improves the delivery of care. Towards this goal, the committee presented several strategies and action plans for the next years (Institute of Medicine, 2001).

Clinical Decision-Making and Patient Laboratory Results Reporting

The dependence of clinical decision-making and patient management processes on laboratory test reporting must emulate laboratory medicine to set higher quality standards. Timely and accurate laboratory results are the main steps toward effective diagnosis and treatment of patients. Like other medical diagnostic areas, laboratory diagnostic is often delivered under an environment of strenuous pressure with complex technologies and innovation, so that it cannot be considered completely safe (Plebian, 2006). Laboratory practice can be divided into 3 phases; (pre-analytical, analytical, and post-analytical). All the 3 phases of the testing process can be focused on individually for improving quality. In fact, laboratory errors can be defined as "failure of a planned action to be completed as intended, or use of a wrong plan to achieve an aim, occurring at any part of the laboratory cycle, from ordering examinations to reporting results and appropriately interpreting

and reacting to them "(International Organization for Standardization, 2005).

Manual results reporting is time consuming with large human error. The computerized system reduces errors and improving patient safety and outcomes. The importance of information system in improving reliability and security of result reporting is widely recognized. Reference range of diseases and medical conditions are important benchmarks for clinical interpretation of laboratory test values. Using the wrong reference range may affect the results interpretation that leads to physicians making errors in their decision-making (Plebian, 2006). This indicates that interpretation provided by laboratory professional with insufficient expertise can be crucial and spotlight the requirement for improvement in standards of interpretation. A study conducted in accident and emergency department to evaluate the delay in clinicians' obtaining emergency biochemistry test results identified unusual events that indicate partial usage of laboratory information system, and 45% of urgent laboratory results have not been accessed (Kilpatrick & Holding, 2001). Sometimes the results released by laboratory may not contain all the needed information or it may contain information considered by clinicians not relevant. However, it has been highlighted that the introduction of new and complex tests might increase the complexity of medical management; this consequently may influence the interpretation of new laboratory tests (Plebian, 2006).

The researcher Lippi and his colleagues published that the errors of total testing process ranges from 0.1% to 3.0% (Lippi, Plebani &Šimundić, 2010). Plebani&Carraro published a paper that described the distribution of mistakes was pre-analytical 68.2%, analytical 13.3% and post-analytical 18.5% (Plebani &Carraro, 1997). In their study on laboratory errors, Plebani and Carraro found that laboratory error rates declined over the 10 years of 1996 to 2006 was 0.47% and 0.33% respectively (Plebani &Carraro, 1997) (Carraro & Plebani, 2007). The decline in the trends of errors rates has been seen more specific in analytical errors due to automation and improved laboratory technology (Plebani, 2007). All available studies concur that a large percentage of laboratory errors occur in the pre-analytical and post-analytical phases and fewer errors occurring during the analytical phase. Furthermore, the quality of clinical laboratory results is strongly influenced by pre-analytical variables. Pre-analytical phase is important component of total lab testing cycle. The pre-analytical phase starts from the test request by clinicians till the sample is ready for testing. The pre-analytical activities include: collection, transportation, preparation (e.g. centrifugation), and storage of specimens. Series of published literature draw attention to the pre-analytical errors which account for the nearly 60-70% of all errors occurring in the clinical laboratory (Lippi et al., 2011). The prevalence of the pre-analytical errors is different among the published studies due to the variation on the study designs and settings. The pre-analytical errors attributed to the mistakes occur during sample collection, handling, preparing for testing and storage. The attentions of laboratory professionals must be focused on the errors that occur outside the laboratory.

Pre-analytical errors includes; hemolysis, incorrect request, patient misidentification, inadequate volume, lipemic among other (Naz, Mumtaz & Sadaruddin, 2012). Hemolysis is the most frequent reason for specimen rejection, as identified by The College of American Pathologists (Jones, Calam & Howanitz, 1997). It leads to leakage of intracellular contents into the plasma and serum then leading to false high results of certain analytes (Laessig, Hassemer, Paskey &Schwartz, 1976). Hemolysis can be caused mainly due to improper blood collection technique and also inappropriate handling, storage and processing of specimen. Moreover, the patient identification errors are major issues, which attributed with the incorrect diagnosis and inappropriate treatment procedures and can lead to fatal consequence in transfusion medicine (Dock, 2005).

BACKGROUND

Medical Errors

Medical errors represent a significant public health issue that would present a threat to patient safety. Since health care institutions were setup "error" as clinical and research became critical concern. The researcher focused on answer the most essential question: what is a medical error? To decrease the incidence of errors, health care providers should determine the mistakes causes, solutions and look at the success of improvement efforts. Furthermore, accurate measurement of the likelihood of errors based on clear and accurate definitions are essential requirements for effective action. Historically, patient safety investigators and researchers examining the impact of errors in the medicine have used numerous definitions of medical error and its terms. They have focused only on patient experiencing injury or damage as a result of medical care (Grober & Bohnen, 2005). In 1950s, the earliest studies on patient safety defined medical errors as "disease of medical progress" and dismissed as "the price we pay for modern diagnosis and therapy" (Barr, 1955). In 1990s, the researchers of Harvard Medical Practice Study have adapted adverse event definition for medical error adverse events: unintended injury to patients caused by medical management that result in measurable disability, prolonged hospitalization or both (Brennan, 1991). (IOM) defined medical error as "The failure of a planned action to be completed as intended or the use of a wrong plan to achieve an aim", it is commonly used definition. An error may or may not cause an adverse event. Adverse events are injuries that results from medical intervention and responsible for harm to patient (death, life-threatening illness, disability etc) (Kohn, Corrigan & Donaldson, 1999). Harvard Medical Practice study in 1991, was land mark study on medical errors and adverse events. The aim of study is to measure the degree of medical mal practice in hospitals of state of New York and compare the results with negligence claims actually registered. First Study conducted for more than 30,121 discharged patients from 51 hospitals in New York in 1984, they found that the adverse events manifest by prolonged hospitalization or disability at the time of discharge or both. Adverse events occurred in 3.7% of hospitalization and 27.6% were due to negligence, about half of the adverse events were judged to have been preventable (Brennan, 1991). A second Harvard medical practice study identified 1133 adverse events in 30,195 patients hospitalized in New York in 1984, the study shows that the drug complications were the most common type of adverse event (19%), followed by wound infections (14%) and technical complications (13%) and Half the adverse events (48%) were associated with an operation. The Negligence was more frequent in patients who had more severe adverse events (Leape et al., 1991). For years, medical and nursing student have been taught Florence Nightingale's dictum- first" do not harm", for this reason the Health care providers trained to be careful and work with high level of proficiency. It is curious that high error rates have not stimulated more concern and efforts at error prevention, this due to the lack of awareness of the severity of the problem and because the serious injuries result from errors are not part of everyday experience of health workers (Leape, 1994). Once the tools of medicine were the physicians' intelligence, the nurses' sympathy and a surgical procedure, there was a tiny cost to be paid for lack of safety system and cooperation. Since the medical tools become more complex, highly specialized teams were needed for health care deliver (Wachter, 2004). The modern intensive care unit (ICU) clearly demonstrates the problem, the average ICU patients encounter 1.7 errors per day, nearly one third of which are life threatening. They concluded that Most of the errors involve communication problems (Donchin et al., 1995).

Quality in Laboratory Testing

Laboratory testing and services have an important role in the health care organization by its great impact on clinical decision making ; up to 70% of the most important decisions of clinicians are based on laboratory test results. The high influence of laboratory testing makes the quality of testing and reporting is of utmost importance (Forsman, 1996). Clinical laboratory work is composed of the technical activities that produce laboratory results for patient care and the management activities that support the technical work. The laboratory technical staff has to perform pre-analytical activities (blood sample collection, transportation, centrifugation); analytical activities (testing, examinations, interpretation); and post-analytical activities (reporting results,) that transform a clinician's order for a laboratory test or examination into the results used by the clinician to diagnose and treat patients (Berte, 2007).

Using quality indicators to collect and analyze the required data through a systematic and consistent approach can ensure evaluation of the quality of laboratory tests. The Institute Of Medicine (IOM) defines the quality of care as "the degree to which health care services for individuals and populations increase the likelihood of desired health outcomes and are consistent with the current professional knowledge'' (IOM, 1990). The Quality Indicator was defined by (IOM) as "an objective measure that evaluates critical health care domains'', (patient safety, effectiveness, equity, patient-centeredness, timeliness, and efficiency) are the main health care domains (Kohn, Corrigan & Donaldson, 1999). The laboratory quality indicators include:

- Test Order Appropriateness;
- Inpatient Wristband Identification Error;
- Patient Satisfaction With Phlebotomy;
- Specimen Inadequacy and Rejection;
- Specimen Container Information Error;
- Proficiency Testing Performance;

- Inpatient Laboratory Results Availability;
- Corrected Laboratory Reports;
- Critical Values Reporting;
- Turnaround Time;
- Clinician Satisfaction With Laboratory Services.

The laboratory quality indicators data must be collected on regular basis to identify the issues and improve the performance of laboratory (Shahangian & Snyder, 2009). Quality and safety in diagnostic laboratory is essential for high quality of services and safe health care, the laboratory department has such a prominent responsibility in patient safety (Lippi & Simundic, 2010). Even though it is difficult to estimate accurately the rate of diagnostic errors in general, it has been reported that prevalence of laboratory errors can be as high as one in every 330-1000 laboratory test (Plebani, 2006).

Laboratory Errors

The great dependence of clinical decision-making and patient management processes on laboratory test reporting must stimulate laboratory medicine to set higher quality standards. Timely and accurate laboratory results are the main steps toward effective diagnosis and treatment of patient. However, the use of laboratory services has grown significantly, recently a survey of UK laboratories it found that 83% increase in requests of tests from primary care between 2000 and 2004 (Beastall, 2004). The promotion of patient centred care should be converted in to a need to investigate any mistakes that occurs in the total testing process or any step of testing that can have negative impact on the patient safety. In fact, any negative outcomes related to laboratory testing should be considered whether the source was analytical, pre-analytical or post- analytical. The mistakes can occur in any steps of test process starting from test request and ending with physician reaction based on laboratory result (Plebani, 2006). The College

of American Pathologists (CAP) has focused on errors in pathology and laboratory medicine since its creation in 1946 and has contributed resources to arranged approaches for reducing or preventing these errors. The CAP has supported worldwide programs that improved the analytic performance of each test through daily quality control (Quality Assurance Service), and proficiency programs (Surveys), provided reagents and documents for use as standards, developed a program of accreditation of clinical laboratories (Laboratory Accreditation Program) and introduced a system of terminology for the electronic health records (SNOMED). In the early 90s CAP initiated supported programs to define frequency of errors throughout all laboratory testing (Q-Probes and Q-Tracks) (Howanitz, 2005). Q-Probes studies are time limited surveys lasting up to 4 months, and Q-Tracks investigations performed yearly (Zarbo et al., 2002).

Analytical Errors

Laboratory errors can be defined as "failure of a planned action to be completed as intended, or use of a wrong plan to achieve an aim, occurring at any part of the laboratory cycle, from ordering examinations to reporting results and appropriately interpreting and reacting to them "(IOS, 2005). A study published in 1947 by Belk et al. estimated the number of analytical errors in clinical laboratories by 162,116 per million laboratory tests. This paper was the origin of quality assessment programs in clinical laboratories (Plebani, 2009). In 1996, group of Australian laboratories published an article that identified the transcription and analytical errors in 14 laboratories by using national quality award criteria for benchmarking indicators. The study indicated 26% of analytical errors and 39% of transcription errors (Khoury, Burnett & McKay, 1996). In the same year CAP conducted Q-Probes in 665 laboratories to estimated analytical errors and its related events, the results showed from 670,489 tests performed in these laboratories reported 9,268 (1.4%) unacceptable results (Steindel, Howanitz & Renner, 1996). In 1997, Plebani & Carraro evaluated the frequency and types of errors in stat laboratory and the results revealed among a total 40,490 laboratory tests, they identified 189 errors, the relative frequency of 0.47% of test results (4700 ppm). The distribution of errors was pre-analytical 68.2%, analytical 13.3% and pos-analytical 18.5% (Plebani & Carraro, 1997). 10 years later, Plebani & Carraro published a paper showed an improvement in the number of laboratory errors. The overall frequency of errors is (3,092ppm) which is significantly lower than result in 1996

(Carraro & Plebani, 1997). The data showed reducing in the number of errors over years; these indicate an evidence of improvement in overall performance and particularly in analytical process. Quality assay, standardization, automation and information technology have improved the quality of analytical step and reduced the contributed errors (Plebani, 2007). The importance role of quality improvement is to be assigned to well defined rules for internal quality control, the introduction of effective external quality assessment schemes and well-trained staff. Nevertheless, the existing reduction in analytical error rate in laboratories can make the laboratory more difficult for single laboratory with few errors to estimate its unacceptable results rate using a traditional metric way. The detection of low error rates required for large database and suitable techniques for detection of errors. There is no difference between the achievable reductions on analytical errors over the few decades and existing evidence that analytical quality is not satisfied when evaluated with sigma scale (Plebani, 2009). Six-sigma is a unique approach that is used to achieve significant improvement in process quality and efficiency. The key elements of six-sigma are: Define Measure, Analyze, and Improve. The statistical technique used for detecting and documenting analytical errors have shown a decrease in the rates of error, but accurate metric should be introduced in laboratories to improve the current status of analytical quality that according to six-sigma approach ranges from 3 to 4 Sigma (Westgard J & Westgard S, 2006).

Post-Analytical Errors

The quality management in laboratory analysis is the main key in laboratory medicine and to manage the quality of the laboratory, it has to consider the whole process of the laboratory analysis. The main step in the laboratory cycle is Post- analytical phase which has a great effect in the overall quality. The post-analytical phase is subdivided into phase performed within the laboratory and another outside the laboratory. The post-analytical procedure performed within laboratory includes; verifying the results, transmitting them to the laboratory information system and communicating them to the clinicians and physicians in various ways. It is done by producing laboratory reports and making necessary oral communication regarding urgent results, the physicians interpret the laboratory reports to make a decision based on the results and other resources (Hawkins, 2012). In representative study by Ross et al., the error rates of post analytical was 47.2% of total errors (Ross & Boone, 1989). Plebani and Carraro demonstrated that the post-analytical error accounts for 18.5% of 4700 laboratory test errors (Plebani and Carraro, 1997). Ten years later, the same researchers did investigations in the stat laboratory to estimate the overall errors, the post-analytical errors were identified with 23.1% of 3092 errors per millions (Carraro & Plebani, 2007). Asten et al. published paper that identified the number of incidents report during 16 months period; the laboratory was responsible for 60% of incidents, where post-analytical phase was involved in 11% of incidents (Astion, Shojana, Hamil, Kim & Ng, 2003).

Pre-Analytical Phase

Pre-analytical phase is an important component of total lab testing cycle. It includes a set of processes, which are not easy to define because they take place in different places at different times. Traditionally, the pre-analytical phase starts from the test request by physician till the sample is ready for testing. The pre-analytical step can be divided into two phases (Plebani, 2006):

- **Pre-Pre-Analytical Phase:** procedures performed outside the laboratory and may not even be under the supervision of laboratory personnel. It starts with test request, patient and specimen identification, blood drawing, sample collection and handling, and then ends with the transportation of specimens to the laboratory.
- **Pre-Analytical Phase:** procedures performed inside the laboratory and the laboratory staffs are responsible for it. This phase involves the specimen preparation, which includes all activities that makes the sample ready and suitable for analysis. This includes, sample log in (recording and numbering), centrifugation, liquating, pipetting, dilution and sorting specimens.

The pre-analytical phase is the main component of a total laboratory quality. Many variables can affect the result of test, including the procedures of collection, handling and processing before analysis of specimen. Narayanan in published article has grouped the variables to physiological, specimen collection and interference factors (Narayanan, 2000).

Physiological variables:

- **Age:** The effect of age on the laboratory result is well recognized and each group has a separate reference interval.
- **Sex:** Sex differences are seen for several analytes and recognized by laboratory staff. This variation is due to the differences in muscle mass and to endocrine and organ-specific differences.
- **Time:** Some analytes fluctuate with differences in time. Circadian rhythm is responsible for diurnal changes seen in levels of some analytes.
- **Pregnancy:** The mean of plasma volume will increase and cause hemodilution in pregnancy.
- **Exercise:** Regular exercise such as running up and down, stairs climbing or workout in gymnasium before specimen collection can strongly affect several biochemical and hematological variables (Narayanan, 2000).

Specimen collection variables:

- **Duration of Fasting:** In some analytes measurement, the patient instructed to fast overnight for at least 12 hours. However, prolonged fasting can affect some laboratory results by decreasing the level of specific analytes (Narayanan, 1993).
- **Time of Specimen Collection:** The time of collection should be kept constant and should not change from day to day to eliminate variation (Narayanan, 2000).
- **Posture during Blood Sampling:** The change of posture during blood collecting may affect the concentration of various analytes. The change in position of patient from supine to sitting position can lead to shift of body fluid from intravascular to interstitial compartment (Narayanan, 1996).
- **Duration of Tourniquet Application:** The using of tourniquet for more than one minute can leads to hemo-concentration, causing increase in the concentration of large molecules. To eliminate the pre-analytical effect of tourniquet application time, it should be released as soon as needle inter to the vein (Narayanan, 1996).

- **Effect of Infusion:** If patient received an infusion, the blood must not be drawn from the site near to the infusion site, it should be obtained from opposite arm (Narayanan, 1993).
- **Anticoagulation Blood Ratio:** The anticoagulant blood ratio is crucial for some laboratory test as it affects the concentration of analytes. Basically, if too little blood is drawn the osmotic effect can leads to cell shrinking and introduce dilution changes in concentration of extracellular analytes (Narayanan, 2000).
- **Specimen Handling and Processing:** The storage time and temperature of specimen and processing steps in preparation of serum, plasma or cell separation can cause a pre-analytical variable (Narayanan, 2000).

Endogenous interferences:

- **Hemolysis and Lypemic:** The endogenous inferences can affect the clinical interpretation of the laboratory data. The most common inferences are hemolysis and turbidity due to hyperlipidemia which interfere with measurement of the analytes (Narayanan, 1996).

Pre-Analytical Errors

The laboratory is an extremely complex service (Plebani, 2006). Nevertheless, significant evidences demonstrate that quality of the laboratory services cannot be assured by focusing only on analytical phase but it should concentrate at the beginning and at the ending of the total testing process. In particular, most errors in laboratory diagnostics occur in the pre-analytical phase. The pre-analytical errors account for 60-70% of all mistakes occurring in the laboratory diagnostics most of which arise from problems in patient preparation and sample collection, transportation, preparation for analysis and storage (Lippi, 2011).

The current available data of the prevalence of pre-analytical errors is heterogeneous, basically depending on the study design and methods of data collection. Mostly, the prevalence of inappropriate specimens can be related to the number of missing tests results, number of specimen inappropriate to analysis, the type of laboratory test requested and to the total number of samples in which each pre-analytical error was relevant (Lippi & Guidi, 2007). Plebani and Carrero in 1997 conducted a study to evaluate the frequency and types of mistakes in stat laboratory to identify the most critical steps in total testing process and plan to corrective strategy, this study discovered that among 40,490 tests, the number of errors 189 mistakes and the pre-analytical shows high percentage of errors with 68.2% (Plebani & Carraro, 2007). Few years later, Stahl et al. conducted a survey to estimate the prevalence of laboratory error in the whole laboratory. They identified 4135 mistakes in 676, 564 tests, the pre-analytical errors accounted for 75% of the total errors (Stahl, Lund & Brandslund, 1998). Verona hospital laboratory' conducted yearlong survey which aimed to estimate the number of errors, 3154 (74%) pre-analytic errors were recorded in the observational period from a total of 423 075 routine blood specimens (Lippi et al., 2006). In 2002, the department of clinical biochemistry at Roskilde hospital began recording all errors in order to monitor their type and frequency. The study reported a total of 1,189 errors; the majority was pre-analytical error with 81% of errors (Szecsi & Ødum, 2009). Plebani and Carrero investigated mistakes in stat laboratory to compare the results with results of study done before 10 years using the same study design. The results were 51,746 errors with the majority of pre-analytical with 61.9% of errors (Carrero & Plebani, 2007).

The unpredictable consequences of laboratory errors may range from no harm to being totally fatal to the patient. The patient safety is considered as primary goal of any health organization. Based on the available data, the risk of inappropriate care due to errors in testing process was ranged from 6.4% to 12%. Beside the immediate risk to patient health, large percentage of 26% to 30% of laboratory errors are associated with physicians being compelled to request for further tests which lead to discomfort and increased cost for unnecessary testing such as (CAT scan, NMR, biopsies etc.) on patients (Plebani, 2006). In a study by Plebani and Carraro 6.4% of errors translated to inappropriate transfusion, modification in heparin infusion, infusion of electrolyte solution and modification in digoxin therapy (Plebani & Carraro, 1997). Pre-analytical errors can be curial to patient safety such as the analysis of potassium analyte due to the role of potassium in body homeostasis. Any false diagnosis of hyperkalemia is usually due to pre-analytical errors such as in vitro hemoloysis, excessive shaking, and delay in separation of blood cell, inadequate clotting, poor transportation especially uncontrolled temperature, or excessive centrifugation affect the sample (Lippi et al., 2006).

The Important Errors in the Pre-Analytical Phase

Hemolysis

Hemolysis is the most frequent reason for specimen rejection as indicated by College of American Pathologists Chemistry Specimen A acceptance Q-Probes study (Jones, Calam & Howanitz, 1997). Hemolysis comes from the Latin hemo (blood) and lysis (breakdown) ; is the release of hemoglobin and other intra-cellular components from erythrocytes to the surrounding plasma, following damage of cell membrane. The upper reference for free hemoglobin is 20 mg/L in plasma and 50 mg/L in serum (Lippi et al., 2008). Hemolysis can occur in both in vivo and in vitro stages, and it is the most cause of pre-analytical errors that affect the accuracy of laboratory tests. In vivo hemolysis is a result of many clinical conditions including several infections, bacteria and parasite. Other causes of in vivo hemolysis

are autoantibodies (such as RH-D or ABO blood group incompatibility), hereditary, heart valves, HELLP (hemolysis, elevated liver enzymes and low platelets syndrome) hemoglobinopathies and drugs (Lippi et al., 2011).

Conversely, In vitro hemolysis can be caused mainly due to improper blood collection technique and also inappropriate handling, storage and processing of specimen. There are many factors that can trigger the in vitro hemolysis, ranging from physiological to anatomical situation. Techniques and methods used during blood collection such as (Bush, 2003):

- Alcohols not dry when contacting the skin.
- Intravenous catheter gauge is too big or too small.
- Pulling syringe plunger back too fast.
- Drawing the blood forcefully from syringe to blood tube.
- Under-filled or filled tubes may cause improper blood additive ratio.
- Long application of Tourniquet.
- Variability in competency level.

Other sources of hemolysis are the three pre-analytical phases: transportation, centrifugation and storage. The transportation of blood sample by using courier for long time or transport under extreme temperature condition can lead to lysis of the cell. In vitro hemolysis has been noticed in the use of some innovative pneumatic tube system (Bowen, 2005). Centrifugation of samples prior transportation can increase the percentage of hemolyzed specimen. The centrifugation is a crucial pre-analytical step, which includes critical conditions such as time between collection and processing, high temperature, high speed, poor separator barrier integrity and re-centrifugation of tubes with gel separators. Inappropriate conditions of storage such as time and temperature can affect the blood cells and cause in vitro hemolysis (Lippi, 2011).

Hemolysis considered as a major challenging problem in the clinical laboratory, which cannot be evident until the complete separation of plasma or serum from the whole blood. The release of hemoglobin of red blood cells and intercellular components of white blood cells to the serum or plasma might falsely elevate the level of same substances in serum or plasma and may cause dilution, which affects the accuracy and reliability of laboratory testing (Laessig, Hassemer, Paskey & Schwartz, 1976). The release of hemoglobin can cause spectrophotometric interference due to increase of optical absorbance or change in blank value especially for laboratory performing measurement at 415 nm, 540 nm and 570 nm (Carraro, Servidio & Plebani, 2000). However, both in vivo and mainly in vitro hemolysis cause pre-analytical variability and interfere with the measurement of some analytes especially, potassium, sodium, calcium, magnesium, bilirubin, haptoglobin, total protein, aldolase, amylase, lactate dehydrogenase, aspartate aminotransferase, alanine aminotransferase, phosphorus, alkaline phosphatase, acid phosphatase, alpha-glutamyltranspeptidase, folate, and iron measurements (Laessig et al., 1976). The blood cell lysis also affect routine coagulation testing, prothrombin time (PT), activated partial thromboplastin time (aPTT), fibrinogen, and dimerized plasmin fragment D (D-dimer) testing (Lippi, Montagnana, Salvagno & Guidi, 2006).

Patient Sample Identification Errors

Correct patient identification is the major concern of patient safety in many health care organizations; it is a necessary requirement for providing safe and effective clinical diagnostic services. Misidentification not only occurs in operating and consulting rooms or inpatient wards but also in the clinical laboratory (Lippi, 2009). The first step in ensuring that laboratory result is for the correct patient is by accurate identification of the patient for phlebotomy. Policies and procedures of specimen collection and handling for accredited clinical laboratory including the identification requirements of each patient from whom a specimen was collected (Howanitz, Renner & Walsh, 2003). Accurate specimen identification is a challenge in all health care organizations while mislabelled specimen in clinical laboratory testing have potential to cause serious consequences for patients. There are many reports of fatal blood transfusion resulted by the misidentification of laboratory specimen, to decrease the risk of curial harm caused by labelling errors some hospitals have implemented zero tolerance laboratory specimen labelling process (Dock, 2005). In many hospitals, the patient wears wristband for ensuring the correct patient identification. The verification done during the specimen collection by phlebotomist includes asking the patient their name and checking again the wristband (Howanitz, 2003).

Identification errors can be classified by three classification systems. The most popular classification system concentrates on the site where errors occurred. The Identification errors caused by staff *outside* laboratory before specimen is received by clinical laboratory are called *pre-laboratory,* such as mislabelling of patient in a doctor's room. Second type is *laboratory errors* where identification errors are caused by laboratory staff, an example is the errors that occur in reference laboratory to which a primary laboratory sends the specimen to. *Post-laboratory errors* are identification errors that happen after a reported result or product has left the laboratory, including verifying results for wrong patient and tested blood product to the wrong patient. The third system of classification concentrates on the type of identification errors. *Patient identification errors* are can be caused by selection of wrong patient from the list or missing of identification information on the wristband. *Specimen identification errors* occur in incorrect specimen identification; this can be result commonly in incorrect specimen labelling. The last classification system focuses on the root cause of identification errors. It can be attributed either to human error, the environment, equipment failure or defective rules and policies (Valenstein & Sirota, 2004).

Misidentification errors are major challenge in the laboratory, particularly in the blood transfusion unit. The prevalence of red blood cells misidentification is significantly high, around 1 in 14,000 while ABO incompatible transfusion results in 1 in 380,000 or once every 2 to 3 years for many of the health care organizations. The morbidity due to the incompatible blood transfusion is not very common, it is about 1 in 1.8 million (Linden, Wagner, Voytovich & Sheehan, 2000). However, the risk of incompatible blood transfusion is higher than the risk of infected blood such as hepatitis B virus, hepatitis C virus and human immunodeficiency virus (HIV) (Luban, 2005). The patient misidentification may occur in one of the blood processing steps: either during specimen collection, laboratory analysis or at the time of blood transfusion. According to a 10 years survey report of New York State, 56% of identification errors occur outside the laboratory and 14 - 20% of these errors occur before the specimen arrives at the clinical laboratory (Linden, 2000). "Wrong blood in tube" errors occur when the sample is labelled with patient's name but the blood in the tube was collected from another patient. Wrong blood in tube can be investigated in the laboratory by checking the patient historical blood type. This kind of investigation cannot be useful if the patient does not have historical blood type or if both patients have the same ABO blood group (Grimm et al., 2010). There are comprehensive data on specimen identification errors available from transfusion medicine. International society of blood transfusion (ISBT) and biomedical excellence for safer transfusion (BEST) committee reported significant incidence rate of misidentification errors. Surveys conducted on 71 hospitals in 10 countries identified mislabelled and '*miscollected*' samples; the rate for mislabelling of the median hospital performance resulted in the rate for mislabelling of 1 in 165 samples while '*miscollected*' samples demonstrated WBIT occurred in rate 1 in every 1986. Mislabelled sample is defined as sample that does not meet the criteria of labelling by lo-

cal laboratory while the *miscollected* sample is defined as sample where the ABO blood group is different from the blood group in the patient's historical blood type file (Dzik et al., 2003). According to the report of serious hazard transfusion based on study between 1996 and 2003, the risk of mistakes happened during transfusion of the blood component is about 1 in 165,000 and receiving an ABO incompatible transfusion at 1 in 100,000 (Stainsby, Russell, Cohen & Lilleyman, 2005). Q-probes study presented the results of comprehensive survey of 122 clinical laboratories in transfusion services, identified a total of 112,112 samples labels were reviewed and 1,258 mislabelled were discovered for overall incidence rate of 1.12% (1 in 89 samples) (Grimm et al., 2010).

The identification errors prevalence rate in transfusion medicine is not proportionate to the errors in the general laboratory samples (hematology, chemistry, microbiology, anatomic pathology) due to greater care existing during the collection of transfusion medicine samples as compared to the routine samples and because the rejection for these specimen are more strict (Lumadue, Boyd & Ness, 1997). With the exception of the transfusion medicine, the rate of identification errors in clinical laboratory is underestimated with less investigation studies (Lippi, 2009). Based on study conducted In 14 Australian laboratories, the transcription error rate was up to 39% while analytical error rate was up to 26% (Khoury, Burnett & Mackay, 1996). Valenstein and Sirota (2004), examined a survey that was conducted by 195 beds medical center in Ohio to identify the identification errors. The paper estimated 529 reports of incorrect labeling specimens during two years, the most common problem were unlabeled specimen, incorrect labeled specimen, and incorrect identification of specimen type (Valenstein and Sirota &2004). In the college of American Pathologists Q-Probes study, performed in 147 clinical laboratories, a total of 3.3 million specimen labels were reviewed, labelling errors were identified at rate of 0.92 per 1000 labels. The most common error was mislabelled specimen (29.9%), partially labelled (22.7%), unlabelled (21.9%) and incomplete labels (20.7%) (Wagar, Stankovic, Raab, Nakhleh & Walsh, 2008). Recent study showed the prevalence rate of identification errors range from 0.2% to 6% for outpatients and from 1% to 2% for inpatients (Lippi & Guidi, 2007).

Many factors may cause identification errors such as wrong practice, workflow issues and methods used in specimen identification. Most of these causes arise during the pre-analytical phase of testing process: incorrect collection of patient data, collection of specimen from incorrect patient, incorrect label information, problem during specimen processing and incorrect entry of results to the right patient. The main causes of physician ordering laboratory tests to incorrect patient is either due to the patient having someone else's identity or physician made a mistake while writing the order. Mistakes can occur as a result of communication barriers or languages. Misidentification may also occur due to collection of specimen from incorrect patient due to incorrect wristband or without wristband (Lippi, 2009). A survey conducted by the College of American Pathologists Q-Track demonstrated the importance of quality and information contained in the wristband. The data collected during two years indicated that missing wristbands accounted for 71.6% of the errors, with wrong wristbands (1.1%) illegible wristbands (7.7%), erroneous ID information (6.8%), missing ID information (9.1%), and conflicting wristbands (3.7%) accounting for the other types of errors (Howanitz, Renner &Walsh, 2002).

Inadequate Sample Volume

The adequacy of specimen volume is a significant factor, which affects the accuracy and reliability of the laboratory test results. Laboratories have guidelines and strict criteria for evaluating specimen delivered to the laboratory for testing. If specimen does not meet adequacy criteria, then drawing another sample from the patient is necessary. In the case of obtaining another specimen from the patient, it leads to delay of the results, patient discomfort, increased workload, and increased cost (Jones, Meier & Howanitz, 1995). The quantity insufficiency of volume is one of the main factors leading to specimen rejection. The main reasons of inadequate volume sample are the malpractice of phlebotomist, difficulty to obtain the blood from paediatric patient, difficult to localize veins in some patients and debilitated cases (Naz, Mumtaz & Sadaruddin, 2012). Insufficient specimen quantity was the second most frequent reasons for specimen rejection in a study done by college of American pathologist Q-probes at 703 clinical laboratories (Jones, Meier & Howanitz, 1995).

Incomplete Laboratory Request Form

One of the main sources of the pre-analytical errors is wrong or incomplete information on the test request form and specimen label. Laboratory test request form is the main problem that affects patient safety and leads to increased workload of laboratory employees. There are few studies reported the magnitude of laboratory request form errors. Transcription errors rate in Khoury et al. study was up to 39% of all request forms, and has error rates of 9% in patient identification data and 17% in data such as sex and date-of-birth (Khoury, 1996). One of the major challenges to the laboratory staff is most of the staff at point of service do not reject the incomplete request form and may not know the significance of missing data. The specific missing information includes; patient identification, physician or ward contact number and misidentification of requested tests. This problem can lead to unwanted consequences such as delay of results, over work load, increased cost when test has to be repeated or duplicated reports are issued (Naz, Mumtaz & Sadaruddin, 2012).

DISSCUSSION

The health care system is highly dependent on clinical laboratory service, the importance of laboratory test reporting in clinical decision-making and patient management processes must emulate laboratory medicine to eliminate the errors. Most of the studies discussed and demonstrated the laboratory errors and their effects on the patient health outcome. The most significant features of the studies on the laboratory mistakes are their limited numbers in this topic and their heterogeneous nature. This means that studies performed and reported in this literature used different data collection approaches (process analysis, questionnaires and collection of rejection forms), the time-span on the collection of data ranged from one month to one year, and have investigated different laboratory sections or activities.

In this chapter, we identified that a large percentage of the laboratory errors occur in the pre-analytical and post-analytical phases with fewer errors occurring in the analytical phase. This is attributed to the advancement in the automation and computer system and adaption of quality control programs particularly in the past 20 years, that led to impressive decline in the occurrence of analytical errors and raised the awareness that analytical errors are not the main factors affecting the quality of clinical laboratory testing and giving more attentions toward the main sources of pre-analytical and post-analytical errors. The distribution of errors as observed by Carraro and Plebani in 1996 was: pre-analytical 68.2%, analytical 13.3% and post-analytical 18.5%. (Szecsi &Ødum, 2009) conducted a survey which demonstrated 81% pre-analytical errors, 10% analytical errors and 9% post-analytical errors, concur. Evidence from these studies demonstrated that a large percentage of laboratory errors occur in the pre-analytical phase. In their study, Carraro and Plebani (2006), the pre-analytical phase still had the highest prevalence of errors with 61.9% followed by 23.1% post-analytical errors and 15%

analytical errors. The study reported significant reduction in the error rates in the same Stat laboratory but distribution of the errors among different phases remained the same.

Furthermore, the frequency of errors could be differing from one institution to another and between departments. This was clearly demonstrated in the study by Carrero and Plebani (1997) where higher frequency of errors was demonstrated in the department of medicine compared with the other departments. The authors did not explain the reasons for the difference. Another important finding is that most of the errors (74-75%) have not affected the patient's health the percentage of (19-24%) can lead to negative clinical outcome, unnecessary repeat of laboratory testing, and associated with inappropriate further investigation which increase the cost of care. In one of the studies (Carrero and Plebani, 1997), the laboratory errors have been attributed to inappropriate treatment of 12 patients.

Data obtained from most of the studies included in this research showed that the most of the problems identified are directly related to specimen collection and transportation as an important cause of pre-analytical mistakes. This includes: hemolyzed specimen, insufficient quantity specimen, clotting specimen, incorrect specimen labeling and incorrect specimen collected. In vitro hemolysis, which means damaging of red blood cell during phlebotomy, remains the main cause of rejection specimens for both inpatient and outpatient which accounted for 53-60% of all unsuitable specimens, nearly five times higher than the second cause of specimen rejection as indicated by bio-chemistry specimen acceptance Q-Probes study (Jones, Calam & Howanitz,1997).

Hemolysis remains a challenging problem in clinical laboratory, affecting the accuracy and reliability tests (Laessig, 1976). The rupture of red blood cells and leakage of hemoglobin and intracellular components to the surrounding fluid leads to false elevation of some analytes or dilution of other analytes. The released proteins, enzymes, lipid and carbohydrates may interfere with the measurement of some analytes (lippi et al., 2008). The issue of hemolyzed specimens can be preventable especially if it is in vitro, hemolysis is usually caused by incorrect collection, handling, transportation and processing of specimens. Furthermore, the complexity of the pre-analytical phase leads to significant variability in the way specimens are collected, transported and processed.

The patient misidentification is not frequent errors in the clinical laboratory, when compared with other significant errors such as hemolysis, quantity insufficient, lipamic among other. In the study of Szecsi and Odum (2009) the frequency of identification errors was accounted for 7.5% of errors from the total laboratory errors, Carraro and Plebani estimated the identification errors 2.6% and 8.8% in their studies. The misidentification errors are underestimated either due to lack of negative outcomes on patients or the errors not being reported. Despite of the low prevalence rate of the patient misidentification errors, these errors are significant healthcare issues as it contributes to the wrong diagnosis and inappropriate treatment procedures of patients. It is also considered as major concern for blood transfusion medicine because it leads to incompatible blood transfusion, which can cause significant patient morbidity or even fatality.

The Q-Probes study (Grimm, 2010) presented the results of comprehensive survey of patient identification and sample labelling in 122 institutions where the frequency rate of mislabelled sample was 1.12% or 1 in 89 samples. Major mislabelled samples were those that were unlabeled, have mismatched information on specimen and requisition or for which the current specimen did not match the historical record on file. The overall rate of rejection of mislabelled rates of samples submitted for ABO blood typing was 80%. The high rejection rate for ABO samples most likely reflects the more strictly labelling requirement applied on transfusion medicine specimens in all

laboratories. Duna and Muga (2010) concluded that specimen misidentification occur most frequently in pre-analytical phase with 73% due to mislabelling during the process of specimen collection.

In the study of Q- probes (Valenstein, Raab &Walsh, 2006) the identification errors were detected before and after test results assessed in 120 institutions. Thus, 85.5% of reported identification errors were detected within the clinical laboratory before results verification while 14.5% of reported errors were detected after results verification. The findings represented laboratories that matched results against pathology requisitions after their verification showed lower pre-verification errors percentage. The results showed that post-verification error rates were lower at institution that had been tracking and monitoring identification errors before starting this survey. This experience makes facility more awareness about identification errors and promoting their detection before results are released.

The study by Carraro and Plebani (2007) has identified a significant link between identification errors and using of information system procedures. The using of hospital computerized order entry system had decreased some errors such as incorrect patient name or wrong ward number and the performance of unrequested laboratory tests. The information system procedures had not eliminated the risk of mismatched patients. These errors come from low compliance with written procedures and indicating some unsatisfactory of information technology.

The difference between inpatients and outpatients in the rate of the laboratory errors was significant in certain studies. There were 0.77% of hemolysis in samples from inpatients and 0.38% of hemolysis errors in samples from outpatients (Lippi et al., 2006). According to study by (Bonini, Plebani, Ceriotti & Rubboli, 2002) two reasons were attributed to this difference: the direct control of samples collection from outpatients by specialized personnel versus blood collecting by nurses or ward personnel who have a high degree of turnover and low skills in blood samples collections. The evidence that most errors and high rejection rate occur for sample collected by non-laboratory staff due to their unawareness of all aspects of specimen collection at higher level, including sample identification.

One the Q-Probes studies (Jones, 1997) showed that the hospital bed size and hospital location had not affected the specimen rejection rates. In the same study, the CAP accreditation and teaching status had no significant association with the specimen rejection rates. A Q-probe study (Wagar, 2008) demonstrated a low rate of labelling errors in laboratory had ongoing quality monitor for specimen identification. Another Q-Probes study (Grimm, et al., 2010) agreed with pervious study, which showed that the laboratories with current ongoing monitoring programs for specimen labelling had a low rate of labelling errors. These laboratories had awareness of the importance of sample labelling and monitoring the proper practice for labelling.

CONCLUSION AND FUTURE DIRECTION

The goal of this study was to enhance our understanding of the pre-analytical errors in the clinical laboratory. The accuracy of test results needs a high quality specimen, and we found that pre-analytical variability had strong influence on laboratory testing and patient outcome. We wanted to understand why and how these errors occurred. Our purpose was also to stimulate ideas of what could be done to prevent the occurrence of adverse events due to the pre-analytical errors. Quality and reliability are the main focus in the clinical laboratory. A change must occur in the traditional view, which focuses only on the quality control of the analytical phase. Much evidence shows that accuracy cannot be achieved in the clinical laboratory by only focus on the quality

control of the analytical phase. The quality system should maintain all steps in laboratory testing to detect any defects. Our findings indicates that a large percentage of laboratory errors occur in the pre-analytical phase which needs more attention and intensive monitoring of its activities.

According to the IOM, most medical errors are attributed to ineffective system and less attributed to the individual malpractice. Medical errors can be reduced through focusing on holistic improvement of the health care delivery system. (Kohn et al.,1999). The important question is about how we could reduce the laboratory errors mainly pre-analytical errors and minimize the effect of pre-analytical variability. Traditionally, the quality of laboratory can be maintained only by direct inspection, quality control and accreditation. These approaches alone could not address and solve the main problems of laboratory errors (Winkelman, Mennemeyer, 1996).

The other lesson we gather from this chapter is that, the diagnosis of patient samples does not only depend on the accuracy and precision of the laboratory test results. The quality of the sample is crucial and hemolysis of specimen was good case example as we examined its adversely affects on the measurement of many analytes. Hemolysis of specimen is a major concern for clinical laboratories worldwide as they are the most frequent pre-analytical errors and lead to multiple testing and misdiagnosis. Further, we have identified that the collecting of quality specimen that yields accurate results needs a high degree of knowledge, expertise, skills and experience (Lippi et al., 2008).

We have identified that misidentification of patients during laboratory testing is a major cause of medical error. It is thus recommended that proper patient identification system is established for ensuring accurate test results and thus prevent wrong diagnosis and improper treatment which lead to unwanted and life threatening consequences. New innovative techniques such as the using of bar-coded wristbands have decreased much of patient identification errors (Howanitz et al.,2003). Nevertheless, despite the use of wristbands, identification errors continue to occur, although at minimal (Lippi et al.,200671). We recommend that when this occurs, immediate feedback about the errors to the admitting clerks must be conducted. However, significant improvement due to ongoing training and education has decreased the rate of wristband errors from 5.5% in 1993 (Renner, Howanitz & Bachner 1993) to 0.1-1% in 2005 (Valenstein, 2005).

Our findings identified that a large percentage of laboratory errors occur outside the laboratory and by non-laboratory personnel. Phlebotomists play a major role in maintaining the quality of the specimen. The educational requirements, background and training policies of phlebotomists differ from one institution to another. Phlebotomists range from employees with no laboratory background to certified technicians. Regardless of the requirements, the management must provide continuous and refresher training programs with certifications to the phlebotomy staff. The certification programs might be playing a major role in increasing the successful phlebotomies and decrease the pre-analytical errors. This will also give more confidence and reduce the turnover of trained staff.

Regardless of the source of errors, the magnitude of medical errors documented demands the need for establishing state-based mandatory report system (Wood & Nash, 2005). This system can be applied in the clinical laboratory to help tackle and monitor the laboratory errors. The errors tracking systems categorizes trends and analyze data to increase knowledge about laboratory errors. The system must use efficient data collection methods techniques for analysis and feedback. The system focuses only on analytical errors that are a minor percentage of the total laboratory errors. Establishing effective tracking and identification system that can identify the errors in the pre-analytical phase is recommended.

It is essential that patient safety, particularly if it relates to services such as in clinical laboratory, be considered as an important component relating to interdepartmental relationship. The cooperation of the laboratory with clinicians, nurses and phlebotomists outside the laboratory is the key elements toward laboratory activities improvement. The availability of expert support system that provides information of the diagnostic efficiency of the laboratory results will play a role in the errors reduction.

Recommendations:

- The conventional view should shift from focusing only on quality control of analytical phase to the quality of pre-analytical activities.
- The clinical laboratory must use standardized policies and procedures for specimen collection, handling, transportation and storage.
- Specimen rejection has to be monitored on regular basis and the significant variables should be identified.
- The clinical laboratory should perform ongoing mentoring program to reduce pre-analytical errors.
- Laboratory technologist should be assigned as a consultant in the hospital wards to provide instructions for specimen collection and handling.
- Minimum identification errors can be achieved by using multiple identifiers to identify the patient specimen.
- Wireless barcode technology to confirm patient identity should be routinely used, where affordable and feasible.
- Assign trained phlebotomists with laboratory background to collect the blood samples.
- Availability of centralized 24/7 phlebotomy services in the inpatient section.

- Using of pre-analytical workstations as a tool for reducing laboratory errors.
- The clinical laboratory has to implement mandatory state based errors reporting system that collects, analyzes and gives a feed back.
- The clinical laboratory has to participate in quality assessment programs such as CAP-Track programs.
- Conduct further studies for estimating the frequency and source of pre-analytical errors using more effective detecting methods.
- Develop a testing protocol that can identify and determine the source of errors.

REFERENCES

Astion, M. L., Shojana, K. G., Hamil, T. R., Kim, S., & Ng, V. L. (2003). Classifying laboratory incidents reports to identify problems that jeopardize patient safety. *American Journal of Clinical Pathology, 120*(1), 18–26. doi:10.1309/8U5D0MA6MFH2FG19 PMID:12866368

Barr, D. P. (1955). Hazards of modern diagnosis and therapy: The price we pay. *Journal of the American Medical Association, 159*, 1452–1456. PMID:13271097

Beastall, G. H. (2004). the impact of the new general medical service contract: National evidence. *The Royal College of Pathologists, 128*, 24.

Berte, L. M. (2007). Laboratory quality management: A roadmap. *Clinics in Laboratory Medicine, 27*(4), 771–790. doi:10.1016/j.cll.2007.07.008 PMID:17950897

Bonini, P., Plebani, M., Ceriotti, F., & Rubboli, F. (2002). Errors in laboratory medicine. *Clinical Chemistry, 48*, 691–698. PMID:11978595

Bowen, R. A., Chan, Y., Ruddel, M. E., Hortin, G. L., Csako, G., Demosky, S. J. Jr, & Remaley, A. T. (2005). Immunoassay interference by a commonly used blood collection tube additive, the organosolicone surfactant silwetL-720. *Clinical Chemistry, 51*(10), 1874–1882. doi:10.1373/clinchem.2005.055400 PMID:16099932

Brennan, T. A., Leape, L. L., Laird, N. M., Hebert, L., Localio, A. R., Lawthers, A. G., & Hiatt, H. H. (1991). Incidence of adverse events and negligence in hospitalized patients: Results of the Harvard Medical Practice Study I. *The New England Journal of Medicine, 324*(6), 370–376. doi:10.1056/NEJM199102073240604 PMID:1987460

Bush, V. (2003). The hemolyzed specimen: Causes, effects, and reduction. *BD Laboratory Notes, 13*, 2–5.

Carraro, P., & Plebani, M. (2007). Errors in a stat laboratory: Types and frequencies 10 years later. *Clinical Chemistry, 53*(7), 1338–1342. doi:10.1373/clinchem.2007.088344 PMID:17525103

Carraro, P., Servidio, G., & Plebani, M. (2000). Hemolyzed specimens: A reason for rejection or a clinical challenge? *Clinical Chemistry, 46*, 306–307. PMID:10657399

Dock, B. (2005). Improving the accuracy of specimen labelling. *Clinical Laboratory Science, 18*, 210–212. PMID:16315737

Dock, B. (2005). Improving the accuracy of specimen labelling. *Clinical Laboratory Science, 18*, 210–212. PMID:16315737

Donchin, Y., Gopher, D., Olin, M., Badihi, Y., Biesky, M. R. N. B., Sprung, C. L., & Cotev, S. et al. (1995). A Look into the Nature and Causes of Human Errors in the Intensive Care Unit. *Critical Care Medicine, 23*(2), 294–300. doi:10.1097/00003246-199502000-00015 PMID:7867355

Dunn, E., & Moga, P. (2010). Patient Misidentification in Laboratory Medicine A Qualitative Analysis of 227 Root Cause Analysis Reports in the Veterans Health *Administration. Archives of Pathology & Laboratory Medicine, 134,* 244–255. PMID:20121614

Dzik, W. H., Murphy, M. F., Andreu, G., Heddle, N., Hogman, C., Kekomaki, R., & Smit-Sibinga, C. T. (2003). Biomedical Excellence for Safer Transfusion (BEST) working party of the International Society for Blood Transfusion. An international study of the performance of sample collection from patients. *Vox Sanguinis, 85*(1), 40–47. doi:10.1046/j.1423-0410.2003.00313.x PMID:12823729

Forsman, R. W. (1996). Why is the laboratory an afterthought for managed care organizations? *Clinical Chemistry, 42,* 813–816. PMID:8653920

Grimm, E., Friedberg, R. C., Wilkinson, D. S., AuBuchon, J. P., Souers, R. J., & Lehman, C. M. J. (2010). Blood Bank Safety Practices Mislabelled Samples and Wrong Blood in Tube–A Q-Probes Analysis of 122 Clinical Laboratories. *Archives of Pathology & Laboratory Medicine, 134,* 1108–1115. PMID:20670129

Grober, E. D., & Bohnen, J. M. (2005). Defining medical error. *Canadian Journal of Surgery, 48*(1), 39–44. PMID:15757035

Hawkins, R. (2012). Managing the Pre- and Post-analytical Phases of the Total Testing Process. *Annals of Laboratory Medicine, 32*(1), 5–16. doi:10.3343/alm.2012.32.1.5 PMID:22259773

Howanitz, P. J. (2005). Errors in laboratory medicine: Practical lessons to improve patient safety. *Archives of Pathology & Laboratory Medicine, 129,* 1252–1261. PMID:16196513

Howanitz, P. J., Renner, S. W., & Walsh, M. K. (2002). Continuous wristband monitoring over 2 years decreases identification errors: A College of American Pathologists Q-Tracks study. *Archives of Pathology & Laboratory Medicine, 126,* 809–815. PMID:12088450

Howanitz, P. J., Renner, S. W., & Walsh, M. K. (2003). Continuous wristband monitoring over 2 years decreases identification errors. A College of American Pathologists Q-TRACKS study. *Archives of Pathology & Laboratory Medicine, 126,* 809–815. PMID:12088450

Institute of Medicine. (2001). *Crossing the Quality Chasm: A New Health Care System for the 21st Century.* Washington, DC: National Academy Press.

International Organization for Standardization. ISO/PDTS 22367. Medical laboratories: reducing error through risk management and continual improvement: complementary element 2005:9 ISO Geneva.

Jones, B., Meier, F., & Howanitz, P. (1995). Complete blood count specimen acceptability: A college of A American Pathology Q-Probes Study of 703 Laboratories. *Archives of Pathology & Laboratory Medicine, 119,* 203–208. PMID:7887772

Jones, B. A., Calam, R. R., & Howanitz, P. J. (1997). Chemistry specimen acceptability: A College of American Pathologists Q-Probe study of 453 labs. *Archives of Pathology & Labratory Medicine, 121,* 19–26.

Jones, B. A., Calam, R. R., & Howanitz, P. J. (1997). Chemistry specimen acceptability: A College of American Pathologists Q-Probe study of 453 labs. *Archives of Pathology & Labratory Medicine, 121,* 19–26.

Jones, B. A., Calam, R. R., & Howanitz, P. J. (1997). Chemistry specimen acceptability: A College of American Pathologists Q-Probes study of 453 laboratories. *Archives of Pathology & Laboratory Medicine, 121,* 19–26. PMID:9111088

Khoury, M., Burnett, L., & Mackay, M. (1996). Error rates in Australian chemical pathology laboratories. *The Medical Journal of Australia, 165,* 128–130. PMID:8709873

Khoury, M., Burnett, L., & McKay, M. A. (1996). Error rate in Australian chemical pathology laboratories. *The Medical Journal of Australia, 165,* 128–130. PMID:8709873

Kilpatrick, E. S., & Holding, S. (2001). Use of computer terminals on wards to access emergency test results: A retrospective study. *British Medical Journal, 322*(7294), 1101–1103. doi:10.1136/bmj.322.7294.1101 PMID:11337442

Kohn, K. T., Corrigan, J. M., & Donaldson, M. S. (1999). *To Err Is Human: Building a Safer Health System.* Washington, DC: National Academy Press.

Laessig, R.H., Hassemer, D.J., Paskey, T.A., & Schwartz, T.H. (1976). The effects of 0.1% and 1.0% erythrocytes and hemolysis on serum chemistry values. *American Journal of Clinical Pathology, 66,* 639–644. PMID:970364

Laessig, R. H., Hassemer, D. J., Paskey, T. A., & Schwartz, T. H. (1976). The effects of 0.1% and 1.0% erythrocytes and hemolysis on serum chemistry values. *American Journal of Clinical Pathology, 66,* 639–644. PMID:970364

Leape, L. L. (1994). Error in medicine. *Journal of the American Medical Association, 272*(23), 1851–1857. doi:10.1001/jama.1994.03520230061039 PMID:7503827

Leape, L. L., Brennan, T. A., Laird, N., Lawthers, A. G., Localio, A. R., Barnes, B. A., & Hiatt, H. H. (1991). The nature of adverse events in hospitalized patients. Results of the Harvard Medical Practice Study II. *The New England Journal of Medicine, 324*(6), 377–384. doi:10.1056/NEJM199102073240605 PMID:1824793

Linden, J. V., Wagner, K., Voytovich, A. E., & Sheehan, J. (2000). Transfusion errors in New York State: An analysis of 10 years' experience. *Transfusion, 40*(10), 1207–1213. doi:10.1046/j.1537-2995.2000.40101207.x PMID:11061857

Lippi, G., Bassi, A., Brocco, G., Montagnana, M., Salvagno, G. L., & Guidi, G. C. (2006). Pre-analytic error tracking in a laboratory medicine department: Results of a 1-year experience. *Clinical Chemistry, 52*(7), 1442–1443. doi:10.1373/clinchem.2006.069534 PMID:16798977

Lippi, G., Blanckaert, N., Bonini, P., Green, S., Kitchen, S., Palicka, V., & Plebani, M. (2009). Causes, consequences, detection, and prevention of identification errors in laboratory diagnostics. *Clinical Chemistry and Laboratory Medicine, 47*(2), 143–153. doi:10.1515/CCLM.2009.045 PMID:19099525

Lippi, G., Blanckaert, N., Bonini, P., Green, S., Kitchen, S., Palicka, V., & Plebani, M. et al. (2008). Haemolysis: An overview of the leading cause of unsuitable specimens in clinical laboratories. *Clinical Chemistry and Laboratory Medicine, 46*(6), 764–772. doi:10.1515/CCLM.2008.170 PMID:18601596

Lippi, G., Chance, J. J., Church, S., Dazzi, P., Fontana, R., Giavarina, D., & Simundic, A. M. (2011). Pre-analytical quality improvement: From dream to reality. *Clinical Chemistry and Laboratory Medicine, 49*(7), 1113–1126. doi:10.1515/CCLM.2011.600 PMID:21517699

Lippi, G., & Guidi, G. (2007). Risk management in the pre-analytical phase of laboratory testing. *Clinical Chemistry and Laboratory Medicine, 45*(6), 720–727. doi:10.1515/CCLM.2007.167 PMID:17579523

Lippi, G., Montagnana, M., Salvagno, G. L., & Guidi, G. C. (2006). Interference of blood cell lysis on routine coagulation testing. *Archives of Pathology & Laboratory Medicine, 130*, 181–184. PMID:16454558

Lippi, G., Plebani, M., & Šimundić, A. M. (2010). Quality in laboratory diagnostics: From theory to practice. *Biochemistry Medicine, 20*, 126–130. doi:10.11613/BM.2010.014

Lippi, G., Salvagno, G., Montagnana, M., Franchini, M., & Guidi, G. (2006). Phlebotomy Issues and Quality Improvement in Results of Laboratory Testing. *Clinical Laboratory, 52*(1), 14. PMID:16812947

Lippi, G., & Simundic, A. M. (2010). Total quality in laboratory diagnostics: It's time to think outside the box. *Biochemical Medicine, 20*, 5–8. doi:10.11613/BM.2010.001

Lohr. (1990). Committee to Design a Strategy for Quality Review and Assurance in Medicare: A Strategy for Quality Assurance. Washington, DC: National Academies Press.

Luban, N. L. (2005). Transfusion safety: Where are we today? *Annals of the New York Academy of Sciences, 1054*(1), 325–341. doi:10.1196/annals.1345.040 PMID:16339681

Lumadue, J. A., Boyd, J. S., & Ness, P. M. (1997). Adherence to a strict specimen-labelling policy decreases the incidence of erroneous blood grouping of blood bank specimens. *Transfusion, 37*(11-12), 1169–1172. doi:10.1046/j.1537-2995.1997.37111298088047.x PMID:9426641

Narayanan, S. (1993). Physiological variables in blood sampling. *Mitteilungen der Deutschen Gesellschaft für Klinische Chemie, 24*, 130–134.

Narayanan, S. (1996). Pre and post analytical errors. *Indian Journal of Clinical Biochemistry, 11*(1), 7–11. doi:10.1007/BF02868404

Narayanan, S. (2000). The Pre-analytic Phase: An Important Component of Laboratory Medicine. *American Journal of Clinical Pathology, 113*, 429–452. doi:10.1309/C0NM-Q7R0-LL2E-B3UY PMID:10705825

Naz, S., Mumtaz, A., & Sadaruddin, A. (2012). Pre-analytical Errors and their Impact on Tests in Clinical Laboratory Practice. *Pakistan Journal of Medical Research, 51*(1), 27–30.

Naz, S., Mumtaz, A., & Sadaruddin, A. (2012). Preanalytical Errors and their Impact on Tests in Clinical Laboratory Practice. *Pakistan Journal of Medical Research, 51*(1), 27–30.

Plebani, M. (2006). Errors in clinical laboratories or error In Laboratory medicine? *Clinical Chemistry and Laboratory Medicine, 44*(6), 750–759. doi:10.1515/CCLM.2006.123 PMID:16729864

Plebani, M. (2007). Laboratory errors: How to improve pre- and post-analytical phases? *Bio chemistry Medicine, 17*, 5–9.

Plebani, M. (2009). Exploring the iceberg of errors in laboratory medicine. *International Journal of Clinical Chemistry and Diagnostic Laboratory Medicine, 404*, 16–23. PMID:19302995

Plebani, M., & Carraro, P. (1997). Mistakes in a stat laboratory: Types and frequency. *Clinical Chemistry, 43*, 1348–1351. PMID:9267312

Renner, S. W., Howanitz, P. J., & Bachner, P. (1993). Wristband identification errors reporting in 712 hospitals: A College of American Pathologists Q-Probe study of quality issues in transfusion practice. *Archives of Pathology & Laboratory Medicine, 117*, 573–577. PMID:8503724

Ross, J. W., & Boone, D. J. (1989). *Institute on critical issues in health laboratory practice.* Wilmington, DE: DuPont Press.

Shahangian, S., & Snyder, S. (2009). Laboratory Medicine Quality Indicator. *American Journal of Clinical Pathology, 131*(3), 418–431. doi:10.1309/AJCPJF8JI4ZLDQUE PMID:19228647

Stahl, M., Lund, E. D., & Brandslund, I. (1998). Reasons for a laboratory's inability to report results for requested analytical tests. *Clinical Chemistry, 44*, 2195–2197. PMID:9761256

Stainsby, D., Russell, J., Cohen, H., & Lilleyman, J. (2005). Reducing adverse events in blood transfusion. *British Journal of Haematology, 131*(1), 8–12. doi:10.1111/j.1365-2141.2005.05702.x PMID:16173957

Steindel, S. J., Howanitz, P. J., & Renner, S. W. (1996). Reasons for proficiency testing failures in clinical chemistry and blood gas analysis: A College of American Pathologists Q-Probes study in 665 laboratories. *Archives of Pathology & Laboratory Medicine, 120*, 1094–1101. PMID:15456173

Szecsi, P., & Ødum, L. (2009). Error tracking in a clinical biochemistry laboratory. *Clinical Chemistry and Laboratory Medicine, 47*(10), 1253–1257. doi:10.1515/CCLM.2009.272 PMID:19663542

Valenstein, P. (2005). *Patient identification accuracy. Q-Tracks (QT1) 2004 annual summary.* Northfield, IL: College of American Pathologists.

Valenstein, P., Raab, S., & Walsh, M. (2006). Identification Errors Involving Clinical Laboratories: A College of American Pathologists Q-Probes Study of Patient and Specimen Identification Errors at 120 Institutions. *Archives of Pathology & Laboratory Medicine, 130*, 1106–1113. PMID:16879009

Valenstein, P. N., & Sirota, R. L. (2004). Identification errors in pathology and laboratory medicine. *The Journal of Laboratory and Clinical Medicine, 24*(4), 979–996. doi:10.1016/j.cll.2004.05.013 PMID:15555752

Wachter, R. (2004). The End of the Beginning: Patient Safety Five Years After 'To Err Is Human. *Health Affairs*, 534–545. PMID:15572380

Wagar, E., Stankovic, A., Raab, S., Nakhleh, R., & Walsh, M. (2008). Specimen Labelling Errors A Q-Probes Analysis of 147 Clinical Laboratories. *Archives of Pathology & Laboratory Medicine, 132*, 1618–1622. PMID:18834220

Westgard, J. O., & Westgard, S. A. (2006). The quality of laboratory testing today. *American Journal of Clinical Pathology, 125*(3), 343–354. doi:10.1309/V50H4FRVVWX12C79 PMID:16613337

Winkelman, J. W., & Mennemeyer, S. T. (1996). Using patient outcomes to screen for clinical laboratory errors. *Clinical Laboratory Management Review, 10*, 134–136. PMID:10172598

Wood, K. E., & Nash, D. B. (2005). Mandatory state-based error-reporting systems: Current and future prospects. *American Journal of Medical Quality, 20*(6), 297–303. doi:10.1177/1062860605281850 PMID:16280392

Zarbo, R. J., Jones, B. A., Friedberg, R. C., Valenstein, P. N., Renner, S. W., Schifman, R. B., & Howanitz, P. J. (2002). Q-tracks: A College of American Pathologists program of continuous laboratory monitoring and longitudinal tracking. *Archives of Pathology & Laboratory Medicine, 126*, 1036–1044. PMID:12204052

KEY TERMS AND DEFINITIONS

Clinical Laboratory: Place where a variety of laboratory tests are performed on the patients' specimens to provide information needed for the diagnosis, treatment, and prevention of disease.

Heamolysis: Breakdown of red blood cells with the release of haemoglobin and the cellular components into the surrounding fluids.

Laboratory Errors: Any mistakes made during performing tests, interpreting data, or reporting the results.

Patient Safety: New healthcare concept aimed to prevent medical errors which often lead to serious healthcare events.

Post-Analytical: Final phase of the laboratory process where results are released to the clinicians for interpretation and makes diagnostic and therapeutic decisions.

Pre-Analytical: First phase of specimen testing process which includes specimen collection, transportation and centrifugation.

Quality: Doing the right thing, at the right time, in the right way, for the right person.

This work was previously published in Transforming Public Health in Developing Nations edited by Mohamud Sheikh, Aziza Mahamoud, and Mowafa Househ, pages 241-263 copyright year 2015 by Information Science Reference (an imprint of IGI Global).

Chapter 62
A Viewpoint of Security for Digital Health Care in the United States:
What's There? What Works? What's Needed?

Steven A. Demurjian
University of Connecticut, USA

Solomon Berhe
University of Connecticut, USA

Alberto De la Rosa Algarín
University of Connecticut, USA

Thomas Agresta
University of Connecticut Health Center, USA

Jinbo Bi
University of Connecticut, USA

Xiaoyan Wang
University of Connecticut Health Center, USA

Michael Blechner
University of Connecticut Health Center, USA

ABSTRACT

In health care, patient information of interest to health providers, researchers, public health researchers, insurers, patients, etc., is stored in different locations via electronic media and/or hard-copy formats. All potential users need electronic access to health information technology systems such as: electronic health records, personal health records, patient portals, and ancillary systems such as imaging, laboratory, pharmacy, etc. Controlling access to information from multiple systems requires granularity levels of privileges ranging from one patient to a cohort to an entire population. In this paper, we present a viewpoint of the state of secure digital health care in the United States, focusing on the resources that need to be protected as dictated by legal entities and regulations, the available approaches in the present state-of-the art, and, the potential needs for the future of security for digital health care. By utilizing a real world scenario, the authors explore the limitations of health information exchange in the United States, and present one possible architecture for secure digital health care that builds on existing technology alternatives.

DOI: 10.4018/978-1-4666-8756-1.ch062

1. INTRODUCTION

Over twenty years ago, two articles related to health care security were published that were noteworthy for the time. In (Biskup, 1990), privacy and confidentiality in medical information systems was explored, advocating a role-based approach, and detailing the state-of-the-art in available systems. In (Ting, 1990), a case study of mental health delivery from information and semantic perspectives was presented, providing scenarios of usage of information by physicians, nurses, etc., and promoting a role-based approach as the most appropriate solution. What is surprising is what has stayed the same and what has changed over the last 20 plus years in the health care domain in terms of tracking patient care (via paper or electronic form) and facilitating secure information exchange as a patient transitions between care settings, more specifically in the United States. For instance, in 1990, would anyone have predicted the introduction of the Health Insurance Portability and Accountability Act[1] of 1996 (HIPAA) Privacy and Security Rules for protected health information? At the time, health care delivery was based more on paper than electronic health records (EHRs). How about the Genetic Information Non-discrimination Act (GINA)[2] of 2008? GINA aims to protect a patient's genetic information against discrimination in health insurance and employment. Or even the Ethical, Legal and Social Implications (ELSI) research program? ELSI was introduced to manage genomic data for personalized medicine. There have also been dramatic changes in patient care, including: EHRs in some medical doctor offices ("implementation rates reached 68% in family practices in 2011"[3] while "just 27% of physicians used EHRs with multi-functional capabilities"[4]); and, personal health records (PHRs) for patients to store their own health information (and download medications from a pharmacy, share data with providers, etc.). Evolving needs for health care delivery include a Patient Centered Medical Home[5] where one provider coordinates care for patients with chronic diseases; an accountable care organization (ACOs)[6] to coordinate providers regarding Medicare patients with chronic conditions; and the upcoming Meaningful Use Stage 2[7] capability for patients to be able to view, download, and transmit their records which will require the development of a standardized transmission of all types of medical information. These three and other evolving initiatives will require secure data collection from multiple health information technology (HIT) systems.

The harsh realities in health care and HIT adoption in the United States are: the limited capabilities of health information exchange (HIE) among all of these various data sources; the high number of providers that are predominately paper based with limited or no access to EHRs or other HIT systems; and, the fact that security is often an afterthought in this process, supported for individual systems for specific providers, but overlooked when one attempts to bring together patient data from multiple electronic sources. In patient centered medical homes, the effective care of a diabetes patient with high blood pressure may involve the family practitioner (who sees the patient regularly), an endocrinologist (if diabetes is complex in its manifestation), a cardiologist (diabetes patients often have heart disease), and a nutritionist (for managing diet or dealing with obesity). These four providers may have different EHRs (or none) and an inability to share data (patient history, lab test results, etc.) to facilitate the required care. The access needs to be integrated (electronic sources), secure (individual sources and across the integrated sources), and collaborative (individuals can view/update same patient record simultaneously). Our main objective in this paper is to enumerate prevalent issues for secure, integrated, and collaborative health care in the United States, requiring us to provide a roadmap for secure digital health care in the not so distant future. Our viewpoint is intended to answer questions such as: what patient information is available for each source, how can information be standardized for ease of use and exchange, how is the local security for that source managed, what needs to be protected from each source, is there a global security policy across the integrated sources, and what security methods are appropriate to employ.

The remainder of this paper has five sections. Section 2 presents background security for digital health care and the involved health information technology systems by focusing on existing United States laws, standards, and emerging models of care spanning clinical, genomic, and phenotypic information. Section 3 provides a scenario on the actual experiences of one co-author in navigating the United States health care system with HIT in use at some level by most providers, but with paper-based records still exchanged via snail mail and fax. Section 4 details a proposed security framework that considers all of the constituent elements of information exchange in the United States, with examples of HIT systems, standards, and applications, as well as their interactions. Using this as a basis, Section 5 proposes a core set of recommendations organized by area that represents our viewpoint of what must be supported for security for digital health care. Finally, Section 6 concludes the paper, and in the process, addressed the applicability of the work herein to other regions of the world.

2. SECURITY FOR DIGITAL HEALTH CARE AND HEALTH INFORMATION TECHNOLOGY

Security for digital health care goes well beyond the needs of compliance of HIPAA, which provides a set of security guidelines in the usage, transmission, and sharing of protected health information. In addition, there is a need to: protect personally identifiable information, including names, addresses, accounts, credit card numbers, etc.; encrypt protected health information and personally identifiable information data and its secure transmission (e.g., using SSL); extensive usage of standards for storage and exchange (Health Level Seven's Clinical Document Architecture[8] and the Continuity of Care Record[9] for administrative, patient demographics, and clinical data); leveraging a wide range of health care standards (e.g., LOINC[10], SNOMED[11], UMLS[12]); and, dealing with data interoperability issues for health information technology systems that use a wide range of data formats (e.g., XML[13], RDF[14], JSON[15], etc.). Instead, to attain security for digital health care in the United States, we will need all of these underlying technologies and standards coupled with a strong understanding of the way that health care data is utilized by the different stakeholders. We must also include the emerging need to manage genomic data for personalized medicine and its potential future integration and/or consolidation with EHRs via ELSI, which is tied to GINA. GINA protects a patient's genetic information against discrimination in health insurance and employment, including: genetic test of patient, his/her family members, fetus of individual or family member, family medical history, and request/receipt of genetic services that may include research trials. HIPAA's rule insures that protected health information is securely maintained with patients retaining rights to their information stored in a personal health record (patient controlled), or to access information from a provider's record (EHR or hard copy). While HIPAA provides guidelines for this, it is important to note that it also allows entities to disclose the information under certain situations. HIPAA's rule defines the "series of administrative, physical, and technical safeguards for covered entities to use to assure the confidentiality, integrity, and availability of electronic protected health information". For ELSI, protection of information must be reconciled across HIPAA and GINA to securely deliver the combination of clinical, genomic, and phenotypic information to researchers, clinical providers, support personnel, insurers, and patients.

Security for digital health care transcends just protecting the information, and must strongly consider the usability of the information by a wide variety of stakeholders using a broad range of HIT systems to effectively and securely leverage different types of patient data, including:

- EHRs (e.g., Allscripts[16], GE Centricity[17], VistA[18], etc.), which are electronic repositories of patient medical records that may exist in provider offices, clinics, and hospitals.
- Personal health records (such as Microsoft HealthVault and webMD) that allow patients to manage their own health care data.
- Patient portals (often part of EHRs) that allow patients to electronically request appointments, prescription refill requests, arranging a referral to another provider, etc.
- Personalized medicine health portals such as Genomas[19], which allows providers to view their own patients' genetic data against their medical record (EHR) in order to bridge the gap between providers and medical researchers.
- Ancillary systems for laboratory results (e.g. blood work), evaluating X-rays, MRIs, CT Scans, etc. to be electronically delivered to providers, pharmacy systems for tracking medication and interactions, etc.
- Patient applications for access to education information and management of chronic diseases, medications, and interactions with providers.
- A clinical research data warehouse that contains de-identified clinical data loaded from medical records for patients with permission to have their data used for medical research, or for public health researchers to do population studies.

Collectively, in the United States, all of these systems target a wide range of patient care and research initiatives. First, *patient centered medical homes* can manage chronic conditions and optimize care by interacting stakeholders (e.g., family practitioner, endocrinologist, cardiologist, and nutritionist example in Section 1); in this situation, there may be a need for the lead provider to access information in other EHRs, PHRs, etc., in a timely manner in order to coordinate effective care. Second, *accountable care organizations* brings together groups of providers, clinics, hospitals, and private insurers in an effort to give coordinated care to a panel of Medicare patients in order to attempt to reduce or eliminate duplicate test and procedures for patients that visit multiple providers and have chronic conditions. Third, *secondary use* of clinical data allows providers and researchers to analyze specific diseases and their treatments across a large patient base via a clinical research data warehouse, seeking events such as adverse drug reactions, infection monitoring, or disease monitoring in a larger population (the flu epidemic in the United States in 2013). Fourth, *meaningful use* is focusing on the adoption and use of HIT within organizations that may lead to improvements in the reporting of care by offering providers incentives to acquire and deploy technology. Fifth, *personalized medicine* is targeting the treatment of an individual based on their unique medical profiles that might include specific types of diseases and focus on the use of a patient's genomic information.

In support of these aforementioned initiatives, health information exchange is vital to insure that the correct data is available at the appropriate time in a usable fashion by a specific stakeholder. In the United States, what is shared in health information exchange is most often determined by the institute that owns the data; it doesn't mean all of the data is shared. In these cases, it is common to see that the data to be shared is off-loaded into another server intended for that purpose so that there is no impact on the real-time usage of an EHR to treat patients. For example, health information exchange allows sharing so that in emergent situations providers can retrieve data on a patient from a system they are not authorized via techniques such as dynamic certification. Alternatively, health information exchange can be used to construct a clinical research data warehouse via an electronic extract, transform, and load (ETL) process from an EHR database, which in turn can provide, for example, workflows and ontologies for managing tissue data including controls for patient consent relating to tissues and boundaries on experimental uses. Health information exchange and other means of extracting clinical and claims (and other) data can also be utilized to support detailed data analysis for secondary use, accountable care organizations, and meaningful use, providing de-identified data to clinical researchers so that best practices can be evaluated across a wide range of clinical settings. This paper considers all of the above factors in order to propose an architecture in Section 4 specifically aimed for the United States health care domain that ideally achieves security across this entire spectrum of standards, regulations, HIT systems and their usage by stakeholders, coupled with health information exchange and supporting a wide range of data analyses.

3. A LACK OF SECURITY AND INFORMATION EXCHANGE IN DIGITAL HEALTH CARE

To better understand health care and the impact of HIT on patient care in the United States, this section along with Figure 1 provides a realistic case study of one co-author navigating through a complex process. Consider that a 54 year old man falls while working in the yard, and breaks his hip; an ambulance (Step 1 in Figure 1) takes him to the emergency room of a small regional hospital (Step 2) where a history is taken using an EHR at the hospital, X-rays are ordered, and a hip fracture is found. After speaking with the emergency room physician, and talking to a physician colleague, the patient decides to transfer by ambulance (Step 3) to a metropolitan area hospital, and his records are sent in hard copy. Upon

arriving at the emergency room of that hospital, another patient history is taken for that hospital's EHR to capture the same information. The same story is told to the emergency room physician, orthopedic resident, etc., and at 2AM in the morning he signs a consent form for either a partial or full hip replacement. At 7AM the transport team arrives to take him to the operating room; at that point, the orthopedic surgeon has another option, to repair the hip with a plate and screws, and the patient, after consulting with his physician colleague, has to re-initial the hardcopy consent form. Surgery is successful, and after three more days in the hospital, the patient is discharged to a rehab facility, (Step 4) with a hard copy of his records. The rehab center is mostly paper-based; they have an electronic system, but the medication list is hard copy as the nurse dispenses meds to patients. After 5 weeks, the patient is discharged (Step 6) to his home, and the Visiting Nurse Association in his area is assigned to monitor his care via a nurse and in home physically therapy.

During the time at rehab and at home, the patient visits the surgeon (Step 5 and Step 7) in order for X-rays to assess the healing, and also meets with his internist (Step 8) for follow up care. The internist has an electronic medical record (EMR) and can download all tests done at an external lab facility, but records at the hospital will have to be faxed and then scanned and put into the EHR as images (unsearchable). Ten weeks after the fracture, the patient is given his release from the orthopedic surgeon (Step 7) with weight bearing, and asks for that care to be managed by a local orthopedist (Step 10). The patient requests that the medical records be sent to the local orthopedist, but 2 weeks later at the appointment, no records have arrived; as a result, new and old X-rays can't be compared. Due to the unusualness of a hip fracture of a 54 year old, the patient is referred to a rheumatologist (Step 9), and brings a hard copy of some of his medical records to the appointment; blood work and a bone scan that determines that the patient has osteoporosis. The rheumatolo-

Figure 1. Illustrating a sample health care process of the United States

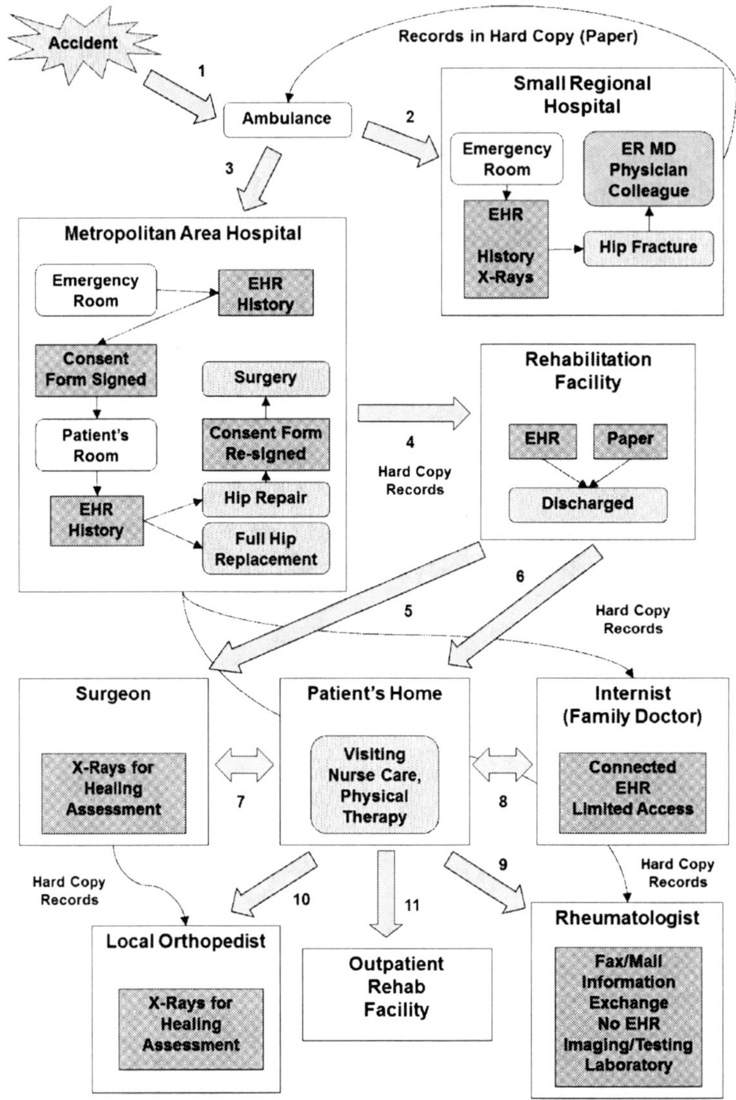

gist's office has no EHR, but can access systems at an imaging facility and testing laboratory; the rheumatologist's also makes a medical record request from hospital. Consider that even with the advance of technology and its availability, fax and snail mail are still playing a dominant role in the way that we transfer healthcare data. How can a rheumatologist without an EHR get all of the information needed from multiple sources in a timely fashion so as not to delay treatment? Clearly, even if we can deal with security for digital health care, there will still be a huge hole in the overall security of patient data with information in so many different and incompatible locations and continued dependence on paper.

Further, suppose that a clinical researcher was interested in conducting a study of males 50-60 who have hip fractures and osteoporosis, and what they may have in common (e.g., low vitamin D, low testosterone, low calcium, etc.). The dramatic push to digitize clinical data via EHRs has led to an unprecedented opportunity for clinical and public health studies (Shea et al., 2010; Wang et al., 2008; Wang et al., 2009; Jha et al., 2009). This growth is being fueled by recent federal legislation that provides generous financial incentives to institutions demonstrating aggressive application and meaningful use of comprehensive EHRs (Shea et al, 2010). Efforts are already underway to link these EHRs across institutions, and standardize the definition of phenotypes for large-scale studies of disease onset and treatment outcome, specifically within the context of routine clinical care (McCarty et al, 2010; Pace et al., 2009; Ritchie et al., 2010). The longitudinal nature of the data contained within EHRs makes them ideal for quantifying outcomes from the utilization of prescription medications (both efficacy and toxicity). More recently, huge efforts have been initiated to link new and existing EHR databases to accelerate research in personalized medicine (McCarty et al, 2010). This is a herculean task in most of the clinical environment with a heterogeneous and poorly integrated informatics infrastructure, since to find enough of a patient cohort, the researcher would need to query multiple hospitals, surgeons, laboratories, internists, and rheumatologists. At the present time in health care in the United States, health information exchange has not advanced to a stage to support such queries in any reasonable time frame. In such a scenario, how can the security issues that span multiple health information technology systems each with their own security control (with local HIPAA compliance) be brought together to securely obtain this data (with a more global HIPAA compliance) into a de-identified clinical research data warehouse to facilitate the research? How is data securely gathered into this data warehouse from paper sources? How is institutional review board approval obtained when the patients may be from multiple institutions? How is HIPAA compliance of hard-paper copies at physician offices that are transferred via fax and/or snail mail protected until they are entered into the clinical research data warehouse repository?

Security for digital health care in the United States must anticipate a future where the medical community has caught up with the use of HIT, and must consider EHR vendors that do not wish to allow their information to be easily shared, as do hospitals, since they deem sharing of data to cause the potential for loss of patients to other hospitals. The EHRs for the regional and metropolitan hospitals do not share data, and may not share data with local providers (e.g., internists, rheumatologists, local orthopedist, etc.). Do we define a solution with the expectation that we are planning for a futuristic scenario where secure sharing and exchange is the norm and HIT is in almost all providers? Is this even realistic in today's medical system in the United States or even within the next 5 years? 10 years?

4. PROPOSED ARCHITECTURE FOR SECURE DIGITAL HEALTH CARE

For successful health information exchange, the security of constituent systems must be integrated and support the application's need. What happens when security privileges of individual systems are in conflict with one another? How do we reconcile these local security policies? Is it possible to define a global encompassing security policy providing a level of guarantee to the local security policies from an enforcement perspective? As today's health care applications continue to become more complex and wide-spread, interacting with many other systems (or applications) using varied technologies, there is a need for some degree of assurance that security for the application (global) is consistent with the sum of the parts (local security) of the constituent systems.

To place our work into its perspective, Figure 2 shows our viewpoint one way that health information technology systems, medical document standards (usually achieved with extensions to XML), and end-user applications interplay with one another to provide an infrastructure for *patient centered medical homes, accountable care organizations, secondary use, meaningful use,* and *personalized medicine* (see Section 2 again). We examine the infrastructure from three viewpoints. The first viewpoint involves the reconciliation of security (local and global) to insure that the required clinical data reaches the providers involved in patient centered medical homes and personalized medicine where data mining and knowledge discovery techniques can be used. The second viewpoint focuses on the availability of de-identified patient data for providers and clinical researchers via privacy-preserving data publishing and sharing in support of accountable

care organizations, secondary use, and meaningful use, that can then in turn be used for data analysis, mining, and clinical decision support to learn what works and what doesn't in terms of treatments of various illnesses and diseases. The third viewpoint facilitates the first two viewpoints via the use of: XML and associated standards for patient and clinical data (Clinical Document Architecture, Continuity of Care Record, etc.); and, ontologies that augment this data with relevant tags that add meaning (SNOMED, LOINC, NDF-RT[20], etc.). The lower left of Figure 2 contains examples of EHR systems (EPIC Lucy[21], OpenEMR[22], PatientOS[23], GE Centricity[24], FreeMED[25]) that share an ability to export patient data, in XML formats or

Figure 2. Proposed health information exchange architecture with information security and analytics in the United States

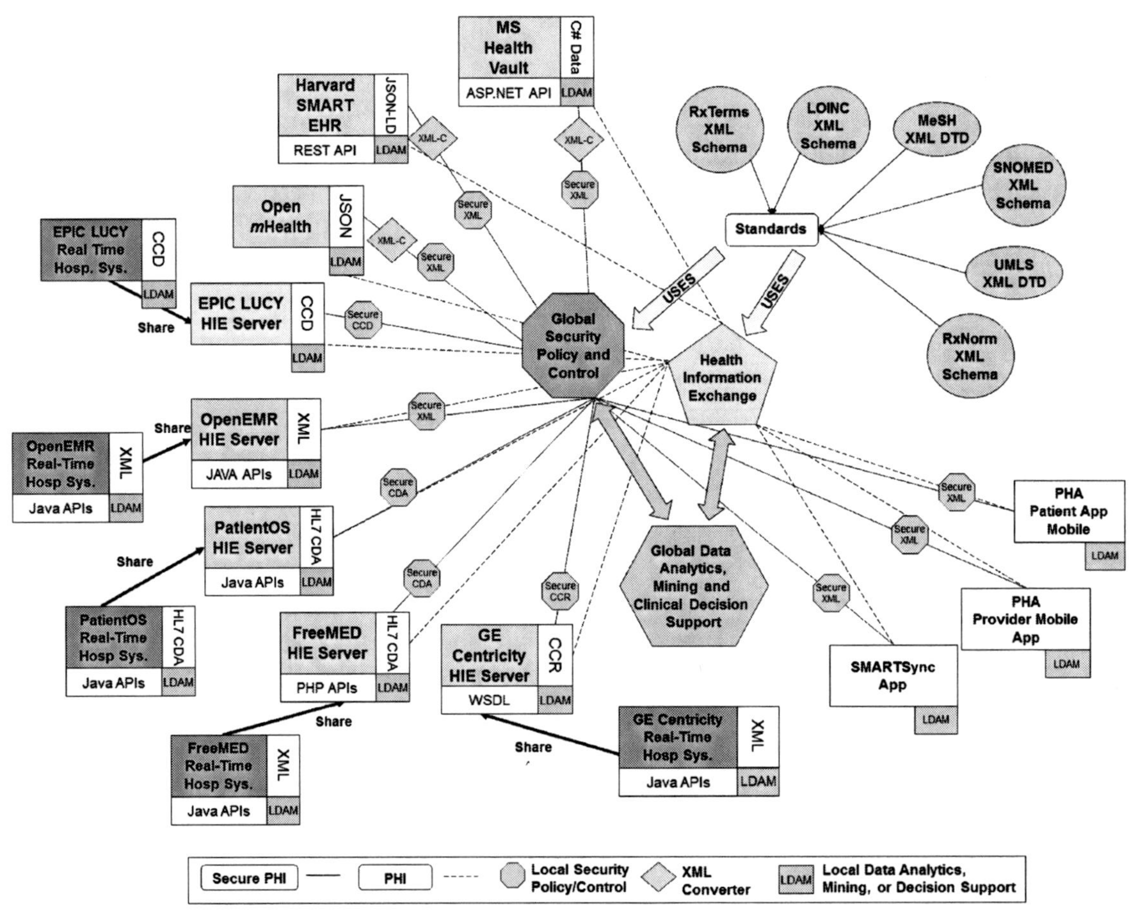

standards, via the use of a proxy server in which data from the EHR has been offloaded. Emerging platforms (Open mHealth[26]to promote mobile health via an open architecture and the Harvard SMART[27] platform for substitutable medical applications that promote reuse) and personal health records (Microsoft HealthVault[28]) are presented in the upper-left of Figure 2. Open mHealth uses JSON to model patient data, while SMART uses RDF/XML and JSON-LD. In order to provide a common layer of document format, these choices of data formats must be converted (as shown by the XML-C diamond) before they can be secured and utilized.

The bottom right of Figure 2 contains examples of medical applications that must be securely managed, PHA and SMARTSync. Personal Health Assistant is an in-house developed mobile (not publicly available) test-bed application for health information management that allows: patients to view and update their personal health record stored in their Microsoft HealthVault account and authorize medical providers to access certain portion of protected health information; and, for providers to obtain the permitted information from their respective patients that they have been authorized to view. The patient version of Personal Health Assistant allows users to perform a set of actions regarding their health information. Users can view and edit their medication list, allergies, observations of daily living, and set security policies for read/write permissions on their medical providers by role as reported in our prior work (De la Rosa Algarín et al., 2013). Security settings can be set at a fine granular level, and each provider gets specific view/update authorizations to the different information components available in Personal Health Assistant. The provider version of Personal Health Assistant allows the users (health professionals) to view and edit the medical information of their patients as long as there are permitted to do so as dictated by the security set by the user (patient).

SMARTSync is an in-house developed (not publicly available) web-based test-bed medication reconciliation application used to create and preserve a patient's medication list through transfers among locations of care, preventing immediate interactions, and avoiding dosage errors in situations where brand and generic drugs are received or multi-component drugs are used. Significant risks include: overmedication when a provider prescribes a new medication (or one from the same class) or when an interacting medication is prescribed; adverse interactions, the result of conflicts between medications, which can change effect strength or serum concentration; and adverse reactions, allergic/other effects, experienced by patients which can result in a patient being wrongly labeled as allergic to a medication, unnecessarily excluding it as a treatment option in the future. To accomplish this, we gathered data form HealthVault and the SMART EHR (Ziminski et al., 2012). The upper right of Figure 2 contains the various standards for medical information, such as RxTerms and RxNorm (services to augment medication information), medical codes (SNOMED), medical nomenclature (UMLS and MeSH), and laboratory codes (LOINC), all of which are used by HIT systems and applications. In addition, local data analytics, data mining, or decision support (blue square component of systems) can be found in institutional HIT systems, patient personal health record solutions or end-point applications (e.g., SMARTSync, Personal Health Assistant). This data analytics component exists in a globalized manner; where researchers external to all of the local components will need access to information found in distributed HIT systems.

The main aspects that allow all the interaction to occur across Figure 2 are presented by the Health Information Exchange component (pentagon), which uses dotted lines to indicate the necessity to share data among HIT end-points. The Global Security Policy and Control (octagon) component provides a centralized representation of which interactions between HIT can occur. The Global Data Analytics, Mining and Clinical Decision Support component (hexagon), which in conjunction with its local counterparts (Local Data Analytics Mining, or Decision Support, LDAM, in each respective system), provides the communication between researchers who seek data to discover hidden knowledge (on a global perspective). Note that while these components are shown in a centralized manner in Figure 2, they aim to represent an abstraction layer between all of the HIT systems. In the United States, the health informatics domain landscape is a federated architecture by nature. Thus, the end result and major challenge presented in Figure 2 is the recognition of a greater need for a comprehensive approach to security at global and local levels operating within an environment that is driven to share data through health information exchange. This comprehensive approach needs to take into consideration the distributed nature of repositories, the fragmentation of patient data across these systems, the discrepancies on sharing and security policies set in each component, as well as the potential usage of parties that do not own the data and are merely borrowing it in a predetermined set of constraints (e.g., time, amount, demographic, etc.).

At a global level, data mining techniques are useful tools in solving security related problems (Lin et al., 1996), permitting the extraction of information or knowledge from collected data or observed examples using statistical algorithms. Data mining methods have applications in intrusion detection, insider analysis, and many other settings (Lin et al., 1996; Zhu et al., 2007). Particularly, for the proposed security infrastructure (Figure 2), the reconciliation of security policies at both global and local levels may benefit from mining large-scale data transition-recording files or security monitoring of log files. The knowledge patterns detected from the mining steps may bring insights into a revision of the existing policies and

a better reconciliation. For instance, cloud computing may become a necessary resource for health information exchange (Khorshed et al., 2011) allowing access to patient data by medical providers who are outside the scope (institution) of an EHR. In a cloud-computing context, insiders may be expanded from organization internal employees and contractors to cloud internal employees and contractors, cloud customers, and cloud third party suppliers. This expansion increases the exposed threats on a healthcare organization's sensitive data, such as protected health information that is being transitioned between and shared among different organizations. Data mining such as cluster analysis, novelty detection, and association rule mining can be used to examine data-access log files and detect abnormal patterns in transactions.

The practice in knowledge discovery from large compiled data also imposes great challenges to security, especially during the process of sharing EHR data. The national and state healthcare agencies in the United States routinely publish patient data from EHRs for secondary data analysis that aims to expand knowledge about disease and treatments in order to enhance healthcare experience for individuals. The access and aggregation of EHRs poses significant concerns about patient privacy and confidentiality. According to HIPAA, de-identified healthcare information may be used and disclosed for secondary analysis and represents the extraction of personal identifiers in a record so that it is difficult to re-link the data to the people mentioned in the original records. To complement this, anonymized means that all of the links between a person and the person's record have been irreversibly broken so that it would be impossible to re-identify the person in the records. However, in large-scale secondary analysis of multiple data sources that involve race, ethnicity, gender, service date, diagnosis codes (ICD-10[29]), or procedure codes, by cross linking these data sets with other publicly available databases, data mining methods may be able to associate an individual with specific diagnoses. For example, one such effort demonstrated that an individual could be re-identified by linking certain attributes in a published data set with a voter registry (Cambridge, MA (Sweeny, 2002)). The reality is that no guarantees can be given in practice.

5. RECOMMENDATIONS FOR SECURE DIGITAL HEALTH CARE

Our major assumption in this section is that a significant barrier for integrated patient care data access in the United States occurs when a stakeholder, who needs to access information from a HIT system, has not been previously authorized to use the required information (in either a routine or emergent situation) and as a result is not easily authenticated to access information from systems that they have not been previously authorized to the individual. We recognize that in order to provide proper security, any recommendations must cover the storage and transmission of protected health information and personally identifiable information data. In this section, we provide our viewpoint of the a set of recommendations across a broad range of system techniques and mechanisms, as well as approaches that require human intervention in the general workflow to monitor and control secure information access. These techniques and mechanisms are readily available for use, and have been extensively deployed in other domains unlike health care. We provide our viewpoint with these recommendations in order to present the case that to provide a proper level of secure digital health care in the United States it will be necessary to leverage existing computational concepts and techniques some of which must be extended and modified for use in the health care domain.

- **Meta Standard for Health Care:** The ability to achieve health information exchange among the myriad variety of HIT is being dramatically hindered by a lack of agreement on one standard coupled with companies that are focused on vendor specific approaches and proprietary formats that inherently limit the ability to share data. The HIT vendor community must adopt practices in their development and deployment technologies that are well accepted in other fields through agreements on standards that allow data to seamlessly flow among different systems. What approaches have been historically utilized in computing to facilitate exchange?

Consider the database field based on the SQL ANSI Standard in 1986 and an ISO standard in 1987. Today, it is trivial to exchange information in database systems (MySQL, SQL Server, Oracle, etc.) with the ability to export an entire database schema (XML) and the entire database repository into XMI instances, at which point the database in that format can be moved from one database platform to another. In programming languages, Java introduced by Sun in 1995 changed the computing landscape with the write-once run anywhere paradigm, revolutionizing the cross platform development and dramatically improving Internet browser capabilities beyond simple html. Java is now dominant in the computing field across all domains and disciplines; it has simply changed the way programming was conceptualized.

These aforementioned examples in computing are the approaches that HIT vendors must adopt – they must be focused on providing a means to export their data from an EHR into a format that can be read and imported by another EHR or an external HIT system. To accomplish this, there needs to be two dramatic changes. First, the definition of a meta-standard that unifies across all of the different existing standards to provide the one single format (schema and structure) that every HIT vendor can import and/or export. Second, the need for a culture change that breaks the boundaries that are in place in regards to hospitals that sharing data will mean losing patients and for vendors that want to lock in hospitals and other medical organizations to solutions that once chosen become extremely difficult or nearly impossible to change. As easy as it is to take a database from Oracle to SQL Server to MySQL, it should be just as trivial to take a patient database from GE Centricity to Allscripts to Epic. The boundaries need to be taken down, and the true owner of the data, the patient, needs to be the one to dictate the way that their health care data is represented, shared, and exchanged; patients are being held hostage in the inability of the health care industry to effectively disseminate data.

The idea of a meta-standard for medical standards is to provide one universal and collective model that allows all types of medical data to be captured in both structure and semantics. Once established, this meta-standard can be the means for one HIT vendor to export data from its product that can then be easily loaded into another product of a different HIT vendor. Instead of focusing on health information exchange on a very low-level basis that considers linking three or four hospitals in a region, we must transcend to an approach that provides a meta-standard that raises the conceptual and abstraction level of information exchange to a place that will seamlessly allow medical providers to share information, change technologies, and adopt new technologies, without facing the overhead of custom integrations among different products. The HIE process must be simplified for effective information sharing that facilitates patient care and is not held hostage to an outmoded business model with vendor proprietary forms that limits sharing or requires custom interfaces between every interacting system.

- **Encryption:** The distributed nature of data storage in healthcare makes it necessary to provide security at storage point, as well as in the point of transmission. An encryption framework must provide a robust level of security for stored information capable of integrating heterogeneous local solutions, in the respective data sources, in a global context. This encryption framework should be extensible to handle new types of data unique to health care (genomic, phenotypic). For secure online data transmission, existing technologies (e.g., HTTPS, SSL, etc.) should be leveraged in order to provide a proper level of protection. The HITECH Act achieves protected health information portability and storage through encryption as applied to hard drives and (portable) systems such as laptops, jump drives, desktops, smart phones, tablets, cloud inter-system links, and user-system links (Mavridis et al., 2001).

- **Certificates:** X.509 certificates and their ability to be extended via certificate attributes can allow, over time, a user to acquire multiple X.509 certificates (each to access a specific system) based on their activity being authorized to utilize different systems. The advantage of multiple certificates (one per work setting) is to minimize the impact for failure; with a single certificate and multiple attribute certificates (one for each work setting) failure may compromise multiple settings, while multiple certificates (one per work setting) should limit the impact of failure. Each work setting can have their own security infrastructure and algorithms to generate a public-private key; the concept of multiple certificates each with multiple attribute certificates attached is akin to a wallet with multiple cards issued from different sources (Mavridis et al., 2001). Related efforts include: a framework for secure e-Health authentication using a multiple factor approach where physicians would provide multiple pieces of information in emergent situations akin to our multiple certificate approach (Boonyarattaphan et al., 2009); and, a framework for adaptive trust negotiation that establishes trust based on attributes other than identity (Ryutov et al., 2005).

- **DIRECT and Health Information Service Provider:** DIRECT[30] allows individuals, providers and organizations to share information with best practices that have trust and privacy considerations that are very consistent to the privacy emphasis of this proposal. A Health Information Service Provider is used to describe the management of security and transport for directed exchange and an organizational model that performs health information service provider functions to allow interactions of HIPAA Covered Entities with the sender or receiver of directed exchange of personally identifiable information, and must include all data collection, use, retention, and disclosure policies. In practice, sender and receiver take sole responsibility for encryption/decryption activities through the use of standardized encryption algorithms. In Figure 2, there would be service providers for each of the data sources (EHRs and personal health records). Health information service providers could use X.509 certificates as previously defined, where a certificate by role could be established for the different role each stakeholder coupd play. Attribute certificates can be associated with various characteristics such as for the data level (HIPPA, FERPA, DE-IDs), the situation (Urgent care, Primary Care, Inpatient Care), the type of data (patient, genomic, de-identified), etc. In an emergent situation where a physician might need access to another EHR, s/he could present her/his X.509 certificates and a process can be initiated by the user to consult among the EHRs with two possible results: access is allowed to the physician based on submitted certificates (with some expiration) or not.
- **Access Control:** Access control models provide the benefit of applying security at different levels of the information exchange scenario. Given the structure of Figure 2, role-based access control (Sandhu et al., 2000) could be used as a cornerstone, but needs extensions for health care. Extension parameters include patient, healthcare facility, task, temporal information, and other stakeholders (Berhe et al., 2010; Caine et al., 2013). Another extension would be the ability to extract local security policies and integrate them into a global one that is enforceable across the health care enterprise (Bhatti et al., 2005; De la Rosa Algarín, 2012; De la Rosa Algarín, 2013). A third extension could be for delegation of authority to facilitate access in an health information exchange setting (Berhe et al., 2010), where a provider often passes on his/her permissions (e.g., patients) to other providers. A fourth extension is the need for secure health information exchange across a wide range of data (e.g., clinical, genomic, and phenotypic) that will involve the co-consideration of HIPAA, GINA, and ELSI, and the exploration of role based access control (RBAC) (Sandhu et al., 2000) and delegation for genomic and phenotypic data.
- **User-Based Security Mechanisms:** There are many security nets in health care in terms of data access that happen after the misuse event has occurred. A clinician role in a hospital would have specific permissions, and an actual user should be further restricted to his/her patients. In practice, clinicians may be able to access more data than they are authorized and monitored in each single system against suspicious patient data retrieval (Barrows et al., 1996), and this is done after the fact via an audit. However, as given in Figure 2, the detection of intruders or system misuse is going to be necessary and will require more sophisticated network monitoring tools against consolidated log files from all of

the constituent HIT systems that are inter-operating. One dominant approach for data access for health information exchange or clinical research data warehouses is the use of an honest broker, an actual individual who is in charge of triggering the clinical (research) data request event to the corresponding HIT system(s) and returning the results to the clinical (researcher) (Silvey et al., 2008). Large hospitals require a dedicated team of patient privacy security officers in charge of enforcing regular password updates, system updates, correct system configuration, hard drive encryption, and other security related tasks; clearly this is more complex in an environment as shown in Figure 2. Often, improving user access means that clinicians must be educated on privacy regulations, procedures, system usage, and configuration, in order to avoid misconfigurations, such as using the same password for the private key, operating system login, and EHR system login that can merely achieved during dedicated seminars (Buckovich et al., 1999).

- **Cloud Computing:** With the emergence of mobile computing, the ability to support mobile access to health care information can be leveraged via cloud computing. The benefit of moving towards cloud-based solutions includes the decreased operational cost of maintaining systems that would otherwise be found in private practices or clinics, their maintenance, and their availability (Wu et al., 2012). The magnitude of this push is evidenced by the 21% growth of the market[31], and the estimated $5.4 billion investment by the year 2017[32]. The computational benefits of moving towards cloud computing in health care are immense and include: continuous patient data monitoring, smart emergency management, always-connected mobile devices, pervasive access to patient data (new

or old), etc. (Dinh et al., 2011). Security must be attained at end-user, processing, and storage layers of an application, and one approach (Zhou et al., 2010) evaluates the security concerns that cloud computing can provide to health care via availability, confidentiality, data integrity, control and audit. For example, as evidenced in (Rodrigues et al., 2013), the security risks not only involved the role-based access control for the end users (e.g. Physicians, Nurses, Administrative Personnel, Patients, etc.), but also the role-based and encryption at the third-party cloud service provider. In support for access control, the work of (Wu et al., 2012) proposes an approach that provides this level of security in selective sharing of EHRs. By aggregating the EHRs from different providers in cloud-based solutions (e.g., OpenEMR, Microsoft HealhtVault, and other shown in Figure 2) and utilizing a modular security policy manager (called the Composite EHR Access broker), role-based enforced information is disseminated. In an attempt to tackle a broader picture of cloud security in healthcare, the work of (Neame, 2013) presents a schema to tackle three main obstacles in EHR sharing: accessibility, privacy, and information functionality assurance. For privacy, the disassociation of the context (names, clinics, etc.) from the content is a simple step to follow that will result in meaningless data when not found in the appropriate respective context. For access control, an augmented security process would be needed and could include smart cards or other unique components that will assure access only from the proper identities. Lastly, in the work of (Alabdulatif et al., 2013), access control to EHRs is improved by restricting the access leveraging encrypted parameters for each user of a cloud data source.

6. CONCLUSION

This paper has looked backwards to the first discussions of privacy and access control for medical settings (Biskup, 1990; Ting, 1990), and more importantly forward to the wide array of emerging HIT systems, applications, and standards, intended to support health information exchange in order to allow varied stakeholders to securely access information in routine and emergent situations. As a result, by focusing in the current state of affairs in health care of the United States, we conclude that security cannot be considered simply from these individual systems, but must take a approach that requires a more global security solution to protect the vast amount of data available for use by medical professionals and data analysis by researchers. Toward this objective, Section 2 presented the changing landscape of medical care, standards, and technologies, that are difficult to support without health information exchange, and is further complicated by the present state (or lack) of medical information exchange in the United States, as illustrated by a scenario of patient care recently experienced by one of the co-authors and detailed in Section 3. Based on this information, in Section 4 and Figure 2, we presented our viewpoint of an architecture that positioned the HIT systems, standards, and applications in the context of health information exchange in the United States, and introducing globalized security enforcement and data mining/analysis components. While these globalized components are shown as internal components of the overall architecture, they aim to represent an abstraction layer that must be considered from the perspective of each constituent system of the health information exchange process. Using this as a basis, the recommendation list in Section 5 is our viewpoint for a first step for a roadmap for considering the security for digital health care that transcends individual systems and must consider the diverse HIT systems, applications, standards, and their interactions currently existing and happening in the United States; using, extending and leveraging traditional security mechanisms (encryption, access control, auditing, etc.) and user based techniques with privacy officers to control access to information via honest brokers and access via emerging platforms (mobile and cloud computing).

It is important to note that in this paper, while we have focused on the landscape on health information technology and information exchange in the United States, initiatives taken by other countries in their domestic health care systems can serve as guides for not only localized health care information technology development, but also for a broader information exchange scenario. Thus, the work presented in this paper also has an impact on EHRs, health information technology, and health information exchange in other countries. One effort of particular note is the US Department of Veterans Affairs' VistA system, which has been deployed in veteran hospitals, outpatient clinics, and nursing homes. VistA is an open source, Java-based EHR that is revolutionary in its adoption across such a wide scope, with linkages to the Department of Defense EHR to allow patients that move between the Department of Defense itself and the Veterans Affairs department with the purpose of having a complete medical history. VistA has expanded to an international setting with the creation of the WorldVistA[33] organization that has exploited VistA outside of the US with extensions for pediatrics, obstetrics, and other areas that are not supported for veterans. As another example, consider the case of the United Kingdom and its National Health Service (NHS) that covers all of the residents (Thomson et al., 2012) with several associated laws that provide: guidelines and enforcement of patient information disclosure (e.g., the Computer Misuse Act 1990[34], Access to Health Records Act 1990[35], The Data Protection Act 1998[36], and others); and, computational standards for information security (e.g., ISO/IEC 27002[37]). In addition, the NHS employs an approach towards a centralized database of patient information with NHS Spine (i.e., a centralized storage of patient data vs. the distributed local EHRs and PHRs in the United States) that has created the NHS Confidentiality campaign (a pro-confidentiality movement aimed at preserving patient information privacy). As another example, consider the Australian health care system that is universal like NHS and covers all residents and temporary-visa holding residents from countries with special relations with Australia (Thomson et al., 2012). The HIT approach of Australia has been focused on a patient-controlled EHR, much like a personal health record found in the United States. The best example is The Personally Controlled eHealth Record System[38], which provides the patient full control over their health information, specifically, what information is part of the health record itself and who can actually access the information[39]. The interested reader is referred to (Thomson et al., 2012) for a comprehensive discussion of health care systems in Australia, Canada, Denmark, England, France, Germany, Iceland, Italy, Japan, Netherlands, New Zealand, Norway, Sweden, Switzerland, and the United States.

REFERENCES

Alabdulatif, A., Khalil, I., & Mai, V. (2013). Protection of electronic health records (EHRs) in cloud. *Engineering in Medicine and Biology Society (EMBC), 2013 35th Annual International Conference of the IEEE* (pp. 4191-4194)

Barrows, R. C., & Clayton, P. D. (1996). Privacy, confidentiality, and electronic medical records. *Journal of the American Medical Informatics Association, 3*(2), 139–148. doi:10.1136/jamia.1996.96236282 PMID:8653450

Berhe, S., Demurjian, S., Saripalle, R., Agresta, T., Liu, J., & Cusano, A. et al. Secure, Obligated and Coordinated Collaboration in Health Care for the Patient-Centered Medical Home. In: *AMIA Annual Symposium Proceedings*. Volume 2010., American Medical Informatics Association (2010) 36

Bhatti, R., Ghafoor, A., Bertino, E., & Joshi, J. B. D. (2005). X-GTRBAC: An XML-based policy specification framework and architecture for enterprise-wide access control. [TISSEC]. *ACM Transactions on Information and System Security, 8*(2), 187–227. doi:10.1145/1065545.1065547

Biskup, J. (1990). *Protection of privacy and confidentiality in medical information systems: Problems and guidelines*. North-Holland.

Boonyarattaphan, A., Bai, Y., & Chung, S. A security framework for e-Health service authentication and e-Health data transmission. In: Communications and Information Technology, 2009. ISCIT 2009. 9th International Symposium on, IEEE (2009) 1213–1218 doi:10.1109/ISCIT.2009.5341116

Buckovich, S. A., Rippen, H. E., & Rozen, M. J. (1999). Driving Toward Guiding Principles: A Goal for Privacy, Confidentiality, and Security of Health Information. *Journal of the American Medical Informatics Association, 6*(2), 122–133. doi:10.1136/jamia.1999.0060122 PMID:10094065

Caine, K., & Hanania, R. (2013). Patients want granular privacy control over health information in electronic medical records. *Journal of the American Medical Informatics Association, 20*(1), 7–15. doi:10.1136/amiajnl-2012-001023 PMID:23184192

De la Rosa Algarín, A., Demurjian, S. A., Berhe, S., & Pavlich-Mariscal, J. (2012). A Security Framework for XML Schemas and Documents for Health Care. *International Workshop on Biomedical and Health Informatics*, (pp. 782–789).

De la Rosa Algarín, A., Ziminski, T. B., Demurjian, S. A., Kuykendall, R., & Rivera Sánchez, Y. (2013). Defining and Enforcing XACML Role-Based Security Policies within an XML Security Framework. *Proceedings of 9th International Conference on Web Information Systems and Technologies, INSTICC*, (pp. 16-25).

Dinh, H. T., Lee, C., Niyato, D., & Wang, P. (2011). *A survey of mobile cloud computing: architecture, applications, and approaches*. Wireless Communications and Mobile Computing.

Jha, A. K., DesRoches, C. M., Campbell, E. G., Donelan, K., Rao, S. R., & Ferris, T. G. et al. (2009). Use of electronic health records in US hospitals. *The New England Journal of Medicine*, *360*(16), 1628–1638. doi:10.1056/NEJMsa0900592 PMID:19321858

Khorshed, M. T., Ali, A. S., & Wasimi, S. A. (2011). Monitoring insider's activities in cloud computing using rule based learning. *2011 IEEE 10th International Conference on Trust, Security and Privacy in Computing and Communications (TrustCom)*, (pp. 757–764).

Kwon, J., & Johnson, M. E. (2012). Security practices and regulatory compliance in the healthcare industry. *Journal of the American Medical Informatics Association*. PMID:22955497

Lin, T. Y., Hinke, T. H., Marks, D. G., & Thuraisingham, B. (1996). Security and data mining. *Database Security*, *9*, 391–399.

Mavridis, I., Georgiadis, C., Pangalos, G., & Khair, M. (2001). Access control based on attribute certificates for medical intranet applications. *Journal of Medical Internet Research*, *3*(1), e9. doi:10.2196/jmir.3.1.e9 PMID:11720951

McCarty, C. A., & Wilke, R. A. (2010). Biobanking and pharmacogenomics. *Pharmacogenomics*, *11*(5), 637–641. doi:10.2217/pgs.10.13 PMID:20415552

Neame, R. (2013). Effective Sharing of Health Records, Maintaining Privacy: A Practical Schema. *Online Journal of Public Health Informatics*, *5*(2), 217. doi:10.5210/ojphi.v5i2.4344 PMID:23923101

Pace, W. D., Cifuentes, M., Valuck, R. J., Staton, E. W., Brandt, E. C., & West, D. R. et al. (2009). An electronic practice-based network for observational comparative effectiveness research. *Annals of Internal Medicine*, *151*(5), 338. doi:10.7326/0003-4819-151-5-200909010-00140 PMID:19638402

Ritchie, M. D., Denny, J. C., Crawford, D. C., Ramirez, A. H., Weiner, J. B., & Pulley, J. M. et al. (2010). Robust replication of genotype-phenotype associations across multiple diseases in an electronic medical record. *American Journal of Human Genetics*, *86*(4), 560–572. doi:10.1016/j.ajhg.2010.03.003 PMID:20362271

Rodrigues, J. J., de la Torre, I., Fernández, G., & López-Coronado, M. (2013). Analysis of the Security and Privacy Requirements of Cloud-Based Electronic Health Records Systems. *Journal of Medical Internet Research*, *15*(8). PMID:23965254

Ryutov, T., Zhou, L., Neuman, C., Leithead, T., & Seamons, K. E. (2005). Adaptive trust negotiation and access control. *Proceedings of the tenth ACM symposium on Access control models and technologies*, ACM, (pp. 139–146). doi:10.1145/1063979.1064004

Sandhu, R., Ferraiolo, D., & Kuhn, R. (2000). The NIST model for role-based access control: towards a unified standard. *Symposium on Access Control Models and Technologies: Proceedings of the fifth ACM workshop on Role-based access control*, (26), (pp. 47–63). doi:10.1145/344287.344301

Shea, S., & Hripcsak, G. (2010). Accelerating the use of electronic health records in physician practices. *The New England Journal of Medicine, 362*(3), 192–195. doi:10.1056/NEJMp0910140 PMID:20089969

Silvey, S. A., Schulte, J., Smaltz, D. H., & Kamal, J. et al. (2008). Honest broker protocol streamlines research access to data while safeguarding patient privacy. *Annual Symposium proceedings/AMIA Symposium*, (pp. 1133).

Sweeney, L. (2002). k-anonymity: A model for protecting privacy. *International Journal of Uncertainty, Fuzziness and Knowledge-based Systems, 10*(05), 557–570. doi:10.1142/S0218488502001648

Thomson, S., Osborn, R., Squires, D., & Jun, M. (2012). *International profiles of health care systems, 2012.* New York: The Commonwealth Fund.

Ting, TC. (199). *Application information security semantics: A case of mental health delivery.*

Wang, X., Chused, A., Elhadad, N., Friedman, C., & Markatou, M. (2008). Automated knowledge acquisition from clinical narrative reports. *AMIA Annual Symposium Proceedings*, (pp. 783).

Wang, X., Hripcsak, G., Markatou, M., & Friedman, C. (2009). Active computerized pharmacovigilance using natural language processing, statistics, and electronic health records: A feasibility study. *Journal of the American Medical Informatics Association, 16*(3), 328–337. doi:10.1197/jamia.M3028 PMID:19261932

Wu, R., Ahn, G. J., & Hu, H. (2012). Secure sharing of electronic health records in clouds. *2012 8th International Conference on Collaborative Computing: Networking, Applications and Worksharing (CollaborateCom)*, (pp. 711-718)

Zhou, M., Zhang, R., Xie, W., Qian, W., & Zhou, A. (2010). Security and privacy in cloud computing: A survey. *2010 Sixth International Conference on Semantics Knowledge and Grid (SKG)*, (pp. 105-112) doi:10.1109/SKG.2010.19

Zhu, D., Premkumar, G., Zhang, X., & Chu, C. H. (2007). Data Mining for Network Intrusion Detection: A Comparison of Alternative Methods*. *Decision Sciences, 32*(4), 635–660. doi:10.1111/j.1540-5915.2001.tb00975.x

Ziminski, T. B., De la Rosa Algarín, A., Saripalle, R., Demurjian, S. A., & Jackson, E. (2012). SMARTSync: Towards Patient-Driven Medication Reconciliation Using the SMART Framework. *International Workshop on Biomedical and Health Informatics*, (pp. 806–813).

ENDNOTES

[1] http://www.hhs.gov/ocr/privacy/

[2] http://www.genome.gov/24519851

[3] http://www.aafp.org/online/en/home/publications/news/news-now/practice-professional-issues/20130201ehradoptrates.html

[4] http://www.informationweek.com/healthcare/electronic-medical-records/ehr-adoption-us-remains-the-slow-poke/240142152

[5] http://pcmh.ahrq.gov/

[6] http://www.innovations.cms.gov/initiatives/ACO/index.html

[7] http://www.cms.gov/Regulations-and-Guidance/Legislation/EHRIncentivePrograms/Meaningful_Use.html

[8] http://www.hl7.org/implement/standards/product_brief.cfm?product_id=7

[9] http://www.astm.org/Standards/E2369.htm

[10] http://loinc.org/

[11] http://www.ihtsdo.org/snomed-ct/

[12] http://www.nlm.nih.gov/research/umls/

[13] http://www.w3.org/XML/

[14] http://www.w3.org/RDF/

[15] http://www.json.org/

[16] http://www.allscripts.com/

[17] http://www3.gehealthcare.com/en/Products/
Categories/Healthcare_IT

[18] http://www.ehealth.va.gov/VistA.asp

[19] http://www.genomas.net/

[20] http://www.nlm.nih.gov/research/umls/
sourcereleasedocs/current/NDFRT/

[21] http://www.epic.com/software-phr.php

[22] http://www.open-emr.org/

[23] http://www.patientos.org/

[24] http://www3.gehealthcare.com/en/Products/
Categories/Healthcare_IT/Electronic_Med-
ical_Records/Centricity_EMR

[25] http://freemedsoftware.org/

[26] http://openmhealth.org/

[27] http://smartplatforms.org/

[28] https://www.healthvault.com

[29] http://apps.who.int/classifications/icd10/
browse/2010/en

[30] http://wiki.directproject.org/

[31] http://www.prweb.com/releases/2013/9/
prweb11146871.htm

[32] http://cloudtimes.org/2013/09/30/the-
healthcare-sector-will-invest-5-4-billion-
in-cloud-computing-by-2017/

[33] http://worldvista.org/

[34] http://www.legislation.gov.uk/ukp-
ga/1990/18/contents

[35] http://www.legislation.gov.uk/ukp-
ga/1990/23/contents

[36] http://www.legislation.gov.uk/ukp-
ga/1998/29/contents

[37] http://webstore.iec.ch/preview/info_
isoiec27002%7Bed1.0%7Den.pdf

[38] http://www.ehealth.gov.au

[39] http://www.ehealth.gov.au/internet/ehealth/
publishing.nsf/Content/ehealth_privacy

*This work was previously published in the International Journal of Privacy and Health Information Management (IJPHIM),
2(1); edited by Muaz A. Niazi, pages 1-21 copyright year 2014 by IGI Publishing (an imprint of IGI Global).*

Chapter 63
Enhancing Emergency Response Management using Emergency Description Information Technology (EDIT):
A Design Science Approach

Michael A. Erskine
Metropolitan State University of Denver, USA

Will Pepper
Better Than Free LLC, USA

ABSTRACT

This paper presents a novel approach toward facilitating the effective collection and communication of information during an emergency. Initially, this research examines current emergency response information workflows and emergency responder dispatch criteria. A process for the optimization of these workflows and criteria, along with a suggested method to improve data collection accuracy and emergency response time using a mobile device application, are suggested. Specifically, a design-science approach incorporating the development of an expert system designed to facilitate efficient and effective sharing of emergency information is applied. The resulting benefits could improve emergency communications during large-scale international gatherings, such as sporting events or festivals, as well as the sharing of industry-specific safety incidents. A process model for conducting analyses of additional emergency response processes is also presented. Finally, future research directions are discussed.

1. INTRODUCTION

Denver, Colorado, a city with a population of over 634,000 individuals, has an emergency-communications network with a failure rate of one-in-every-five emergency calls. Dispatchers failed to meet emergency response time standards more than 1,070 times. Additionally, addresses of incidents had been misreported, crucial emergency location information was never received, and dis-

DOI: 10.4018/978-1-4666-8756-1.ch063

patcher mistakes have led to at least one wrongful death lawsuit due to a failure "to supervise and train its emergency-communications operators and police dispatchers" (Osher, 2013). Such communication failures are not unique to Denver and impact emergency call centers globally.

According to the National Emergency Number Association (NENA), there are over 6,000 public-safety answering points (PSAPs) in the United States alone (NENA, 2014). Public safety representatives suggest that a large number of emergency calls cannot be completed, as the current generation of wireless communication technology cannot adequately determine the position of a caller (Fung, 2014a). Additionally, of one thousand PSAPs, only 187 report a 'great deal' of confidence when receiving data from wireless carriers (Fung 2014a). Furthermore, it has been stated that only 2% of all PSAPs can receive and interpret short messaging service (SMS) data. Yet, over 70 percent of the 400 thousand individuals in the United States that call PSAPs each day connect via mobile devices. Most of these mobile devices likely had the capability to transmit SMS data. While the United States Federal Communications Commission (FCC) recently voted to mandate that all cellular service providers must support the capability of mobile devices to connect to PSAPs using SMS, it is still unclear how incident location information will be provided to dispatchers (Fung 2014b).

While PSAPs are challenged by technical constraints, they must also deal with human communication barriers, including excess background noise, language barriers, caller hysteria, or the inability to precisely describe the incident location. As these challenges exist during normal PSAP operation, large-scale public events further highlight the need for an improved process and technology. For instance, public events, such as the London Olympics, the Munich Oktoberfest and the Vienna Donauinselfest attract 680 thousand international visitors, 6.4 million total visitors and over 1 million international visits, respectively (Office for

National Statistics, 2012; Oktoberfest, 2013; Die Presse, 2014). International visitors to such large-scale public events may not be familiar with local emergency telephone numbers, may not know the local language sufficiently to explain details of an emergency, and may not be familiar enough with a city to adequately describe the emergency location. Surprisingly, the information systems literature barely addresses such issues. One exception is Yang, Su, and Yuan (2012) who researched fire disasters at major public events, including the 2008 Beijing Olympics, and stated that a key to their design was to understand user requirements. Thus, this research project approaches the design of an improved communication technology from the perspective of emergency communications operators who rely on accurate and detailed emergency information to make life-saving decisions.

The purpose of this research is to conceptualize, design and develop a mobile expert system to optimize emergency reporting. The development of such a system aligns with the global initiative of modernizing government services to support contemporary technologies. Surprisingly, the information systems scholarship, and more specifically the e-government research area, has largely avoided addressing the reporting, collecting and disseminating emergency information. For example, between 2003 and 2013, the 'basket of eight' top information systems journals address this issue in only six relevant studies (Venkatesh, 2013). See Table 1 for more information on these studies.

This paper addresses this research gap by evaluating key requirements for a mobile application to optimize the sharing of emergency information with local emergency response resources, as well as developing a prototype of such an application. An understanding of how individuals can benefit from an intelligent system to ensure accurate collection and communication of emergency data provides a unique exploration opportunity for the information systems scholarship. For instance, while numerous systems designed to collect public

Table 1. References to 'emergency services' (and similar) in top is journals based on AIS senior scholars' rankings between 2003 and 2013

Journal	Relevant Studies
European Journal of Information Systems	Allen, Karanasios and Norman, 2013; Ferneley and Light, 2006
Information Systems Journal	*None*
Information Systems Research	Yang, Su, and Yuan, 2012
Journal of AIS	*None*
Journal of Information Technology	*None*
Journal of MIS	Fruhling and Vreede, 2006; Xu, Teo, and Agarwal, 2009
Journal of Strategic Information Systems	Boonstra, Broekhuis, Offenbeck, and Wortmann, 2011; Leidner, 2009
MIS Quarterly	Chen, Sharman, Roa, and Upadhyaya, 2013

safety-data exist, such systems can only provide a benefit if the collected information is accurate (Shah, Bao, Lu, & Chen, 2011). Such a system could be integrated with other e-government initiatives that address improved emergency resource dispatching and citizen communications. In addition to sharing public safety information, other examples such systems include safety-reporting technology in the construction, manufacturing, logistics and aviation sectors.

By utilizing a process-based design science approach this research aims to leverage information technology research to reduce errors in the collection of emergency incident information and to optimize the reporting of an emergency incident. Design science research has been defined as an attempt to develop tools that serve humans and human purposes in order to try to understand the environment around us. The two axes of design science research include research activities (theorizing, building, evaluating, and justifying) and research outputs (constructs, frameworks, methodologies, and concrete supporting evidence)

as suggested by March and Smith (1995). Furthermore, while traditional design projects focus on the contribution of utility, a design science approach contributes to the knowledge base as well as the utility (Hevner, Park, and Ram 2014). The specific research questions considered through the design science approach of this paper include: Can a mobile expert system effectively guide witnesses or victims of an emergency incident? Can a mobile expert system improve emergency reporting to be more efficiently than by placing a voice telephone call? Can responses to essential questions be collected optimally allowing emergency dispatchers to make better-informed decisions and allocate resources more effectively? The process-based, design science approach addresses these research questions in the hypothetical context of an automobile accident.

2. RESEARCH METHOD

The benefits of using empirical research with a design science approach include (1) progress in the information systems scholarship, (2) an investigation into commonalities between current or past situations and theory, (3) solutions for known or unknown problems, (4) results that influence and build potentially new solutions to problems, (5) and the use of empirical research in new environments to test results in a method involving solutions for future problems (Hevner, March, Park, and Ram 2004; Neuman 2006; Anderson, Donnellan, and Hevner 2011; Gregor and Baskerville 2012; Bider, Johannesson, and Perjons 2013). Furthermore, it is suggested that design science research address a conceptual, research and developmental dimension (Gregg, Kulkarni, and Vinzé 2001). This paper contributes to all three dimensions through the novelty of augmenting traditional voice-only emergency communication, a formal gathering of existing communications challenges and the development of a prototype mobile application, respectively.

Following with the well-established principles of design science research, the first component of this research project was an empirical investigation into the primary information required by emergency dispatchers. This data was gathered through an open-ended questionnaire asking emergency services dispatchers to state the four to five information items that are required to successfully dispatch appropriate personnel. Contacts for this phase of the study were solicited via e-mail from addresses found via Google searches of county and municipal emergency services, as well as posting the question to emergency dispatcher community groups on LinkedIn and Facebook. The results gathered from emergency experts working in twenty-three areas of various sized and geographic location revealed five succinct questions. These questions, which were asked verbally, were then applied to a user-friendly application that presented these questions to a caller visually, allowing for a brief amount of time to pass in order to generate sufficient answers, and then automatically placing a voice call to the correct local emergency number.

While many communities have invested heavily into emergency call centers and supporting infrastructure, evidence suggests that more can be done to ensure efficiencies of such systems responses. For example, language or cultural barriers may prevent voice calls, operators may have difficulty identifying key information due to noise and other distractions, tense situations may cause communication challenges, and sometimes information is incorrectly interpreted resulting in inefficient responses. When a traumatic event, such as an accident, occurs people go through various emotions that can potentially be exasperated through adrenaline that clouds communication and judgment (Howie, 2008). This state of emotion could lead to information that is unusable, convoluted, or time delayed, thus affecting the dispatcher's ability to effectively assign first responders. Studies have also addressed the misinterpretation between callers and dispatchers caused by hysteria, emotion and anger (Tracy and Tracy, 1998; Whalen and Zimmerman, 1998; Garcia and Parmer, 2011).

An additional concern is that non-emergency calls can place a burden on responders (Snooks, Williams, Crouch, Foster, Hartley-Sharpe, and Dale, 2002). Palumbo, Kubincanek, Emerman, Jouriles, Cydulka, and Shard (1996) found that in 74 percent of emergency call cases dispatchers and physicians disagreed on whether emergency medical services with basic or advanced life support should be dispatched. Through the use of an expert system to ascertain whether a perceived emergency incident necessitates emergency responders, the burden placed on emergency responders for non-emergency calls could be reduced.

Globally, there are numerous emergency telephone number standards and various levels of awareness. In addition, regional or international visitors may not be familiar with such numbers outside their home regions. In the United States the designated universal emergency number is 911, while in the European Union this number is 112, or 000 in Australia. Providing an expert system that can accurately determine the correct emergency number could be extremely useful in a natural disaster situation. For instance, at a global tourist destination such as Paris, where the local number is 112, a visitor from Mexico may incorrectly dial 066, which is the emergency number that would be more familiar. Travelers may also encounter language barriers when contacting emergency services. Mobile expert systems could gather pertinent information in the native language and share such information with the closest emergency dispatcher in the language of the PSAPs geographic area. Prototyping an application that can connect individuals with the proper emergency response infrastructure, based on need and location, could overcome several barriers, such as a lack of awareness regarding local emergency numbers, language or other communications barriers and automatically transmitting key information such as location coordinates.

The required information for first responders begins with an inquiry of the location and a description of the emergency incident. This basic information can already determine which type of emergency response may be necessary. Examples of situations meriting different responders would be that the information of "intersection of 4th and Main streets" and "shooting" would result in the allocation of the nearest police cruiser, whereas "127 Jerome Street" and "choking" would result in the allocation of an ambulance and paramedics. While this early information would allow emergency services to be instantly deployed, as additional information is acquired, additional units, specialized equipment or auxiliary personnel could be added. For instance, for the "shooting" example an ambulance could be added as more information is gathered. An example of an accident decision-tree is presented in the Figure 1. As community emergency response resources vary, such workflows must be designed and evaluated for various municipalities and regions independently.

While the benefits of existing emergency response systems are substantial, an alternative to traditional voice-only calls could provide additional benefits. Recent advances in mobile technology present a unique opportunity to address these drawbacks. Particularly contemporary smartphones with large displays and various sensors could provide additional benefits not previously available. While the global trend of consumers moving from fixed telephone systems to mobile devices presents communication challenges (Sayed, Tarighat and Khajehnouri, 2005; FCC, 2014), there could also be significant benefits. The impact of mobile devices on emergency call centers is already evident, as for example, of the approximately 240 million emergency calls made in the United States each year, nearly one third are placed from mobile devices (NENA, 2014; CTIA, 2014). This is not surprising considering that as of December 2012, 38.2% of U.S. households were wireless only and that the U.S. penetration of wireless devices had reached 102.2% (CTIA, 2014).

In the United States, 61 percent of all mobile subscribers utilize a smartphone (Nielsen, 2013). In 2014 all of Western Europe, Australia, South Korea, Japan and Canada will also achieve a greater than 50 percent smartphone penetration,

Figure 1. Example automobile accident workflow

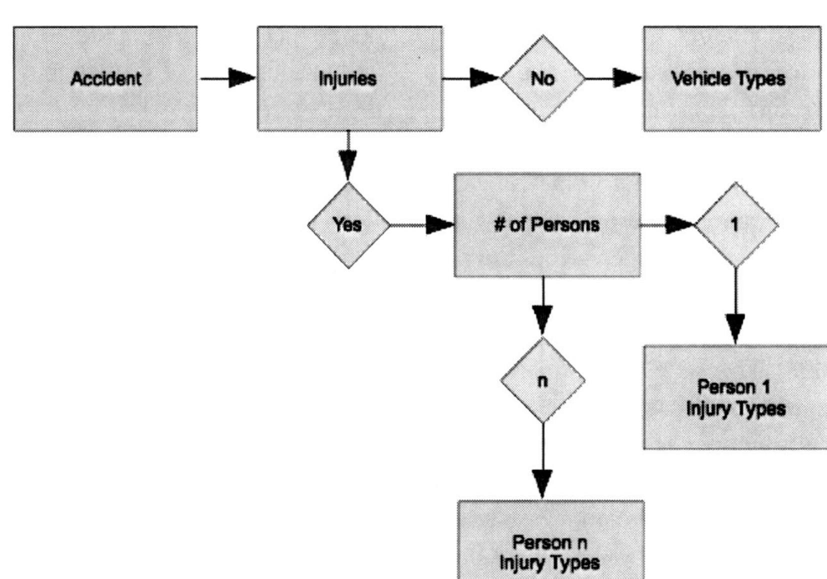

and by 2017 the global smartphone penetration is expected to reach 50 percent (eMarketer, 2013). This continued trend toward global adoption of smartphone technology presents a unique opportunity to enhance emergency services data collection by leveraging the capabilities of such devices instead of relying solely on voice and limited SMS capabilities. The benefits of similar systems, such as vehicle telematics that can place calls based on environmental conditions, such as an airbag deployment or collision detection, have already reduced the amount of time between an incident and a call (911.gov, 2014).

One of the core requirements to dispatch emergency services to the site of an emergency, is to identify the exact location of the emergency. Specifically, the Federal Communications Commission (FCC) in the U.S. and the Directive for Mobile Communication in the E.U. require the capability to determine a caller's location (Junglas and Watson, 2008).

In addition to the automatic communication of location information, critical medical information could also be transmitted. For instance, medial allergies or pre-existing medical conditions could be transmitted automatically along with the dispatch communication. This would be the equivalent of a digital medical bracelet. It has been documented that emergency medical services (EMS) providers often do not have sufficient access to pre-existing medical information when responding to incidents (Finnell and Overhage, 2010). While there has been an effort to link such data to EMS services, these may only be available locally or regionally. When travelling internationally it would become increasingly difficult to notify a dispatcher of specific pre-existing medical conditions.

In addition to medical information, details regarding psychiatric conditions could be transmitted as well. This could be especially helpful, as previous studies have discovered significant benefits of responding with a specialized crisis team to deal with psychiatric emergency services. For instance, such a response can provide a positive

intervention and can reduce the need for hospitalization (Scott, 2000; Sabnis and Glick, 2012).

While the global implementation of such a system would take substantial resources and planning, implementations for large-scale, international events such as the FIFA World Cup or the Olympic games could provide immediate value. Such events would be ideal test environments for such a system as a) a heavy emphasis is placed on safety, b) visitors may not be familiar with local emergency response numbers and c) because visitors may represent a variety of cultures and languages that such a tool must accommodate. Additionally, such a system could be deployed specifically to deal with emergency communications during a large-scale disaster. The benefits of mobile decision support systems to aid disaster response have been demonstrated and explored in several studies (Thompson, Altay, Green & Lapetina, 2006; Erskine & Gregg, 2012; Erskine, Sibona & Kalantar, 2013). In addition to facilitating post-disaster emergency information sharing, such systems can also be used to predict natural-disaster emergency situations (Brovelli & Cannata, 2004; Cannata, Marzochhi, & Molinari, 2012; Suri & Hofierka, 2004).

3. OPTIMIZING THE COMMUNICATION OF EMERGENCY INFORMATION

To better understand the key information necessary to successfully dispatch the appropriate resources in an emergency, key patterns in such situations were analyzed. While this ongoing research area will benefit from the gathering of data from actual emergencies, this initial research project uses qualitative research methods that rely on an inductive, discovery methodology to utilize determine vital information, allowing latent knowledge gaps to be addressed (Heredero, Berzosa, and Santos, 2010; Myers, 1997). This type of approach has already informed the development of information systems, such as those systems that rely on communal assistance (Dedrick and West 2005). The first step was a Google search using the term 'county 911' which produced over 696,000 suggested results. As many of these suggested sites were duplicate or class/sub-class sites (e.g., Genesee County 911 Consortium Index Page, Genesee County 911 Consortium - Active Events), the results needed to be narrowed down. From the initial search, fifty-five emergency agencies were evaluated for any educational material to assist callers. Data was collected, transcribed, summarized into descriptive codes to organize the observations and then categorized as patterns emerged. Then the codes were refined based on the patterns and interactions among the concepts. Linkages were reported that further support the need to formulate a theory that will support the development of a model assisted with observed facts (Myers, 2009).

In response to the initial findings the design science approach was expanded to develop a prototype mobile application to deliver a more efficient data-gathering tool. Most of the initial information gathered from websites helped determine how to appropriately classify a actual emergency versus a non-emergency situation. For instance, a suspicious vehicle in your neighborhood should simply be reported to police, but not necessarily by dialing the emergency dispatch center. A few websites provide answers to common citizen questions and others, such as Wood County 911, provide instructional material of what to do in an emergency (Wood County 911, 2014). However, such educational materials provide little benefit in an emergency as someone may not have read the information or have forgotten it during the stress of an actual emergency situation.

Of the fifty-five websites evaluated, thirty-nine emails were sent to the individual in the position equivalent to manager of the dispatchers (i.e., Division Manager, Head of Operations). Outside of the formalities of a traditional e-mail communication, the message consisted of one open-ended question: "What are the 4 or 5 questions that a caller needs to be prepared to answer upon calling 911?" Of those contacted, only five responded with answers, though others did respond with the intent to respond at a later time. To retrieve additional responses, the same question was posted to various LinkedIn and Facebook groups of which emergency call center dispatchers and managers were members. This approach led to the most feedback. Comments such as "I wish they would just educate people about the overall system itself", "in an emergency, you do what you have been trained to do. Train yourself now; when it counts, you will not have time to think about it", "as bad as the situation is, the caller must remember to listen to the operator" and "the caller must listen to what the dispatcher is asking. I find that many times the caller is so agitated they don't pay attention." These comments, as well as answers to the five questions developed from these communications, suggest that a practical solution is needed to communicate crucial emergency information. Due to the various contact methods, there is no meaningful way to present response rates for this portion of the study.

When former and current emergency dispatchers were asked the five most important pieces of information a caller needs to relay in a crisis, the response was unanimous with the key piece of information being the location of the incident. Those interviewed for this portion of the study represented twenty-three counties and cities in the United States. Some locations were as small as Chartham, MA (pop. 6,625) to as large Detroit (pop. 706,585) and Franklin County, Ohio (pop. 1,179,000). Of the twenty-four interviewed subjects, "location" or "where" was in one of the five answers twenty-two times, with the response being the number one more than any other answer (seventeen times). The second most important piece of information was "what", "what's wrong", or "what's the problem/situation" (fourteen times). Coming in third is "who", "name(s)", and "parties involved" (ten times), with fourth being a phone number in case of the call is dropped or background noise interference (five times). Interestingly, the fifth most popular answer may be asked more for the benefit of the first responders: are there any weapons at the scene (six times)?

Design science theory addresses problems that are either "unsolved" and must be addressed in innovative ways, or "solved" problems that can be improved through more efficient techniques (Hevner and Chatterjee 2010). Considering this, a prototype application was developed to demonstrate the proposed effectiveness of an expert system to reduce communications errors in emergency situations.

4. PROTOTYPE DEVELOPMENT

While the prototype was developed to focus on an auto accident emergency event, such a system could be expanded to address more sophisticated events including medical emergencies and natural disasters. The prototype application developed presents the first implementation of an emergency description information technology (EDIT) designed to collect essential information from citizens in stressful emergency situations.

One of the first steps is to capture the existing response workflows and utilize the opportunity to optimize such workflows. Next, the workflow is applied to the application development process and integrated into the existing PSAP workflow. See Figure 2 for a visual presentation of this workflow.

The EDIT prototype was developed using MySQL, HTML5, CSS, jQuery mobile, PHP, and

tested using various mobile platforms including iOS and Android. The prototype also utilized an external web server to host the application. Future enhancements will include the development of native applications to improve responsiveness and reduce the quantity of communications between the client and server.

EDIT must provide succinct information in a timely fashion while working in crisis environment. Upon first launching the application on a mobile device, the exact position of the mobile device would be determined using the native positioning services (e.g., global positioning system). This location data will be transmitted immediately, providing essential location information to the emergency resources dispatcher. Next, the expert system will provide a series of simple, 'yes' or 'no' questions initially based on broad circumstances that drill-down to greater granularity in order to guide the first responders. Finally, the application sends all of the collected information to the closest relay station and then automatically dials the appropriate regional emergency number. This allows for the application to provide initial incident information and allows the dispatcher to ask for specific additional information. The application would need to be customizable for different agencies and municipalities due each department's data flow schema, and the collected information would need to be coded properly to match existing data classification and prioritization schemas. An example of this would be that residents of coastal areas, such as Miami, may deal with nautical emergencies, while people in interior areas, such as Mexico City, would not.

Figure 2. Continuous development workflow

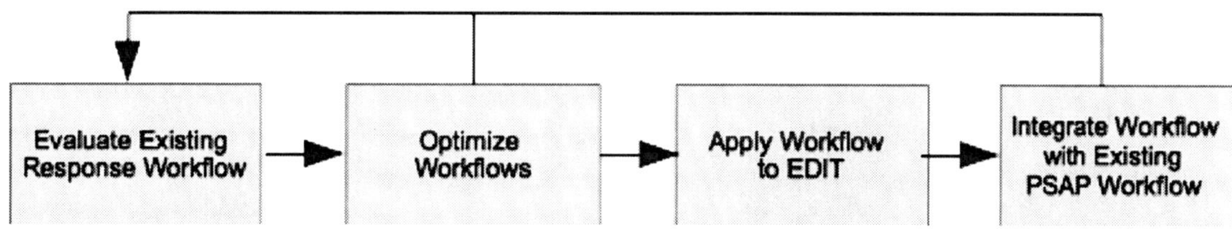

Thus, residents of Miami may need to collect and share unique information concerning nautical emergencies with appropriate entities.

An important consideration during the visual design of the application was the development of a concise and calming layout. Highly stressful situations often cause individuals to easily loose concentration. Thus, simple questions were developed to allow witnesses and victims to concisely provide key information. Additionally, the color scheme of the application interface includes various shades of green, a color that has been found to ease a nervous individual or an individual in a high-pressure situation (Rousseau, 2008). While research also supports that shades of the color blue are calming, they can also evoke feelings of sadness, which may impact the way a person responds while utilizing the expert system. As a green color scheme evokes a calming effect, relieves stress and improves reading ability, this color scheme was selected for the EDIT application (Color Psychology, 2014). See Figure 3 for a visual representation of the concise and calming interface using a green color scheme.

5. RESULTS OF DESIGN SCIENCE APPROACH

This research paper suggested a novel process-based approach to providing efficiency in an emergency situation. While an initial prototype has been developed, significant work will need to continue to develop a production-ready implementation.

Figure 3. Concise and calming interface

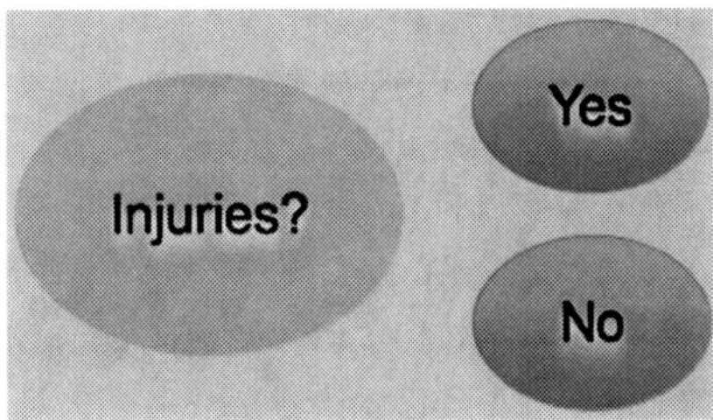

This paper has several implications on the information systems and e-government scholarships. Specifically, researchers can benefit from the specific process-based design science approach applied to the examination of emergency communications that incorporates existing knowledge from literature and empirical studies as well as the collection of new evidence. This approach can be used to identify problems in other information systems and e-government research domains. By choosing to use a design science approach, future research can benefit from the application of theory and empirical evaluations (Hevner, March, Park, and Ram 2004; Venable, Pries-Heje, and Baskerville 2014). Second, this paper addresses a hybrid communications approach that is not often examined in existing research. This hybrid approach allows the benefits of each communication type (e.g., voice, data) to be leveraged, creating a more efficient communication channel. Third, this paper introduces an interface design language specifically for mobile applications used in highly stressful situations, such as emergencies. A greater understanding of the use of mobile applications in such situations could inform human-computer interaction research related to disaster response systems, safety management systems and other technologies used in highly stressful situations. Each of these implications provides significant future research opportunities.

Furthermore, this paper suggests several practical implications. First, an extensive body of global emergency dispatch communications problems is presented. Second, this paper suggests that EDIT could be utilized to enhance communications in emergency situations. Specifically, developers of emergency response systems are presented with an enhanced communications method over traditional voice-only communications. The results of this study suggest that contemporary mobile devices could augment voice communication with text-based information and data collected automatically through sensors. While this study applies the EDIT concept to augment emergency communications, such technology could be used to aid in communicating when language barriers are present or when information is better presented visually. Such technology could provide significant benefits to emergency managers at large-scale events. Third, the benefits of developing workflows for specific emergency incidents are described. For instance, such workflows can be leveraged to automate responses without the need for dispatcher intervention. Fourth, mobile application designers and developers may benefit through the utilization of concise and calming interfaces when developing tools to be used by individuals in highly stressful situations. Finally, an integration workflow is suggested for incorporating EDIT into existing PSAP workflows. Organizations and individuals who create technologies related to emergency response management may benefit from these findings.

6. FUTURE RESEARCH

The next step of this project will be to perform simulations of recreations of emergency events using traditional telephone dispatch and the prototyped expert system. The authors expect that using a laboratory setting to record the information acquisition times of the prototyped software verses a simulated emergency phone will result in software acquiring crucial information more rapidly than the traditional verbal communication. Previous research supports that data communications can provide the same information as verbal communications, but more efficiently (Pepper, Aiken, & Garner, 2011). Another research step would be to utilize actual emergency dispatch information and call transcripts and compare these to use of the mobile expert system in order to quantify efficiencies. Additionally, benefits and drawbacks based on environmental and user characteristics could be explored to determine how versatile such a system would be in actual use. Furthermore, exploration will need to be performed

in determining how to most effectively integrate such a system into an actual dispatch facility or how such a system should behave outside a compatible region. Specifically, the effectiveness of integrating with or simply augmenting an existing computer aided call handling (CACH) systems will need to be examined.

While there are initiatives to support the transmission of emergency information using short message service (SMS) communications, organizations such as the FCC, CTIA and NENA continue emphasize the importance of voice communication in emergencies unless there are significant reasons that prohibit someone from doing so (CTIA, 2014; FCC, 2014; NENA, 2014). Thus, it will be essential for such a system to demonstrate viability and positive improvements before gaining acceptance and endorsements from organizations that represent emergency response services.

Furthermore, the collected data attributes from existing emergency dispatch transcripts could be analyzed in real-time and analyzed for patterns using decision-support systems. The use of such technology has been demonstrated to allow decision-makers to predict large-scale disasters. Furthermore, the use of crowd-sourced information has been suggested to aid decision makers with determining appropriate responses to natural disasters (Erskine and Gregg, 2012; Horita and Albuquerque, 2013; Horita et al. 2013). Such systems could have a greater capability of detecting disasters by analyzing real-time digital emergency communications, as would be provided by EDIT.

7. CONCLUSION

This paper utilizes a design-science approach to address a global problem: the efficient collection and effective communication of data that is essential to those in and responding to an emergency. This capability would closely align with other e-government initiatives that leverage contemporary technologies to enhance government processes.

By focusing on retrieval of pertinent information about emergency incidents in an extremely efficient manner (e.g., including mobile device decision-trees that gather user information while automatically sending location variables), such optimization processes may decrease response time, diminish lost or undecipherable verbal incident descriptions, and address the many other communication issues that arise from traditional voice-based emergency response systems.

Benefits to scholarly research include an examination of information systems literature in the context of emergency services. Specifically, important studies that inform the design science process of emergency information communications were presented. Additionally, a significant research gap demonstrates the need for e-government and information systems scholars to further examine how emergency management workflows can be improved.

Industry implications include the development of a prototype expert system that augments voice communication. Beyond safety or emergency information, such technology could allow various mobile communications to occur regardless of technical and communications barriers. Furthermore, the importance of considering color schemes to reduce stress and confusion when communication was suggested. Application developers may consider such color schemes when designing systems for use in situations that may influence high levels of anxiety.

This study includes several limitations. For instance, this study has only contributed through the development of a mobile device platform and has not yet addressed simulated or actual emergency communications. Future research that provides a simulation of emergency events is suggested to further validate EDIT. Furthermore, while mobile communication networks have experienced significant growth, there are many remote areas that continue to lack the necessary infrastructure.

This research considers that there are many organizational, sociological, and technical challenges that may arise from developing a new method in collecting emergency information, however the benefit of using EDIT for collecting specific electronic data prior to a voice call could outweigh the significant implementation barriers (Churchman, 1979; Walls, Widmeyer, and El Sawy, 1992; Markus, Majchrzak, and Gasser 2002; Manoj and Baker 2007).

REFERENCES

Allen, D. K., Karanasios, S., & Norman, A. (2013). Information sharing and interoperability: The case of major incident management. *European Journal of Information Systems*.

Ammenwerth, E., Buchauer, A., Bludau, B., & Haux, R. (2000). Mobile information and communication tools in the hospital. *International Journal of Medical Informatics*, *57*(1), 21–40. doi:10.1016/S1386-5056(99)00056-8 PMID:10708253

Anderson, J., Donnellan, B., & Hevner, A. (2011). Exploring the relationship between design science research and innovation: A case study of innovation at Chevron. *Communications in Computer and Information Science*, (286): 116–131.

Bider, I., Johannesson, P., & Perjons, E. (2013). Using empirical knowledge and studies in the frame of design science research, *Proceedings of the 8th International Conference on Design Science at the Intersection of Physical and Virtual Design*, 463-470. doi:10.1007/978-3-642-38827-9_38

Boonstra, A., Broekhuis, M., Offenbeek, M. V., & Wortmann, H. (2011). Strategic alternatives in telecare design: Developing a value-configuration-based alignment framework. *The Journal of Strategic Information Systems*, *20*(2), 198–214. doi:10.1016/j.jsis.2010.12.001

Brovelli, M. A., & Cannata, M. (2004). Digital Terrain model reconstruction in urban areas from airborne laser scanning data: The method and an example for Pavia (Northern Italy). *Computers & Geosciences, 30*(4), 325–331. doi:10.1016/j.cageo.2003.07.004

Cannata, M., Marzocchi, R., & Molinari, M. (2012). Modeling of landslide-generated tsunamis with GRASS. *Transactions in GIS, 16*(2), 191–214. doi:10.1111/j.1467-9671.2012.01315.x

CCA. (2014). About CCA, Retrieved September 27, 2014, from https://competitivecarriers.org/about/about-rca-2/914473

Chen, R., Sharman, R., Rao, H. R., & Upadhyaya, S. J. (2013). Data model development for fire related extreme events: An activity theory approach. *Management Information Systems Quarterly, 37*(1), 125–147.

Churchman, C. W. (1979). *The Systems Approach.* New York: Dell.

Color Psychology. (2014). Retrieved September 27, 2014, from http://psychology.about.com/od/sensationandperception/a/colorpsych.htm

CTIA. (2014). Wireless quick facts. Retrieved September 27, 2014, from http://www.ctia.org/your-wireless-life/how-wireless-works/wireless-quick-facts

Dedrick, J., & West, J. (2003). "Why firms adopt open source platforms: a grounded theory of innovationand standards adoption," In Proceedings of the workshop on standard making: A critical research frontier for information systems, pp. 236-257.

911. Dispatch. (2014). Required emergency information, Retrieved September 27, 2014, from http://www.911dispatch.com/info/calltaking/calltaker.html

eMarketer. 2013. Smartphone adoption tips past 50%," URL: http://www.emarketer.com/Article/Smartphone-Adoption-Tips-Past-50-Major-Markets-Worldwide/1009923

Erskine, M. A., & Gregg, D. G. (2012). Utilizing volunteered geographic information to develop a real-time disaster mapping tool: a prototype and research framework, In *Proceedings of the Conference on Information Resource Management (CONF-IRM 2012)*, Vienna.

Erskine, M. A., Sibona, C., & Kalantar, H. (2013). Aggregating, analyzing and diffusing natural disaster information: a research framework, In *Proceedings of the Nineteenth Americas Conference on Information Systems*, Chicago.

FCC. (2014). Retrieved September 27, 2014, from http://www.fcc.gov/guides/wireless-911-services

Ferneley, E., & Light, B. (2006). Secondary user relations in emerging mobile computing environments. *European Journal of Information Systems, 15*(3), 301–306. doi:10.1057/palgrave.ejis.3000620

Finnell, J. T., & Overhage, J. M. (2010). Emergency medical services: the frontier in health information exchange, In *American Medical Informatics Association Annual Symposium Proceedings 2010*, 222.

Fitzgerald, G., & Russo, N. L. (2005). The turnaround of the London ambulance service computer-aided dispatch system (LASCAD). *European Journal of Information Systems, 14*(3), 244–257. doi:10.1057/palgrave.ejis.3000541

Fruhling, A., & Vreede, G. J. D. (2006). Field experiences with eXtreme programming: Developing an emergency response system. *Journal of Management Information Systems, 22*(4), 39–68. doi:10.2753/MIS0742-1222220403

Fung, B. (2014a) Cellphone calls to 911 prove hard to trace, *Washington Post*, April 27, 2014.

Fung, B. (2014b). FCC is requiring broad support of text-to-911, *Washington Post*, August 9, 2014.

Garcia, A. C., & Parmer, P. A. (1999). Misplaced mistrust: The collaborative construction of doubt in 911 emergency calls. *Symbolic Interaction*, 22(4), 297–324. doi:10.1525/si.1999.22.4.297

Gill, A., Alam, S., & Eustace, J. (2014). Using Social Architecture to Analyzing Online Social Network Use in Emergency Management.

911. gov. (2014). Current 911 data collection, Retrieved September 27, 2014, from http://www.911.gov/pdf/Current911DataCollection-072613.pdf

Gregg, D. G., Kulkarni, U. R., & Vinzé, A. S. (2001). Understanding the philosophical underpinnings of software engineering research in information systems. *Information Systems Frontiers*, 3(2), 169–183. doi:10.1023/A:1011491322406

Gregor, S., & Baskerville, R. (2012). The fusion of design science and social science research. *Information Systems Foundation Workshop*, Canberra, Australia.

Heredero, C., Berzosa, D., & Santos, R. (2010). The implementation of free software in firms: An empirical analysis. *The International Journal of Digital Accounting Research*, 10, 113–130.

Hevner, A. R., & Chaterjee, S. (2010). *Design Research in Information Systems* (pp. 14–18). New York: Springer. doi:10.1007/978-1-4419-5653-8

Hevner, A. R., March, S. T., Park, J., & Ram, S. (2004). Design science in information systems research. *Management Information Systems Quarterly*, 28(1), 75–105.

Horita, F. E., & de Albuquerque, J. P. (2013). An approach to support decision-making in disaster management based on volunteer geographic information (VGI) and spatial decision support systems (SDSS). In *Proceedings of the 10th International Conference on Information Systems for Crisis Response and Management*, Baden-Baden, Germany, 12-15.

Horita, F. E. A., Degrossi, L. C., de Assis, L. F. G., Zipf, A., & de Albuquerque, J. P. (2013). The use of volunteered geographic information (VGI) and crowdsourcing in disaster management: a systematic literature review, In *Proceedings of the Nineteenth Americas Conference on Information Systems*, Chicago.

Howie, C. (2008). What to do after a car accident, CNN, Retrieved September 27, 2014, from http://www.cnn.com/2008/LIVING/wayoflife/05/09/car.accident/

Junglas, I. A., & Watson, R. T. (2008). Location-based services. *Communications of the ACM*, 51(3), 65–69. doi:10.1145/1325555.1325568

Leidner, D. E., Pan, G., & Pan, S. L. (2009). The role of IT in crisis response: Lessons from the SARS and Asian Tsunami disasters. *The Journal of Strategic Information Systems*, 18(2), 80–99. doi:10.1016/j.jsis.2009.05.001

Lindsey, B. (2011). Social media and disasters: Current uses, future options, and policy considerations. *Congressional Research Service*, 7(5700), 1–10.

Manoj, B. S., & Baker, A. H. (2007). Communication challenges in emergency response. *Communications of the ACM*, 50(3), 51–53. doi:10.1145/1226736.1226765

March, S. T., & Smith, G. F. (1995). Design and natural science research on information technology. *Decision Support Systems*, 15(4), 251–266. doi:10.1016/0167-9236(94)00041-2

Markus, M. L., Majchrzak, A., & Gasser, L. (2002). A design theory for systems that support emergent knowledge processes. *Management Information Systems Quarterly, 26*(3), 179–212.

Myers, M. (1997). *Qualitative research in information systems.* MIS Quarterly Discovery. doi:10.2307/249422

Myers, M. (2009). *Qualitative Research in Business and Management.* London: Sage.

NENA. (2014). 911 Statistics, Retrieved September 27, 2014, from https://www.nena.org/?page=911Statistics

Neuman, W. L. (2006). *Social Research Methods. Qualitative and Quantitative Approaches.* Pearson.

Nielsen. (2013). Mobile Majority, Retrieved September 27, 2014, from http://www.nielsen.com/us/en/newswire/2013/mobile-majority--u-s--smartphone-ownership-tops-60-.html

Office for National Statistics. (2012). London 2012 Olympic & Paralympic Games attracted 680,000 overseas visitors, Retrieved September 27, 2014, from http://www.ons.gov.uk/ons/dcp29904_287477.pdf

Oktoberfest. (2013). The Oktoberfest 2013 roundup. Retrieved September 27, 2014, from http://www.oktoberfest.de/en/article/About+the+Oktoberfest/About+the+Oktoberfest/The+Oktoberfest+2013+roundup/3734/

Osher, C. N. (2013). Operator error: how emergency calls are managed by dispatchers can be problematic, *The Denver Post*, Retrieved September 27, 2014, from http://www.denverpost.com/ci_22500950/denvers-911-call-performance-audits-reveal-problems

Palumbo, L., Kubincanek, J., Emerman, C., Jouriles, N., Cydulka, R., & Shade, B. (1996). Performance of a system to determine EMS dispatch priorities. *The American Journal of Emergency Medicine, 14*(4), 388–390. doi:10.1016/S0735-6757(96)90056-X PMID:8768162

Pepper, W., Aiken, M., & Garner, B. (2011). Usefulness and usability of a multilingual electronic meeting system. *Global Journal of Computer Science and Technology, 11*(5), 34–40.

Rousseau, L. (2008). The essential principles of graphic design, In Color, (pp. 14-16), F+W Publications, Cincinnati.

Sabnis, D., & Glick, R. L. (2012). Innovative community-based crisis and emergency services. In *Handbook of Community Psychiatry* (pp. 379–387). Springer New York. doi:10.1007/978-1-4614-3149-7_31

Sayed, A. H., Tarighat, A., & Khajehnouri, N. (2005). Network-based wireless location: Challenges faced in developing techniques for accurate wireless location information. *Signal Processing Magazine, IEEE, 22*(4), 24–40. doi:10.1109/MSP.2005.1458275

Scott, R. L. (2000). Evaluation of a mobile crisis program: Effectiveness, efficiency, and consumer satisfaction. *Psychiatric Services (Washington, D.C.), 51*(9), 1153–1156. doi:10.1176/appi.ps.51.9.1153 PMID:10970919

Shah, S., Bao, F., Lu, C. T., & Chen, I. R. (2011). Crowdsafe: crowd sourcing of crime incidents and safe routing on mobile devices. In *Proceedings of the 19th ACM SIGSPATIAL International Conference on Advances in Geographic Information Systems* (pp. 521-524). ACM. doi:10.1145/2093973.2094064

Snooks, H., Williams, S., Crouch, R., Foster, T., Hartley-Sharpe, C., & Dale, J. (2002). NHS emergency response to 999 calls: Alternatives for cases that are neither life threatening nor serious, *BMJ. British Medical Journal, 325*(7359), 330–333. doi:10.1136/bmj.325.7359.330 PMID:12169513

Suri, M., & Hofierka, J. (2004). A new GIS-based solar radiation model and its application to photovoltaic assessments. *Transactions in GIS, 8*(2), 175–190. doi:10.1111/j.1467-9671.2004.00174.x

Sutton, J., Palen, L., & Shklovski, I. (2008). Backchannels on the front lines: emergent uses of social media in the 2007 southern California wildfires, In *Proceedings of the 5th International ISCRAM Conference*, (pp. 624-632), Washington, DC.

Thompson, S., Altay, N., Green, W. G. III, & Lapetina, J. (2006). Improving disaster response efforts with decision support systems. *International Journal of Emergency Management, 3*(4), 250–263. doi:10.1504/IJEM.2006.011295

Tracy, K., & Tracy, S. J. (1998). Rudeness at 911 reconceptualizing face and face attack. *Human Communication Research, 25*(2), 225–251. doi:10.1111/j.1468-2958.1998.tb00444.x

Venable, J., Pries-Heje, J., & Baskerville, R. (2014). FEDS: A framework for evaluation in design science research. *European Journal of Information Systems*, 1–13.

Venkatesh, V. (2013). Rankings based on AIS Senior Scholar's Basket Of Journals, Retrieved September 27, 2014, from http://www.vvenkatesh.com/isranking/

Walls, J. G., Widmeyer, G. R., & El Sawy, O. A. (1992). Building an information system design theory for vigilant EIS. *Information Systems Research, 3*(1), 36–59. doi:10.1287/isre.3.1.36

Whalen, J., & Zimmerman, D. H. (1998). Observations on the display and management of emotion in naturally occurring activities: The case of hysteria in calls to 9-1-1. *Social Psychology Quarterly, 61*(2), 141–159. doi:10.2307/2787066

Winroither, E., & Kocina, E. (2014). Donauinselfest will Gäste aus dem Ausland. Retrieved September 27, 2014, from http://diepresse.com/home/kultur/popco/Festivals/donauinselfest/3827487/Donauinselfest-will-Gaeste-aus-dem-Ausland

Wood County 911. (2013). Retrieved September 27, 2014, from http://www.woodcounty911.com/calling.htm

Xu, H., Teo, H. H., Tan, B. C., & Agarwal, R. (2009). The role of push-pull technology in privacy calculus: The case of location-based services. *Journal of Management Information Systems, 26*(3), 135–174. doi:10.2753/MIS0742-1222260305

Yang, L., Su, G., & Yuan, H. (2012). Design principles of integrated information platform for emergency responses: The case of 2008 Beijing Olympic games. *Information Systems Research, 23*(3), 761–786. doi:10.1287/isre.1110.0387

Yuan, Y., & Zhang, J. (2003). Towards an appropriate business model for m-commerce. *International Journal of Mobile Communications, 1*(1/2), 35–56. doi:10.1504/IJMC.2003.002459

This work was previously published in the International Journal of Electronic Government Research (IJEGR), 11(2); edited by Vishanth Weerakkody, pages 51-65 copyright year 2015 by IGI Publishing (an imprint of IGI Global).

Chapter 64

Improving the Treatment Outcomes for ADHD Patients with IS/IT:
An Actor–Network Theory Perspective

Bader Binhadyan
RMIT University, Australia

Indrit Troshani
University of Adelaide, Australia

Nilmini Wickramasinghe
RMIT University, Australia

ABSTRACT

The key role for IS/IT in e-health has now been well established; however, within e-health the area of e-mental health is still new and emerging and scholars and practitioners alike are dubious as to the role for IS/IT and its benefits. We propose using Actor-network Theory (ANT) to assist in understanding the enabling role in e-mental health and we focus on one area of mental health, adults with Attention Deficit Hyperactivity Disorder (ADHD). We focus on Saudi Arabia. Attention to ADHD has begun to gain growing attention from Saudi Arabia healthcare providers and researchers. Currently, there is an estimated 15% of school age children suffering from ADHD. More than half of these children are expected to continue to show the symptoms of ADHD through their adolescence and adulthood. ADHD impacts the quality of life these individuals. Technology has the potential to improve mental health services this can be seen in enabling early intervention or treatment for people with mental health issues. Saudi Arabia is investing heavily in e-health and aiming to build a complete patient electronic record by 2020.

DOI: 10.4018/978-1-4666-8756-1.ch064

1. INTRODUCTION

The rapid developments of the Internet and mobile technologies during the last two decades have enabled healthcare providers and services globally to adapt these technologies in order to facilitate better service delivery (Eysenbach 2001). Recently, the mental health sector is realising the benefit of using technologies. This is because these technologies promise to improve efficiency, accessibility and the opportunities for early intervention and treatment of for many people with mental illnesses (Christensen et al. 2002); such as Attention Deficit Hyperactivity Disorder (ADHD). Although Saudi Arabia has invested billions of dollars to improve the quality and the delivery of e-health in the last 10 years (Altuwaijri 2010), less focus has been given to e-mental health. This is a key void and one this paper sets out to address.

ADHD in Saudi Arabia affects approximately 15% of children (Munshi 2014). ADHD symptoms include hyperactivity and impulsiveness, inattention or both (Barkley 1998) and more than half of these children with ADHD will carry over these ADHD symptoms into adulthood (Rucklidge & Tannock 2002). These symptoms will seriously impact the quality of life for children, teens or adults (Barkley et al. 1990). The most effective treatments of ADHD include medication, education, therapy, and coaching/counselling; the multimodal framework recommended by Canadian Attention Deficit Hyperactivity Disorder Resource Alliance (CADDRA) (CADDRA 2011). The need for better services and increased awareness for people with ADHD in Saudi Arabia has inspired groups of clinicians to establish the Saudi ADHD Society (AFTA Society) in 2009.

AFTA Society is a NFP (Not-For-Profit) organisation with a particular focus on increasing the quality of life of people with ADHD and to educate/train clinicians/parents about the disorder. Their emphasis is on school age children with ADHD. Less attention has been paid to ADHD in Saudi Arabia by researchers and healthcare providers (Taleb & Farheen 2013; Alqahtani 2010), which has resulted in a lack of public awareness and information regarding ADHD in adults.

The emphasis of this research will be on assisting the current state of ADHD treatment and management in Saudi Arabia, and how the IS/IT solution that is being designed and developed in an Australian context, might be transferred to the Saudi Arabian context. In this research, AFTA Society was chosen to be the case study and Actor-network Theory will be used to assist with the investigation. The research question guiding this study is: How can an IS/IT solution be designed to enable better support in the treatment of ADHD in adults in Saudi Arabia?

2. RELATED LITERATURE

This section provides a brief background of the use of IS/IT in healthcare in general and then specifically in Saudi Arabia, followed by a definition of e-health and the use of technology in mental health services in general, and ADHD in particular. Finally, the relevance of ADHD in adults and what current non-pharmaceutical treatments are used to treat and manage ADHD in adults is presented.

2.1. Background

Technology in healthcare has the potential to assist developed and developing countries to solve many issues they are facing, such as creating easy access to information and services, coping with changing population health patterns and satisfaction and safety of stakeholders and specific population groups. Healthcare is becoming technology-driven (Moumtzoglou 2011) with the possibility of superior healthcare delivery with the adoption of e-business in the form of e-health (Eysenbach 2001).

E-Health covers a broad area in healthcare (Eysenbach 2001). E-mental health is one of the areas that e-health covers. E-mental health is a relatively new area of e-health and hence few, if any, policies or strategic directions currently exist. Even though the use of technologies in mental healthcare is relatively new, there is a positive trend towards using technologies among different age groups, for different mental illness preventions and treatments (Ben-Zeev et al. 2012; Proudfoot et al. 2010; Whittaker et al. 2012). Technology has the potential to improve efficiency, accessibility, quality and the opportunities for early intervention and treatment for individuals with different mental illness (Anthony et al. 2010; Christensen et al. 2002), especially in treating young adults with ADHD (Beck et al. 2010; Wang & Hsieh 2013).

Technological tools and methods, such as Internet-based interventions and mobile-based application or Short Message Services (SMS) therapy are used for the treatment of people with mental illness like depression and anxiety (Anthony et al. 2010; Christensen & Petrie 2013; Whittaker et al. 2012). They can also target young adults seeking mental health attention (Christensen et al. 2002).

2.2. Saudi Arabia E-Health

"Saudi Arabia offers a picture of spectacular progress in health care.... Although many nations have seen sizable growth in their health care systems, probably no other nation of large geographic expanse and population has, in comparable time, achieved so much on a broad national scale, with a relatively high level of care made available to virtually all segments of the population" (Gallagher 2002, p. 182).

In the last decade, the Saudi Arabian government made the development of healthcare systems a high priority and has invested billions of dollars to improve the delivery and quality of health services. For example, the Ministry of Health (MoH) has also allocated just over US$1 billion to develop and improve e-health programme for public sector between 2008-2011 (Qurban & Austria 2008).Because of these huge investments

and the high level of care and attention, the Saudi population's health services has improved significantly (Almalki et al. 2011).

Due to a number of challenges that the Saudi Arabian health sector is facing, such as vast growth, vast geography, and emergence of lifestyle diseases (Ministry of Health Portal 2011), MoH quickly started to adapt and implement the e-health concept. E-health focus and strategies in Saudi Arabia concentrate on patient centric care (Figure 1) by building a significant nationwide e-health network that will allow more than 3500 e-healthcare facilities to use a single patient record by 2020 (Ministry of Health Portal 2011; Nuviun Digital Health 2014).

The national e-health programme of Saudi Arabia aims to achieve the following:

- Interoperable Electronic Health Record (iEHR) for every patient.
- Patient health information will be available to clinicians in all healthcare services.
- Deliver an efficient system to transfer patients between healthcare services.
- Offer electronic services to all healthcare facilities.

The National e-health programme roadmap will cover the mental health sector in year 4-6 with no further details of mental health programmes or using IT mental health (Ministry of Health Portal 2011) even though the Saudi King, King Abdullah bin Abdul-Aziz Al Saud, has giving his order to allocate over US$4 billion to establish 22 health projects, which includes three health centres for children's growth and behaviour disorders (Ministry News 2013).

Information technology, such as the Internet, has become a key component of the daily lives of a large part of the Saudi population, which makes them the largest internet user population in the Arab world, with an internet services penetration rate of 59.24% (Simsim 2011; Internet Live Stats 2014). Eighty percent of Internet users are between ages 16 and 35 (Al-Tawil 2001).

Figure 1. Saudi e-health strategies adapted from (Ministry of Health Portal 2011)

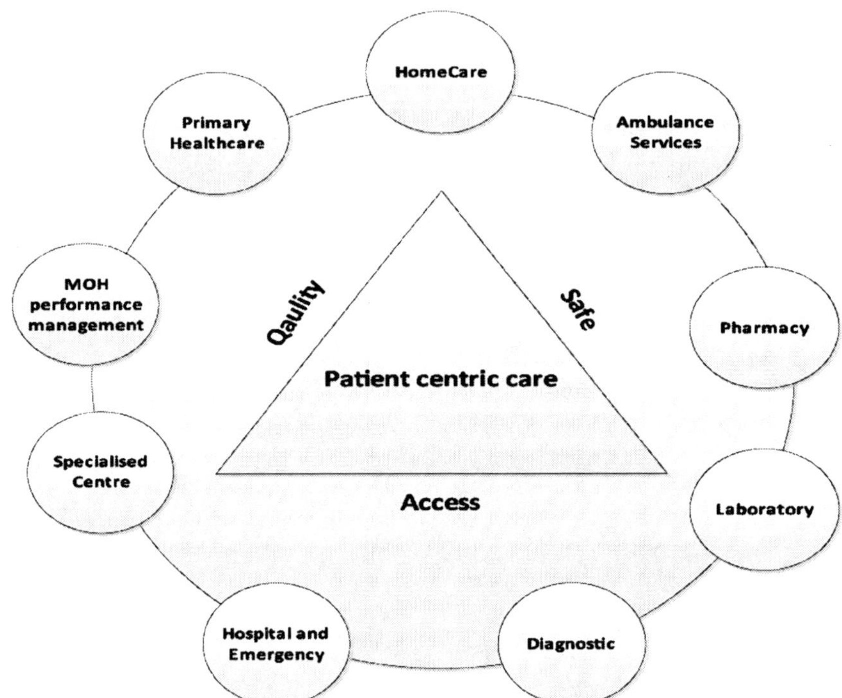

2.3. ADHD

Globally, ADHD is considered one of the major public health issues which affects approximately 5% of children (Polanczyk et al. 2007). Over of 50% of these children will carry this disorder throughout their adolescence to their adulthood with a worldwide-pooled frequency of adulthood ADHD around 2.5% (Rucklidge & Tannock 2002).

The hyperactivity symptoms in adults are more refined than in childhood, which presents itself as restlessness, racing thoughts, unreasonable talking, or trying to do many things at once (Mannuzza et al. 1993; Barkley et al. 2008; Murphy et al. 2002). Despite the similarity of symptoms between children and adults with ADHD, adults with ADHD symptoms are likely to experience the following:

- Have obtained less formal education, (Mannuzza et al. 1998 ; Pope 2010);

- Family functioning, difficulties with self-control which leads to risk taking and substance abuse, and/or trouble with the law (Barkley et al. 1990);
- Difficulty to remain focused, lack attention to details, follow instruction, or finish or meet deadlines (Barkley et al. 2008).

2.4. Saudi Arabia and ADHD

Recent studies indicated that about 15% of children suffer from ADHD in Saudi Arabia (Arab News 2014; Munshi 2014). As less attention has been paid to this issue in Saudi Arabia (Alqahtani 2010) and insufficient studies have focused on the issue (Taleb & Farheen 2013), there is a lack of information regarding adults with ADHD, and this forced some individuals to form a community group for ADHD.

However, given there is less attention paid to ADHD issues in Saudi Arabia (Alqahtani 2010) and insufficient studies have focused on the issues (Taleb & Farheen 2013), it is difficult for the research to find official data or information regarding adult with ADHD in Saudi Arabia.

2.5. AFTA Society

ADHD Saudi Society was established in in 2004, under King Faisal Specialist Hospital supervision, which later in 2008 held the first ADHD conference in the Middle East. In 2009, this society became a NFP organisation called AFTA Society that runs under the supervision of the Ministry of Social Affairs, Saudi Arabia. Their main mission is to increase the quality of life of people with ADHD by providing better services and increasing awareness.

Since its establishment, AFTA has introduced a number of projects to increase awareness and improve diagnoses and treatments as well as educate targeted people or specialists. AFTA held the first Middle Eastern symposium on ADHD, which aimed to promote understanding of ADHD among social workers, teachers, and parents (King Faisal Specialist Hospital Research Centre 2004). There are only a small number of clinicians who are trained or specialised to treat ADHD comparing to the population of ADHD in Saudi Arabia (Arab News 2014) AFTA is going to open the first charitable diagnosis and treatment centre for children with ADHD. AFTA also uses internet tools such social media to promote for the work. Because it is the first NFP in the Middle East and they have started from the scratch, ADHD is only slowly starting to generate a small amount of attention from healthcare authorities.

2.6. Treatment and Management of ADHD

The recommended treatment/management for ADHD symptoms in adults should contain combinations of coaching/counselling, education therapy and medication (Canadian Attention Deficit Hyperactivity Disorder Resource Alliance (CADDRA) 2011; Department of Human Services Victoria n.d.; The Royal Australian College of Physicians 2009). Such an approach is called the Multimodal framework.

- **Therapies:** The therapies that have been useful for treating ADHD in adults include Cognitive Behavioural Therapy (CBT) (Ramsay 2012; Ramsay & Rostain 2011), Neurofeedback Therapy (Arns et al. 2008; Gevensleben et al. 2009), Working Memory Training (WMT) (Klingberg et al. 2005; Gropper et al. 2014).
- **Education:** Education is centred on informing the individual about their mental illness and includes information on intervention related to educational accommodations, support, and management (Swartz et al. 2005; Wilens et al. 2008).
- **Coaching:** Coaching is centred on life mentoring and guiding which includes improving time management, studies, and social skills at university (Goldstein 2005; Prevatt et al. 2011; Swartz et al. 2005; Zwart & Kallemeyn 2001).

2.7. The Use of Technology in the Multimodal Framework

This research will assist the current state of ADHD treatment and management in Saudi Arabia, and how the IT solution that is being designed and developed in an Australian context can be transferred to a Saudi Arabian context. The e-Multimodal framework (Figure 2) that is designed for an Australian context will be adapted to see how it can be transferred to Saudi Arabia.

There are a number of technology tools that have been identified in the literature to treat ADHD in adults; namely, for coaching; e.g.: smartphone (Prevatt et al. 2011), therapy; e.g.: Neurofeedback Therapy (Arns et al. 2009) internet-based CBT

Figure 2. The e-multimodal framework

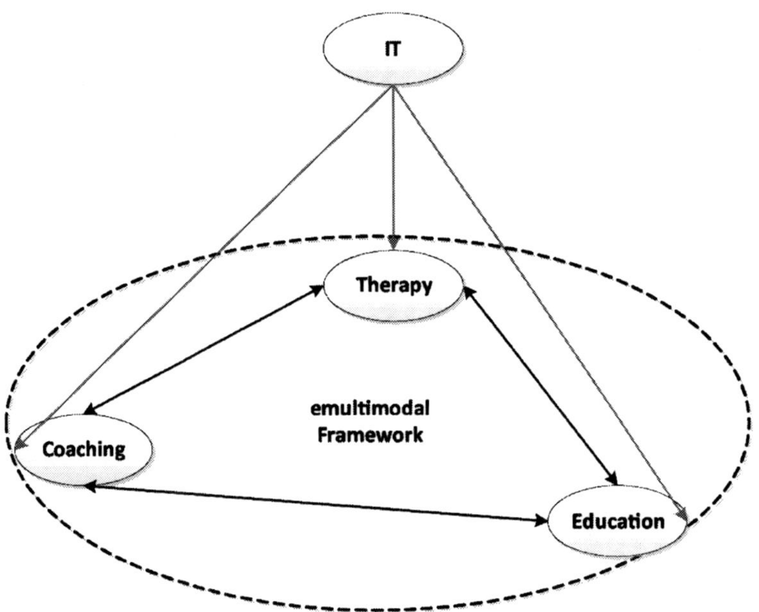

(Pettersson et al. 2014), computerized WMT (Gropper et al. 2014), and education; e.g.: Social media (CADDRA 2011). The major tools that use IT to deliver the treatment, managing, or prevention of ADHD are shown in Table 1.

3. METHOD AND RESEARCH DESIGN

Because this area of study has not been explored before and the e-mental health in Saudi Arabia does not have defined characteristics, an exploratory qualitative research method is the most suitable method and a single case study is used (Yin 2009). At this stage of the research, the answer to the research question of "How can an IT solution be designed to enable better support treatment of ADHD in adults in Saudi Arabia?" will be examined and explored.

This research design will use an instrumental case study as a tool of investigation found in numerous fields, especially evaluation, in which the researcher develops an in-depth analysis of a case (Creswell 2013). According to Stake (1995) there are three types of case study research; intrinsic, instrumental, and collective case studies. To gain

Table 1. Technological tools found in the treatment of ADHD

	The Multimodal Framework Components	Tools	Place
1	Coaching/Education	• Email counselling • Informative Website • Real live time chat	http://www.kidshelp.com.au/teens
		• Informative Website	http://www.betterhealth.vic.gov.au/
2	Therapy	• Neurofeedback • Working Memory Training	Operates at specialised psychopathology clinics

more insight and knowledge into this research topic, an instrumental case study has been chosen.

In general, case study methodology is not strictly planned but the researchers will be guided by what they will see in the field, given a planned field study with specific steps with data collection and analyses (Fidel 1984). This flexibility provides the researchers with the ability to deal with unexpected results; however, to reduce the risks that might appear during the observation and analyses of this research, a framework that was developed by Eisenhardt (1989) who states that case study involve of eight steps will employed. The eight steps include:

3.1. Getting Started

In this step, after reviewing and outlining the literature the research question will be developed and defined. A priori constructs will be examined for further measuring.

3.2. Selecting the Case Study

AFTA Society is chosen as the single case study that will be examined against the e-multimodal framework.

3.3. Crafting the Instruments and Protocols

Observation is the main method adopted to collect data for this research. Observation is a fundamental and highly important method in all qualitative inquiry (Yin 2009). As mentioned earlier, research and information in regards to adults with ADHD in Saudi Arabia, observing and examining AFTA online projects and methods that have been used to deliver their services as this will be the most stable method at this stage of the research. Tools, like Nvivo and MS Visio, will be used to facilitate this stage of the research to explore the relationships and identify differences in both contexts. Some of the aspects that will be observed and taken into consideration include the culture and how the role of IT in mental health will be different in a Saudi Arabian context.

3.4. Entering the Field

In this stage, the data will be collected. Data collection and analysis overlap and research can go back and forth until the main theory emerges.

3.5. Data Analysis

The case study approach allows the researcher to move back and forth from data collection and analysis, and it will continue until the main theory starts to develop. The data is analysed by using within-case analysis (Yin 2009). The data collected will be inspected for common characteristics that represent categories or themes (Boyatzis 1998). For instance, the important data or information collected will be divided into categories that will later involve a group of sub categories after more in depth analysis occurs.

3.6. Hypotheses Formulation

The relationship will be validated and the categories will be refined. Most likely in this stage, all findings will be considered and the overall theory can be shaped and tested. The relationships and findings will be verified among the unique and specific constructs and aspects identified, for instance cultures and languages.

3.7. Enfolding Literature

In this level, the findings will be compared with similar and conflicting literature.

3.8. Recommendation

Based on the outcomes of the data analysis and findings and the literature, a recommendation will be proposed.

In addition, this research will draw upon actor-network theory as a rich theoretical lens of analysis.

4. ACTOR-NETWORK THEORY (ANT)

ANT constitutes a framework for investigating how technical artefacts come into being (Callon 1991; Latour 1999; Allen 2004; Bijker et al. 1987). It addresses the role of technology in social settings and the processes by way of which it affects or is affected by social elements in a setting over time (Mähring et al. 2004). It focuses on actors and their attempts to secure their interests by forming and strengthening alliances in actor-networks which, in turn, generate technical artefacts (e.g. a pervasive e-health application) (Akrich 1992). As the actor-networks that generate these artefacts become stabilized, the technical artefacts are said to become taken for granted or "irreversible" (Denis et al. 2007).

Actors are human or non-human entities that can make their presence individually felt by other actors (Law 1987). ANT offers a symmetrical treatment between the technical and the social aspects of technology, in that both human and non-human actors are treated alike. That is, technical artefacts are treated as genuine actors, in that, while just merely physical, technical artefacts constitute a dynamic embodiment of human actors' subjectivities, including their motives, intentions, interests and prejudices (Faraj et al. 2004, p. 189). Using ANT can be advantageous particularly for investigating the development of complex technology such as e-health. ANT allows investigation to be focused on the nature of an actor-network as a representation of complex social interactions consisting of entrepreneurial political activities and negotiations that occur in order to enrol supporting actors or allies. Successful enrolment in a network represents the alignment of the otherwise diverse interests of its actors (McLoughlin 1999; Walsham 1997).

There are two pivotal concepts underpinning ANT, inscription and translation. Inscription means that actors that develop an artefact seek to inscribe their interests into it. When inscribed, interests may be manifested as specific anticipations and restrictions concerning future usage patterns of the artefact (Hanseth & Monteiro 1997). The artefact, thus, becomes a genuine actor that has the ability to impose the inscribed interest onto other actors, i.e. the users of the artefact. Therefore, the technical aspects of artefacts, their roles and constitutions are profoundly social (Mähring et al. 2004).

Translation constitutes a variety of negotiation methods whereby different actors' interests are continually aligned to achieve a stable actor-network that is dedicated to constructing a technical artefact (Rodon et al. 2008; Callon 1986a). Translation comprises problematisation, interessement, enrolment, and mobilization. During problematisation one (or more) initiating actor(s), also known as a focal actor, defines and constructs a problem and articulates the manner in which it affects its interests (Lee & Oh 2006). The focal actor also identifies other actors whose interests are consistent with its own and attempts to establish itself as an indispensable resource for them to resolve the identified problem (Callon 1986b). The aim of problematisation is to frame the identified problem in a way such that different actors draw mutually compatible understandings concerning the way the problem and its solution affect their interests rather than make all interests that same (Denis et al. 2007; Troshani & Lymer 2010; Troshani & Wickramasinghe 2014; Callon 1986b).

Interessement consists of processes that attempt to "lock in" other actors as allies or supporters in the actor-network. During interessement, the focal actor attempts to convince others that the interests defined during problematisation are aligned with its own. Successful interessement "confirms (more or less completely) the validity of the problematisation and the alliances it implies"

(Callon 1986b, pp. 209-210). During enrolment focal actors attempt to define and coordinate roles aiming to stabilize and strengthen the emerging network. It involves "multilateral negotiations, trials of strength and tricks that accompany the interessement and enable them [focal actor(s)] to succeed" (Callon 1986b, p. 211). Successful enrolment in networks represents the alignment of the otherwise diverse interests of its actors (Walsham 1997).

During mobilization the focal actor employs methods for ensuring that allies operate in accordance with their agreement and do not betray its interests (Callon 1986b). Although temporarily, stability may be achieved in an actor-network when allies are mobilized at which point "the underlying ideas have become institutionalized and are no longer seen as controversial" (Mähring et al. 2004, p. 214).

With ANT researchers "follow the actors" and explore how these actors themselves define unfolding events in their attempts to develop technology solutions (e.g. pervasive e-health applications) to solve healthcare problems (Latour 1987a; Latour 2005). When an actor-network achieves stability or agreement with respect to a technical solution, network actors are said to be aligned. In the healthcare settings, this means that relevant human actors, including patients, clinicians, policy makers, and non-human actors, including diagnostic equipment and software, codes of practice, have become aligned and their network solidified. That is, the emerging pervasive e-health applications that these actor-networks are attempting to generate have become taken for granted or "irreversible" (Denis et al. 2007; Timpka et al. 2007; Steen 2010; Greenhalgh & Stones 2010).

4.1. Using ANT to Tackle eMental Health Complexity

ANT provides a useful vehicle to capture actor involvement in the development of pervasive e-health and e-mental health solutions for many reasons (Sohn & Lee 2007). First, by focusing on actor-networks as the fundamental building blocks for developing pervasive e-health solutions, ANT looks at the relationships between actors as complex social interactions comprising entrepreneurial and political activities and negotiations (Latour 1987; Garud & Rappa 1994). That is, it examines the manner in which actors form, strengthen, and maintain networks of actor alliances in relation to pervasive e-health and e-mental health solutions, and how their goals are locked into patterns of interactions and in processes of ongoing alignment of dynamic interests (Mähring et al. 2004). By focusing on the evolving process of their construction, as opposed to focusing on pre-defined or fixed elements, insight can be generated concerning the effectiveness of the operation of pervasive e-health and e-mental solutions and the shape that they will (or will not) take in addition to drawing attention to both anticipated and unanticipated consequences of their use in healthcare settings (Robert et al. 2010; Broer et al. 2010). Therefore, ANT allows investigating such questions as how and why pervasive e-health and e-mental solutions "come into being and how users and other actors conform, ignore, modify, or usurp the original designers' interests" (Faraj et al. 2004, p. 189). In doing so, ANT can help investigate the fluidity of the healthcare reality and the underlying complex actor interactions as they unfold (Cresswell 2010; Walsham 1997; Lee & Oh 2006; Hanseth et al. 2004; Latour 1987).

This is important for two reasons: i) ANT takes an "action-oriented or formative" (Broer et al. 2010) process-based qualitative approach which opens up the healthcare 'black-box' which is critical if the requirements of pervasive e-health and e-mental health solutions are to be fully understood; and, ii) there is agreement in the literature that there is a "need to recognize that different actors can play multiple roles in multiple networks at multiple time points" (Cresswell et al. 2010, pp. 4-5). Thus, by recognizing healthcare fluidity, ANT facilitates formative assessments to studying pervasive e-health and e-mental solutions while recognizing the co-existence of multiple realities in actor-networks thereby challenging predictability assumptions of traditional summative outcome-oriented or causal approaches (Mol 1998; Cresswell 2010; Broer et al. 2010; Bate & Robert 2002).

Second, ANT offers a rich language that allows pervasive e-health researchers "not to distinguish a priori between [the] social and technical" (Hanseth & Monteiro 1997, p. 185), thereby encouraging "a detailed description of the concrete mechanisms at work which glue the [actor] network together – without being distracted by the means, technical or non-technical, of actually achieving this" (Hanseth & Monteiro 1997, p. 185). That is, by considering non-human actors in healthcare settings, such as e-health hardware devices or pervasive e-health software applications, ANT examines how these can affect the behavior of human actors and are affected by them. This is important because technical objects are "no longer viewed as passive "black box" containers of information, but as playing an active role that is determined by their position in the ever-changing network" (Cresswell et al. 2010, p. 4). By providing a lexicon that blurs the boundaries between the (non-human) technical and human actors, ANT helps achieve depth and richness in capturing the true complexity of healthcare relationships, and consequently, crystallize requirements of pervasive e-health solutions (McLean & Hassard 2004).

Third, ANT can be particularly useful in helping direct analysis toward improving the understanding of unfolding action. This includes identifying and distinguishing the categories of participating actors and their interests, as well as crucial developments concerning pervasive e-health solutions and actions undertaken by actors based on their interests to react to and affect such developments (Ramiller 2005; Ramiller 2007). Furthermore, with ANT, multiple human actors belonging to the same organization can be collec-

tively deemed as a single actor and their underlying stable networks can be included or excluded from analysis as necessary. According to Hanseth and Monteiro (1997)), this is justified as ANT "has a scalable notion of an actor" (p. 190), meaning that it "does not distinguish between a macro- and micro-actor because opening one (macro) black-box, there is always a new actor-network" (p. 190). Actors enrolled in and committed to the (micro-level) actor-networks within actant organizations can be considered to be spokespersons and representative of the interests of other actors in their organizations (Callon & Latour 1981).

This is consistent with ANT assumptions concerning the use of sociological levels (e.g. individual, group, organization) as units of analysis. Specifically, "ANT focuses on the identification of networks of actors, where the networks themselves are seen to become actors, as the scope of analysis widens. This affords a flexible framework that makes the "levels" in implementation research a matter of empirical discovery rather than stipulation, and that helps thereby to foster a greater realism in capturing the action that takes place." (Ramiller 2005, p. 53). This approach enables researchers to draw together actors from both micro- and macro contexts. In doing so, ANT focuses on micro-contexts, i.e. how actors interact with one another to shape pervasive e-health solutions, and uses findings to draw conclusions about macro contexts, i.e. political and institutional environments where actors are embedded (Cresswell 2010).

A number of studies have been found where ANT has been effectively used to research a number of issues in healthcare. For example, ANT has been employed to examine the development and adoption of electronic patient records (Greenhalgh & Stones 2010; Robert et al. 2010), the development of indoor smoke-free regulation in relation to tobacco use policy (Young et al. 2010), development of quality improvement collaboratives in mental health care (Broer et al. 2010), development of information infrastructures in psychiatric rehabilitation services (Timpka et al. 2006), and the development of genetic testing technologies (Williams-Jones & Graham 2003).

5. CHALLENGES OF USING ANT IN E-MENTAL HEALTH RESEARCH

Whilst ANT is criticized for its inherent limited capability for providing empirically verifiable evidence (Cresswell 2010), by offering a rich vocabulary, ANT can help both with explanation and interpretations of healthcare phenomena which can help refine information and requirements specification of pervasive e-health e-mental health solutions (Law & Hassard 1999). In this section, we discuss critical issues concerning the valid production of ANT accounts, including the achievement of symmetry which is necessary in order to strengthen explanation and interpretation in ANT accounts (McLean & Hassard 2004).

5.1. The Inclusion/Exclusion Issue

With ANT, one must closely "follow the actors" to understand how actor-network negotiations influence the shape that technical artefacts will take (Callon 1986a; Law 1991; Latour 1987). In practice, snowballing can be used to identify actors in pervasive e-health solutions networks (Aaker & Day 1990). To decide "who to include and who to exclude" (McLean & Hassard 2004, p. 499) investigative work can be directed at contextualizing a particular pervasive e-health solution as the assemblage that researchers wish to chart (Miller 1996). While following the actors, one can stop when the contextualisers (e.g. pervasive e-health solutions negotiations, interactions, alliances) stop, i.e. as references to these contextualisers or specific actors "melt from view" (Law 1991, p. 11).

5.2. The Humans/Non-Humans Issue

All actors including social and technical actors, rely on spokespersons to speak on their behalf (Pels 1995). Spokespersons can symmetrically speak for both "people and things, but only humans can act (can be permitted to act) as spokespersons" (Pels 1995, p. 138). Focusing on human interpretations only can provide a social bias of the technical which can adversely affect symmetry between the two (Collins & Yearley 1992). In response to this, researchers can follow Callon (1986b)) who argues that "no point of view is privileged and no interpretation is censored" (p. 200). Thus, researchers can follow all those involved in doing relevant work concerning pervasive e-health solutions, irrespective of how many and heterogeneous they are (Latour 1987). Heterogeneous actors can provide different perspectives which account for multiple realities. This offers triangulation whilst reducing the possibility of interpretations being locked in one mindset.

5.3. The Privileging and Status Issue

Technical actors (e.g. pervasive e-health applications) can be conceptualized as those whose interests they represent and inscribe (Walsham 1997) and which are shaped as "a consequence of the relations in which they are located and performed; that is, in, by and through these relations"(McLean & Hassard 2004, p. 507). E-health researchers can follow Callon and Latour (1992)) who argue that in the process of developing pervasive e-health solutions, both the social and the technical are "analytically composite" (p. 348) and "twin results" (p. 348) of network building processes and thus, no attempts should be made to analytically favour these solutions (Collins & Yearley 1992). Therefore, the emerging pervasive e-health solutions are indeed actors, but in same manner as other actors, they are susceptible to shaping and constraint (Ramiller 2007).

6. DISCUSSION

This research aims to investigate how an IS/IT solution that is designed to facilitate the treatment of adults with ADHD in an Australia context can be applied to a Saudi Arabian context. This will be done through observing and analysing the status of current treatments of adults with ADHD in Saudi Arabia and examining the cultural similarity and differences between Saudi Arabia and Australia.

On a micro level, this research will be seen in three different areas. This includes; human resources for the general mental health and wellbeing for ADHD individuals, and Saudi Arabia mental health services in their e-health development program. As mentioned earlier, ADHD impacts the quality of life of people and might even cause them to be in trouble with the law or take risks (Dalteg et al. 1998). Adults with ADHD have lower chances of completing a tertiary degree in comparison to their peers, and often they have higher drop out or failure to complete a university degree which also be thought of as a waste of resources (Lamberg 2003).

The outcome of this research will not only assist adults to have a better quality of life, but also help health providers such as AFTA Society to deliver its mission to help individuals with their general happiness, mental health and wellbeing, and sense of achievement. Technology will help the AFTA Society to provide better treatment of ADHD of people in Saudi Arabia.

By 2020 Saudi Arabia aims to develop a nationwide e-health programme that will cover all services and facilities of healthcare which will allow these services and facilities to use one single patient record; therefore, this research will contribute to this development, which will also aide in the introduction of e-mental health services and will provide high quality results that will assist both adults with ADHD and mental health providers.

7. CONCLUSION

E-health constitutes the use of digitally enabled technologies to facilitate the exchange of clinical, administrative, and transactional data ubiquitously in healthcare settings and has the potential to offer enormous value for all actors operating in healthcare including patients and healthcare providers (Ha & Lee 2008; Sohn & Lee 2007). Yet, taking advantage of the benefits that pervasive e-health and more specifically e-mental health can provide to improve the delivery of effective quality services in healthcare remains elusive for e-health entrepreneurs. At least in part this is attributed to the complexity of modern healthcare settings where pervasive e-health applications are expected to operate (Cho et al. 2008). In attempts to enhance current understanding concerning underlying contextual e-health complexity factors, this paper presents an argument concerning how e-health complexity can be tackled using ANT as an appropriate investigative lens. Specifically, it can help specify the requirements of pervasive e-health services that are expected to operate in fluid healthcare settings with fuzzy boundaries where causal and predictable behaviours can be elusive. This is important because ANT can help capture the multiple realities of actor-networks thereby potentially enhancing pervasive e-health effectiveness.

Additionally, ANT can assist in the generation of the currently absent comprehensive, multifaceted, and unified body of knowledge necessary to conduct healthcare activities in a manner addressing present inequalities through a consistent knowledge-based effort rather than, as it is presently done, through the erratic application of ever increasing funds. An existing case that serves to underscore this is the NHS Connecting for Health (a national e-health solution for the UK) that had to be abandoned on the 31st March 2013 after costing millions of pounds. While not a guarantee of success, we believe the adoption of an ANT analysis at the onset of this project would have helped to avoid many of the problems and crisis points experienced in this project. However, before it can be effectively applied it is vital that a deeper understanding of the critical issues, barriers, facilitators and key success factors be identified. In using ANT we realize that the theory has been criticized by several scholars (Latour 2005). However these criticisms are connected to its appropriateness as an ontology and/or epistemology. We believe that as a lens for facilitating a deeper understanding of complex operations it is most invaluable.

This research in progress has been developed to explore the possibilities to adapt an IS/IT solution, which is designed to treat and manage ADHD in adults in an Australian context, in the Saudi Arabian context. This investigation will assist mental health providers in Saudi Arabia to facilitate the treatment and management of ADHD in adults. In particular, it recommends that such a IS/IT solution can enable adults with ADHD to improve their quality of life and also better manage their ADHD. This investigation will inspire researchers and mental health providers to conduct research and analysis that seeks to enhance healthcare and health outcomes, and support the introduction of an e-mental health strategy in Saudi Arabia. This research also will contribute to e-health practice in Saudi Arabia as well as support policy development associated with e-mental health.

In closing, we believe that the use of ANT generally to shed light on the complexities of various pervasive e-health and e-mental health solutions at both macro and micro levels is a prudent use of this theory and we call for more research in this area.

REFERENCES

Aaker, D. A., & Day, G. S. (1990). *Marketing Research* (4th ed.). New York: Wiley.

Akrich, M. (1992). The de-scription of technical objects. In W. E. Bijker, J. Law, & M. I. T. Press (Eds.), *Shaping technology/building society: studies in sociotechnical change* (pp. 205–224). Cambridge, MA.

Al-Tawil, K. M. (2001). The Internet in Saudi Arabia. *Telecommunications Policy, 25*(8), 625–632. doi:10.1016/S0308-5961(01)00036-2

Allen, J. P. (2004). Redefining the network: Enrollment strategies in the PDA industry. *Information Technology & People, 17*(2), 171–185. doi:10.1108/09593840410542493

Almalki, M., Fitzgerald, G., & Clark, M. (2011). Health care system in Saudi Arabia: An overview. *Eastern Mediterranean Health Journal, 17*(10), PMID:22256414

Alqahtani, M. M. (2010). The comorbidity of ADHD in the general population of Saudi Arabian school-age children. *Journal of Attention Disorders, 14*(1), 25–30. doi:10.1177/1087054709347195 PMID:19850953

Altuwaijri, M. 2010, 'Supporting the Saudi e-health initiative: the Master of Health Informatics programme at KSAU-HS', EMHJ, vol. 16, no. 1.

Anthony, K., Nagel, D. M., & Goss, S. 2010, *The use of technology in mental health: Applications, ethics and practice*, Charles C Thomas Pub Limited. Arab News, *1.6 million children in KSA suffer from ADHD* Available from: <http://www.arabnews.com/news/553851>. [01/07].

Arns, M., de Ridder, S., Strehl, U., Breteler, M., & Coenen, A. (2009). Efficacy of neurofeedback treatment in ADHD: the effects on inattention, impulsivity and hyperactivity: a meta-analysis. *Clinical EEG and Neuroscience, 40*(3), 180–189. doi:10.1177/155005940904000311 PMID:19715181

Arns, M., Gunkelman, J., Breteler, M., & Spronk, D. (2008). EEG phenotypes predict treatment outcome to stimulants in children with ADHD. *Journal of Integrative Neuroscience*, *7*(03), 421–438. doi:10.1142/S0219635208001897 PMID:18988300

Barkley, R. A. (1998). *Attention deficit hyperactivity disorder: A handbook for diagnosis and treatment* (2nd ed.). New York: Guilford.

Barkley, R. A., Fischer, M., Edelbrock, C. S., & Smallish, L. (1990). The adolescent outcome of hyperactive children diagnosed by research criteria: I. An 8-year prospective follow-up study. *Journal of the American Academy of Child and Adolescent Psychiatry*, *29*(4), 546–557. doi:10.1097/00004583-199007000-00007 PMID:2387789

Barkley, R. A., Murphy, K. R., & Fischer, M. (2008). *ADHD in adults: What the science says*. New York: Guilford.

Bate, P., & Robert, G. (2002). Studying health care "quality" qualitatively: The dilemmas and tensions between different forms of evaluation research within the U.K. National Health Service. *Qualitative Health Research*, *12*(7), 966–091. doi:10.1177/104973202129120386 PMID:12214681

Beck, S. J., Hanson, C. A., Puffenberger, S. S., Benninger, K. L., & Benninger, W. B. (2010). A controlled trial of working memory training for children and adolescents with ADHD. *Journal of Clinical Child and Adolescent Psychology*, *39*(6), 825–836. doi:10.1080/15374416.2010.517162 PMID:21058129

Ben-Zeev, D., Davis, K. E., Kaiser, S., Krzsos, I., & Drake, R. E. (2012). *Mobile technologies among people with serious mental illness: Opportunities for future services* (pp. 1–4). Administration and Policy in Mental Health and Mental Health Services Research.

Bijker, W. E., Hughes, T. P., & Pinch, T. J. (1987). *The Social Construction of Technological Systems*. Cambridge, MA: MIT Press.

Boyatzis, R. E. (1998). Transforming qualitative information: Thematic analysis and code development. *Sage (Atlanta, Ga.)*.

Broer, T., Nieboer, A. P., & Bal, R. A. (2010). Opening the black box of quality improvement collaboratives: An Actor-Network theory approach. *BMC Health Services Research*, *10*(1), 1–9. doi:10.1186/1472-6963-10-265 PMID:20825648

CADDRA. 2011, Canadian Attention Deficit Hyperactivity Disorder Resource Alliance (CADDRA): Canadian ADHD Practice Guidelines, ed.^eds Third, CADDRA, Toronto ON.

Callon, M. (1986a). The sociology of an actor-network: the case of the electric vehicle. In M. Callon, J. Law, & A. Rip (Eds.), *Mapping the dynamics of science and technology* (pp. 19–34). London: Macmillan Press.

Callon, M. (1986b). Some elements of sociology translation: domestication of the scallops and the fishermen of St Brieuc Bay. In J. Law (Ed.), *Power, action & belief. A new sociology of knowledge?* (pp. 196–229). London: Routledge & Kegan Paul.

Callon, M. (1991). Techno-economic network and irreversability. In J. Law (Ed.), *A sociology of monsters. Essays on power, technology and domination* (pp. 132–164). London: Routledge.

Callon, M., & Latour, B. (1981). Unscrewing the Big Leviathan: how actors macrostructure reality and how sociologists help them to do so. In K. D. Knorr-Cetina & A. V. Cicourel (Eds.), *Advances in Social Theory and Methodology: Toward an Integration of Micro- and Macro-Sociologies* (pp. 277–303). Boston, Mass: Routledge and Kegan Paul.

Callon, M & Latour, B 1992, 'Don't throw the baby out with the bath school! A reply to Collins and Yearley', *Science as practice and culture*, vol. 343, p. 368.

Canadian Attention Deficit Hyperactivity Disorder Resource Alliance (CADDRA). (2011). *Canadian ADHD Practice Guidelines* (3rd ed.). Toronto, ON: CADDRA.

Cho, S., Mathiassen, L., & Nilsson, A. (2008). Contextual dynamics during health information systems implementation: An event-based actor-network approach. *European Journal of Information Systems*, *17*(6), 614–630. doi:10.1057/ejis.2008.49

Christensen, H., Griffiths, K. M., & Evans, K. 2002, e-Mental health in Australia: Implications of the Internet and related technologies for policy, Commonwealth Department of Health and Ageing Canberra, Canberra.

Christensen, H., & Petrie, K. (2013). State of the e-mental health field in Australia: Where are we now? *The Australian and New Zealand Journal of Psychiatry*, *47*(2), 117–120. doi:10.1177/0004867412471439 PMID:23297367

Collins, H., & Yearley, S. (1992). Epitemological chicken. In A. Pickering (Ed.), *Science, Practice and Culture*. Chicago, IL: University of Chicago Press.

Cresswell, K. M. (2010). Actor-Network Theory and its role in understanding the implementation of information technology developments in healthcare. *BMC Medical Informatics and Decision Making*, *10*(67), 1–11. PMID:21040575

Cresswell, K. M., Worth, A., & Sheikh, A. (2010). Actor-Network Theory and its role in understanding the implementation of information technology developments in healthcare. *BMC Medical Informatics and Decision Making*, *10*(1), 67. doi:10.1186/1472-6947-10-67 PMID:21040575

Creswell, J. W. (2013). *Research design: Qualitative, quantitative, and mixed methods approaches* (4th ed.). London: Sage Publications, Incorporated.

Dalteg, A., Gustafsson, P., & Levander, S. (1998). Hyperactivity syndrome is common among prisoners. ADHD not only a pediatric psychiatric diagnosis. *Lakartidningen*, *95*(26-27), 3078–3080. PMID:9679423

Denis, J.-L., Langley, A., & Rouleau, L. (2007). Strategizing in pluralistic contexts: Rethinking theoretical frames. *Human Relations*, *60*(1), 179–215. doi:10.1177/0018726707075288

Department of Human Services Victoria. *Attention deficit hyperactivity disorder - adults*. Available from: <http://www.betterhealth.vic.gov.au/bhcv2/bhcarticles.nsf/pages/Attention_deficit_hyperactivity_disorder_and_adults#>. [03/01].

Eisenhardt, K. M. (1989). Building theories from case study research. *Academy of Management Review*, *14*(4), 532–550.

Eysenbach, G. (2001). What is e-health? *Journal of Medical Internet Research*, *3*(2), e20. doi:10.2196/jmir.3.2.e20 PMID:11720962

Faraj, S., Kwon, D., & Watts, S. (2004). Contested artifact: Technology sensemaking, actor-networks, and the shaping of the web browser. *Information Technology & People*, *17*(2), 186–209. doi:10.1108/09593840410542501

Fidel, R. (1984). The case study method: A case study. *Library & Information Science Research*, 6(3), 273–288.

Gallagher, E. B. 2002, 'Modernization and health reform in Saudi Arabia, Chapter 4', Health care reform around the world. London, Auburn House, pp. 181-197.

Garud, R., & Rappa, M. A. (1994). A socio-cognitive model of technology evolution: The case of cochlear implants. *Organization Science*, 5(3), 344–362. doi:10.1287/orsc.5.3.344

Gevensleben, H., Holl, B., Albrecht, B., Vogel, C., Schlamp, D., & Kratz, O. et al. (2009). Is neurofeedback an efficacious treatment for ADHD? A randomised controlled clinical trial. *Journal of Child Psychology and Psychiatry, and Allied Disciplines*, 50(7), 780–789. doi:10.1111/j.1469-7610.2008.02033.x PMID:19207632

Goldstein, SE 2005, 'Editorial: Coaching as a treatment for ADHD'.

Greenhalgh, T., & Stones, R. (2010). Theorising big IT in health care: Strong stucturation theory meets actor-network theory. *Social Science & Medicine*, 70(9), 1285–1294. doi:10.1016/j.socscimed.2009.12.034 PMID:20185218

Gropper, R. J., Gotlieb, H., Kronitz, R., & Tannock, R. (2014). Working memory training in college students with ADHD or LD. *Journal of Attention Disorders*, 1087054713516490. PMID:24420765

Ha, K., & Lee, J. 2008, 'U-health and regulatory implications in Korea', Portland International Center for Management of Engineering and Technology (PICMET 2008 Proceedings).

Hanseth, O., Aanestad, M., & Berg, M. (2004). 'Actor-network theory and information systems. What's so special?'. *Information Technology & People*, 17(2), 116–123. doi:10.1108/09593840410542466

Hanseth, O., & Monteiro, E. (1997). 'Inscribing behavior in information infrastructure standards', *Accounting. Management & Information Technology*, 7(4), 183–211. doi:10.1016/S0959-8022(97)00008-8

Internet Live Stats. *Internet Users by Country (2014) - Internet Live Stats*. Available from: <http://www.internetlivestats.com/internet-users-by-country>. [09/07].

King Faisal Specialist Hospital Research Centre. *First Middle Eastern Symposium on Attention Deficit Hyperactivity Disorder (ADHD)*. Available from: <http://www.kfshrc.edu.sa/symposia/html/adhd.html>. [17/07].

Klingberg, T., Fernell, E., Olesen, P. J., Johnson, M., Gustafsson, P., & Dahlström, K. et al. (2005). Computerized training of working memory in children with ADHD-A randomized, controlled trial. *Journal of the American Academy of Child and Adolescent Psychiatry*, 44(2), 177–186. doi:10.1097/00004583-200502000-00010 PMID:15689731

Lamberg, L. (2003). ADHD Often Undiagnosed in Adults: Appropriate Treatment May Benefit Work, Family, Social Life. *Journal of the American Medical Association*, 290(12), 1565–1567. doi:10.1001/jama.290.12.1565 PMID:14506100

Latour, B. (1987). *Science in action*. Cambridge, MA: Harvard University Press.

Latour, B. (1987a). *Science in Action: How to Follow Scientists and Engineers Through Society*. Cambridge, Massachusetts: Harvard University Press.

Latour, B. 1999, 'On recalling ANT', in Actor-network Theory and After, eds J Law & J Hassard, Blackwell/Sociological Review, Oxford.

Latour, B. (2005). *Reassembling the Social: An Introduction to Actor-Network Theory*. Oxford: Oxford University Press.

Law, J. (1987). Technolong and heterogenous engineering: the case of Portugese expansion. In W. E. Bijker, T. P. Hughes, T. J. Pinch, & M. I. T. Press (Eds.), *The social construction of technological systems: new directions in the sociology and history of technology* (pp. 111–134). Cambridge, MA.

Law, J. (1991). Introduction. In J. Law (Ed.), *A Sociology of Monsters: Essays on Power, Technology, and Domination*. London: Routledge.

Law, J., & Hassard, J. (1999). *Actor-network theory and after*. Oxford, England: Blackwell.

Lee, H., & Oh, S. (2006). A standards war waged by a developing country: Understanding international standard setting from the actor-network perspective. *The Journal of Strategic Information Systems*, *15*(3), 177–195. doi:10.1016/j.jsis.2005.10.002

Mähring, M., Holmström, J., Keil, M., & Montealegre, R. (2004). Trojan actor-networks and swift translation: Bringing actor-network theory to IT project escalation studies. *Information Technology & People*, *17*(2), 210–238. doi:10.1108/09593840410542510

Mannuzza, S., Klein, R., Bessler, A., Malloy, P., & LaPadula, M. (1998). Adult psychiatric status of hyperactive boys grown up. *The American Journal of Psychiatry*, *155*(4), 493–498. PMID:9545994

Mannuzza, S., Klein, R. G., Bessler, A., Malloy, P., & LaPadula, M. (1993). Adult outcome of hyperactive boys: Educational achievement, occupational rank, and psychiatric status. *Archives of General Psychiatry*, *50*(7), 565. doi:10.1001/archpsyc.1993.01820190067007 PMID:8317950

McLean, C., & Hassard, J. (2004). Symmetrical absence/symmetrical absurdity: Critical notes on the production of actor-network accounts. *Journal of Management Studies*, *41*(3), 493–519. doi:10.1111/j.1467-6486.2004.00442.x

McLoughlin, I. (1999). *Creative technological change: the shaping of technology and organisations*. London: Routledge. doi:10.4324/9780203019870

Miller, P. (1996). The multiplying machine. *Accounting, Organizations and Society*, *21*(7/8), 615–630.

Ministry News. *King Abdullah Approves of Allocating SR 15 Billion to Establish 22 Health Projects*. Available from: <http://www.moh.gov.sa/en/Ministry/MediaCenter/News/Pages/News-2013-04-24-003.aspx>. [15/07].

Ministry of Health Portal. *National e-Health Strategy*. Available from: <http://www.moh.gov.sa/en/Ministry/nehs/Pages/Overview-of-eHealth.aspx>. [12/07].

Mol, A. 1998, 'Ontological politics. A word and some questions', The Sociological Review, vol. 46, no. S, pp. 74-89.

Moumtzoglou, A. 2011, 'E-Health: A Bridge to People-Centered Health Care', E-health Systems Quality and Reliability: Models and Standards, p. 47.

Munshi, A. M. A. (2014). Knowledge and misperceptions towards diagnosis and management of attention deficit hyperactive disorder (ADHD) among primary school and kindergarten female teachers in Al-Rusaifah district, Makkah City, Saudi Arabia. *International Journal of Medical Science and Public Health*, *3*(4), 3–4. doi:10.5455/ijmsph.2014.120220141

Murphy, K. R., Barkley, R. A., & Bush, T. (2002). Young adults with attention deficit hyperactivity disorder: Subtype differences in comorbidity, educational, and clinical history. *The Journal of Nervous and Mental Disease*, *190*(3), 147–157. doi:10.1097/00005053-200203000-00003 PMID:11923649

Nuviun Digital Health. *Saudi Arabia is Building a Massive Nationwide eHealth Network*. Available from: <http://nuviun.com/content/blog/saudi-Arabia-eHealth>. [14/07].

Pels, D. (1995). The politics of symmetry. *Social Studies of Science, 26*(2), 277–304. doi:10.1177/030631296026002004

Pettersson, R., Söderström, S., Edlund-Söderström, K., & Nilsson, K. W. (2014). Internet-Based Cognitive Behavioral Therapy for Adults With ADHD in Outpatient Psychiatric Care A Randomized Trial. *Journal of Attention Disorders*, 1087054714539998. PMID:24970720

Polanczyk, G., de Lima, M., Horta, B., Biederman, J., & Rohde, L. (2007). The worldwide prevalence of ADHD: A systematic review and metaregression analysis. *The American Journal of Psychiatry, 164*(6), 942–948. doi:10.1176/appi.ajp.164.6.942 PMID:17541055

Pope, D. J. (2010). The impact of inattention, hyperactivity and impulsivity on academic achievement in UK university students. *Journal of Further and Higher Education, 34*(3), 335–345. doi:10.1 080/0309877X.2010.484053

Prevatt, F., Lampropoulos, G. K., Bowles, V., & Garrett, L. (2011). The use of between session assignments in ADHD coaching with college students. *Journal of Attention Disorders, 15*(1), 18–27. doi:10.1177/1087054709356181 PMID:20019381

Proudfoot, J., Parker, G., Pavlovic, D. H., Manicavasagar, V., Adler, E., & Whitton, A. (2010). Community attitudes to the appropriation of mobile phones for monitoring and managing depression, anxiety, and stress. *Journal of Medical Internet Research, 12*(5), e64. doi:10.2196/jmir.1475 PMID:21169174

Qurban, M., & Austria, R. 2008, 'Public Perception on E-Health Services: Implications of Preliminary Findings of the King Fahd Military Medical Complex for Military Hospitals in the Kingdom of Saudi Arabia', in *European and Mediterranean Conference on Information Systems (EMCIS), Dubai*.

Ramiller, N. C. (2005). Applying the sociology of translation to a system project in a lagging enterprise. *Journal of Information Technology Theory and Application, 7*(1), 51–76.

Ramiller, NC 2007, 'Constructing safety: system designs, system effects, and the play of heterogeneous interests in a behavioral health care setting', *International Journal of Medical Informatics*, vol. 76S, no. Supplement 1, pp. S196-S204.

Robert, G., Greenhalgh, T., MacFarlane, F., & Peacock, R. (2010). Adopting and assimilating new non-pharmaceutical technologies into health care: A systematic review. *Journal of Health Services Research & Policy, 15*(4), 243–250. doi:10.1258/jhsrp.2010.009137 PMID:20592046

Rodon, J, Pastor, JA, Sese, F & Christiaanse, E 2008, 'Unravelling the dynamics of IOIS implementation: an actor-network study of an IOIS in the seaport of Barcelona', *Journal of Information Technology*, vol. 23, no. 97-108.

Rucklidge, J. J., & Tannock, R. (2002). Neuropsychological profiles of adolescents with ADHD: Effects of reading difficulties and gender. *Journal of Child Psychology and Psychiatry, and Allied Disciplines, 43*(8), 988–1003. doi:10.1111/1469-7610.00227 PMID:12455921

Simsim, M. T. (2011). Internet usage and user preferences in Saudi Arabia. *Journal of King Saud University-Engineering Sciences, 23*(2), 101–107. doi:10.1016/j.jksues.2011.03.006

Sohn, M., & Lee, J. 2007, 'U-health in Korea: opportunities and challenges', Portland International Center for Management of Engineering and Technology (PICMET 2007 Proceedings).

Stake, RE 1995, 'The art of case study research'.

Steen, J. (2010). Actor-network theory and the dilemma of the resource concept in strategic management. *Scandinavian Journal of Management*, *26*(3), 324–331. doi:10.1016/j.scaman.2010.05.003

Swartz, S. L., Prevatt, F., & Proctor, B. E. (2005). A coaching intervention for college students with Attention Deficit/Hyperactivity Disorder. *Psychology in the Schools*, *42*(6), 647–656. doi:10.1002/pits.20101

Taleb, RAA & Farheen, A 2013, ' A Descriptive Study of Attention Deficit Hyperactivity Disorder in Sabia City, Saudi Arabia ', *Int J Cur Res Rev*, vol. 5, no. 11.

The Royal Australian College of Physicians. (2009). *Australian Guidelines on Attention Deficit Hyperactivity Disorder (ADHD) (draft)*. Canberra: NH&MRC.

Timpka, T., Bång, M., Delbanco, T., & Walker, J. (2007). Information infrastructure for inter-organizational mental health services: An actor-network theory analysis of psychiatric rehabilitation. *Journal of Biomedical Informatics*, *40*(4), 429–437. doi:10.1016/j.jbi.2006.11.001 PMID:17182285

Timpka, T., Bånga, M., Delbanco, T., & Walker, J. (2006). Information infrastructure for inter-organizational mental health services: An actor-network theory analysis of psychiatric rehabilitation. *Journal of Biomedical Informatics*, *40*(4), 429–437. doi:10.1016/j.jbi.2006.11.001 PMID:17182285

Troshani, I., & Lymer, A. (2010). Translation in XBRL standardization. *Information Technology & People*, *23*(2), 136–164. doi:10.1108/09593841011052147

Troshani, I., & Wickramasinghe, N. 2014 Tackling Complexity in E-Health with Actor-network Theory, *Proceedings of 47th Hawaii International Conference on System Sciences (HICSS 2014)*, 6-9 January, Waikoloa, Hawaii. doi:10.1109/HICSS.2014.372

Walsham, G. (1997). Actor-network and IS research: current status and future prospects. In A. S. Lee, J. Liebenau, & J. I. DeGross (Eds.), *Information Systems and Qualitative Research* (pp. 466–480). London: Chapman & Hall. doi:10.1007/978-0-387-35309-8_23

Wang, J.-R., & Hsieh, S. (2013). Neurofeedback training improves attention and working memory performance. *Clinical Neurophysiology*, *124*(12), 2406–2420. doi:10.1016/j.clinph.2013.05.020 PMID:23827814

Whittaker, R., Merry, S., Stasiak, K., McDowell, H., Doherty, I., & Shepherd, M. et al. (2012). MEMO–A mobile phone depression prevention intervention for adolescents: Development process and postprogram findings on acceptability from a randomized controlled trial. *Journal of Medical Internet Research*, *14*(1), e13. doi:10.2196/jmir.1857 PMID:22278284

Wilens, T. E., Adler, L. A., Adams, J., Sgambati, S., Rotrosen, J., & Sawtelle, R. et al. (2008). Misuse and diversion of stimulants prescribed for ADHD: A systematic review of the literature. *Journal of the American Academy of Child and Adolescent Psychiatry*, *47*(1), 21–31. doi:10.1097/chi.0b013e31815a56f1 PMID:18174822

Williams-Jones, B., & Graham, J. E. (2003). Actor-network theory: A tool to support the ethical analysis of commercial genetic testing. *New Genetics & Society*, *22*(3), 271–296. doi:10.1080/1463677032000147225 PMID:15115034

Yin, R. K. (2009). Case study research: Design and methods. *Sage (Atlanta, Ga.)*.

Young, D., Borland, R., & Coghill, K. (2010). An actor-network theory analysis of policy innovation for smoke-free places: Understanding change in complex systems. *American Journal of Public Health, 100*(7), 1208–1217. doi:10.2105/AJPH.2009.184705 PMID:20466949

Zwart, L. M., & Kallemeyn, L. M. (2001). Peer-Based Coaching for College Students with ADHD and Learning Disabilities. *Journal of Postsecondary Education and Disability, 15*(1), 1–15.

Chapter 65
Human and Organizational Factors of Healthcare Data Breaches:
The Swiss Cheese Model of Data Breach Causation And Prevention

Faouzi Kamoun
Zayed University, UAE

Mathew Nicho
University of Dubai, UAE

ABSTRACT

Over the past few years, concerns related to healthcare data privacy have been mounting since healthcare information has become more digitized, distributed and mobile. However, very little is known about the root cause of data breach incidents; making it difficult for healthcare organizations to establish proper security controls and defenses. Through a systematic review and synthesis of data breaches literature, and using databases of earlier reported healthcare data breaches, the authors re-examine and analyze the causal factors behind healthcare data breaches. The authors then use the Swiss Cheese Model (SCM) to shed light on the technical, organizational and human factors of these breaches. The author's research suggests that incorporating the SCM concepts into the healthcare security policies and procedures can assist healthcare providers in assessing the vulnerabilities and risks associated with the maintenance and transmission of protected health information.

INTRODUCTION

Personal health records (PHR) and electronic health records play an important role in managing health information and enhancing the qual-ity of patients' healthcare through enhanced collection, compilation, storage, tracking and dissemination of health records among health-care providers (Kierkegaard, 2012). The health sector is characterized by a wealth of ever grow-

DOI: 10.4018/978-1-4666-8756-1.ch065

ing information that is dispersed throughout the healthcare organization and its downstream chain of business associates (BA) which includes any person or entity that creates, receives, maintains, or transmits protected health information (PHI) in fulfilling certain functions or activities for the health organization (HHS, 2013a). At the same time, as the healthcare sector is shifting from paper-based to electronic records, electronic data archives are accumulating in healthcare facilities and administrative agencies (O'Keefe & Connolly, 2011). The exchange of electronic protected health information (ePHI) and electronic health records (EHR) further accentuated the need to protect patients' health information, while guaranteeing easy access and a smooth flow of this information among the authorized entities.

Health information is believed to be among the most sensitive and confidential personal data, with the result that confidential data hemorrhage is exposing healthcare providers to unprecedented legal and financial risks (Johnson, 2009).

According to Johnson (2009) data hemorrhages come from many different sources like ambulatory healthcare providers, acute-care hospitals, physician groups, medical laboratories, insurance carriers, back-offices of health maintenance organizations, and outsourced service providers such as billing, collection, and transcription firms. The effects of data breaches on these parties are manifold. The improper disclosure or misuse of health information can cause serious reputational harm such as discrimination, stigmatization, loss of insurance and/or employment (Kulynych & Korn, 2002). The financial costs of data breaches, which include both direct costs, such as "clean-up" costs, and indirect costs, such as loss of revenues from reputational harm, are perhaps the most damaging factors from an organizational perspective. Data breaches can also lead to privacy violations, medical identity fraud, financial identity theft (such as forged taxation, fake health insurance and drug prescription claims) and identity theft

(Johnson, 2009). Thus healthcare information security and privacy is a major ethical and legal issue (Appari & Johnson, 2010). In particular, the ethical principle of personal autonomy suggests that individuals have the right to control all matters related to their own body, including their personal health information (Neame, 2012).This right translates into public expectations and legal requirements that healthcare providers shall secure the privacy and confidentiality of patients' health records. We should note however that regulatory compliance and adoption of privacy policies are not strong indicators of adequate patient privacy protection (e.g. Antón et al., 2007, Antón et al., 2010; Bhatti & Grandison, 2010; Grandison & Bhatti, 2010; Massey et al., 2010).

Despite the ethical and legal obligations of healthcare providers to protect the confidentiality of patients' health records, the past few years have witnessed an increase in the number and scope of reported healthcare data breach incidents. This is due to many factors, including (1) the fact that breach reporting became mandatory in September 2009, (2) the ease at which the healthcare sector can be penetrated, and (3) the wealth of sensitive personal information available and accessible to criminals in a patient's health record. For example, a PHR may reveal personal information (such as name, dates of birth, social security number, address, employer and phone numbers), financial and insurance information (such as bank account, credit card numbers, and insurance numbers) and health information (such as diagnosis results, medications, allergies, addiction problems and treatment types).

Despite all forms of legislations, data encryption, and security technologies made available during the past years, one fundamental question remains that is still not fully addressed: "why do data breaches[1] still occur in the healthcare sector?" While a thorough answer is not evident, this research aims to shed light on the possible causes that might contribute to healthcare data breaches.

Few studies have been conducted to investigate the root cause of healthcare data breaches. For example, a recent study, conducted by the Ponemon Institute (Ponemon (2012a)) showed that over 78 percent of the 709 surveyed IT practitioners blamed employee behavior, both malicious and negligent, as the major cause of data breaches. In particular, careless employees losing laptops or other mobile devices, mishandling of data at rest and in motion and malicious employees or other insiders have been identified as the root causes of most of the reported data breaches. However, one might question whether these survey results were biased towards the *"careless worker"* myth that tends to put the blame on people and hence focuses on changing their behavior. One might also conjecture that other potential latent organizational factors may play an equally important role in healthcare data breaches.

This work is motivated by the fact that a good understanding of the root causes of data breach incidents is critical for instituting an effective data breach risk management and security governance. The objectives of this paper are to:

1. Propose a framework to integrate reported healthcare data breaches into a comprehensive model that provides a better understanding of data breach causation and prevention.
2. Identify the constituent components of the proposed framework within the context of healthcare data breaches.
3. Apply the framework to better understand the causes of healthcare data breaches and outline effective risk mitigation strategies.

This paper is organized as follows:

In section 2, we begin by surveying recently reported healthcare data breach incidents. The relevant literature is reviewed and the research contribution is highlighted in section 3. Next, in sections 4 and 5, we provide a quick review of human error theory, with a special emphasis on the Swiss cheese model and its relevance to this research. In section 6, we describe our research methodology and outline the data collection approach of this study. In section 7, we demonstrate how to apply the Swiss cheese model to better understand the factors behind healthcare data breaches. Finally, in section 7, we summarize the usefulness of our proposed model and outline its practical implications.

Healthcare Data Breaches and Notification Laws

The growing concerns over data privacy violations and identity thefts led to the enactment of several privacy and security breach notification laws. For example, in the United States, California was the first state to enact in 2002 a data breach notification law, the Senate Bill 1386 (SB 1386), also known as the California Security Breach Notification Act. SB 1386 requires state agencies and other entities to notify residents of California in the event of unauthorized access to unencrypted personal information. California also enacted Senate Bill 13 in 2005, which requires that state agencies may not disclose personal information to researchers at the University of California or other nonprofit institutions, unless they get the approval of the Committee for the Protection of Human Subjects for the California Health and Human Services Agency. In 2007, California passed Assembly Bill 1298 (AB 1298) to expand SB 1386 to cover the protection of medical and health insurance information. Following California's lead, several other U.S states have enacted their own data security notification laws. At the federal level, the Health Insurance Portability and Accountability Act (HIPAA) provided the first national standard in the U.S for safeguarding personal health information by establishing privacy and security guidelines to regulate the use and disclosure of PHI. The Health Information Technology for Economic and Clinical Health (HITECH) act of 2009 provided additional requirements pertaining to the privacy and security of the electronic transmission of PHI. For instance, HITECH introduced breach notification requirements, new enforcement provisions, and tightened the sanctions against privacy violations of PHI. Furthermore, to enforce security when PHI is accessed or exchanged among organizations, HITECH extends HIPAA's security, privacy and liability rules to cover the business associates of the covered entities[2].

Despite all the above mandates and regulations, and as highlighted hereafter, there is ample evidence in the literature that many health organizations are nonetheless unprepared to prevent, cope with or respond to a data breach:

According to the Privacy Rights Clearing House, three of the six most significant data breaches were in the healthcare sector. In 2011, out of the 7,288,453 records in the Privacy Rights Clearing House database, 199 records were made public, fitting the criteria of healthcare medical providers. These breaches included (1) unintended disclosure of sensitive information posted publicly on a website, mishandled or sent to the wrong party via email, fax or mail; (2) hacking, spyware or malware; (3) payment card fraud; (4) insider threats; and (5) physical loss or stealing of non-electronic records, portable devices or stationary electronic devices (PRCH, 2012).

The Identity Theft Resource Center revealed that 133 out of the 399 reported data breaches in 2012 (as of the 28th of November 2012) were health-related, divulging 2,190,845 medical records (ITRC, 2012)

A recent study, conducted by the Ponemon Institute, showed that reported healthcare data breaches have increased by 32% from 2010 to 2011 (Ponemon, 2011). Furthermore, nearly 60% of healthcare organizations have experienced at least one data breach (Sessions & Kobus, 2012) These statistics, however, do not necessarily reflect actual increase in data breaches, as they might be the likely consequence of the new US reporting mandates that were introduced in 2009. In 2011, it is estimated the average per capita cost of a healthcare data breach was $240 for each stolen or lost record (Ponemon, 2012b). This organizational cost comprises (1) the lost revenue from turnover of existing patients/customers; (2) opportunity cost; (3) detection, escalation and notification costs; and (4) post data breach expenses (including the cost associated with special forensic and remediation activities, legal expenditures, discount offerings for future products and services, and regulatory interventions).

Table 1. Common causes of data breaches involving more than 500 individuals (HHS, 2011)

Cause	Number of reported incidents	Number of affected individuals	Additional details
Theft of paper or electronic media records	99	2,979,121	Includes theft of backup tapes, laptops, desktop computers, portable electronic devices, and network servers.
Loss of electronic media or paper records, containing PHI	33	1,156,847	Includes loss of portable devices (backup tapes, compact discs, memory cards, flash derives, smart phones, laptops), paper records, and network hard drives.
Unauthorized access to, or uses or disclosures of PHI	31	1,006,393	Includes hacking, unauthorized employees accessing PHI, and authorized employees engaged in unauthorized use of PHI.
Human or technological errors	19	78,663	Includes misdirected mailings
Improper disposal of PHI	11	70,279	Includes the mishandling of PHI by business associates.

The U.S. Department of Health and Human Services (HSS) reported in its 2011 annual report to Congress that from September 23, 2009 (the date the HITECH breach notification requirements became effective), to December 31, 2010, over 30,000 instances of healthcare data breaches have been reported, affecting 7.8 million patients (HHS, 2011). In particular, in 2010 less than 1% of the reported healthcare data breaches involved 500 or more individuals, yet these large breaches affected more than 99% of the 5.4 million exposed individuals. The causes of these reported incidents are summarized in Table 1.

In 2010, the HHS received more than 25,000 reports of "smaller" breaches involving fewer than 500 individuals. These smaller breaches affected more than 50,000 individuals. Most of these reported breaches were due to misdirected communications and impacted just one individual. Furthermore, in 2010, the greatest number of reported breaches originated from human or technological errors and often these incidents involved the PHI of one or two individuals (HHS, 2011).

Recent studies have also shown that, besides employees' abuse of access privilege, negligence is still a major source of data breaches (Kobus, 2012), as evident from the following statistics:

1. In a study conducted by the Ponemon Institute, 39% of the data breach incidents involved a negligent employee or contractor (Ponemon, 2012a).
2. In the UK, figures released to the privacy campaign group Big Brother Watch revealed that 806 healthcare data breaches took place at 152 National Health Service trusts between 2008 and 2011. These breaches included 23 incidents of PHI being posted on social networking sites by medical staff, 129 cases of employees illicitly searching for PHI about colleagues and family members, and 57 incidents were related to the theft or loss of unencrypted PHI. These reported data breaches resulted in the dismissal of 102 health service employees (Laja, 2011).
3. In Europe, recent studies have shown that most of the healthcare data breaches were due to the lack of encryption and employee carelessness, as opposed to hackers. In particular, negligence and carelessness of hospital employees in handling sensitive medical records were identified as the leading cause of healthcare data breaches, accounting for 41 percent of all data breaches (Kierkegaard, 2012).
4. Employee negligence has also been cited by Johnson and Willey (2011) who demonstrated with concrete examples how peer-to-peer (P2P) file-sharing networks contained leaked files that had significant PHI content.

While the majority of earlier studies have mostly focused on individual errors as the major cause of healthcare data breaches, we argue that other important organizational factors needs to also be taken into account. In fact, a more thorough analysis of healthcare data breach incidents suggests that these breaches are not usually caused by a single failure and mistake, but can be traced back to a chain of errors. Hence, in order to mitigate the risks of data breaches, we must enhance our understanding of how data breach accidents do occur. This is particularly significant since learning from reported data breaches can be better accomplished if we better comprehend the root causes of these events.

Literature Review and Research Contribution

We conducted a systematic review of the extant literature from the health informatics and Information Systems security research. Our review focused on identifying the anatomy, events, statistics, and taxonomies related to healthcare data breaches, with special focus on theoretical models that could help us better understand the nature and root causes of these breaches. This review enabled us to recognize that the lack of theoretical models that can explain the root causes of healthcare data breaches is a major gap in the existing literature. Accordingly, we looked at ways to integrate the various collected healthcare data breach literature contributions into a coherent model that would better explain the causes of data breach incidents.

To date. very limited research has been conducted to investigate the root causes of data breach incidents, as most of the earlier studies focused on outlining taxonomies of organizational data breaches, without delving deeper into the underlying causation factors. For example, based on the data breaches reported by the Privacy Rights Clearinghouse (PRCH, 2012) and the Data Loss DB (OSF, 2012), Neame (2012) classified data breaches into three main categories and seven sub-classes, as highlighted in Figure 1.

Neame (2012) proposed several preventive measures to address each of the above seven data breach threat categories. Collins et al (2011) applied the Situational Crime Prevention (SCP) methodology to strengthen the security procedures and reduce the number of data breaches. They highlighted the fact that much of the available literature on data breaches had focused more on the technical perspectives, related to advanced computer-based defenses, and seemed to neglect the underlying human and organizational factors.

To our knowledge, no prior study has been conducted to better understand the underlying human and organizational factors of healthcare data breaches. In fact, to date no comprehensive model has been developed to better explain the

Figure 1. Neame's taxonomy of data breaches (Neame, 2012)

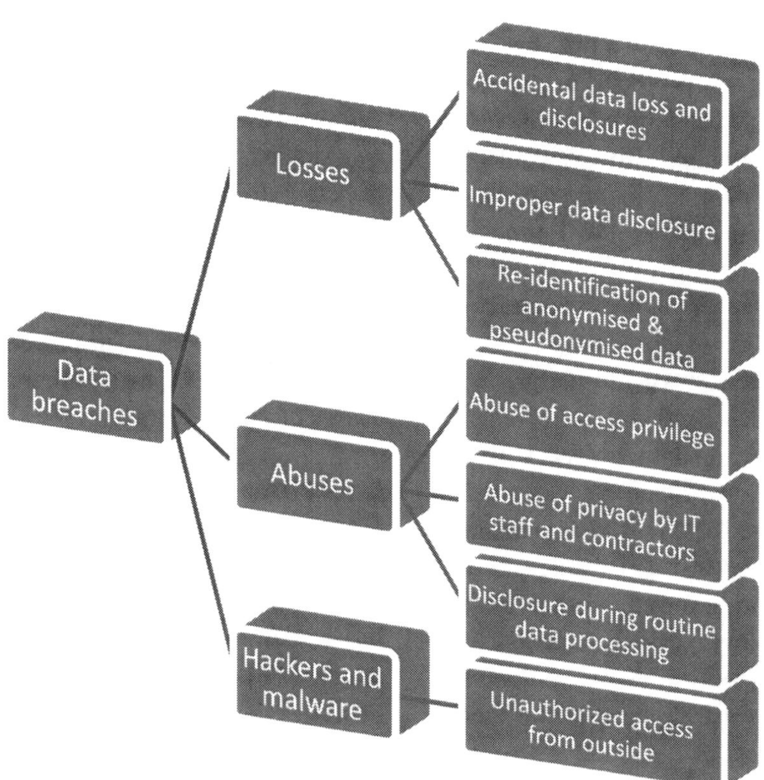

causes of data breaches. Thus, the aim of this study is to address this gap and contribute to healthcare data breach literature by exploring the multifaceted roots of healthcare data breaches. More precisely, this contribution aims to add to the existing body of knowledge about healthcare data breaches by proposing an analytical theory, based on the SCM, to shed light on the human, organizational, and technical perspectives of healthcare data breach causation and prevention. In particular, this contribution provides a more holistic approach to uncover the root causes of human-induced healthcare data breaches that go beyond individual errors, omissions, or malicious acts to include potential latent organizational and technical deficiencies. This integrated approach to data breach causation and prevention can enhance the readiness of healthcare organizations to proactively manage future data breaches.

Human Error Theory

In this section, we provide a brief summary of the key concepts in the human error theory that are relevant to this research. Some of these concepts will be revisited in section 7.

Various models and theories have been developed to explain human errors. For example, Reason (1990) distinguishes between:

1. **Design Versus Human-Induced Errors:** For example, while fingers are often pointed at healthcare professionals, following a data breach, poor data management policies and processes (design errors) might be the root cause of the breach.
2. **Variable Versus Constant Errors:** Variable errors are random in nature and difficult to predict, while constant errors follow some kind of consistent (yet risky) pattern that can be predicted and hence controlled. For example, among the top significant data breaches reported by the Privacy Rights Clearing House (ITRC, 2012) is the theft of

laptop and desktop computers. In particular leaving laptops that contain unencrypted PHI unattended in employee vehicles has been a constant and recurring error that has led to numerous data breaches.

Based on the intention, errors can also be classified as *slips, lapses, mistakes and violations* (Reason, 1990).

1. Slips are actions that were not performed as intended or planned.
2. Lapses are missed actions or omissions caused by the lack of attention.
3. Mistakes are errors emanating from faulty plans or intentions.
4. Violations are errors that result from intentional or deliberate actions that are often against the established rules and regulations. These can be categorized as *routine, situational and optimizing violations*. Routine violations are errors that became the normal way of doing things, such as shortcuts to established procedures. Situational violations are the result of particular circumstances, such as time pressure or the difficulty to comply with the rules under the given circumstances. Optimizing violations involve breaking established rules for self-gratification (fun, curiosity, and thrill) or personal benefit.

Another key concept in human error theory is the "defenses in depth" approach towards error management (Reason, 1990). This concept is based on the principle that there are many stages where errors can occur, and hence various stages where defenses can be built to prevent them.

The Swiss Cheese Model (SCM)

The Swiss cheese model (Reason, 1990) of accident causation and response is a widely accepted model that brought major contribution to the discipline of organizational and human error management. This model reflects on contemporary attempts towards better understanding the complexity of the socio-technical systems. The SCM has been used in risk analysis and management of human systems, including aviation, emergency, engineering and medical safety. For instance, the International Civil Aviation Organization (ICAO) has formally adopted the SCM to better understand the human factors behind airplane crashes. The SCM depicts human systems as multiple slices of Swiss cheese that are stacked together. Each slice represents one layer of human system defense against failure.

Reason (1990) argues that most organizational errors can be traced to four or more levels, including organizational influences (such as lack of funding and training), unsafe supervision, preconditions for unsafe acts (such as mental fatigue and poor communication/coordination practices), and the unsafe acts themselves.

The holes in the cheese slices represent weaknesses in the individual parts of the system, and they continuously evolve by opening, shutting, and shifting their positions. When holes momentarily line up, a "trajectory of accident opportunity" is created, allowing the hazard to penetrate all the holes of the defense layers, leading to failure. The SCM endorses the concept of causation chain, which recognizes that most accidents happen when all windows of error opportunities, across all levels of the organization, align. The SCM also suggests that by putting more defensive layers (slices) and by keeping fewer/smaller holes, one can minimize the occurrence of potential errors. Reason (1990) noticed that investigators often focused their efforts on the unsafe act of the operators that led to the accident, while inadvertently neglecting other important factors. In fact, an important concept embedded in the SCM is the causal sequence of human failures which recognizes that holes in the defenses happen for two reasons, namely active (operational) failures and latent (organizational) failures.

Active failures are the unsafe acts committed by people who are in direct contact with the system and that can be directly related to the accident. They can take various forms such as slips, lapses, fumbles, mistakes, and procedural violations (Reason, 1990).

Latent failures are dormant weaknesses in the system (aka "resident pathogens") that, when manifested, combine with active failures to penetrate the layers of defenses and contribute to the accident. They often arise from strategic and top-level decisions, and occur because of poor regulations, unworkable procedures, poor documentation, inadequate tools, and bad decisions made by the top management. Latent failures can trigger two types of undesirable effects. First, they can develop towards error-provoking conditions such as time-pressure, inadequate training, fatigue, and inadequate equipment. Second, they can create ongoing holes in the defense lines (Reason, 1990).

Compared to active failures, latent failures can be anticipated, identified and remedied much easier, thus promoting a proactive risk management approach.

Reason's SCM advocates that human error problems can be viewed from two perspectives: the person approach and the system approach (Reason, 2000).

The person approach emphasizes the individuals' errors and procedural violation, blaming people for carelessness, inattention, poor motivation, negligence and recklessness. The counter-measures in this approach are mainly geared towards reducing unwanted variability in human behavior by raising safety awareness, refining existing procedures, and taking the necessary disciplinary actions (Reason, 2000).

The system approach recognizes that human errors are unavoidable and can be expected even in high reliability organizations and that these mistakes are consequences rather than causes. Therefore, the approach turns its focus on the conditions under which the individuals work. It argues that errors are rooted deep in "upstream systematic factors". These include recurrent error traps and the underlying weaknesses that are often rooted in the organization's processes, culture, attitude towards risk-taking, and its aptitude to learn from past mistakes. The counter-measures in the system approach focuses on changing the conditions under which people work and on building safeguards and system defenses to mitigate errors (Reason, 2000). Reason (2000, p769) noted that:

Two important features of human error tend to be overlooked. First, it is often the best people who make the worst mistakes – error is not the monopoly of an unfortunate few. Second, far from being random, mishaps tend to fall into recurrent patterns. The same set of circumstances can provoke similar errors, regardless of the people involved. The pursuit of greater safety is seriously impeded by an approach that does not seek out and remove the error-provoking properties within the system at large.

As a conceptual model, the SCM suggests that no one failure, human or technical, is sufficient to cause a mishap. Rather, accidents are the outcomes of a combination of several causal factors arising at different levels of the system (Reason et al., 2006).

Research Methodology and Data Collection

To get deeper insights into the technical, human and organizational factors of healthcare data breaches we gathered and analyzed an extensive list of reported data breaches from various credible sources, as illustrated in Table 2. This data collection activity has been conducted over a period of eight months (September 2012-April 2013).

In our case, we refined our queries to search for data breaches within the medical sector only. We also made use of the literature analysis methodology by conducting a systematic review of previous research on data privacy and security where healthcare data breach incidents were cited. In particular, we made use of the earlier work of Kobus (2012), Laja (2011), Johnson and Willey (2011), Walker (2011), Baker et al (2011), and Kierkegaard (2012). Further, as highlighted previously, earlier conceptual research, in the form of data breach taxonomies has also guided us in establishing our model for healthcare data breach causation and prevention.

Our preliminary analysis of the reported healthcare data breaches indicated that many data breach incidents were rooted in factors that go beyond the control of the individual healthcare

Table 2. Healthcare data breach sources

Organization	Description
Open Security Foundation (OSF, 2012)	Non-profit organization that specializes in searching for and archiving data loss incidents, including those that were not reported by the media
US Department of Health and Human Services (HHS, 2013b)	The Secretary of Health and Human Services provides a list of breaches of unsecured protected health information affecting 500 or more individuals, as required by section 13402(e)(4) of the HITECH Act. The list consists of brief descriptions of the breach cases that the office of civil rights has investigated and closed, as well as the names of private practice providers who have reported healthcare data breaches to the Secretary.
Privacy Right Clearinghouse (PRCH, 2012)	A nonprofit consumer advocacy and education center based in San Diego that maintains a comprehensive website with resources that include an online complaint submission form, numerous articles, and an online Chronology of Data Breaches since 2005.
Big Brother Watch (BBW, 2012)	British civil liberties and privacy pressure group whose research and online published reports uncovered hundreds of incidents whereby patient medical records were compromised

worker. Based on our literature review and after an in-depth analysis of the reported healthcare data breach incidents, we were able to synthesize the fragmented body of knowledge on data breach causation and prevention and then apply Reason's Swiss cheese model to better understand how healthcare data breach incidents occur. This is discussed in the next section.

Application of the SCM to Healthcare Data Breaches

Based on the literature review and our analysis of healthcare data breach incidents, we propose in Figure 2 the Swiss cheese model for data breach causation and prevention. The model suggests that most healthcare data breaches can be traced to one or more of four levels of failures (slices). These levels consist of organizational influence factors, inadequate security defenses, precursors of unsafe data handling, and the unsafe act of data handling. This model advocates that the data breach incidents occur when holes in the four slices lineup, resulting in a trajectory of data breach opportunity.

In order to better understand and describe the holes in the cheese layers from a practical rather than a speculative perspective, we have re-examined the reported cases of healthcare data breaches to gain practical insights into the failed or absent defenses in each of the four layers.

SCM Layer Description

Organizational Influence

Many reported healthcare data breach incidents suggest that latent organizational weaknesses and failures have assisted data breach hazards to penetrate the layers of defenses:

1. The lack of training for healthcare employees on how to best handle and protect PHI is reflected in many reported data breach incidents. For example, in 2011, thousands of X-rays were stolen from St. Joseph Medical Center in Towson by a thief who successfully tricked hospital employees into believing that he was a contractor for a radiological film destruction company to gain access to the

Figure 2. The SCM for data breach causation and prevention (adapted from (Reason, 1990))

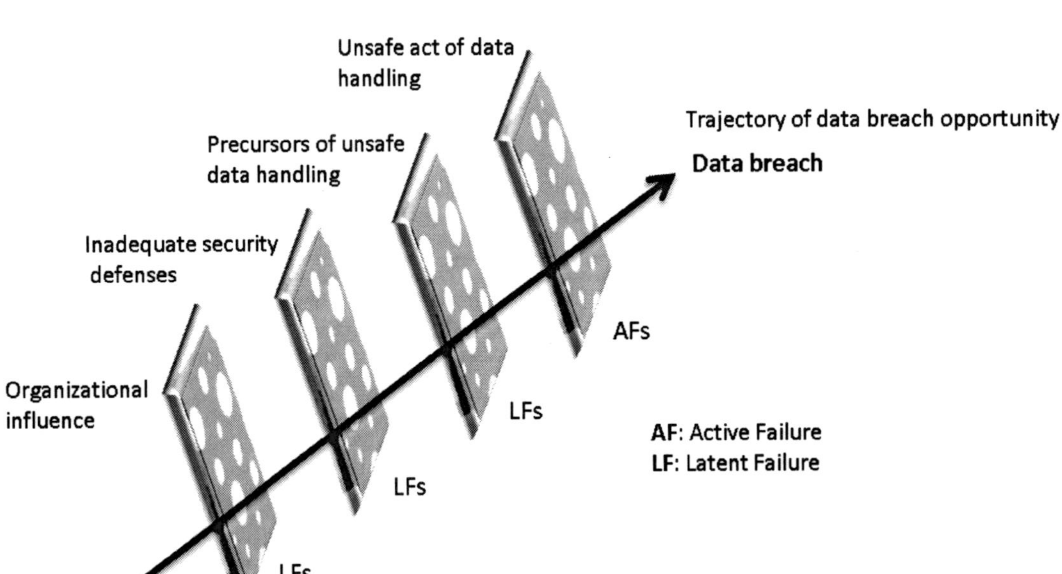

X-rays. It is believed that the X-ray films, which included private health information, were stolen for their silver content (Walker, 2011). In another incident, a "phishing" scam led a healthcare employee to share the login information for an email inbox, potentially jeopardizing the ePHI of 610 patients (HHS, 2011). One can argue that such incidents might have been mitigated if the hospital employees were trained to recognize and deal with social engineering tricks.

2. Poor or unforced data protection security policies and procedures can be inferred from many data breach incidents. For example, there is evidence that many healthcare organizations are lacking policies that dictate the separation of personal emails and data from organizational emails and PHI. For example, Kobus (2012) cited several incidents whereby healthcare employees posted on their Facebook and Twitter accounts information related to their patients' therapy. In another incident, one employee emailed unencrypted medical records to a personal email account, putting the PHI of more than 2,000 patients at risk (HHS, 2011). Johnson & Willey (2011) found medical settlement spreadsheets that contained names, addresses, dates of birth, social security numbers, phone numbers, diagnosis codes, and insurance information on peer-to-peer file-sharing networks. In another reported incident, attackers were able to hack the Utah Department of Technology Services computer server on March 30, 2012 and access over 780,000 Medicaid claim records, because the servers were not configured according to normal policies and procedures (Gibson, 2012). A study conducted by the Ponemon Institute (Ponemon, 2012a) on the human factors of data protection, revealed that the bad practice of healthcare employees carrying unnecessary sensitive information on their laptops while traveling, was among the top ten data breach risky practices. The same study also found that the lack of physical access control policies led to situations where the healthcare employees left their computers, containing PHI, unattended after work. Another key finding of the Ponemon study (Ponemon, 2012a) is that 81 percent of the survey respondents allowed "Bring Your Own Device" (BYOD) to access organizational data and that 54% said they were not sure if these devices were secure. Hence, the lack of in-depth understanding the security risks of a BYOD policy and the lack of employees' education on the usage of personal mobile devices such as smartphones and tablets to access organizational data can enable a trajectory for a data breach incident.

3. Poor employment termination policy is another organizational flaw that was reflected in the case reported in (HHS, 2011) wherein one employee who was no longer employed had access to a password-protected website containing the PHI of more than 400,00 individuals.

4. According to the 2012 Redspin Breach Report (Redspin, 2012) more than half (57%) of all PHR breaches in the U.S involved a business associate. A particular major data breach incident was reported on September 14, 2011 in which the backup tapes containing ePHI of about 4.9 million patients were stolen out of the military contractor's car in San Antonio (PRCH, 2012). This incident is yet another indication that an organizational faux pas (poor selection, assessment and/or audit of business associate to ensure PHI protection and HIPAA-compliance) can be a latent facilitator of a data breach incident.

Inadequate Security Defenses

Many reported data breach incidents suggest that the damage of data exposure could have been mitigated if remedies against latent weaknesses in the security defenses were implemented in the first place.

1. The de facto lack of data encryption is perhaps the most noticeable flaw in the security defenses that, when combined with data theft or loss, amplifies the damages of a data breach. For instance, from the sample of data breach incidents listed in Table 3, the impact could have been lessened if the data was adequately encrypted.

2. The lack of proper physical security mechanisms is another sign of inadequate security defenses that has been cited in many reported healthcare data breach incidents. For example, in 2009, an intruder managed to steal 57 hard drives which contained ePHI of more than 1 million patients from BlueCross BlueShield of Tennessee (Johnson, & Willey, 2011). In another incident, an intruder managed to gain access to a locked office in Temple Community Hospital in Los Angeles and stole a computer that contained the names of 600 patients, their hospital account numbers and their individual CT scans (LA, 2012).

3. The December 2012 security breach at the Carolinas Medical Center-Randolph illustrates how the lack of technical security safeguards can facilitate a trajectory of data breach opportunity. In this case, an unauthorized electronic intruder managed to access incoming and outgoing emails from a provider's account without the provider's or the hospital's knowledge, thus impacting approximately 5,600 patients (Walsh, 2012). In another 2012 security incident, the ePHI of patients from the Surgeons of Lake County in Libertyville, Ill., were kept hostage by hackers who penetrated the computer network, encrypted the data server and sent a ransom note, requesting payment in return for access to the ePHI (Robertson, 2012). In January 2011, hackers breached a server containing social security numbers and medical codes of around 230,000 Seacoast Radiology patients. The breach was initiated by gamers who were just looking for servers (space bandwidth) to play a best-selling video game (Goodin, 2011). In July 2009, the Alberta Health System was infected with the Coreflood virus which infiltrated the network via email. The virus relayed the ePHI of 11,582 patients back to the hacker (OSF, 2012). The lack of security safeguards was also reflected in the failure to properly clean hard disks and securely wipe the data before disposal. This was reflected for instance in

Table 3. Data breach incidents involving unencrypted ePHI

Data breach incident	Reference
Unencrypted tapes containing the PHI of more than 19,000 patients were lost	(HHS, 2011)
Desktop computer with unencrypted data was stolen from Sutter Medical Foundations, Sacramento, CA.	(PRCH, 2012; Baker et al., 2011)
Unencrypted backup tapes were stolen from a car, exposing the health and personal information of more than 4.9 million patients.	(PRCH, 2012)
On August 25, 2009, a Blue Cross and Blue Shield laptop containing unencrypted ePHI of more than 800,000 physicians was stolen from an employee at the company's headquarter in Chicago	(OSF, 2012)
In 2003, a psychiatric Hospital in Aarhus (Denmark) sent an unencrypted email to a doctor, containing PHI. A Virus on the doctor's computer caused the email to be forwarded to unauthorized recipients.	(Kierkegaard, 2012)
An employee at the secure mental health unit of the Scottish hospital lost USB stick containing unencrypted EPHI, including the criminal record of some violent patients being treated at the Tryst Park unit of Bellsdyke psychiatric hospital	(Kierkegaard, 2012)

the Affinity Health Plan Inc. data breach incident reported in (HHS, 2011) whereby hard drives, in more than twenty leased photocopiers, that might contain ePHI of up to 344,579 patients were returned intact to lessor.

Precursors of Unsafe Data Handling

Some reported healthcare data breach incidents can be traced down to some prior signs of poor communication and coordination, unclear instructions, or mental overload due to fatigue, distractions and stress.

1. In May 2012, the Aneurin Bevan Health Board in Wales received a £70,000 fine for breaching the Data Protection Act, following the release of sensitive personal data to the wrong person. The breach was attributed to poor communication between a doctor and his secretary who was not provided with enough details to correctly identify the patient to whom a letter should be sent. This resulted in PHI being mailed to a patient with a very similar name (NHS, 2012).
2. According to the U.S. Department of Health and Human Services (HHS, 2011), the most common human error that resulted in data breaches in 2010 was the misdirection of mailing involving paper records, where individuals received another patient's PHI because of the wrong mailing address. Misdirected emails and faxes were also cited as common data breach factors. For example, in June 2011, the Information Commissioner's Office has imposed a £120,000 fine on Surrey County Council as it repeatedly sent unencrypted ePHI to the wrong email recipients (ICO, 2011). While no study has been conducted to shed light on the root causes of PHI misdirection, the human factor theory seems to suggest that, besides the possibility of employee negli-

gence, their lack of focus due to stress, fatigue and distractions might be contributing factors as well. In fact, a survey conducted by HealthLeaders Media for Kronos Inc. revealed that nurse fatigue is prevalent in the healthcare industry and is directly linked to on-the-job errors (Kronos, 2013). Further, according to the Joint Commission review of research on healthcare workers, employee fatigue is directly linked to many adverse effects, like confusion, the inability to stay focused, and slower or faulty information processing and judgment; all of which can potentially be preconditions for unsafe handling and management of PHI (Joint, 2011). Lockley et al (2007) demonstrated how extended work hours lead to fatigue-related errors among healthcare workers.

Unsafe Act of Data Handling

The unsafe act of the individual who is in direct contact with the PHI and that led to the data breach constitutes an active failure that is directly related to the data breach. According to the human error theory, as discussed in section 4, these failures can take various forms such as slips, lapses, mistakes, and violations (routine, situational, or optimizing violations). Table 4 illustrates, via sample reported healthcare data breach incidents, each of these four error categories.

"Defenses in Depth" Approach to Healthcare Data Breaches

The "defenses in depth" concept is deeply rooted in Reason's approach towards human error management (Reason, 1990). This principle has also been adopted in physical security (see for example (Ward & Smithy, 2002)) where multiple rings (deter, detect, delay, respond and deny) act as safeguards within the physical asset's security perimeter.

Table 4. Taxonomy of human errors that led to healthcare data breaches

Error category	Sample Cases
Slip	• On May 3, 2010, a business associate working for the Aramark Healthcare Support Services, Inc. sent an email to multiple patients where the names and email addresses were visible to all the 937 email recipients (HHS, 2011). • On October 2, 2012, a licensed clinical social worker at Town Council of Chapel Hill accidentally attached confidential patient information to an email that was forwarded to the town council colleagues (PRCH, 2012). • During the period 2007-2009, doctors' offices in Tennessee have been accidentally sending confidential patient information to an Indiana businessman's fax machine, instead of the Tennessee Department of Human Services (OSF, 2012). • On April 29, 2006, a programmer's error on the Valley Baptist Medical Center website exposed names, dates of birth, and SSNs of healthcare workers (OSF, 2012).
Lapse	• On March 9, 2009, an employee from the Massachusetts Physician Organization Inc. left PHI records of 192 patients of Mass General, including patients with HIV/AIDS, on a subway train while commuting to work (Kierkegaard, 2012). • In May 2010, an NHS worker at the secure mental health unit of the Scottish hospital lost USB stick containing unencrypted EPHI, including the criminal record of some violent patients at the Tryst Park unit of Bellsdyke psychiatric hospital (Kierkegaard, 2012). • On June 3, 2006, an insurance company employee at Humana downloaded a file containing customers' personal information into a hotel computer and then forgot to delete the files (OSF, 2012).
Mistake	• In February 2010, a healthcare employee uploaded records of 9,000 patients to an unsecured website (HHS, 2011). • In June 2010, a doctor from the California Center for Development and Rehabilitation left office cleaning to his sons, who dumped 1,000 patient files at the West Mecklenburg Recycling Center. The files contained names, addresses, dates of birth, SSNs, drivers' license numbers, insurance account numbers, and health information of 1,600 patients (Kierkegaard, 2012; PRCH, 2012). • In December 2010, an employee at Adventist Behavioral Health mistakenly sent sensitive patient documents to a recycling facility instead of a shredding facility (PRCH, 2012). • In February 2011, a member of staff at the University Hospital and Coventry & Warwickshire NHS Trust accidentally disposed of the medical records of 18 patients (along with other rubbish) in a his communal waste bin at a residential apartment block (PRCH, 2012)
Routine / Situational violation	• On April 23, 2012, a Naugatuck Valley Community College instructor used, without permission, patient X-rays from St. Mary's Hospital to teach radiology technology. The X-rays contained PHI. The instructor told students not to reveal the practice (PRCH, 2012). • On March 27, 2012, a physician at the Affordable Medical and Surgical Services dumped over 1,000 abortion records in a dumpster without attempting to properly destroy them (PRCH, 2012). • On January 10, 2013, an employee at Good Health Systems, a third-party contractor for Utah's Medicaid, saved beneficiary personal information of around 6,000 patients onto an unencrypted thumb drive that he subsequently lost while driving between Salt lake City, Denver, and Washington D.C (Gibson, 2013).
Optimizing violation	• A curious medical staff was caught examining the health records of friends and family members (Baker et al., 2011). • On November 10, 2009, two employees at the Massachusetts Eye and Ear Infirmary, who had access to the PHI of 1,076 individuals, misused patient credit information for personal gain (HHS, 2011). • On March 1, 2013, a therapist at the South Miami Hospital, Baptist Health disclosed and sold Social Security numbers, dates of birth, patient names, and other data to another party later used them to file fraudulent tax returns (PRCH, 2012). • On March 11, 2010, an employee at the University of Pittsburgh Student Health Center stole and then destroyed documents containing PHI of approximately 8,000 individual (HHS, 2011). • On April 2009, a patient registration secretary at John Hopkins was suspected of identity theft that affected as many as 49 patients (Johnson & Willey, 2011).

As suggested by Reason (2000), we recognize that each hole in the SCM of Figure 2 represents an individual weakness in the healthcare system that can potentially lead to a data breach. At the same time, each slice can act as a defensive layer against potential breaches. Accordingly, to curtail the likelihood of potential data breaches, we outline herein some preliminary results pertaining to some counter-measures that can potentially act as defensive layers and contribute towards minimizing or reducing the size of the individual holes. In doing so, we recognize that the efforts made to compile these safeguards are ongoing and that further research is warranted. We also note that some of the proposed counter-measures were suggested or justified by earlier research, while other safeguards are based on the authors' knowledge, personal opinion and experience.

Organizational Influence

A data safety culture, coupled with strong organizational policies, practices, leadership and oversight can act as a strong defensive layer against data breaches:

1. Building and maintaining an organizational culture of compliance to protect the patients' privacy rights is a key step towards data breach prevention. Such a culture should recognize that data breach incidents are often inevitable and accordingly should deeply internalize data safety within the healthcare organization and its BAs, based on all applicable data privacy regulations and mandates. An information security culture includes all the socio-technical measures that support technical security methods (Schlienger & Teufel, 2003). In fact, most of the processes needed to protect information assets are, to a large extent, dependent on human behavior (Van Niekerk & Von Solms, 2010). Hence an organizational approach to data breach prevention should put special emphasis on employee behavior, as the organization's success or failure is closely related to the things that its employees do or fail to do (Da Veiga & Eloff, 2010). Accordingly, and in congruence with Reason's safety culture model (Reason, 1997), there is a need for:

    a. An *informed culture*, where supervisors and healthcare employees have sound knowledge and awareness about the technical, human and organizational factors that have influence on the safety of personal health records.

    b. A *reporting culture*, where healthcare employees are willing to promptly report data breach incidents.

    c. A *Just culture*, where data breach incidents are seen as opportunities to learn from in order to enhance the organizational preparedness against potential future breaches.

2. It is important that healthcare organizations adopt best IT governance practices. These include top management support, establishing a data protection team, securing adequate resources, conducting compliance auditing and monitoring, performing regular data inventories, establishing data classification schemes, conducting security clearance, adhering to well-established IT security frameworks, and appointing a security officer in charge of PHI protection (Ponemon, 2012b).

3. It is compulsory for covered entities to develop, document, and maintain clear and effective policies and procedures governing the handling of personal and health records, both at rest and in motion, and from acquisition to disposal. These policies and procedures should be revised, strengthened and publicized to cover (1) the usage of social media and file-sharing sites (Kobus, 2012), (2) access authorization, (3) PHI disposal, (4) acceptable/ethical usage and sanctions, (5) mandatory training, (6) internal monitoring and auditing, (7) data breach response procedures, (8) separation of personal emails and data from organizational emails and data, and (9) effective password management.

4. It is important to educate, train and retrain the medical staff and all employees who are in direct contact with PHI on the importance of protecting this information and on how to safely and securely handle devices that contain ePHI. Training should cover common risky PHI handling practices, while highlighting best practices to respond to

common security threats, including social engineering tricks.

5. There is a strong need for the covered entities to carefully select and assess their vendors and business associates to ensure the proper handling of PHI so that data privacy is protected. In fact earlier studies (see for example (Khalfan, 2004)) have shown that organizations need to exercise diligence when selecting a business or outsourcing partner. Accordingly, BA's contracts should be carefully drafted and revised if necessary to further emphasis the protection of PHI, including the requirement for a third-party vulnerability assessment of the BA security measures.

6. A sound risk management program plays a central role in reducing data breach vulnerabilities to an adequate level. The presence of a robust risk management process is also a privacy mandate under the HIPPA. At the core of this process lies the risk assessment phase, where a structured and thorough assessment of potential threats to the confidentiality, availability and integrity of the PHI need to be conducted. Data breach risk assessment should also make use of unstructured approaches such as considering specific scenarios of common data breach patterns to understand how these may occur, and outline what can be done to thwart them. As suggested by Straub & Welke (1998), effective risk management also requires managers to be aware of the full array of security controls that are available and to implement those most ones.

Inadequate Security Defenses

Information security technologies and physical security controls can add an extra layer of defense against potential data breaches.

The recent data healthcare data breach incidents involving the loss and inappropriate disposal of paper records and electronic devices containing PHI suggest that the damages could have been minimized if the following security safeguards were implemented:

1. Shredding obsolete medical paper records and wiping hard drives before disposal.
2. Adopting encryption technologies on hard drives and memory sticks.
3. Separating personal information data from medical records (Neame, 2012).
4. Moving PHI from paper and legacy systems (such as spreadsheet, ad hoc databases, and word processing files) to secured enterprise-class health record systems (Johnson & Willey, 2011).
5. Adopting password locking and remote data wiping security solutions.

Physical safeguards and controls can also play an important role in protecting electronic storage media containing PHI. These safeguards include the appropriate usage of identity and access management solutions, including locked doors, badge access, alarm systems, physical locks for computer devices, biometric access controls, and CCTV security cameras.

Other security technologies can contribute towards protecting ePHI from loss, unauthorized access or alteration. These solutions include Virtual Private Networks (VPNs), firewalls, encryption solutions, endpoint security management software, file integrity monitoring solutions and intrusion detection and prevention systems.

Precursors of Unsafe Data Handling

To mitigate the threat of unsafe data handling due to potential employee fatigue, healthcare organizations should strive to set and enforce policies that set limits on the number of working hours. Ensuring adequate staffing to reduce overload can facilitate in achieving such a goal. It is also helpful to educate employees who are in direct contact with PHI on fatigue management, limitations of human performance and short-term memory, and impact of pressure and stress on the safety of PHI.

CONCLUSION

This paper contributes to healthcare data breach prevention by proposing an analytical theory, based on the SCM that integrates the human, organizational and technical factors of healthcare data breach causation and prevention. The SCM is found to be a useful theoretical model to elucidate the multifaceted origins of healthcare data breaches, as we seek a better understanding of the reasons behind healthcare data breaches. In particular, the model brings forwards the latent conditions of data breach incidents that have often being neglected in the literature.

Our research advocates that individual characters and behaviors such as carelessness, malice and unawareness are not the only contributing factors to data breaches. In other words, data breaches are sometimes the outcomes of circumstances that are beyond the control of those who were directly linked to the breach incident. Hence, because humans are fallible, organizational and technological systems must be designed to prevent data breaches, taking into account the imperfection of human performance.

What does this research imply for healthcare professionals and managers? This research suggests that instead of trying to simply pass the blame of data breaches on employees, healthcare providers should set up proper IT governance, policies, practices and information security technologies to account for data breach risks and minimize them. In fact, we argue that data breaches are the inevitable outcomes of not only human imperfection, but also poor organizational and technical systems design. At the same time, this research suggests that human and organizational aspects of data breach prevention need to be taken into account alongside the technical

factors as well. Hence, this paper highlights the need to revisit the causal factors of healthcare data breaches from a broader socio-technical perspective.

Since the SCM endorses the "defenses in depth" security approach, it can assist healthcare organizations develop a more comprehensive and systematic approach to reduce data breach risks. In particular, the SCM suggests inserting additional layers into the healthcare data handling system can prevent future data breach incidents.

As a future research, we plan to explore further countermeasures and safeguards in order to implement the "defenses in depth" approach to healthcare data breaches, as suggested by the SCM.

ACKNOWLEDGMENT

The authors would like to thank editor-in-chief and the anonymous referees for their constructive and helpful comments which led to the improvement of this paper.

REFERENCES

Antón, A. I., Earp, J. B., Vail, M. W., Jain, N., Gheen, C. M., & Frink, J. M. (2007). HIPAA's effect on Web site privacy policies. *IEEE Security & Privacy*, 5(1), 45–52. doi:10.1109/MSP.2007.7

Antón, A. I., Earp, J. B., & Young, J. D. (2010). How Internet users' privacy concerns have evolved since 2002. *IEEE Security & Privacy*, 8(1), 21–27. doi:10.1109/MSP.2010.38

Appari, A., & Johnson, M. E. (2010). Information security and privacy in healthcare: Current state of research. *Int. J. Internet and Enterprise Management*, 6(4), 279–314. doi:10.1504/IJIEM.2010.035624

Baker, A., Vega, L., DeHart, T., & Harrison, S. (2011). Healthcare and security: Understanding and evaluating risks. In M. M. Roberston (Ed.), Ergonomics and health aspects of work with computers (pp. 99-108). LNCS, Berlin Heidelberg, Germany: Springer-Verlag.

BBW. (2012). *Big brother watch*. Retrieved December 3, 2012 from, http://www.bigbrotherwatch.org.uk/

Bhatti, R., & Grandison, T. (2010). Improving security policy coverage in healthcare. In A. Chryssanthou, I. Apostolakis, & I, Varlamis (Eds.), Certification and security in health-related web applications: Concepts and solutions (pp. 66-83). IGI Global.

Collins, J. D., Sainato, V. A., & Khey, D. N. (2011). Organizational data breaches 205-2010: Applying SCP to the healthcare and education sectors. *International Journal of Cyber Criminology, 5*(1), 794–810.

Da Veiga, A., & Eloff, J. H. P. (2010). A framework and assessment instrument for information security culture. *Computers & Security, 29*(2), 196–207. doi:10.1016/j.cose.2009.09.002

Gibson, S. (2012). 'Configuration error' leads to breach of nearly 780,000 records. *Healthcare Tech Review,* April 12, 2012, Retrieved from, http://healthcaretechreview.com/configuration-error-leads-to-breach-of-nearly-780000-records/

Gibson, S. (2013). Lost USB drive leads to breach of 6,000 patient records. *Healthcare Tech Review,* 24 January 2013. Retrieved from http://healthcaretechreview.com/data-breach-lost-usb-drive/

Goodin, D. (2011). Gamers raid medical server to host Call of Duty: 230,000 patient records exposed. *The Register,* 14 January 2011. Retrieved from http://www.theregister.co.uk/2011/01/14/seacoast_radiology_server_breach/

Grandison, T., & Bhatti, R. (2010). Regulatory compliance and the correlation to privacy protection in healthcare. *International Journal of Computational Models and Algorithms in Medicine, 1*(2), 37–52. doi:10.4018/jcmam.2010040103

HHS. (2011). *U.S. Department of Health & Human Services, Annual report to congress on breaches of unsecured protected health information for calendar year 2009 to 2010.* Retrieved December 20, 2012, from http://www.hhs.gov/ocr/privacy/hipaa/administrative/breachnotificationrule/breachrept.pdf

HHS. (2013a). *U.S. Department of Health & Human Services, Standards for privacy of individually identifiable health information.* Retrieved September 16, 2013 from, http://aspe.hhs.gov/admnsimp/final/PvcPre02.htm

HHS. (2013b). *U.S. Department of Health & Human Services, breaches affecting 500 or more individuals.* Retrieved December 3, 2012, from http://www.hhs.gov/ocr/privacy/hipaa/administrative/breachnotificationrule/breachtool.html

ICO. (2011). ICO issues monetary penalty over misdirected emails. *Information Commissioner Office Council Release.* Retrieved from http://www.ico.org.uk/~/media/documents/pressreleases/2011/monetary_penalty_surrey_council_release_20110609.ashx

ITRC. (2012). *Identity Theft Research Center: 2012 Data breach stats.* Retrieved November 11, 2012, from http://www.idtheftcenter.org/ITRC%20Breach%20Stats%20Report%202012.pdf

Johnson, M. E. (2009). Data hemorrhages in the health-care sector. []. LNCS, Berlin Heidelberg: Springer-Verlag.]. *Financial Cryptography and Data Security, 5628,* 71–89. doi:10.1007/978-3-642-03549-4_5

Johnson, M. E., & Willey, N. (2011, January 4-7). Will HITECH heal patient data hemorrhages? In *Proceedings of the 44th Hawaii International Conference on Systems Sciences* (pp. 1-10).

Joint. (2011). *The Joint Commission, healthcare worker fatigue and patient safety, The Joint Commission Sentinel Event Alert*, 48, Dec 14, 2011. Retrieved from http://www.jointcommission.org/assets/1/18/sea_48.pdf

Khalfan, A. M. (2004). Information security considerations in IS/IT outsourcing projects: A descriptive case study of two sectors. *International Journal of Information Management, 24*, 29–42. doi:10.1016/j.ijinfomgt.2003.12.001

Kierkegaard, P. (2012). Medical data breaches: Notification delayed is notification denied. *Computer and Security Review, 28*, 168–183.

Kobus, T. J. (2012). The A to Z of healthcare data breaches. *Journal of Healthcare Risk Management, 32*(1), 24–28. PubMed doi:10.1002/jhrm.21088

Kronos. (2013). *Kronos survey reveals nurse fatigue is pervasive in the healthcare industry and directly linked to on-the-job errors.* Kronos Inc. Press Release, March 2013. Retrieved from http://www.kronos.com/pr/kronos-survey-reveals-nurse-fatigue-is-pervasive-in-the-healthcare-industry-and-directly-linked-to-on-the-job-errors.aspx

Kulynych, J., & Korn, D. (2002). The effect of the new federal medical-privacy rule on research. *The New England Journal of Medicine, 346*(3), 201–204. PubMed doi:10.1056/NEJM200201173460312

LA. (2012). Patient data stolen from Temple Community Hospital. *Los Angeles Times*, Aug 31, 2012. Retrieved from http://latimesblogs.latimes.com/lanow/2012/08/patient-data-stolen-from-temple-community-hospital-.html

Laja, S. (2011). NHS staff breach personal data 806 times in three years. *Guardian Professional*, Oct 28 2011. Retrieved December 3, 2012, from http://www.guardian.co.uk/healthcare-network/2011/oct/28/nhs-staff-breach-personal-data-806-times

Lockley, S. W., Barger, L. K., Ayas, N. T., Rothschild, J. M., Czeisler, C. A., & Landrigan, C. P. (2007). Effects of healthcare provider work hours and sleep deprivation on safety and performance. [PubMed]. *Joint Commission Journal on Quality and Patient Safety, 33*(11), 7–18. PMID:18173162

Massey, A. K., Otto, P. N., Hayward, L. J., & Antón, A. I. (2010). Evaluating existing security and privacy requirements for legal compliance. [Springer-Verlag.]. *Requirements Engineering Journal, 15*(1), 119–137. doi:10.1007/s00766-009-0089-5

Neame, R. (2012). Practical measures for keeping health information private. *Electronic Journal of Health Informatics, 7*(2), 1–10.

NHS. (2012). £70,000 fine for Aneurin Bevan health board after data breach. *NHS News,* 30 April 2012. Retrieved from http://www.nhis.info/news/nhs-news/%C2%A370000-fine-for-aneurin-bevan-health-board-after-data-breach/327/

O'Keefe, C. M., & Connolly, C. (2011). Regulation and perception concerning the use of health data for research in Australia. *Electronic Journal of Health Informatics, 6*(2), 1–13.

OSF. (2012). *Open security foundation, data loss DB.* Retrieved December 19, 2012, from http://datalossdb.org/

Ponemon. (2011). *Second annual benchmark study on patient privacy and data security.* 2011 Ponemon Research Report. Retrieved November 14, 2012, from http://www2.idexpertscorp.com/assets/uploads/PDFs/2011_Ponemon_ID_Experts_Study.pdf

Ponemon. (2012a). *The human factor in data protection*. Ponemon Research Report. Retrieved October 12, 2012, from http://www.trendmicro.com/cloud-content/us/pdfs/security-intelligence/reports/rpt_trend-micro_ponemon-survey-2012.pdf?ClickID=anpnsknps09tprya9k9ovzpzrnvrln99wrl

Ponemon. (2012b). *2011 cost of data breach: United States*. Ponemon Research Report, March 2012. Retrieved December 20, 2012 from, http://www.ponemon.org/local/upload/file/2011_US_CODB_FINAL_5.pdf

PRCH. (2012). *Privacy rights clearing house, Chronology of data breaches 2005- present*. Retrieved October 8, 2012, from http://www.privacyrights.org/data-breach/new

Reason, J. (1990). *Human error*. Cambridge, MA: Cambridge University Press. doi:10.1017/CBO9781139062367

Reason, J. (1997). *Managing the risks of organizational accidents*. Aldershot, UK: Ashgate.

Reason, J. (2000). Human errors: Models and management. *British Medical Journal, 320*(7237), 768–770. PubMed doi:10.1136/bmj.320.7237.768

Reason, J., Hollnagel, E., & Paries, E. J. (2006). Revisiting the "Swiss Cheese" model of accidents. *EUROCONTROL Experiment Center (EEC) Note No. 13/06*, Oct 2006. Retrieved December 3, 2012, from, http://www.eurocontrol.int/eec/gallery/content/public/document/eec/report/2006/017_Swiss_Cheese_Model.pdf

Redspin. (2012). Protected health information. *Redspin Breach Report* 2012, 2013 Feb. Retrieved from http://www.redspin.com/docs/Redspin_Breach_Report_2012.pdf

Robertson, J. (2012). Hackers steal, encrypt health records and hold data for ransom. *Bloomberg Report*, 10 Aug 2012. Retrieved from http://go.bloomberg.com/tech-blog/2012-08-10-hackers-steal-encrypt-health-records-and-hold-data-for-ransom/

Schlienger, T., & Teufel, S. (2003, July 9-11). Information security culture: From analysis to change. In *Proceedings of the Third Annual IS South Africa Conference*, Johannesburg, South Africa.

Sessions, L., & Kobus, T. J. (2012). The anatomy of healthcare data breach. *AHLA Connections*, 38-42. Retrieved December 20, 2012, from http://www.bakerlaw.com/files/Uploads/Documents/News/Articles/HEALTHCARE/Sessions.pdf

Straub, D. M., & Welke, R. J. (1998). Coping with systems risk: Security planning models for management decision making. *Management Information Systems Quarterly, 22*(4), 441–469. doi:10.2307/249551

Van Niekerk, J. F., & Von Solms, R. (2010). Information security culture: A management perspective. *Computers & Security, 29*(4), 476–486. doi:10.1016/j.cose.2009.10.005

Walker, A. K. (2011). Thousands of X-rays stolen from St. Joseph hospital: Police believe film was targeted for silver. *The Baltimore Sun*, Nov 4, 2011. Retrieved December 3, 2012, from http://articles.baltimoresun.com/2011-11-04/health/bs-hs-stolen-xrays-20111104_1_x-rays-film-hospital

Walsh, B. (2012). Email intruder causes N.C. hospital data breach. *Clinical Innovation + Technology*, Dec 11, 2012. Retrieved from http://www.clinical-innovation.com/topics/privacy-security/email-intruder-causes-nc-hospital-data-breach

Ward, P., & Smith, C. L. (2002). The development of access control policies for information technology systems. *Computers & Security, 21*(4), 356–371. doi:10.1016/S0167-4048(02)00414-5

ENDNOTES

[1] For the purpose of this study, and consistent with the definition of breach in section 13400(1)(A) of the HITECH Act, we define "healthcare data breach" as the acquisition, access, use, or disclosure of protected health information which compromises the security or privacy of this information.

[2] Under the HIPAA Privacy Rule, a covered entity includes a health plan (e.g. Health insurance issuers, Health Maintenance Organizations, and Medicare insurers), a healthcare clearinghouse (e.g. billing services, community health management systems), or a healthcare provider (e.g. doctors, clinics, nursing homes, pharmacies) who transmits any health information in electronic form.

This work was previously published in the International Journal of Healthcare Information Systems and Informatics (IJHISI), 9(1); edited by Joseph Tan, pages 42-60 copyright year 2014 by IGI Publishing (an imprint of IGI Global).

Chapter 66

How an Actor Network Theory (ANT) Analysis Can Help Us to Understand the Personally Controlled Electronic Health Record (PCEHR) in Australia

Imran Muhammad
RMIT University, Australia

Nilmini Wickramasinghe
Epworth Healthcare, Australia & RMIT University, Australia

ABSTRACT

Australia has designed, developed, and now implemented its national e-health solution known as the Personally Controlled Electronic Healthcare Record (PCEHR). This is a unique system as it subscribes to a shared governance model between patients and providers. To date, though, as with other national e-health solutions, there is poor uptake and much concern regarding the success of this multi-million dollar project. The authors contend that while these implementations and adoptions of e-health solutions are necessary, it is essential that an appropriate lens of analysis should be used in order to maximise and sustain the benefits of Information Systems/Information Technology (IS/IT) in healthcare delivery. Hence, in this chapter, the authors proffer Actor-Network Theory (ANT) as an appropriate lens to evaluate these various e-health solutions and illustrate in the context of the Personally Controlled Electronic Health Record (PCEHR), the chosen e-health solution for Australia.

INTRODUCTION

Globally, governments are increasingly investing in health information technology particularly in digitalising health records as well as other e-health solutions. This is in response to immense pressures of changing patient demographics, health, financial implications, work force shortages, advancements in medical technologies and their impact on healthcare demand and delivery as well as a

DOI: 10.4018/978-1-4666-8756-1.ch066

move towards a system where interaction between healthcare providers and consumers can achieve maximum output with limited human and financial resources (Wickramasinghe and Schaffer 2010).

It is well established that healthcare is an information rich industry (ibid). The underlying assumption in support of the introduction of IT(information technology) in healthcare service delivery is that by improving the ways of accessing and sharing information across healthcare systems and moving away from pen, paper and human memory towards a new environment, where key stakeholders (for example: service providers, consumers, government agencies and healthcare managers) can reliably and securely share information electronically, will significantly improve health outcomes and quality of care (Mort et al. 2007), help with cost savings, improve patient involvement and produce useable secondary data for further research and training (Car et al., 2008). However, such a transformation is not a straightforward proposition and is sometimes faced with many known and unknown hurdles such as (technological, organisational, financial and people issues) because of the complex and multifaceted environment of healthcare service delivery where different human and non-human actors interact with each other in multiple ways (Ammenwerth et al., 2006;Catwell and Sheikh, 2009; Cresswell et al. 2010; Lorenzi et al., 2009; DesRoches et al. 2008; André et al. 2008).

Further, given the inherent complexities of healthcare operations, it has been argued that these kinds of interventions are challenging and need to be evaluated with theoretically informed techniques (Wickramasinghe and Schaffer, 2010). One approach identified in the literature, to facilitate correctly and accurately capturing the complexities and levels of interventions in healthcare operations, is to use a Socio-Technical Systems (STS) perspective (Wickramasinghe, Bali, & Lehaney, 2009; Yusof et al., 2007; Aarts et al., 2004). A Socio-Technical system is described as a system where technical dimensions and social dimen-

sions of a system are interrelated (Cresswell et al. 2010). To determine the functionality of a system, it is important to understand a better fit between technical sub-systems and social sub-systems in an organisation (Mitchell & Nault 2008). This emphasis then is on not only studying the impact of the technology on organisations and their work processes but also the impact of social and people issues on technology and processes (Cresswell et al. 2010). For this reason, it is also important to understand the inter-relationship and interactions of the two between each other (Coiera, 2004).

To provide an even richer and more accurate picture of key healthcare operations as well as the impact of technology on these scenarios several scholars have argued that Actor-Network Theory (ANT) should be used together with an STS perspective (Wickramasinghe, Bali, & Lehaney, 2009; Yusof et al., 2007; Aarts et al., 2004; Cresswell et al. 2010). Hence, this paper reflects on the use of Actor-Network Theory to evaluate the Personally Controlled Electronic Health Record (PCEHR) in the Australian context in an attempt to demonstrate the merits of such an approach.

THE PERSONALLY CONTROLLED ELECTRONIC HEALTH RECORD (PCEHR)

Before discussing the PCEHR and its benefits, it is important to first understand that there are many different terminologies and vocabularies used interchangeably for clinical communication and electronic record handling and storage. In general all these terms typically make up the myriad of e-health solutions currently discussed in most countries. The ambiguity in the use and significance of the terms used can become an obstacle in the progress of ehealth adoption. If the definition of the term used for the system is not clear, this can complicate the contractual matters along with policy expectations and directives and expected features of product. It further

Table 1. Nomenclature and terminologies

Term	Description	Reference
Electronic Medical Record (EMR)	Any electronic record maintained by a private practitioner or family health teams locally within their clinics computer systems is referred to as an EMR. Service providers can access patient's visit history, health record, previous diagnosis, plans of care and lab reports and their placement orders with in their clinical practice with-out any integration with other providers or hospital systems and with very limited scope.	(Nagle 2007; Fisher,1999)
Electronic Patient Record (EPR)	The EPR is an electronic record maintained and managed by healthcare organisations at large. These healthcare organisations like hospitals can share this record with in their jurisdiction if shared infrastructure is available along with same vendor solutions. The ownership of the record is held by the organisation and access is typically restricted to the authorised users and user groups within the organisation's healthcare circle. Patients cannot access this record electronically and their GPs can request information.	(Mohd & Mohamad 2005; Nagle 2007).
Electronic Health Record (EHR)	The Electronic Health Record is a comprehensive health record that consists of information collected from different service providers and point-of-service systems such as pharmacies and diagnostic centres for all healthcare encounters an individual may have with them. Within the larger concept of EHR, health information is proprietary to the person whom it relates to and other service providers within or outside the jurisdiction can access this information only with proper access rights.	(Nagle 2007; Neves et al. 2008)
Personal Health Record (PHR)	The PHR can be defined by its attributes including, but not limited to, the nature of information and its scope in the PHR, the source of information, the party who owns the record, the functionary of the system, data reposition location and type, approaches towards privacy and security, and definition of access roles. It can be differentiated from other systems by its maintenance, ownership and access rules. Depending on the type of PHR users can draw information from different sources including healthcare providers, medical devices, wellness promoter systems or websites, research institutions and government websites.	(Halamka et al. 2007; Krohn 2007; Thompson & Brailer 2004; Detmer et al. 2008; Jones et al. 2010).

can instigate confusion in developing polices and regulations or legislation. For this reason, we look at publications in the past 10 years in order to understand the nomenclature and terminologies used for a better understanding of the meanings of the term (refer to Table 1).

The terminology adopted in Australia for electronic record keeping and its e-health solution is known as the Personally Controlled Electronic Health Record (PCEHR) which sits between individually-controlled health records and healthcare provider health records (NEHTA and DoHA 2011; Figure 1). Thus, the PCEHR has a shared use and mixed governance model (NEHTA and DoHA 2011; Figure1).

Specifically, the PCEHR is a person-centric secure repository of electronic health and medical records of individual's medical history that would act as a hub for linking hospital, medical and pharmaceutical systems using a patient unique identifier (NHHRC, 2009:134). One of its key features is that it captures information from different systems and presents this information in a single view to consumers and authorised service

Figure 1. The position of the PCEHR in the e-health solution spectrum

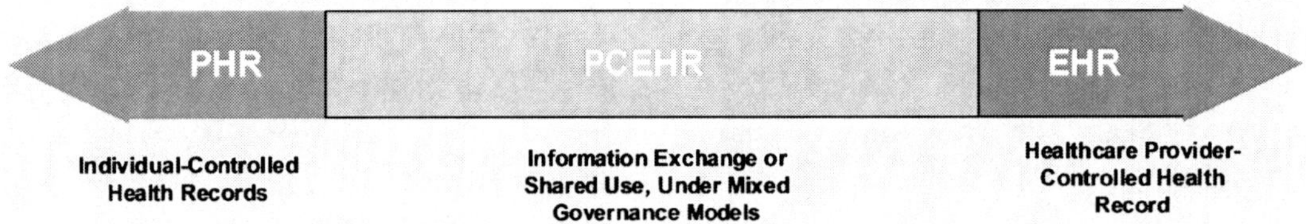

Table 2. PCEHR features (NEHTA and DoHA 2011)

> - It will provide patients health information including medication, medical history referrals, lab test results, prescriptions, discharge summaries, allergies and immunisations.
> - Rigorous governance and privacy procedures.
> - Fast and reliable access of patient's health information for both consumers and service providers remotely via fast Internet connection to enhance decision making for diagnoses and treatments and preventive actions.
> - Provide high quality data for policy development as-well-as research and planning to government bodies.
> - Provide all activity history of any actions preformed on the PCEHR by any service provider and/or consumer.
> - Individuals can make enquires and complaints about the management of their information.
> - Easy access to health literacy information via a direct link.
> - Can collect information from consumer devices such as blood pressure monitors or blood glucose monitors.

providers for better decision making about health and service delivery (NEHTA & DoHA 2011). This is a hybrid health information system that integrates web based personal health records with a clinical electronic health record system and allows shared access to both consumers and healthcare providers based on a shared responsibilities and mixed governance model. (Leslie 2011). The proposed PCEHR will have the key features as presented in Table 2.

Unlike most other eHealth solutions to date, the proposed PCEHR in Australia has a unique point of difference. Specifically, this PCEHR requires the patient (citizen) to authorise any additional information to be included in his/her record. This includes giving the access rights to providers with the exception of an emergency situation where a provider can access records other than those labelled as "no access" (NEHTA and DoHA, 2011). These records would be identified by Individual Health Identifiers (IHI) assigned by Medicare Australia, in which, IHIs will be created automatically but can be activated only at the request of the individual. More importantly, this system will operate on the principal of an "opt-in" model. That is an entirely voluntary basis, in which a user can "opt-in" or "opt-out" any information they wish to be included and can even withdraw from the system at any time. In addition, individuals would also have the final authority to allow and deny access of any service provider or organization (NEHTA & DoHA, 2011).

Further, this system will also include a reporting service, which can be used for the analysis of the information from multiple sources for better decision-making. Moreover, as this system matures many more types of reports would evolve and may help with research and training.

The benefits of ICT use in the healthcare sector may be enormous, however the uptake and diffusion of ICT in healthcare service and delivery is still a major challenge for healthcare service providers, governments and developers (Showell 2011; Leslie 2011; Hordern et al. 2011; Boonstra & Broekhuis 2010; Liu et al. 2011; Trudel 2010; Bernstein et al. 2007; HFMA 2006; Tang et al. 2006). There are very high stakes involved in health information system adoption and implementation for service providers and governments as well as system developers in the shape of financial, clinical and organisational risks (Westbrook & Braithwaite 2010; Karsh et al. 2010). This makes it imperative to identify the challenges that the healthcare service sector is facing in the adoption of e-health solutions, especially from the PECHR perspective. The following section examines the key constraints to the PCEHR development, adoption, implementation and diffusion of the new eHealth solution. In so doing, it is possible to appreciate the complex nature of healthcare operations as well as the importance of people, process and technology issues.

CONSTRAINTS TO THE DEVELOPMENT, ADOPTION, IMPLEMENTATION AND DIFFUSION OF PCEHR TECHNOLOGY

A large number of health information systems have been implemented around the globe with mixed results. Despite the claims that eHealth solutions can play a significant role in efficiency and effectiveness of healthcare service delivery, literature still provides evidence of failed clinical systems and lack of adoption by users (Protti & Smit 2006; Basch 2005; DesRoches et al. 2008).

Challenges and barriers to develop, adopt and implement eHealth solutions have been extensively debated. Researchers have divided these barriers into different categories ranging from environmental, social, technical and organisational (André et al. 2008) and note that these categories play crucial roles in the decision-making processes of technology adoption (Huang & Palvia 2001). In this study, we believe that the barriers identified by André et al. (2008) while important and a necessary condition may not be all-inclusive or sufficient. The primary reason for this being that in a healthcare service context where organisations are now required to work as a networked framework, health information technology implementation and adoption becomes an even more complex and challenging endeavour because of the different business processes, available infrastructure, compatibility issues, decision centres, authorization mechanisms and hierarchies, enterprise systems and data semantics (Avgerou 2008; Liu et al. 2011; Trudel 2010).

In the Australian context, social issues are considered a significant topic in healthcare IT transformation. This includes topics relating to individual privacy, legal, health information security and ethics issues. Individual privacy is considered as the private property of a person to whom this information is relating, so information privacy is defined as the ability of an individual to control the access to personal information (Culnan

& Armstrong 1997). The breach of privacy is a common concern among Australian consumers and privacy advocates despite the draft's (Personally Controlled Electronic health Record Act 2011) emphasis on the security and privacy of an electronic health record of individuals as well as any information that is protected by law. Further, the placement of these requirements and standards as well as the fact that the language is vague only serves to add more confusion and raise concerns among both healthcare providers and consumers (Hoffinan & Podguski 2008). It is noted that standardisation is important to set security and access rules of the system (Hoffinan & Podguski 2008) and this has been identified as a policy issue. In addition, there is a need for direct involvement of citizens in consultation about the development and implementation of the PCEHR system not just interest groups and citizen privacy and information security groups that have been emphasised as policy issues and to date this has proved challenging and contentious (Showell 2011).

Secondly, financial issues have been identified as a big hurdle in the adoption and implementation of health information technology especially an electronic health record (Aaronson et al. 2001; Aarts et al. 2004; Aarts & Koppel 2009; Abbott 2005; André et al. 2008; Bernstein et al. 2007; Boonstra & Broekhuis 2010; Culnan & Armstrong 1997; HFMA 2006; Kennedy 2011; Liu et al. 2011; Thweatt & Kleiner 2007; Trudel 2010; Ashish 2009; Bahensky et al. 2008; Bates 2005; Bath 2008; Weimar 2009; Kaplan & Harris-Salamone 2009). These issues range from start-up costs to software upgrades and staff training. It is observed that for sole practitioners; the capital cost is very high and not considered as a good investment for returns (Ashish 2009). Lack of incentives, budget over runs and high time costs are other financial concerns (DePhillips 2007; Cohn et al. 2009; Boonstra & Broekhuis 2010; Liu et al. 2011; Trudel 2010). This in turn makes the embracement of ICTs in healthcare problematic.

Thirdly, organizational issues have also been extensively reported in the literature. For example, poor governance, organisational culture and poor management of the change process harm the flow of transformation (Hoffinan 2009; Greenhalgh & Stones 2010; Kennedy 2011; Bernstein et al. 2007). Technological issues can also exacerbate the resistance to the adoption of health information technology and complicate the diffusion of PCEHR technology. Furthermore, the lack of infrastructure, standards and protocols which in turn results in fragmented healthcare information systems could further complicate a very complex situation for coordination (Davidson & Heslinga 2006; Hoffinan & Podguski 2008; Kralewski et al. 2010; Vitacca et al. 2009; HFMA 2006; Kennedy 2011; Trudel 2010).

Fourthly, technology issues such as the lack of interpretability between different healthcare delivery and management systems can hinder the penetration of this technology and its sustainability (André et al. 2008; Kennedy 2011; Liu et al. 2011). Pre-implementation and post-implementation vendor support is another key concern for organisations (Kralewski et al. 2010; Cohn et al. 2009; Kennedy 2011; Liu et al. 2011; Trudel 2010; Tang et al. 2006). Lack of technical resources and experience with information technology implementation within healthcare settings is another problem faced by many (Torda et al. 2010; Trudel 2010; Liu et al. 2011; Kennedy 2011; André et al. 2008; Bath 2008; DePhillips 2007; Davidson & Heslinga 2006; McReavy et al. 2009). The accuracy of data obtained through the information system and its ability of sorting, querying and validating data in some cases is very poor and is considered as a big barrier for HIT adoption (Rosenbloom et al. 2006; Rosebaugh 2004; Kimaro & Nhampossa 2007).

Lastly, people issues are yet another big concern ranging from user acceptance (Frame et al. 2008; Agarwal & Prasad 1997), perceived ease of use (Al-Azmi et al. 2009), lack of knowledge about the system (Bath 2008; Elrod & Androwich

2009; Kaplan & Harris-Salamone 2009; André et al. 2008; Liu et al. 2011), lack of training , lack of stake holder consultation (Showell 2011), lack of willingness to assimilate the technology into daily routines and processes (Cash 2008; Ross et al. 2010; Davidson & Heslinga 2006; Kaplan & Harris-Salamone 2009), conflict between system and user embedded values (Cash 2008; Kaplan & Harris-Salamone 2009), complex and complicated user interfaces (Yusof et al. 2007), conflict between physician activities and training schedules (André et al. 2008; Yusof et al. 2007; Kaplan & Harris-Salamone 2009).

Given the complex nature of the healthcare system and the challenges and barriers described relating to the adoption and implementation of ICTs into healthcare contexts, the importance of conceptualising and framing the critical factors for evaluating the proposed PCEHR system cannot be over emphasised. Hence, the next section presents our conceptual model that attempts to capture all the key considerations as discussed above for further analysis.

CONCEPTUAL MODEL

Based on the literature discussed in the previous sections some key factors important for the successful implementation of a PCEHR have been identified and served to develop the proposed conceptual modal as shown in Figure 2. This conceptual model will serve to capture all the important aspects of the barriers and facilitators for the prediction of the successful adoption and implementation of the PCEHR. The proposed model identifies the network of different actors interconnected to each other. These actors include social, people, technology, finance, and organization. Based on the literature review, their interactions presented a very complex picture of relationships. To study this complex network of interactions of humans with technology in organisations and certain individual levels a

Figure 2.

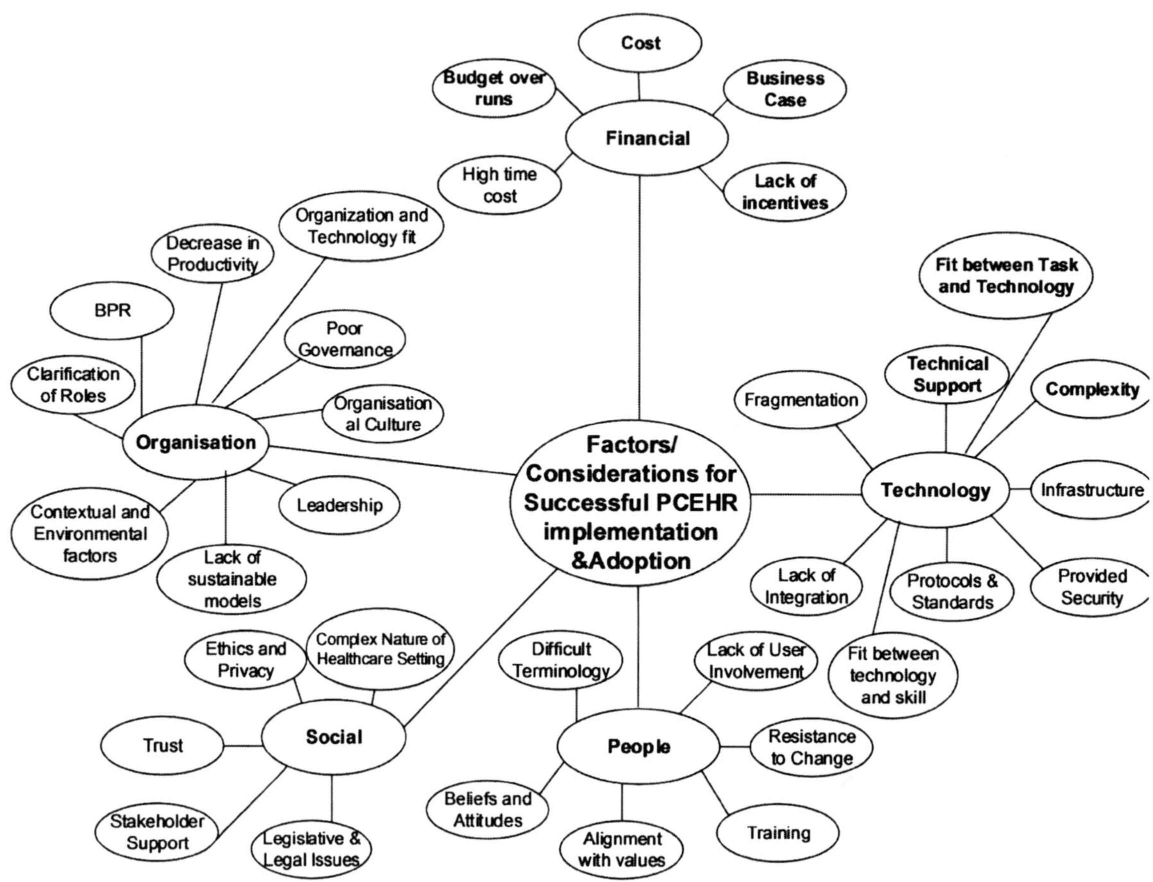

Socio-Technical System (STS) perspective is proposed(Cresswell et al. 2010).

A Socio-Technical System is described as a system where technical dimensions and social dimensions are interrelated (Cresswell et al. 2010). To determine the functionality of a system, it is important to understand that a better fit between technical sub-systems and social sub-systems in an organisation is presented (Mitchell & Nault 2008). As seen in the conceptual model, it appears that this study is complex and consists of hybrid entities of both human and non-human elements such as organisation, people and social dimensions. Thus, to better understand this study an appropriate lens of analysis to use is Actor-network Theory (ANT) (Wickramasinghe & Bali 2009). This choice is consistent with many other researchers' view that

ANT can help to understand the socio-technical nature of information systems in health care settings (Walsham 1997; Tobler 2008; Greenhalgh & Stones 2010; Cresswell et al. 2010; Timpka et al. 2007; Wickramasinghe & Bali 2009).

ACTOR-NETWORK THEORY

Actor-Network Theory (ANT) is based on a recursive philosophy (Latour 1992). Its fundamental stand is that technologies and people are linked in a network. ANT tries to bridge the gap between a socio-technical divide by denying the existence of purely social or technical relations. In doing so it takes a very radical stand and assumes that each entity (such as technologies, organisation) are actors therefore have the potential to transform and mediate social relationships (Cresswell et al. 2010). It also emphasises the concept of heterogeneous networks because of the non-similar nature of elements and their relationship in network makes these networks open and evolving systems (Hanseth 2007). Therefore Actor- networks are highly dynamic and inherently unstable in their nature; and a better understanding of how alignment between people, technology, their roles, routines, values, training and incentives as well as understanding of the role of technology that how it can facilitate or negatively impact the work processes and tasks in an organisation can stabilise these network to some extent (Greenhalgh & Stones 2010; Wickramasinghe et al. 2011). For this reason, ANT can be a material-semiotic approach and can provide an appropriate lens to study the ordering of scientific, technological, social, and organisational processes and events (Wickramasinghe et al. 2011). To realise the importance of the application of ANT into the study of PCEHR evaluation it is important to understand the key concepts of ANT and map them to the critical issues of the PCEHR development in Australia.

An initial assessment of these key concepts and their mapping is provided in Table 3.

Three Stages of ANT

In addition to the key concepts of ANT described above (Table 3) there are three critical stages of ANT which need to be considered as presented in Figure 3.

Stage 1: Inscription

A process of creating technical text and communication artifacts to protect actor's interests in a network is described as an inscription (Leila 2009; Wickramasinghe & Bali 2009; Latour 2005). This is a term used for all texts and communications in different mediums including but not limited to journal articles, conference papers and presenta-

tions, grants proposals and patents. The idea of Inscription also relates to the notion of durability; for instance a general discussion would be less durable as compared to a recorded meeting. Therefore, the idea behind Inscription is to enhance the durability of the network by associating them with durable material. Actors can use Inscription as a path to gain credibility in enrolment and the co-optation process during translation.

Stage 2: Translation

Translation is a very important and vital concept in ANT. This term is used to explain the process of creation of Actor-Networks and the formation of ordering effects (Callon 1986; Law 1992). This stage can help researchers in providing the insight into how the software system (PCEHR) can be integrated into the very complex environment of healthcare. The process of Translation can also be called the process of negotiation because after the creation of the network in the presence of many actors a strong or primary actor would translate interests of other actors into his/her own by negotiating with them. At this stage all actors decide to be part of network if it is worth while to build it (Wickramasinghe & Bali 2009).

The process of Translation of Actors/Actants is achieved through a series of four moments of translations (Callon, 1986). Figure 3 depicts the key ANT concepts along with these four moments of Translation.

Stage 3: Framing

Framing is an operation that can help to define actors and distinguish different actors and goods from each other (Callon, 1986). This last and final stage in the ANT process can help network to stabilise. At this stage key issues occurred throughout the PECHR should already have been negotiated within the network and technologies can become more stable over time (Wickramasinghe & Bali 2009).

Table 3. Key concepts of ANT and their mapping with the PCEHR

Key Constructs of ANT	Initial Mapping of the PCEHR with ANT
Actor/Actant: Actors are the web of participants in the network including all human and non-human entities. Because of the strong biased interpretation of the word actor towards human; a word actant is commonly used to refer both human and non-human actors. Examples are human, information systems, technical artifacts, work process and graphical representation (Wickramasinghe et al. 2011).	In PCEHR context Actor/Actant are different stakeholders in healthcare delivery settings such as Technology (Web 2.0, Databases, Graphical User Interfaces, IHI and different Computer hardware and Software) and People (service providers, healthcare funders, healthcare service recipients, healthcare organisations, suppliers and private health insurers as well as clinical administrative technologies, work process and health records in the form of paper or electronic.
Heterogeneous Network: Is a network of aligned interests formed by the actors. This is a network of materially heterogeneous actors that is achieved by a great deal of work that both shapes those various social and non-social elements, and "disciplines" them so that they work together, instead of "making off on their own" (Latour, 1996, Latour, 2005; Wickramasinghe et al. 2011).	The PCEHR technology here is clearly a network of different applications in this context. But it is important to understand that the heterogeneous network in ANT requires conceptualising the network as aligned interest including people, organisations, standards and protocols and their interaction with technology. The key here is a better alignment and representation of the interests so that the healthcare delivery can be improved.
Tokens/Quasi Objects: Are created through the successful interaction of actors/actants in a network and are passed between actors within the network. As the token is increasingly transmitted or passed through the network, it becomes increasingly punctualised and also increasingly reified. When the token is decreasingly transmitted, or when an actor fails to transmit the token (e.g., disconnection of patient portal from PCEHR Server), punctualisation and reification are decreased as well (Wickramasinghe et al. 2011).	In PCEHR context this translate to successful cost effective and efficient healthcare delivery, such as for GPs treating patient by having a capability of sharing health information with other service providers and for patients who are on long term medications having capability to print prescription from home issued by their doctor through the PCEHR portal. It is important to understand that to maintain the integrity of the network at all times is very important because if wrong information is passed through the network, the errors would be devastating and can propagate quickly and will multiply.
Punctualisation: The concept of ANT is pretty much based of punctualisation. Within the domain of ANT every actor in the web of relations is connected to others and as a whole it will be considered as a single object or concept same as the concept of abstraction is treated in Object Oriented Programming. These sub-actors are sometime hidden from the normal view and only can be viewed in case of the network break-down; this concept is often referred as a depunctualisation. Because ANT require all actors or sections of network to perform required tasks and therefor maintain the web of relations. In case of any actor cease to operate or maintain link the entire Actor-Network would break down resulting in ending the punctualisation. Punctualisation is a process and cannot be achieved indefinitely rather is a relational effect and is recursive that can reproduce itself (Law 1997).	For example, a computer on which one is working would be treated as a single block or unit. Only when it breaks down and one needs help with spare parts can reveal the hidden chain of network consist of different actors made up of (People, Computer parts and organisations). Similarly in a PCEHR context, uploading the health record of a patient is in reality a consequence of the interaction and coordination of many sub-tasks. This will only reveal itself if some kind of breakdown at this point occurs and depunctualisation of the network happens and all sub-tasks then would need to be carefully examined.
Obligatory Passage Point (OOP): Broadly refers to a situation that has to occur in order for all the actors to satisfy the interests that have been attributed to them by the focal actor. The focal actor defines the OPP through which the other actors must pass through and by which the focal actor becomes indispensable (Callon, 1986).	In PCEHR context, we can illustrate this by taking the example of access rights. The interface of the system is developed in a way that no service can access any record without using their IHI, which in this case constitute an obligatory passage point through which they have to pass for their everyday activities.
Irreversibility: Callon (1986, p. 159) states that the degree of irreversibility depends on (i) the extent to which it is subsequently impossible to go back to a point where that translation was only one amongst others and (ii) the extent to which it shapes and determines subsequent translations.	In the context of a very complex nature of healthcare operations irreversibility is very less likely to occur and would be more dependent on social networks and the nature of the interaction between human and non-human actors in the network. Here it is important to remember though the chain of events needs to be monitored carefully so the future events can be addressed in the best possible manners.

Figure 3.

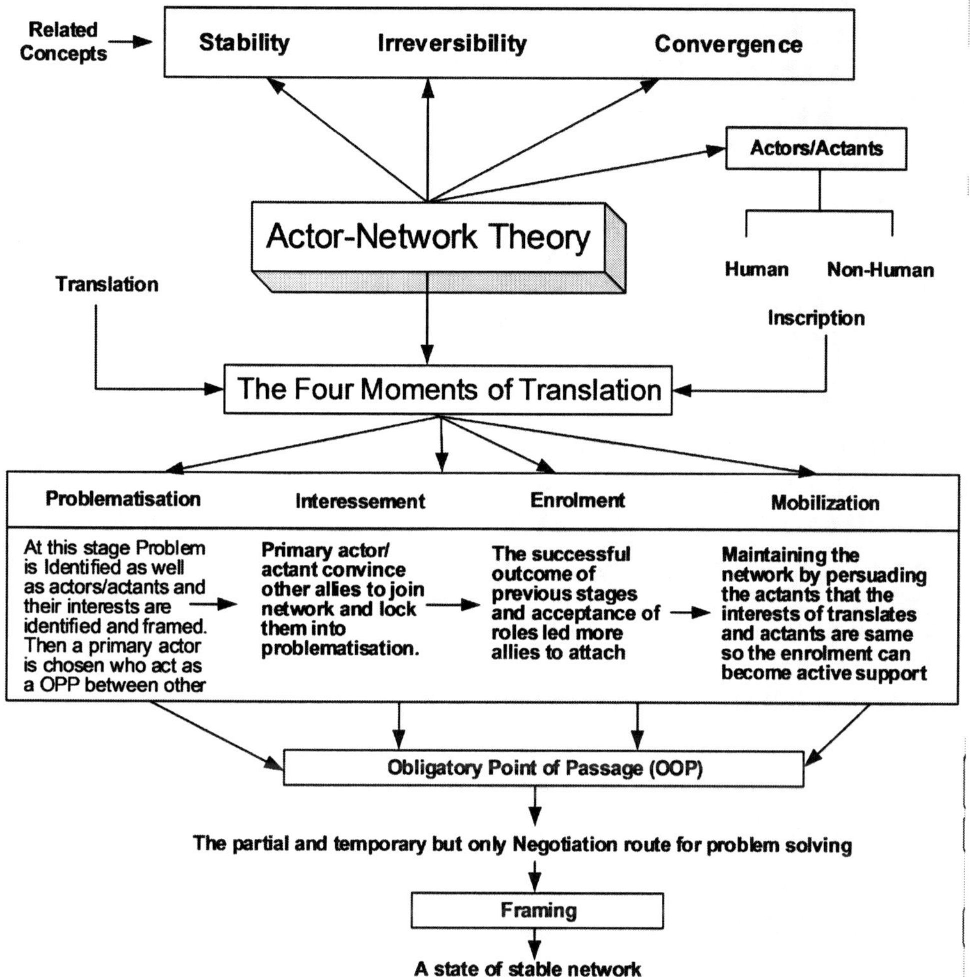

THE ACTOR-NETWORK THEORY APPROACH TO EVALUATE IT IN HEALTHCARE

ANT is considered an appropriate choice to analyse the PCEHR evaluation study because it can identify and acknowledge any impact of human and non-human social or policy issues within the healthcare setting (Latour et al. 1996). Moreover, it is robust enough to accurately capture all the complexities, nuances and richness of healthcare operations. In so doing, it can also help to investigate and theorise the question of why and how networks come into existence, what sort of associations and impact they can have on each other, how they move and change their position in a network, how they enrol and leave the network and most importantly how these networks can achieve stability (Doolin & Lowe 2002; Callon 1986; McLean & Hassard 2004). ANT's assumption is that if any new actor is enrolled in the network or an old actor leaves the network it would affect whole network (Cresswell et al. 2010; Doolin & Lowe 2002). These considerations are naturally relevant in the context of the PCEHR.

In addition, ANT also can help to understand the active role of objects in shaping social realities by challenging assumptions of the separation between non-human and human worlds (Walsham 1997; Greenhalgh & Stones 2010; Tobler 2008; Law & Hassard 1999; Rydin 2010). This helps researchers to study the complexities of the relationships between human and non-human actors, the sustainability of power relationships between human actors and what kind of influence artefacts can have on human actors relationships in transforming healthcare (Cresswell et al. 2010).

The rationale to choose ANT to evaluate the PCEHR system is thus the strength of ANT to identify and explore the real and perceived complexities involved in Australian healthcare service delivery. Although ANT has been applied in the implementation and adoption of different healthcare innovation studies (Berg, 2001; Cresswell et al. 2010; Cresswell et al. 2011; Bossen, 2007; Hall, 2005); It is important to note however, that ANT has also been criticised for its limitations (Williams, 2007; Walsham, 1997; Cresswell et al. 2010; Cresswell et al. 2011; Greenhalgh and Stones, 2010).

Some of the key limitations identified in the literature include: ANT's lack of ability to pay proper attention to broader social structures (Walsham, 1997), its lack of ability to pay attention to macro-environmental factors (McLean and Hassard, 2004), ANT's inability to explain the relationship formations between actors and changes of events in network (Greenhalgh and Stones, 2010; Cresswell et al. 2011; Kaghan and Bowker, 2001). To overcome the ANT's limitations, many researchers have suggested that ANT can be combined with other theoretical lenses such as Structuration theory (ST), Strong Structuration Theory (SST), Theory of Practice (ToP) and Social Shaping of Technology (SSoT) (Trudel, 2010; Cresswell et al. 2011; Greenhalgh and Stones, 2010; Walsham, 1997).

CONCLUSION

The need for IT based interventions in the healthcare services delivery to improve information and communication flow is well recognised all around the globe. Different e-health solutions are being implemented with mixed success to address this challenge (Protti & Smit 2006; Basch 2005; DesRoches et al. 2008; Greenhalgh and Stones, 2010). It is, therefore important to evaluate these technologies with theoretically informed approaches in an attempt to enjoy more successful outcomes.

We believe it is important to develop a deeper understanding constraint to the development, adoption, implementation and diffusion of these various ehealth solutions. Specifically, we suggest that a socio-technical ANT based approach can inform and facilitate such evaluations and we illustrate this by presenting an initial analysis and conceptual model for the PCEHR development in Australia. We are confident that this approach can be beneficial to both practitioners and researchers.

This paper has served to outline the key concepts of ANT that are relevant in the context of the PCEHR adoption and implementation and discussed the appropriateness of an ANT based theoretical lens for the evaluation of PCEHR in very complex environment of healthcare service delivery. We have also noted that ANT has been criticised by several scholars on the basis of its appropriateness as an ontology and/or epistemology (Latour, 2005). Therefore we recommend that to reduce the negative impact of these limitations the use of Structuration Theory be incorporated. To further strengthen our study, we plan to combine ANT with structuration theory to analyse the PCEHR in Australia. We close by calling for more confirmatory follow up research in this vital area.

REFERENCES

Aaronson, J. W., Murphy-Cullen, C. L., Chop, W. M., & Frey, R. D. (2001). Electronic medical records: the family practice resident perspective. *Family Medicine*, *33*(2), 128–132. PMID:11271741

Aarts, J., Doorewaard, H., & Berg, M. (2004). Understanding Implementation: The Case of a Computerized Physician Order Entry System in a Large Dutch University Medical Center. *Journal of the American Medical Informatics Association*, *11*, 207–216. doi:10.1197/jamia. M1372 PMID:14764612

Aarts, J., & Koppel, R. (2009). Implementation of computerized physician order entry in seven countries. *Health Affairs (Project Hope)*, *28*(2), 404–414. doi:10.1377/hlthaff.28.2.404 PMID:19275996

Abbott, T. (2005). *The adoption of eHealth in Australia*. Paper presented at the Health Informatics Conference Melbourne 2005. Melbourne, Australia.

Agarwal, R., & Prasad, J. (1997). The Role of Innovation Characteristics and Perceived Voluntariness in the Acceptance of Information Technologies. *Decision Sciences*, *28*(3), 557–582. doi:10.1111/j.1540-5915.1997.tb01322.x

Al-Azmi, S., Al-Enezi, N., & Chowdhury, R. (2009). Users' attitudes to an electronic medical record system and its correlates: A multivariate analysis. *The HIM Journal*, *38*(2), 33–40. PMID:19546486

Ammenwerth, E., Iller, C., & Mahler, C. (2006). IT-adoption and the interaction of task, technology and individuals: A fit framework and a case study. *BMC Medical Informatics and Decision Making*, 6. PMID:16451720

André, B., Ringdal, G. I., Loge, J. H., Rannestad, T., Laerum, H., & Kaasa, S. (2008). Experiences with the implementation of computerized tools in health care units: A review article. *International Journal of Human-Computer Interaction*, *24*(8), 753–775. doi:10.1080/10447310802205768

Armstrong, B. K. et al. (2007). Challenges in Health and Health Care For Australia. *The Medical Journal of Australia*, *187*(9), 485–489. PMID:17979607

Ashish, K. (2009). Use of electronic health records in U.S. hospitals. *Medical Benefits*. doi: 101056NEJMsa0900592, 25

Avgerou, C. (2008). Information systems in developing countries: A critical research review. *Journal of Information Technology*, *23*, 133–146. doi:10.1057/palgrave.jit.2000136

Bahensky, J. A., Jaana, M., & Ward, M. M. (2008). Health care information technology in rural America: Electronic medical record adoption status in meeting the national agenda. *The Journal of Rural Health*, *24*(2), 101–105. doi:10.1111/j.1748-0361.2008.00145.x PMID:18397442

Basch, P. (2005). Electronic Health Records and the National Health Information Network: Affordable, Adoptable, and Ready for Prime Time? *Annals of Internal Medicine*, *143*(3), 227–228. doi:10.7326/0003-4819-143-3-200508020-00009 PMID:16061921

Bates. (2005). Physicians And Ambulatory Electronic Health Records. *Health Aff*, *24*, 1180-1189.

Bath, P. (2008). Health informatics: Current issues and challenges. *Journal of Information Science*, *34*(4), 501. doi:10.1177/0165551508092267

Berg, M. (2001). Implementing information systems in health care organizations: Myths and challenges. *International Journal of Medical Informatics*, *64*(2-3), 143–156. doi:10.1016/ S1386-5056(01)00200-3 PMID:11734382

Bernstein, M. L., McCreless, T., & Côté, M. J. (2007). Five constants of information technology adoption in healthcare. *Hospital Topics*, *85*(1), 17–25. doi:10.3200/HTPS.85.1.17-26 PMID:17405421

Boonstra, A., & Broekhuis, M. (2010). Barriers to the acceptance of electronic medical records by physicians from systematic review to taxonomy and interventions. *BMC Health Services Research*, *10*(1), 231. doi:10.1186/1472-6963-10-231 PMID:20691097

Bossen, C. (2007). Test the artefact – Develop the organization: The implementation of an electronic medication plan. *International Journal of Medical Informatics*, *76*(1), 13–21. doi:10.1016/j.ijmedinf.2006.01.001 PMID:16455299

Callon, M. (1986). *Some elements of a sociology of translation: Domestication of the scallops and the fishermen of St. Bricue Bay*. Academic Press.

Car, J., Anandan, C., Black, A., Cresswell, K., Pagliari, C., & McKinstry, B. et al. (2008). *The Impact of eHealth on the Quality & Safety of Healthcare: A Systematic Overview and Synthesis of the Literature*. NHS Connecting for Health Evaluation Programme.

Cash, J. (2008). Technology can make or break the hospital-physician relationship. *Healthcare Financial Management*, *62*(12), 104–109. PMID:19069330

Catwell, L., & Sheikh, A. (2009). Evaluating eHealth Interventions: The Need for Continuous Systemic Evaluation. *PLoS Medicine*, *6*(8), e1000126. doi:10.1371/journal.pmed.1000126 PMID:19688038

Cohn, K., Berman, J., Chaiken, B., Green, D., Green, M., Morrison, D., & Scherger, J. (2009). Engaging physicians to adopt healthcare information technology. *Journal of Healthcare Management*, *54*(5), 291. PMID:19831114

Coiera, E. (2004). Four rules for the reinvention of health care. *BMJ (Clinical Research Ed.)*, *328*(7449), 1197–1199. doi:10.1136/bmj.328.7449.1197 PMID:15142933

Cresswell, K., Worth, A., & Sheikh, A. (2011). Implementing and adopting electronic health record systems: How actor-network theory can support evaluation. *Clinical Governance: An International Journal*, *16*(4), 320–336. doi:10.1108/14777271111175369

Cresswell, K. M., Worth, A., & Sheikh, A. (2010). Actor-Network Theory and its role in understanding the implementation of information technology developments in healthcare. *BMC Medical Informatics and Decision Making*, *10*, 67. doi:10.1186/1472-6947-10-67 PMID:21040575

Culnan, M., & Armstrong, P. K. (1997). *Information Privacy Concerns, Procedural Fairness and Impersonal Trust: An Empirical Investigation*. Retrieved from http://citeseer.ist.psu.edu/viewdoc/summary?doi=10.1.1.40.5243

Davidson, E., & Heslinga, D. (2006). Bridging the IT - Adoption Gap for Small Physician Practices: An Action Research Study on Electronic Health Records. *Information Systems Management*, *24*(1), 15. doi:10.1080/10580530601036786

DePhillips, H. A. (2007). Initiatives and Barriers to Adopting Health Information Technology: A US Perspective. *Disease Management & Health Outcomes*, *15*(1). doi:10.2165/00115677-200715010-00001

DesRoches, C. M., Campbell, E. G., Rao, S. R., Donelan, K., Ferris, T. G., & Jha, A. et al. (2008). Electronic health records in ambulatory care—A national survey of physicians. *The New England Journal of Medicine*, *359*(1), 50–60. doi:10.1056/NEJMsa0802005 PMID:18565855

Detmer, D., Bloomrosen, M., Raymond, B., & Tang, P. (2008). Integrated Personal Health Records: Transformative Tools for Consumer-Centric Care. *BMC Medical Informatics and Decision Making*, *8*(1), 45. doi:10.1186/1472-6947-8-45 PMID:18837999

DoHA. (2010). *Building a 21st Century - Primary Health Care System - Australia's First National Primary Health Care Strategy*. Australian Government Department of Health and Ageing. Retrieved from http://www.yourhealth.gov.au/internet/ yourhealth/publishing.nsf/Content/Building-a-21st-Century-Primary-Health-Care-System-TOC

Doolin, B., & Lowe, A. (2002). To reveal is to critique: Actor-network theory and critical information systems research. *Journal of Information Technology*, 69–78. doi:10.1080/02683960210145986

Elrod, J., & Androwich, I. M. (2009). Applying human factors analysis to the design of the electronic health record. *Studies in Health Technology and Informatics*, *146*, 132–136. PMID:19592822

Fisher, J. S. (1999). *Electronic Records in Clinical Practice*. Cinical Diabetes.

Frame, J., Watson, J., & Thomson, K. (2008). Deploying a culture change programme management approach in support of information and communication technology developments in Greater Glasgow NHS Board. *Health Informatics Journal*, *14*(2), 125–139. doi:10.1177/1081180X08089320 PMID:18477599

Greenhalgh, T., & Stones, R. (2010). Theorising big IT programmes in healthcare: Strong structuration theory meets actor-network theory. *Social Science & Medicine*, *70*(9), 1285–1294. doi:10.1016/j. socscimed.2009.12.034 PMID:20185218

Halamka, J. D., Mandl, K. D., & Tang, P. C. (2007). Early experiences with personal health records. *Journal of the American Medical Informatics Association*, *15*(1), 1–7. doi:10.1197/jamia.M2562 PMID:17947615

Hall, E. (2005). The 'geneticisation' of heart disease: A network analysis of the production of new genetic knowledge. *Social Science & Medicine*, *60*(12), 2673–2683. doi:10.1016/j. socscimed.2004.11.024 PMID:15820579

Hanseth, O. (2007). Integration-complexity-risk: The making of information systems out-of-control. In *Risk, Complexity and ICT*. Oslo: Edward Elgar. doi:10.4337/9781847207005.00005

Hartman, M. et al. (2009). National health spending in 2007: Slower drug spending contributes to lowest rate of overall growth since 1998. *Health Affairs*, *28*(1), 246. doi:10.1377/hlthaff.28.1.246 PMID:19124877

Häyrinen, K., Saranto, K., & Nykänen, P. (2008). Definition, structure, content, use and impacts of electronic health records: A review of the research literature. *International Journal of Medical Informatics*, *77*(5), 291–304. doi:10.1016/j. ijmedinf.2007.09.001 PMID:17951106

Hennington, A. H., & Janz, B. (2007). *Information systems and healthcare XVI: Physician adoption of electronic medical records: Applying the UTAUT model in a healthcare context*. Academic Press.

Heslop, L. (2010). *Patient and health care delivery systems in the US, Canada and Australia: A critical ethnographic analysis*. LAP LAMBERT Academic Publishing.

HFMA. (2006). *Overcoming Barriers to Electronic health Record adoption: Results of Survey and Roundtable Discussions Conducted by the Healthcare Financial Management Association*. Retrieved from http://mhcc.maryland.gov/ electronichealth/mhitr/EHR%20Links/overcoming_barriers_to_ehr_adoption.pdf

Hillestad, R. et al. (2005). Can electronic medical record systems transform health care? Potential health benefits, savings, and costs. *Health Affairs*, *24*(5), 1103. doi:10.1377/hlthaff.24.5.1103 PMID:16162551

Hoffinan, L. (2009). Implementing electronic medical records. *Communications of the ACM.* doi: 10114515927611592770

Hoffinan, S., & Podguski, A. (2008). *Finding a cure: The case for regulation and oversight of electronic health record systems.* Academic Press.

Hordern, A., Georgiou, A., Whetton, S., & Prgomet, M. (2011). Consumer e-health: An overview of research evidence and implications for future policy. *The HIM Journal, 40*(2), 6–14. PMID:21712556

Huang, Z., & Palvia, P. (2001). ERP implementation issues in advanced and developing countries. *Business Process Management Journal, 7*(3), 276–284. doi:10.1108/14637151010392773

Jones, D. A., Shipman, J. P., Plaut, D. A., & Selden, C. R. (2010). Characteristics of personal health records: Findings of the Medical Library Association/National Library of Medicine Joint Electronic Personal Health Record Task Force. *Journal of the Medical Library Association, 98*(3), 243–249. doi:10.3163/1536-5050.98.3.013 PMID:20648259

Kaghan, W., & Bowker, G. (2001). Out of machine age? Complexity, sociotechnical systems and actor network theory. *Journal of Engineering and Technology Management, 18*, 253–269. doi:10.1016/S0923-4748(01)00037-6

Kaplan, B., & Harris-Salamone, K. D. (2009). Health IT success and failure: Recommendations from literature and an AMIA workshop. *Journal of the American Medical Informatics Association, 16*(3), 291–299. doi:10.1197/jamia.M2997 PMID:19261935

Karsh, B.-T., Weinger, M. B., Abbott, P. A., & Wears, R. L. (2010). Health information technology: Fallacies and sober realities. *Journal of the American Medical Informatics Association, 17*(6), 617–623. doi:10.1136/jamia.2010.005637 PMID:20962121

Kennedy, B. L. (2011). *Exploring the Sustainment of Health Information Technology: Successful Practices for Addressing Human Factors.* Northcentral University.

Kimaro, H., & Nhampossa, J. (2007). *The challenges of sustainability of health information systems in developing countries: Comparative case studies of Mozambique and Tanzania.* Academic Press.

Kralewski, J., Dowd, B. E., Zink, T., & Gans, D. N. (2010). Preparing your practice for the adoption and implementation of electronic health records. *Physician Executive, 36*(2), 30–33. PMID:20411843

Krohn, R. (2007). The consumer-centric personal health record–It's time. *Journal of Healthcare Information Management, 21*(1), 21.

Latour, B. (2005). *Reassembling the social: An introduction to Actor-Network Theory.* Oxford University Press.

Latour, B., Harbers, H., & Koenis, S. (1996). *On actor-network theory: A few clarifications.* Academic Press.

Latour, B., & Law, J. (1986). *The Powers of Association: Power, Action and Belief.* Academic Press.

Latour, B., Mauguin, P., & Teil, G. (1992). A note on socio-technical graphs. *Social Studies of Science, 22*(1), 33. doi:10.1177/0306312792022001002

Law, J. (1991). *A Sociology of monsters: Essays on power, technology, and domination.* Routledge.

Law, J. (1997). *Heterogeneities, published by the Centre for Science Studies.* Lancaster University. Retrieved from http://www.biomedcentral.com/1472-6947/10/67/

Law, J., & Hassard, J. (1999). *Actor network theory and after.* Wiley-Blackwell.

Leila. (2009). The Bug's Blog: Bruno Latour, Action-Network-Theory, and Dismantling Heirarchies: Actor-Network-Theory: Terms and Concepts. *The Bug's Blog*. Retrieved from http://latourbugblog.blogspot.com/2009/01/actor-network-theory-terms-and-concepts.html

Leslie, H. (2011). *Australia's PCEHR Challenge | Archetypical*. Retrieved from http://omowizard.wordpress.com/2011/08/30/australias-pcehr-challenge/

Liu, L. S., Shih, P. C., & Hayes, G. R. (2011). Barriers to the adoption and use of personal health record systems. In *Proceedings of the 2011 iConference* (pp. 363–370). Academic Press.

Lorenzi, N. et al. (2009). How to successfully select and implement electronic health records (EHR) in small ambulatory practice settings. *BMC Medical Informatics and Decision Making, 9*, 15. doi:10.1186/1472-6947-9-15 PMID:19236705

McLean, C., & Hassard, J. (2004). Symmetrical Absence/Symmetrical Absurdity: Critical Notes on the Production of Actor-Network Accounts. *Journal of Management Studies, 41*(3), 493–519. doi:10.1111/j.1467-6486.2004.00442.x

McReavy, D., Toth, L., Tremonti, C., & Yoder, C. (2009). *The CFO's role in implementing EHR systems: the experiences of a Florida health system point to 10 actions that can help CFOs manage the revenue risks and opportunities of implementing an electronic health record*. Retrieved December 16, 2011, from http://findarticles.com/p/articles/mi_m3257/is_6_63/ai_n35529545/

Mitchell, V., & Nault, B. (2008). *The emergence of functional knowledge in sociotechnical systems*. Academic Press.

Mohd, H., & Mohamad, S. M. S. (2005). Acceptance model of electronic medical record. *Management, 2*(1), 75.

Mort, M., Finch, T., & May, C. (2007). Making and unmaking telepatients: identity and governance in new health technologies. *Science, Technology & Human Values, 34*(1), 9–33. doi:10.1177/0162243907311274

Nagle, L. M. (2007). EHR versus EMR versus EPR. *Nursing Leadership, 20*(1), 30–32. doi:10.12927/cjnl.2007.18782 PMID:17472137

NEHTA & DoHA. (2011). *Concept of Operations: Relating to the introduction of a Personally Controlled Electronic Health Record System*. Retrieved from http://www.yourhealth.gov.au/internet/yourhealth/publishing.nsf/Content/CA2578620005CE1DCA2578F800194110/$File/PCEHR%20Concept%20of%20Operations.pdf

Neves, J. et al. (2008). Electronic Health Records and Decision Support Local and Global Perspectives. *WSEAS Transactions on Biology and Biomedicine, 5*, 8.

NHHRC. (2009). *A Healthier Future for All Australians: National Health and Hospitals Reform Commission - Final Report June 2009*. Retrieved from http://www.health.gov.au/internet/main/publishing.nsf/Content/nhhrc-report

Protti, D., & Smit, C. (2006). The Netherlands: Another European Country Where GPs Have Been Using EMRs for Over Twenty Years. - Google Scholar. *Healthcare Information Management & Communications, 30*(3).

Rhodes, J. (2009). Using Actor-Network Theory to Trace an ICT (Telecenter) Implementation Trajectory in an African Women's Micro-Enterprise Development Organization. *Information Technologies & International Development, 5*(3), 1–20.

Rogers, E. (2003). *Diffusion of innovation*. New York: Free Press.

Rosebaugh, D. (2004). Getting ready for the software in your future. *Home Health Care Management Practice*. doi: 1011771084822303259877

Rosenbloom, S. T. et al. (2006). Implementing Pediatric Growth Charts into an Electronic Health Record System. *Journal of the American Medical Informatics Association, 13*, 302–308. doi:10.1197/jamia.M1944 PMID:16501182

Ross, S. E., Schilling, L. M., Fernald, D. H., Davidson, A. J., & West, D. R. (2010). Health information exchange in small-to-medium sized family medicine practices: Motivators, barriers, and potential facilitators of adoption. *International Journal of Medical Informatics, 79*(2), 123–129. doi:10.1016/j.ijmedinf.2009.12.001 PMID:20061182

Rydin, Y. (2010). Actor-network theory and planning theory: A response to Boelens. *Planning Theory, 9*, 265–268.

Showell, C.M. (2011). Citizens, patients and policy: A challenge for Australia's national electronic health record. *Health Information Management Journal OnLine, 40*(2).

Tang, P. C., Ash, J. S., Bates, D. W., Overhage, J. M., & Sands, D. Z. (2006). Personal health records: Definitions, benefits, and strategies for overcoming barriers to adoption. *Journal of the American Medical Informatics Association, 13*(2), 121–126. doi:10.1197/jamia.M2025 PMID:16357345

Thompson, T. G., & Brailer, D. J. (2004). *The decade of health information technology: Delivering consumer-centric and information-rich health care. Framework for Strategic Action, Office for the National Coordinator for Health Information Technology (ONCHIT).* Department of Health and Human Services, and the United States Federal Government.

Thweatt, E. G., & Kleiner, B. H. (2007). New Developments in Health Care Organisational Management. *Journal of Health Management, 9*(3), 433–441. doi:10.1177/097206340700900308

Timpka, T. et al. (2007). Information infrastructure for inter-organizational mental health services: An actor network theory analysis of psychiatric rehabilitation. *Journal of Biomedical Informatics, 40*(4), 429–437. doi:10.1016/j.jbi.2006.11.001 PMID:17182285

Tobler, N. (2008). *Technology, organizational change, and the nonhuman agent: Exploratory analysis of electronic health record implementation in a small practice ambulatory care.* The University of Utah.

Torda, P., Han, E. S., & Scholle, S. H. (2010). Easing the adoption and use of electronic health records in small practices. *Health Affairs (Project Hope), 29*(4), 668–675. doi:10.1377/hlthaff.2010.0188 PMID:20368597

Trudel, M. C. (2010). *Challenges to personal information sharing in interorganizational settings: Learning from the Quebec Health Smart Card project.* The University of Western Ontario.

Vitacca, M., Mazzù, M., & Scalvini, S. (2009). Socio-technical and organizational challenges to wider e-Health implementation. *Chronic Respiratory Disease, 6*(2), 91–97. doi:10.1177/1479972309102805 PMID:19411570

Walsham, G. (1997). Actor-network theory and IS research: Current status and future prospects. In *Information Systems and Qualitative Research: Proceedings of the IFIP TC8 WG 8.2 International Conference on Information Systems and Qualitative Research.* Academic Press.

Weimar, C. (2009). Electronic health care advances, physician frustration grows. *Physician Executive, 35*(2), 8–15. PMID:19452840

Westbrook, J. I., & Braithwaite, J. (2010). Will Information and Communication Technology Disrupt the Health System and Deliver on Its Promise? *The Medical Journal of Australia, 193*(7), 399–400. PMID:20919970

Wickramasinghe, N., & Bali, R. K. (2009). The S'ANT Imperative for Realizing the Vision of Healthcare Network Centric Operations. *International Journal of Actor-Network Theory and Technological Innovation*, *1*(1), 45–58. doi:10.4018/jantti.2009010103

Wickramasinghe, N., Bali, R. K., & Lehaney, B. (2009). *Knowledge Management Primer*. Taylor & Francis.

Wickramasinghe, N., & Schaffer, J. (2010). *Realizing Value Driven e-Health Solutions*. IBM centre for the Business of government.

Wickramasinghe, N., Tatnall, A., & Goldberg, S. (2011). The Advantages Of Mobile Solutions For Chronic Disease Management. *PACIS 2011 Proceedings*. Retrieved from http://aisel.aisnet.org/pacis2011/214.

Williams, R. (2007). Managing complex adaptive networks. In *Proceedings of the 4th International Conference on Intellectual Capital, Knowledge Management & Organizational Learning* (pp. 441–452). Academic Press.

Yusof, M., Stergioulas, L., & Zugic, J. (2007). *Health information systems adoption: Findings from a systematic review*. Academic Press.

KEY TERMS AND DEFINITIONS

EMR (Electronic Medical Record): A medical record that is written, stored and maintained in a digital format usually by a clinician.

EPR (Electronic Patient Record): An electronic record of patient related facts maintained and managed by healthcare organisations at large.

HER (Electronic Health Record): A comprehensive health record that consists of information collected from different service providers and point-of-service systems such as pharmacies and diagnostic centres for all healthcare encounters an individual may have with them.

Individual Health Identifiers: Unique numbers given to each user of the PCEHR so that their record remains unique at all times.

PCEHR (Personally Controlled Electronic Health Record): The Australian national e-health solution that has an unique shared governance model.

This work was previously published in Technological Advancements and the Impact of Actor-Network Theory edited by Arthur Tatnall, pages 15-34 copyright year 2014 by Information Science Reference (an imprint of IGI Global).

Chapter 67

A Social Work Approach in High–Tech Neurosurgery and Social Work Research Approaches in Health Care

Colin Pritchard
Bournemouth University, UK

ABSTRACT

Psychiatric social work is inherently inter-disciplinary with an interactive bio-psycho-social model of behaviour. This chapter mainly focuses upon an innovative study in neurosurgery. Sub-arachnoid haemorrhage (SAH) is a life-threatening condition and survivors are often left with serious cognitive impairment. Patients and their carers led the design of a two-year controlled prospective study of a patient and family support service, using the Specialist Neurovascular Nurse (SNVN) to speed rehabilitation and family readjustment. Cost-effective measures found the SNVN group gained significant psychosocial and fiscal benefits when compared to the control group, thus highlighting the effectiveness of a social work approach in neurosurgery. Other studies in healthcare, including surgical patient safety, effectiveness in reducing mortality, cultural influence on suicide rates and implications for prevention, and the implications of the changing patterns of neurological mortality in Western nations, are briefly described.

INTRODUCTION

Psychiatric social work has always considered itself to have an interdisciplinary approach, especially in relation to health care. In part, this is because of the interactive model of the bio-psycho-social approach to the nature of human behaviour. The following studies illustrate the value of such an approach in health care because social work, as a practice-based discipline, is a science-based art which can bring the insights of a psychosocial perspective into different areas of health care. The contexts of health care practice to be explored are hospital and after-care for neurosurgery patients and suicide prevention in mental health. The author's research suggests that it is helpful to have a social work-based service for patients and their caregivers integrated with

DOI: 10.4018/978-1-4666-8756-1.ch067

any health care offered. Ideally, it is recommended that there be at least one social worker in every health care team developing such services. These services are developed using social work principles and practices which by their nature are holistic, collaborative, information sharing, and responsive to patients and their families' needs.

SOCIAL WORK APPROACH IN HIGH-TECH NEUROSURGERY

This chapter begins with an innovative project in high-tech neurosurgery dealing with patient cohorts of sub-arachnoid haemorrhage (SAH), a life-threatening condition. To understand a person and their family's response to a SAH, some background and discussion of what happens to those involved is necessary.

There are probably few conditions more dramatic than that of a SAH in which, generally without warning and no previous symptoms, an aneurysm on one of the major rings of arteries in the brain bursts. Because the skull is a hard box and the brain a soft vital organ, anything that takes up extra space, be it a tumour or a bleed (haemorrhage) such as a stroke, and SAH is a type of stroke, immediately creates a potential life-threatening or seriously disabling condition. The size and position of the bleed will affect the patient physiologically and, therefore, psychosocially but will be different in virtually every patient. It impacts often dramatically because of the suddenness with which it comes upon an individual's family and their social circumstances.

A little more than 50 years ago, almost 90% of SAH patients died within days, and before modern neurosurgery many of the survivors were left with neurological damage which might include loss of speech or sensation, or paralysis ranging from one to all four limbs. At the worst, it involved a traumatic dementia. Today, whilst about 5-10% of SAH are fatal within days, if the patient is

stabilised, one of two treatments is effective. The long-standing treatment is a craniotomy, which involves a surgical opening of the skull, finding the aneurysm, and then clipping it. Whilst this is quite an invasive procedure, this is considered a total cure assuming there are no other aneurysms, although there may be varied degrees of physical weakness and impairment.

A more recent treatment is endovascular in which lines are passed through the femoral artery and up into the brain where a coil is placed within the damaged artery. Since this approach is less invasive it is used more often but as it is not always feasible craniotomies are still performed. Whichever treatment is used, if there are no other aneurysms, the patient's life-threatening condition is cured (Frazer, Ahuja, Watkins, & Cipolitti, 2007; Molyneux et al., 2009). However, mention is seldom made of the fact that 3% of all coiled patients have a re-bleed and die. This suggests that the endovascular approach still requires development as less than 1% of craniotomies have a re-bleed from a failed clip. Nonetheless, in both the retrospective and prospective studies to be described, we found that irrespective of treatment approach, there was no difference in the immediate psychosocial impact on the family of suddenly finding their loved ones in a neurosurgical unit fighting for their lives (Janes et al., 2013; Mezue, Matthew, Draper, & Watson, 2004; Pritchard, Foulkes, Lang, & Neil-Dwyer, 2001, 2004).

Following treatment, many patients develop what is now recognised as a post-traumatic stress disorder (PTSD) reaction (Noble et al., 2011; Visser-Meiley, Rhebergen, Rinkel, van Zandvoort, & Post, 2009), which had long been thought inevitable by virtue of the shock of being confronted with a sudden traumatic life-threatening disease (Buchanan, Elias, & Goplen, 2000). This was summed up by one neurosurgeon in responding to a ward sister's question, "if SAH patients are clinically cured, why do they keep returning to the neurosurgical unit?" He replied,

Whilst the treatment was life-saving and now after clipping they're cured but of course they'll be knocked-off. They've had a massive assault to the brain [the bleed] requiring major treatment. I tell patients they can expect to be off work months, and some are for years. Some never go back because their confidence is destroyed. (Anonymous, personal communication, February, 2000)

Background to the Project

The author was invited by neurosurgical professionals to explore the problems faced by the post-treatment group, but at the time the professionals had not identified what questions were to be addressed. Two groups of twelve former patients were invited to the unit to discuss their experience and in effect became a focus group. The patients all readily agreed but there was still no hypothesis and the author met them with an open mind, although with a degree of irritation because the neurosurgical professionals had not specified the questions to be asked.

The first patient and her husband told such a terrible story of isolation, fearfulness, anxiety, and family tensions, that it did not seem ethical to ask much more but rather offer a listening ear. The next pair (patient and carer) told a similar unhappy story and I realised I was dealing with people in quite severe PTSD states, which at the time was not recognised by those in neurosurgery who rather saw the psycho-cognitive distress as an almost inevitable sequel to the physical impact of the SAH. In brief, I had ceased being a researcher and had moved into a counsellor role as this appeared to be what they needed. It had become clear that the patents and their carers "wanted to tell their story" and it seemed an important story that needed to be told.

In the light of this, it was decided to design a survey about patient and carer experience and the interviewees were invited to comment upon and contribute to a draft questionnaire. All interviewees took an active part, crucially acknowledging that the whole treatment and post-discharge experience would be different for the patient and their carer.

Against the author's judgement, the participants insisted that we included the widest coverage of their experience as well as demographics in the questionnaire. The questionnaire was to be postal and self-administered, aimed at those patients and their families discharged over the previous two years. Former patients and families were asked to indicate a degree of agreement/disagreement on a series of structured statements developed by the patient focus group, using a five-point Lickert Scale which evaluated their experience of the service as inpatients and post-discharge. In effect, the patients and their carers designed the questionnaire from their perspective, rather than from that of the professionals, to include everything they thought important.

There were open-ended qualitative questions giving respondents the opportunity to raise issues important to them. These embraced what was "best" and "worst" about their SAH experience both within and after discharge from hospital. The key question which emerged was: "Based on your experience, what if anything would you teach the doctors and nurses?"

The statements and demographic clinical information together yielded 79 questions. With so many questions it was not expected to attract a good response rate especially because it was retrospective. However, the patient and carer focus groups were pressing and very persuasive so it was important that as much as possible from their own words should be included in the questionnaire.

In the event, the strength and relevance of the essentially patient-family designed questionnaire was reflected in a 77% response rate from a two year cohort of treated SAH patients, yielding 142 paired patient and carer respondents. Their results reflected current and standard care in this and other neurosurgical units and were, therefore, designated the "Treatment-as-Usual" (TAU) group, when we undertook a prospective study.

The reason for the high response rate became clear on reading the open-ended responses as many people wrote reams and often with accompanying letters. It also became apparent that many patients were still in a PTSD state, and the patient-centred questionnaire was obviously more relevant to their experience than any questionnaire designed from the professional's perspective. Whilst the majority of patients had had a very good clinical recovery, even after two years many were still cognitively and psychologically distressed.

Below are three cases that typify SAH patient experiences and the psychological aftermath of their condition even after excellent life-saving surgery, as there was virtually no follow-up care to deal with the psychosocial impact of a SAH. To place these experiences in context, it is noteworthy that 54% of patients were less than 50 years old, meaning that the SAH occurred at the height of their professional and family life when they had responsibilities to partners, children, and employers. The case examples are anonymised.

The Case of "John"

John was a 35 year old entrepreneur, who had just been awarded a major contract that would double his business from 10 to 20 employees. He had observed that he was well on the way to becoming a millionaire. He rang his wife to tell her the good news and planned a romantic dinner, but whilst driving home he suddenly experienced the most intense headache, at first thinking he had been struck from behind. Fortunately, he was able to steer his car off the motorway before becoming totally unconscious. His first subsequent memory occurred a week later when he found his wife crying beside his bed. He made a very good post-operative recovery and was discharged home in less than two weeks. However, he continued to feel distressed, could not concentrate, experienced panic attacks, feared another stroke, and was unable to face returning to work. His identity centred on his career as he was the business. Because of his

time off work, the business failed and he and his family lost everything. John had seen his general practitioner (GP) but because SAH is relatively rare, the GP had little experience of the condition. As John's wound healed well with virtually no physical disability associated with stroke, the community nurse felt he had no further need of assistance and follow-up care. As a family, John, his wife, and his children (who were aged 10 and 12 years), felt even more isolated.

Continuing and longer-term problems remained, with John experiencing periods of depression and an inability to judge what was "physically normal" along with continued cognitive disruption. After a year facing these issues, the pressure on his relationship with his wife meant that his marriage was faltering. Prior to the SAH, he and his wife had led an active sex life but after the SAH, he began to have sexual difficulties because of alarm at his rising blood pressure. Crucially, no one had explained to him that as there were no other aneurysms he was cured. His anxiety, therefore, remained.

The Case of "Mary"

Mary was a 48 year old senior social worker. During an argument with her "stroppy teenage" daughter, she suddenly felt a massive blow inside her head. As her vision deteriorated, she felt her daughter was disappearing before her eyes, and as she fell to the ground, the last thing she heard was her daughter screaming, "Mam, mam, I've killed you!" A week later, she remembered becoming aware of being in the neurosurgical unit, terrified by what was going on around her. She made a good clinical recovery and was discharged home but there was little effective follow-up other than being given the standard booklet explaining the nature of SAH. Mary considered this booklet somewhat useful but insufficient as it "told us little of what it meant to our situation". One family consequence was that Mary's husband had to take time off work to look after his wife, causing considerable difficulty at work. Mary had a minor weakness in her left leg though there were no other physical problems. The wound healed well so the community care stopped. Mary thought she was "going mad", whilst her teenage daughter went into depression, convinced she had caused her mother's illness. The daughter began to miss school preferring to stay at home with her mother to ensure her mother was safe. As a result, her education deteriorated. Family tensions also arose, with the threat of either the daughter or the husband leaving. Her husband's employers were unsympathetic and he faced losing his position because of the time he had spent as a carer. After a month, he had no choice but to return to work. Mary felt deserted and quite unable to go back to an emotionally demanding job. Her employers, whilst a little more sympathetic, had to temporarily backfill her position while she was away. This meant that Mary lost the opportunity for a promotion and in despair she resigned, compounding the situation at home.

The Case of "Margaret"

Margaret, aged 58, was a very successful head teacher in a large secondary school, known for her omni-competence, running her home and family, and meeting the numerous demands of her job. Sitting in the garden one summer evening, she bent down to smell a rose and experienced a painful explosion in her head and lost consciousness. As is typical of the above SAH experience, she recalled, "My world was turned upside down. I came away from neurosurgery a trembling wreck; couldn't distinguish any minor ache from the threat of another attack". After six months of barely improved anxiety and total loss of confidence, though she had virtually no physical disability, Margaret decided to take early retirement from a job to which she was previously passionately committed.

The above case examples typify the title of Wertheimer's (2008) book, *A Dented Image: Journeys of Recovery from a Subarachnoid Haemorrhage*. The book describes what happens to many post-discharged SAH receiving standard TAU. For months or years afterwards, all participants felt that, whilst their lives had been saved, they had been irredeemably shattered.

Patient and Caregiver Designed Research: TAU Outcomes

The initial TAU results, published in the *British Journal of Neurosurgery* (Pritchard et al, 2001), added to the grim picture surrounding the post-operative SAH experience of other researchers (for example, Buchanan et al., 2000; Mezue et al., 2004). However, the uniqueness of this study was that by identifying the patients and their carers' problems, our open-ended qualitative questions enabled them to recommend a solution based upon what they felt they needed.

On the positive side, 25% of the patients said they only had mild or no stress, but the majority (53%) disclosed having severe socially disabling stress. Nearly half (45%) said that they had poor general health but relatively few reported physical weaknesses associated with stroke, although 10% had speech difficulties and 30% reported memory difficulties. There was an overwhelming complaint regarding the lack of support and sense of isolation. One theme throughout was the high level of anxiety (52%) and depression (38%) and a feeling of not knowing what is normal any more.

The social consequences of SAH were quite drastic. 9% lost their jobs; and of those of working age, 82% of the cohort had time off work, 48% were still off work up to two years post-SAH, and only 20% had returned to work in less than three months post-SAH. The actual cost to the families ran into the tens of thousands of pounds and although many middle-class occupations provide full pay for the first six months of sick leave this was soon exhausted, with the cost of being away from work transferred to the employer and the wider economy. Whilst the cost of high-tech neurosurgery is not borne by British people, since the national publicly funded health scheme (NHS) treats without charge at the point of need, it is often forgotten that there is considerable economic cost to families because of the time off work. At the extreme, patients risk becoming unemployed or being under-employed, a theme to which we shall return.

The results of this research detailing the social costs of the condition shocked the surgeons in the Unit who admitted to not giving thought to the consequences of being off work, simply pleased that the patients made clinical recovery. Clinical recovery is the surgeon's primary goal and provides their major source of job satisfaction (Pritchard, Brackstone, & MacFie, 2010). Fortunately, the neurosurgeons recognised that something had to be done and the answer became apparent from the patients' and carers' replies. They had described how isolated in the community they felt as many general practitioners and community nurses had little experience of SAH, an uncommon condition with a life-time prevalence of 1 in a 100,000 people (Lindsay, Bone, & Fuller, 2010) and in the UK only about 2,200 cases a year (Royal College of Surgeons of England, 2006).

Patients and their caregivers, therefore, needed someone from the unit who understood the condition to respond to their family-specific queries. In other words, they needed someone like the "traditional" hospital social worker, who was well-informed about their particular hospital ward's conditions, and who if they did not know, knew someone who did. They could offer appropriate support and counselling where necessary to assist the patient's rehabilitation, including any necessary family re-integration in the community upon discharge from hospital.

As a result, the unit neurosurgeons, concerned for their patients, pressed the Hospital Trust to provide patients with a family support service in a funded two year prospective study. The ward sister developed her counselling skills and became the specialist neurovascular nurse (SNVN) in a new post to be evaluated in the two year prospective study to see if such a service met the needs of patients and families in a reasonably cost-effective way. The prospective patients' outcomes would be compared against the results from the TAU group to determine any statistically significant differences.

A Social Work Approach in Neurosurgery: A Comparative Longitudinal Controlled Study

The two year retrospective TAU cohort attracted a response rate of 77% of people posted, but the two year prospective study, which yielded 184 patients and carers, had a remarkable 92% response rate from families who had received help from the neurosurgical unit-based SNVN (Pritchard, Foulkes, et al., 2004).

In terms of clinical background, site of bleed, and on a range of standardised measures, such as the Glasgow Coma Score, there was little to choose between the TAU and SNVN cohorts, although among the SNVN patients there was a small but significantly greater number of larger bleeds than the TAU, suggesting that the SNVN group were slightly more physically damaged. Overall, the cohorts were a good match in terms of age, social class background, number of children, and gender. Participants were predominantly female at 67%.

Qualitative Findings: TAU vs. SNVN Groups Follow Up

Key statistical significant differences in replies to the structured questionnaire (from a series of chi square tests) concerned patients' stay in hospital as well as post-discharge. Of the TAU patients, 28% said they were discharged too soon to SNVN's 16%; frightened 51% to 24%; in pain 47% to 24%; and crucially with unanswered questions about prognosis, TAU 48% to SNVN 20%. Whilst a fair proportion of the SNVN patient group continued to have some psychosocial problems, these were virtually half the rate of the TAU group, indicating the early accumulative value of the SNVN making contact in the neurosurgical unit prior to discharge.

Patients' post-discharge findings were also markedly different, with SNVN having a significantly more satisfactory outcome than TAU on virtually every psychosocial measure. For example, personal stress 43% (TAU) to 19% (SNVH); stress on the family 77% to 29%; family member off work because of SAH 56% to 32%; making unnecessary calls to the GP 32% to 10%; feeling frightened 40% to 11%; and depressed 35% to 21%. Thus, whilst patients in contact with the SNVN were not without problems, they were markedly less distressed than the TAU group, which as we will see, has practical and economic implications.

The carers' post-discharge findings were even more markedly different between the two groups, although there were differences between patients' and carers' perceptions, indicating the different nature of the burden of the condition and how it affected them differently.

Only 20% of TAU carers said there was no further stress from the SAH compared to 72% of the SNVN carers, and 13% of TAU to 54% of SNVN reported they "had all the support they needed". Moreover, 51% of TAU carers to 11% of SNVN carers made "unnecessary calls to the GP"; and "worries about my relative affected my work", was true for 77% of TAU carers to 39% of SNVN carers. These findings provide another indication of the value of social work input of the SNVN service to the carers as well as patients.

When patients and carers of the SNVN group were asked about the service, 88% said the service was a vital link between home and hospital. Only 9% were critical, 76% being highly satisfied, and 54% said the GP should be more willing to take advice from the SNVN. More than 80% of patients and carers said the SNVN was an "invaluable support to the family".

The Costs of Being Absent from Work

In terms of patients losing their jobs due to the SAH, this occurred in 11% of TAU patients to 1% SNVN. Whilst 28% of TAU patients were on sick leave less than three months to 41% of SNVN, 47% TAU to 16% SAH carers were off work for six or more months due to their SAH. In regard to carers who had been off work less than a month, the results were: TAU 47% to 74% SNVN carers; being off work more than 17 weeks occurred in 26% of the TAU to only 2% SNVN carers.

Based upon the respondents' type of employment, it was possible to estimate the cost to families of the disruption to employment. For TAU patients, this cost averaged £9,076 compared to £4,011 for SNVN patients. For TAU carers, this cost was £3,193 to £888 for SNVN carers. This loss of income for patients and the families of patients is an issue often forgotten. Serious illnesses can have considerable economic costs to families and the wider economy. Thus, overall the TAU families loss of potential earnings exceeded £748,000 when compared to the SNVN £491,000. This represents a "hidden" saving of £257,000 to the families who received psychosocial support which was more than six times the cost of employing the SNVN over the two years.

These figures above do not include any fiscal estimate of the benefit of the improved psychosocial state of the SNVN families. There were slight but significant reductions in length of stay in hospital, reduced use of consultants in outpatient clinics taken by the SNVN, and reduction in GP time in the SNVN families. The service, therefore, had monetary savings of £4,165 per patient receiving a SNVN service.

The Wessex SNVN service was the first of its kind in neurosurgery. The ground-breaking research relating to the importance of a psychosocial approach to rehabilitation with patients and caregivers was a model for other hospital units to follow. Today, of the 33 neurosurgical units in the UK and Ireland, 13 units now have family support services.

Commonality of the Role of the SNVN and Hospital Social Worker

The development of the SNVN fitted within the social work tradition of being holistic and patient-centred, viewing the patient and their family within the wider context of their community. This meant that upon the patient's admission, the SNVN made herself available to the patient and their caregivers, although often in the first few days the patient was not able to respond. However, the simple presence of the SNVN and her availability to the carers at this moment of need in the face of traumatic events engendered for the family the beginning of hope. Whilst no false assurances were given, the SNVN began to talk with the family about what would be needed when the patient was discharged from hospital to return home.

Initially, the SNVN did a home visit but being a regional service this quickly became impractical, so both patients and carers were seen on the hospital ward. Regular telephone and internet contact was maintained after discharge. An important feature was that because the families had telephone access, they seldom used the telephone other than by the agreed appointment. Moreover, the SNVN developed a patients' and carers' support and psycho-education group which she facilitated, providing wider and mutual support. Details of this group can be found elsewhere (Pritchard, Lindsay, Cox, & Foulkes, 2011). Typical of effective social work outcomes, it was the quality of the SNVN client/family relationship that was more important to patients and their caregivers. This was the active ingredient that contributed to the significantly better SNVN outcomes.

This theme associated with superior SVNM outcomes was succinctly outlined by a senior military person, aged 48, who returned to full time duties. He said,

Unusually I remember much of my inpatient experience. I was fortunate to have had surgery at the very highest international level. But the second outstanding feature was the SNVN. She was available to deal with all those little questions which if they had not been dealt with would have become major barriers to my recovery, adding to my family's distress [emphasis added]. (Anonymous, personal communication, January, 2004)

This comment is a reminder of the constant interaction between the individual patient and their family and how dealing with the sum of the whole improves the quality of life for each individual member.

Whilst the post-operative cognitive deterioration associated with SAH has long been known, it was assumed to be almost inevitable (Baisch, Schenk, & Noble, 2011; Buchanan et al., 2000; Mezue et al., 2004; Noble et al., 2011). This study shows this is not the case and such distress can be substantially reduced in many patients, if not totally avoided. The situation of TAU patients whose PTSD is largely left unaddressed also ignores the impact on the family, but a social work type approach can bring about major measurable positive changes even in a high-tech neurosurgery ward.

INFLUENCING NATIONAL POLICY FOR SAH PATIENTS AND FAMILIES

Potential National Impact

The above study led to an invitation from the British Society of Neurological Surgeons to re-evaluate their national data (Royal College of Surgeons of England, 2006) on 2,450 SAH patients and to estimate what the effect would be if every

Neurosurgery unit had a SNVN. The clinical and demographic data of TAU and SNVN Wessex cohorts were matched and projected onto the UK cases of SAH yielding a comparative sample of 2,380 patients (Pritchard et al., 2011). The composition of this sample indicates that the Wessex SAH sample was fairly typical of SAH patients in the UK during the period under review.

The results when scaled up nationally were dramatic. The 2,380 matched patients consisted of 66% females. At a national level, the SAH patients aged under 44 years were estimated to have 895 school-aged children, and of patients aged between 45-54 there were a further 1,285 school-aged children who would likely have been affected by their parents life-threatening illness. Estimates of length of stay found the projected TAU group would have had 34,850 hospital days compared with the estimated SNVN 30,685 days, a 13% saving (Pritchard et al., 2011).

In 2008, a neurosurgical bed cost £544 per day but most SAH patients would have spent at least one day/night in the Intensive Therapy Unit at £1000 per day (Pritchard et al., 2011). A cautious estimate of reduced neurosurgical beds alone would, therefore, have yielded a potential "saving" of £2,176,000 to the NHS through provision of a social work service. The "saving" for families was estimated at £6,014 million for patients and £2,083 for carers because of the substantially reduced "time-off" work for those who would have received SNVN support.

When economists and politicians discuss the cost of modern health care provision, such sums seem to be presented as if these costs were an economic loss, albeit for a desirable public and moral good. This ignores the fact that many patients of working age return to full time employment and, therefore, in the case of Britain's NHS continue to pay income tax and social security payments which fund the NHS.

Breaking the national sample down by age and accounting for annual age-related mortality and projecting estimate years of productive work, we found that over their expected life-time, at 2008 prices, former working-aged SAH patients could, if making a good psychosocial recovery as did the SNVN, yield a contribution of £162 million to the wider economy (Pritchard & Hickish, 2011). This shows that successful integrated neurosurgery not only saves lives and rehabilitates but brings economic benefit.

Evaluating PTSD in Neurosurgery: Elective and Emergency Surgery and Spin-Off Social Work-Led Research in Surgery

The original study attracted the attention of Ear-Nose-Throat (ENT) surgeons who worked in neurosurgery on a chronic condition known as Acoustic Neuroma (AN), a slow growing benign tumour. They were interested to discover whether their elective AN patients had similar problems to SAH patients as an elective craniotomy is the mode of treating AN.

From the two-year retrospective survey of 102 patients and caregivers, it was found that the AN cohort had substantially fewer psychosocial problems than the SAH patients, even though initially AN patients had slightly more physical problems in the first six-months post-discharge. This led us to conclude that the greater degree of PTSD amongst the retrospective SAH cohort was in part due to the traumatic and acute nature of the SAH (Pritchard, Clapham, Davis, Lang, & Neil-Dwyer, 2004; Pritchard, Clapham, Foulkes, Lang, & Neil-Dwyer, 2004; Pritchard, Foulkes, et al., 2004). These results gave us further confidence in the need for a post-operative psychosocial family centred service to deal with the unresolved PTSD.

PATIENT-RELATED-OUTCOME-MEASURES (PROM) AND PATIENT SAFETY

This social work led research in neurosurgery coincided with national concerns about patient safety in operating theatres. The Chief Medical Officer (2007) recommended that there should be a revalidation of consultant surgeons every five years and their assessment should include "Patient-Related-Outcome-Measures" (PROM). The above patient-carer-centred studies were the first of their kind in neurosurgery and led to an invitation to the author to serve on the Research and Peer Review Sub-Committee of the Royal College of Surgeons in the development of the revalidation criteria.

The Committee was an unusual setting for a Research Professor of Psychiatric Social Work who learned much about the expertise and also the often divergent focus of surgeons, recognising that they needed a more holistic focus to include patients, families, and the society in which they live. Because the Chief Medical Officer's (2007) focus was upon "failures" in the operating theatre or when things go wrong, the author challenged the negative media and political portrayal that many surgeons had uncritically appeared to accept. In the discussions, it became apparent that the Chief Medical Officer's criticisms were a little unfair, and as John McVie, professor of surgery at the University of Hull, asked, "How can we hear the voice of the surgeon?" (Personal communication, June, 2008). This led to a quantitative and qualitative anonymous and non-attributable survey of all members of the Association of Surgeons of Great Britain and Ireland on the issues concerned with patient safety in theatre.

A 27% online response rate yielded 549 consultant surgeons and outlined the interaction of problems and resources, staffing theatre teams, and crucially, the dichotomy between surgeons' and managers' priorities (Pritchard & Brackstone, 2009; Pritchard, Brackstone & MacFie, 2010).

In the survey, the author and team examined the rate of "Patient Adverse Events", and we had a higher rate than those complained of by the Chief Medical Officer (2007), showing the integrity and honesty of our respondents. Nevertheless, the rates from the Association of Surgeons of Great Britain and Ireland were contrasted against a major systematic analysis from North America (de Vries, Ramrattan, Smorenburg, Gouma, & Boermeester, 2008) to find that the Association's rates were considerably lower.

Perhaps the most encouraging outcomes emerged from the qualitative open-ended questions on job satisfaction, as 100% of the respondents indicated that their work was about facilitating a positive outcome for patients. The worst aspect of their work was identified as a poor outcome for the patient indicating the strong patient-centeredness of these 549 surgeons. In considering sweeping criticism of the British NHS, however, the nation's health outcomes do need to be judged in the light of comparable countries, something to which I now turn.

COST-EFFECTIVENESS OF NHS IN REDUCING CANCER DEATHS COMPARED TO OTHER WESTERN COUNTRIES

The author was accused by a consultant surgeon of being an "ivory towered academic", that surgeons, by contrast, "are at the table every day to see the problems". But it was suggested to him that surgeons "don't see the big picture" which is essential for developing evidence-based policy. Two studies compared the UK and twenty "Other-Western-Countries" (OWC) on the ultimate health outcome, Total Adult (15-74) Mortality and, because of specific criticisms of the UK, these were compared with adult Cancer Mortality Rates (Pritchard & Hickish, 2011; Pritchard & Wallace, 2011).

Tables 1 to 3 show the updated results from the study that outline the analysis to 2008. Ten death rates per million indicate a reduction in Total Adult deaths and Cancer Mortality Rates and show that the 21 Western countries have made major achievements. However, in terms of actual falls, divided by the % GDP spent on health to produce a cost-effective ratio, the UK was one of the most effective and efficient in the Western world. The UK had some of the biggest reductions between 1980-2010 in both Total Adult Mortality and Cancer Mortality, indicating that the NHS achieves more with proportionately less (Pritchard & Hickish, 2011; Pritchard & Wallace, 2011).

Readers from the 21 countries will be able to assess the degree of success of their own country. Indeed, some might find it surprising that in terms of money spent on health and reduced deaths, the USA was one of the least effective and efficient.

I will now proceed to a discussion regarding research into social work's role in ameliorating suicide in mental health contexts.

SOCIAL WORK RESEARCH'S CONTRIBUTION TO SUICIDE STUDIES

Durkheim has been described as the "father of sociology" and his seminal work related to social factors in suicide (Durkheim, 1897). Psychiatric social work, whilst inherently multidisciplinary, is based essentially in the social and behavioural sciences which can be valuable in health care as it builds upon an underlying sociological and empirical approach.

Britain decriminalised suicide in 1962 but the Roman Catholic Church still asserts that suicide is a mortal sin. Islam's Quran is quite explicit – suicide is considered to be an act of murder. The author interviewed a depressed Islamic woman who required a translator but the translator would not translate gently-asked questions about the client's despair and whether she ever thought of "hurting herself". This led to a study with an Islamic colleague to explore the theoretical position that there would be disproportionate high rates of "Undetermined Deaths" (UnD) thought to be the sources of "Under-Reported-Suicides" (Cantor, Leenaars, & Lester, 1997; Stanistreet, Taylor, Jeffrey, & Gabby, 2001).

The author and his team examined reported suicides and UnD in 17 "Islamic" countries where, such as Pakistan, suicide is still a crime. We found that suicide rates in six countries were over 100 per million (pm), five of which had higher rates for males than the UK. Conversely, 10 nations had rates of less than 20pm but 12 countries had UnD rates of more than 130pm, with nine Islamic countries having an odds ratio of more than 3:1 UnD to suicides, strongly indicating a high level of under-reporting (Pritchard & Amanullah, 2007).

After publication, a number of psychiatrists from Islamic countries expressed appreciation that the issue had been raised, for when one researcher highlighted the impact of untreated mental illness (Khan & Hyder, 2006), he, like the Islamic author, was then severely criticised for bringing Islam into disrepute. To this came the reply taken from the Prophet in the Hidith: "the most important men in the world are men of knowledge and the best are those who seek new knowledge" (Fadiman & Frager, 1997, p. 157).

These results led us to ask about those Catholic countries where religious doctrine still condemns suicide. We recognised that countries such as Ireland and Portugal have only relatively recently reported more realistic suicide rates, whilst in the more traditional Catholic countries in Latin America the stigma associated with suicide still exists (Cantor et al., 1997; Curlin, Nwodim, Vance, Chin, & Lantos, 2008). We, therefore, adopted a feminist perspective, recognising that countries that have relatively limited women's rights in the form of restricted access to family planning add significant additional pressures to women's lives (Carrol, 2007; Langer, 2002; Sedgh, Henshaw, Singh, Ahman, & Shah, 2007).

Table 1. All-Causes-of- Deaths (15-74 years) UK v OWC 1980-82 to 2008-10, rates per million, ratios of change. UK: OWC Odds Ratio, chi square tests. # indicates UK poorer outcome (ranked by highest current ACD).

Country & Ranks. Index v Baseline Years	Reduced ACD - Ratio	UK: OWC Odds Ratio	UK v Others X2 - p Value
1 – 9. USA 1979-81 2005-07	8621 5832 – 0.68	1:1.26	70.40 <0.000
2 – 8. Denmark 1980-82 2004-06	8778 5475 – 0.62	1:1.11	13.01 <0.001
3 – 4. Germany 1981-83* 2008-10	9390 4978 – 0.53	1:1.06	6.1144 <0.025
4 – 6. Portugal 1980-82 2008-10	9083 4955 – 0.55	1:1.10	13.03 <0.001
5 – 7. Finland 1980-82 2008-10	9057 4875 – 0.54	1:1.08	9.4021 <0.005
6 – 2. UK 1979-81 **2003-05** **2004-06** **2005-07** **2006-08** **2007-09** **2008-10**	**9425** **5364 – 0.57** **5281 – 0.56** **5100 – 0.54** **4998 – 0.53** **4804 – 0.51** **4696 – 0.50**	**N/a**	**N/a**
7 – 5. Belgium 1979-81 2005-07	9279 5017 – 0.54	1:1.0	0.6595 n.sig
8 – 13. Canada 1979-81 03-05	8092 4694 – 0.58	1:1.16	7.5273 <0.01
9 – 1. Ireland 1979-81 2007-09	9975 4615 – 0.46	1:0.90	21.32 ## <0.0001
10 – 18. Greece 1979-8` 2007-09	7023 4609 – 0.66	1:1.29	80.73 <0.0001
11 – 14. France 1979-81 2006-08	7963 4576 – 0.57	1:08	5.1716 <0.025
12 – 12. New Zealand 1979-81 2007-09	8125 4276 – 0.51	1:1.02	0.2397 n.sig
13 – 19. Spain 1980-82 2007-09	6925 4266 – 0.62	1:1.22	41.69 <0.0001
14 – 17. Netherlands 1979-81 2008-10	7417 4246 – 0.57	1:1.14	27.98 <0.0001
15 – 11. Italy 1979-81 2006-08	8131 4104 – 0.50	1:0.94	3.6263 <0.1 trend #
16 – 3. Austria 1979-81 2008-10	9440 4069 – 0.43	1:0.86	31.32 ## <0.0001
17 – 17. Norway 1980-82 2008-10	7600 3967 – 0.52	1:1.04	3.0794 <0.1trend
18 – 18. Switzerland 1979-81 2004-06	7592 3920 – 0.52	1:0.93	9.7978 ## <0.01
19 – 19. Sweden 1979-81 2008-10	6345 3884 – 0.61	1:1.22	57.78 <0.0001

continued on following page

Table 1. Continued

Country & Ranks. Index v Baseline Years	Reduced ACD - Ratio	UK: OWC Odds Ratio	UK v Others X2 - p Value
20 – 20. Australia 1979-81 2004-06	8230 3783 – 0.46	1:0.82	69.19 ## <0.0001
21 – 21. Japan 1979-81 2007-09	6272 3747 – 0.60	1:1.18	34.06 <0.0001
OWC Average 1979-81 OWC Average 2008-10	8167 4494 – 0.55	1:1.10	

n.sig = not significant

Table 2. Cancer Mortality (15-74 years) UK v OWC 1979-2010, rates per million, ratios of change. UK: OWC Odds Ratios, chi square tests. # indicates UK poorer outcome (ranked by highest current rates)

Country Baseline v Index Years & Ranks	Reduced CD - Ratio	OWC: UK Odds Ratio	UK v Others X2 - p Value
1 – 1 Denmark 1980-82 2004-06	2908 2312 – 0.80	1:1.11	5.7406 <0.025
2 – 5 France 1979-81 2006-08	2607 2029 – 0.78	1:1.10	5.4531 <0.025
3 – 4 Netherlands 1979-81 2008-10	2637 2021 – 0.77	1:1.12	6.7442 <0.01
4 – 2 Belgium 1979-81 2005-07	2874 2015 – 0.71	1:1.00	0.1524 n.sig
5 – 6 Germany 1981-83* 2008-10	2585 2010 – 0.78	1:1.13	8.6084 <0.005
6-3. UK 1979-81 **2003-05** **2004-06** **2005-07** **2006-08** **2007-09** **2008-10**	**2800** **2128 – 0.76** **2021 – 0.72** **1995 – 0.71** **1977 – 0.71** **1950 – 0.70** **1925 – 0.69**	**n/a**	**N/a**
7 – 12 Canada 1979-81 2003-05	2456 1964 – 0.80	1:1.06	1.4883 n.sig
8 – 9 Ireland 1979-81 2007-09	2542 1937 – 0.76	1:1.09	4.556 <0.05
9 – 8 Italy 1979-81 2006-08	2574 1894 – 0.74	1:1.04	0.9571 n.sig
10 – 19 Portugal 1979-81 2008-10	1993 1875 – 0.94	1:1.36	51.57 <0.0001
11 – 17 Spain 1980-82 2007-09	2104 1861 – 0.88	1:1.25	30.39 <0.0001
12 – 13 USA 1979-81 2005-07	2372 1856 – 0.78	1:1.10	4.8246 <0.05
13 - 7 Austria 1979-81 2008-10	2584 1832 – 0.71	1:1.03	0.5830 n.sig

continued on following page

Table 2. Continued

Country Baseline v Index Years & Ranks	Reduced CD - Ratio	OWC: UK Odds Ratio	UK v Others X2 - p Value
14 – 10 New Zealand 1979-81 2007-09	2525 1823 – 0.72	1:1.03	0.7155 n.sig
15 – 18 Greece 1979-81 2007-09	2076 1787 – 0.86	1:1.23	23.51 <0.0001
16 – 11 Switzerland 1979-81 2004-06	2510 1652 – 0.66	1:0.92	21.34 ## <0.05
17 – 15 Norway 1980-82 2008-10	2272 1649 – 0.73	1:1.06	1.5276 n.sig
18 – 14 Australia 1979-81 2004-06	2295 1624 – 0.71	1:0.99	0.2062 n.sig
19 – 18 Japan 1079-81 2007-09	2020 1601 – 0.79	1:1.13	8.4088 <0.005
20 – 21 Sweden 1979-81 2008-10	1967 1575 – 0.80	1:1.16	11.51 <0.001
21 – 16 Finland 1980-82 2008-10	2145 1516 – 0.71	1:1.02	0.3812 n.sig
OWC Average 1979-81 OWCAverage 2008-10	2402 1842 – 0.77	1:1.12	

n.sig = not significant

The study focused on suicide in Latin America amongst female youths (aged 15-24) compared with the older female age bands to find strong indicative evidence of major under-reporting of suicide (Pritchard & Hean, 2008; Pritchard, Roberts & Pritchard, 2013). Crucially, quite unlike Western European Catholic countries, young women in most Latin American countries had disproportionately higher suicide UnD rates and far higher suicide and UnD rates than in older women. Another important association was the higher Latin American rate of suicides or UnD with higher birth rates. This perhaps is not surprising as most Latin American countries have restricted access to family planning (Carroll, 2007; Langer, 2002).

These studies indicate the influence of cultural factors even between countries who nominally share the same Catholic doctrine. The one Latin American exception, Cuba, whose suicide rates were found to be considerably higher than their UnD, matched the pattern found in both Western and European Catholic countries. This cultural influence is linked to another issue, namely the legality and social acceptance of family planning which is general throughout Catholic Western countries, although Ireland and Portugal, which are the latest European Catholic countries to accept contraception, do have the highest rate of female youth suicide in Europe (Pritchard, Roberts, & Pritchard, 2013).

This pervasive cultural influence on suicide (Kelleher, Chambers, Corcoran, Williamson, & Keeley, 1998) was recently demonstrated in a study that used Durkheim's 1878 original suicide data in 11 European countries. This showed that whilst suicide rates moved up and down, often related to unemployment, in the periods 1972-74, 1984-86, and 2004-06, the differential rates between the countries during the period 1878-2006 hardly altered. This shows that there was a consistency in suicide rates over more than a 100 years (Hansen & Pritchard, 2008).

Table 3. Cost-effectiveness ratios GDP expenditure-on-health expenditure to Reduced Cancer Mortality (15-74) rates per million p.a. (ranked by greatest cost-effective ratio)

Country & Years	Reduced rpm	Cost - Effective Ratio
1. UK 2003-05	672	1:92
2004--6	779	1:107
2005-07	805	1:110
2006-08	823	1:113
2007-09	856	1:116
2008-10	875	1:120
2. Switzerland 2004-06	858	1:93
3. Belgium 2005-07	859	1:98
4=. New Zealand 2007-09	702	1:89
4=. Ireland 2007-09	648	1:89
6. Australia 2004-06	671	1:87
7. Italy 2006-08	680	1:83
8. Finland 2008-10	629	1:82
9. Austria 2008-10	752	1:79
10. Norway 2008-10	623	1:77
11. Netherlands 2008-10	616	1:72
12. Denmark 2004-06	596	1:68
13=. France 2006-08	578	1:60
13=. Germany 2008-10	575	1:60
15. Japan 2007-09	419	1:57
16. Canada 2003-05	492	1:55
17. Sweden 2008-10	392	1:45
18. USA 2005-07	516	1:39
19. Greece 2007-09	289	1:36
20. Spain 2007-09	243	1:33
21. Portugal 2008-10	118	1:15
Average OWC	562	1:66

I now turn to a research study of changing patterns of mortality due to social changes.

IDENTIFYING CHANGING MORTALITY INDICATING IMPACT OF SOCIAL CHANGES

During a clinical review, it was realised that there were four recorded cases of Motor Neurone Disease (MND) within a three year period. Whilst it could have been a statistical artefact, it was surprising as the textbooks suggest a mortality of about 1 in 100,000, the equivalent of 10 per million annually (Lindsay et al., 2010). At the same time the Department of Psychiatry at the University of Southampton was dealing with the relatively new phenomena of early-onset-dementia.

This led to two studies of the changing patterns of neurological mortality in the Western world, based upon WHO (2013) data, to find that compared with all causes of deaths, there were major disproportionate increases in adults under 74 years and in effect the dementias were starting 10 years earlier (Pritchard & Hean, 2008; Pritchard, Mayers, & Baldwin, 2013).

Some argued that the reason for these increases might be due to the Gompertzian hypothesis that people are now living longer to develop diseases they previously would not have developed (Chio, Magnani, & Schiffer, 1995; Riggs & Schochet, 1992). Whilst there may be an element of truth in this, we and others demonstrated that this was not the main cause, not least because of the variation between the countries and the sexes. In most countries, women's health outcomes have worsened compared to men's. This is linked to the fact that women's life styles have changed considerably over the past 30 years as they have increasingly entered the workplace in areas which had been a male preserve. Thus, they have been relatively more exposed to the major multi-environmental changes found across the world (Callaghan B., Feldman, D., Gruis, K., & Feldman, 2011; Johansen, 2004; Pritchard & Hickish, 2011; Pritchard, Mayers, & Baldwin, 2013; Retsky, Swartzendruber, Bame, & Wardwell, 1994)

A new analysis for this chapter (Table 4) shows comparison of All Causes of Deaths (ACD) and Combined Neurological Deaths for the 55-74 year olds, with Odds ratios calculated the Combined Neurological deaths have increased proportionate to ACD. Spain has the biggest change 1:3.39, followed by the USA 1:2.75, with Germany, Italy, and the UK on 1:2.69. Only the Netherlands, France, and Japan did not double their Odds ratio, and the smallest change, Japan at 1:1.67, is the equivalent of neurological deaths increasing by 67% over ACD.

When the latest paper was published (Pritchard, Mayers, & Baldwin, 2013), the CEO of a new charity, "Young-Dementia UK", rang to express appreciation that the study was raising the issue. When asked the age of the majority of the charity's caseload, she pointed to those mainly in their late

40s and early 50s. A finding of dementia being a disease of midlife would have been unthinkable 30 or more years ago.

When considering clinical studies, a contributory cause of these increases at national levels is indicative of environmental factors. A micro study, triggered by social work practitioners in a rural English country of a cluster of MND, found a local rate four times that of the country and double that of the UK rates (Pritchard & Silk, 2014). This hypothesis-stimulating study was of a village with under 5000 people aged 55+, a village next to a busy airport and surrounded by significantly high Electro-Magnetic-Fields from radar and mobile phone masts on the downs surrounding the village. Again, this finding indicates a possible environmental impact upon human health. Despite reductions in cancer deaths in the Western countries, the incidence of cancer continues to rise, albeit slower than in the past but again pointing to the influence of environmental factors, strongly suggesting epigenetic factors (Pritchard & Hickish, 2011).

SOME METHODOLOGICAL CONSIDERATIONS

In our earlier chapter, Richard Williams and I discussed the relative paucity of quantitative outcome studies in British social work, and a brief perusal of the last three years of the *British Journal of Social Work* shows quantitative outcomes were very much in the minority, most research studies being "qualitative" in research design. As the above studies demonstrate, those that started from a qualitative research design were able to be triangulated with quantitative methods, allowing the results to be more widely generalised across larger populations. We urge a melding of research methods where appropriate, so that valuable social work perspectives can contribute to the wider field of health.

*Table 4. All Causes Deaths, Combined Neurological Deaths by sex rates per million [rpm] and Final Odds Ratios of ACD to Combined Neurological deaths 1979-81 v 2008-10. 55-74 years old. Ranked by highest Combined Gender Odds Ratio. Significantly Female ratios higher than Males **

Country, Latest Years & 79-81 Latest Combined Rank	Total Deaths Males	Total Deaths Females	Combined Neurological Males	Combined Neurological Females	Odds Ratios ACD: Neuro Both Sexes
1. Spain 1979-81 2006-08	22469 14571	11746 6164	283 510	204 424	
Ratio of change	0.65	0.52	**1.80**	**2.08 ***	1:3.39
2. USA 1979-81 2005-07	26981 16288	14370 10635	360 595	261 530	
Ratio of change	0.60	0.74 *	**1.65**	**2.03 ***	1:2.75
4=. UK 1979-81 2008-10	31146 14005	17153 9131	425 518	327 461	
4=. Ratio of change	0.45	0.53 *	**1.22**	**1.41 ***	1:2.69
4=. Germany 1990-92 2008-10	25734 16360	17926 7191	444 457	247 333	
Ratio of change	0.64	0.40	**1.03**	**1.35 ***	1:2.69
4=. Italy 1979-81 2006-08	27257 13522	13669 7044	**359** **454**	**245** **362**	
Ratio of change	0.50	0.52 *	**1.26**	**1.48 ***	1:2.69
7=. Canada 1979-81 2002-2004	24799 14278	12696 8845	411 510	300 461	
Ratio of change	0.58	0.69 *	**1.24**	**1.54 ***	1:2.18
7=. Australia 1979-81 2004-06	26087 12061	13286 7092	403 397	**290** **338**	
Ratio of change	0.46	0.53 *	0.99	**1.17 ***	1:2.18
8. Netherlands 1979-81 2008-10	25615 13017	12092 8375	424 422	**318** **389**	
Ratio of change	0.51	0.69 *	1.00	**1.22 ***	1:1.87
9. France 1979-81 2006-08	26049 14776	11948 6651	599 542	421 416	
Ratio of change	0.57	0.56	0.90	0.99 *	1:1.68
10. Japan 1979-81 2007-09	20066 12700	11018 5501	243 226	159 138	
Ratio of change	0.63	0.50	0.93	0.87	1:1.67
Average 1979-81 2008-10	25620 14158	13591 6195	395 463	277 383	
Ratio of change	0.55	0. 46	**1.17**	**1.38 ***	1:2.13

CONCLUSION

Is this chapter a long way from social work research and practice? I do not think so. All social work theory as it is translated into practice draws heavily upon social science, but it does not become too detached and "ivory towered" because social workers rarely lose sight of the individual or the vulnerable person, be they consultant surgeon, or surgical patient.

It is argued that social work practitioners should have greater confidence in social work outcomes as they are skilled at working at the interface of complex and often conflicting margins and boundaries of different health and welfare agencies and departments. We believe that we need to have more quantitative findings to support this view, as Richard Williams and I have indicated in our earlier chapter on social work outcomes. Ultimately, there is only one question that matters in the human services, whether it be social work, medicine, or some other agency. That question is, "has the intervention or policy made a positive contribution to the individual and society?"

The social work discipline, built upon a passion for social justice, is one of the few to see the individual within the context of their family and society and is, therefore, uniquely placed to contribute to other disciplines. Social work practitioners should have the confidence in their work to demonstrate its worth.

REFERENCES

Baisch, S. B., Schenk, T., & Noble, A. J. (2011). What is the cause of post-traumatic stress disorder following subarachnoid haemorrhage? Post-ictal events are key. *Acta Neurochirurgica*, *153*(4), 913–922. doi:10.1007/s00701-010-0843-y PMID:20963450

Buchanan, K. M., Elias, L. J., & Goplen, G. B. (2000). Differing perspectives on outcome after subarachnoid hemorrhage: The patient, the relative, the neurosurgeon. *Neurosurgery*, *46*, 831–838. Retrieved from http://journals.lww.com/neurosurgery/pages/default.aspx PMID:10764256

Callaghan, B., Feldman, D., Gruis, K., & Feldman, E. (2011). The association of exposure to lead, mercury, and selenium and the development of amyotrophic lateral sclerosis and the epigenetic implications. *Neurodegenerative Diseases*, *8*(1-2), 1–8. doi:10.1159/000315405 PMID:20689252

Cantor, C. H., Leenaars, A. A., & Lester, D. (1997). Under-reporting of suicide in Ireland 1960-1989. *Archives of Suicide Research*, *3*(1), 5–12. doi:10.1080/13811119708258251

Carroll, R. (2007, October 8). Killer law. *Guardian*. Retrieved from http://www.theguardian.com/society/2007/oct/08/health.lifeandhealth

Chief Medical Officer. (2007). *Towards a safer surgery*. London: HMSO.

Chio, A., Magnani, C., & Schiffer, D. (1995). Gompertzian analysis of amyotrophic lateral sclerosis mortality in Italy, 1957-1987: Application to birth cohorts. *Neuroepidemiology*, *14*(6), 269–277. doi:10.1159/000109802 PMID:8569998

Curlin, F. A., Nwodim, C., Vance, J. L., Chin, M. H., & Lantos, J. D. (2008). To die, to sleep: US physicians' religious and other objections to physician-assisted suicide, terminal sedation, and withdrawal of life support. *The American Journal of Hospice & Palliative Medicine*, *25*(2), 112–120. doi:10.1177/1049909107310141 PMID:18198363

de Vries, E. N., Ramrattan, M. A., Smorenburg, S. M., Gouma, D. J., & Boermeester, M. A. (2008). The incidence and nature of in-hospital adverse events: A systematic review. *Quality & Safety in Health Care*, *17*(3), 216–223. doi:10.1136/qshc.2007.023622 PMID:18519629

Durkheim, E. (1897). *Suicide: A study in sociology* (J. A. Spaulding & G. George Simpson, Trans.). New York: Free Press.

Fadiman, J., & Frager, R. (1997). *Essential Sufism.* San Francisco: Harper Collins.

Frazer, D., Ahuja, A., Watkins, L., & Cipolitti, L. (2007). Coiling versus clipping for the treatment of aneurysmal subarachnoid hemorrhage: A longitudinal investigation into cognitive outcome. *Neurosurgery, 60*(3), 434–441. doi:10.1227/01. NEU.0000255335.72662.25 PMID:17327787

Hansen, L., & Pritchard, C. (2008). Consistency in suicide rates in twenty-two developed countries by gender over time 1874-78, 1974-76, and 1998-2000. *Archives of Suicide Research, 12*(3), 251–262. doi:10.1080/13811110802101153 PMID:18576206

Janes, F., Gigli, G. L., D'Anna, L., Cancelli, I., Perelli, A., Canal, G.,...& Valente M. (2013). Stroke incidence and 30-day and six-month case fatality rates in Udine, Italy: A population-based prospective study. *International Journal of Stroke, 8*(Suppl. A100), 100-105. doi:10.1111/ijs.12000

Johansen, C. (2004). Electromagnetic fields and health effects: Epidemiological studies of cancer, diseases of the central nervous system and arrhythmia-related heart disease. *Scandinavian Journal of Work, Environment & Health, 30*(Suppl. 1), 1–30. Retrieved from http://www. sjweh.fi/ PMID:15255560

Kelleher, M. J., Chambers, D., Corcoran, P., Williamson, E., & Keeley, H. S. (1998). Religious sanctions and rates of suicide worldwide. *Crisis, 19*(2), 78–86. doi:10.1027/0227-5910.19.2.78 PMID:9785649

Khan, M. M., & Hyder, A. A. (2006). Suicides in the developing world: Case study from Pakistan. *Suicide & Life-Threatening Behavior, 36*(1), 76–81. doi:10.1521/suli.2006.36.1.76 PMID:16676628

Langer, A. (2002). El embarazo no deseado: Impacto sobre la salud y la sociedad en América Latina y el Caribe [Unwanted pregnancy: Impact on health and society in Latin America and the Caribbean]. *Revista Panamericana de Salud Pública, 11*(3), 192–205. doi:10.1590/S1020-49892002000300013 PMID:11998185

Lindsay, K. W., Bone, I., & Fuller, G. (2010). *Neurology & neurosurgery illustrated.* Edinburgh: Churchill Livingstone.

Mezue, W., Matthew, B., Draper, P., & Watson, R. (2004). The impact of care on carers of patients treated for aneurysmal subarachnoid haemorrhage. *British Journal of Neurosurgery, 18*(2), 135–137. doi:10.1080/02688690410001680984 PMID:15176554

Molyneux, A. J., Kerr, R. S., Birks, J., Ramzi, N., Yarnold, J., Sneade, M., & Rischmiller, J. (2009). Risk of recurrent subarachnoid haemorrhage, death, or dependence and standardised mortality ratios after clipping or coiling for intracranial aneurysm in the international subarachnoid aneurysm trial (ISAT): Long-term follow-up. *Lancet Neurology, 8*(5), 427–433. doi:10.1016/S1474-4422(09)70080-8 PMID:19329361

Noble, A. J., Baisch, S., Covey, J., Mukerji, N., Nath, F., & Schenk, T. (2011). Subarachnoid hemorrhage patients' fears of recurrence are related to the presence of posttraumatic stress disorder. *Neurosurgery, 69*(2), 323–332. doi:10.1227/NEU.0b013e318216047e PMID:21415779

Pritchard, C., & Amanullah, S. (2007). An analysis of suicide and undetermined deaths in 17 predominately Islamic countries contrasted with the UK. *Psychological Medicine, 37*(3), 421–430. doi:10.1017/S0033291706009159 PMID:17176500

Pritchard, C., & Brackstone, J. (2009). "The voice of the surgeon" on patient safety: The ASGBI survey. Newsletter (Association of Surgeons of Great Britain & Ireland), 28, 34-36.

Pritchard, C., Brackstone, J., & MacFie, J. (2010). Adverse events and patient safety in the operating theatre: Perspectives of 549 surgeons. *Bulletin of the Royal College of Surgeons of England, 92*(6), 1–4. doi:10.1308/147363510X507972

Pritchard, C., Clapham, L., Davis, A., Lang, D. A., & Neil-Dwyer, G. (2004). Psycho-socio-economic outcomes in acoustic neuroma patients and their carers related to tumour size. *Clinical Otolaryngology and Allied Sciences, 29*(4), 324–330. doi:10.1111/j.1365-2273.2004.00822.x PMID:15270817

Pritchard, C., Clapham, L., Foulkes, L., Lang, D. A., & Neil-Dwyer, G. (2004). Comparison of cohorts of elective and emergency neurosurgical patients: Psychosocial outcomes of acoustic neuroma and aneurysmal sub arachnoid hemorrhage patients and carers. *Surgical Neurology, 62*(1), 7–16. doi:10.1016/j.surneu.2004.01.018 PMID:15226061

Pritchard, C., Foulkes, L., Lang, D. A., & Neil-Dwyer, G. (2001). Psychosocial outcomes for patients and carers after aneurysmal subarachnoid haemorrhage. *British Journal of Neurosurgery, 15*(6), 456–463. doi:10.1080/02688690120097679 PMID:11813996

Pritchard, C., Foulkes, L., Lang, D. A., & Neil-Dwyer, G. (2004). Two year prospective study of psychosocial outcomes and a cost-analysis of "treatment-as-usual" versus an "enhanced" (specialist liaison nurse) service for aneurysmal sub arachnoid haemorrhage (ASAH) patients and families. *British Journal of Neurosurgery, 18*(4), 347–356. doi:10.1080/02688690400004993 PMID:15702833

Pritchard, C., & Hean, S. (2008). Suicide and undetermined deaths among youths and young adults in Latin America: Comparison with the 10 major developed countries – A source of hidden suicides? *Crisis, 29*(3), 145–153. doi:10.1027/0227-5910.29.3.145 PMID:18714911

Pritchard, C., & Hickish, T. (2011). Comparing cancer mortality and GDP health expenditure in England and Wales with other major developed countries from 1979 to 2006. *British Journal of Cancer, 105*(11), 1788–1794. doi:10.1038/bjc.2011.393 PMID:21970877

Pritchard, C., Lindsay, K., Cox, M., & Foulkes, L. (2011). Re-evaluating the national subarachnoid haemorrhage study (2006) from a patient-related-outcome-measure perspective: Comparing fiscal outcomes of treatment-as-usual with an enhanced service. *British Journal of Neurosurgery, 25*(3), 376–383. doi:10.3109/02688697.2011.566379 PMID:21513445

Pritchard, C., Mayers, A., & Baldwin, D. (2013). Changing patterns of neurological mortality in the 10 developed countries: 1979-2010. *Public Health, 127*(4), 357–368. doi:10.1016/j.puhe.2012.12.018 PMID:23601790

Pritchard, C., Roberts, S., & Pritchard, C. E. (2013). "Giving a voice to the unheard"? Is female youth (15-24 years) suicide linked to restricted access to family planning? Comparing two Catholic continents. *International Social Work, 56*(6), 798–815. doi:10.1177/0020872812441645

Pritchard, C., & Silk, A. (2014). A case-study survey of an eight-year cluster of motor neurone disease (MND) referrals in a rural English village: Exploring possible aetiological influences in a hypothesis stimulating study. *Journal of Neurological Disorders, 2,* 147. doi:10.4172/2329-6895.1000147

Pritchard, C., & Wallace, M. S. (2011). Comparing the USA, UK and 17 Western countries' efficiency and effectiveness in reducing mortality. *Journal of the Royal Society of Medicine Short Reports*, *2*(60), 1–10. doi:10.1258/shorts.2011.011076 PMID:21847442

Retsky, M. W., Swartzendruber, D. E., Bame, P. D., & Wardwell, R. H. (1994). Computer model challenges breast cancer treatment strategy. *Cancer Investigation*, *12*(6), 559–567. doi:10.3109/07357909409023040 PMID:7994590

Riggs, J. E., Schochet, S. S., Jr. (1992). Rising mortality due to Parkinson's disease and amyotrophic lateral sclerosis: A manifestation of the competitive nature of human mortality. *Journal of Clinical Epidemiology*, *45*, 1007-1012. doi:(92)90116-510.1016/0895-4356

Royal College of Surgeons of England. (2006). *The national subarachnoid haemorrhage evaluation study: Final report of an audit carried out in 34 neurosurgical units in the UK and Ireland between 14 September 2001 to 13 September 2002*. London: British Society of Neurological Surgeons, Royal College of Surgeons. Retrieved from http://www.rcseng.ac.uk/publications/docs/nat_study_subarachnoid_haem_feb2006.html

Sedgh, G., Henshaw, S., Singh, S., Ahman, E., & Shah, I. H. (2007). Induced abortion: Estimated rates and trends worldwide. *Lancet*, *370*(9595), 1338–1345. doi:10.1016/S0140-6736(07)61575-X PMID:17933648

Stanistreet, D., Taylor, S., Jeffrey, V., & Gabby, M. (2001). Accident or suicide? Predictors of coroners' decisions in suicide and accident verdicts. *Medicine, Science, and the Law*, *41*, 111–115. doi:10.1177/002580240104100205 PMID:11368390

Visser-Meiley, J. M. A., Rhebergen, M. L., Rinkel, G. J. E., van Zandvoort, M. J., & Post, M. W. M. (2009). Long-term health-related quality of life after aneurysmal subarachnoid haemorrhage: Relationship with psychological symptoms and personality characteristics. *Stroke*, *40*(4), 1526–1529. doi:10.1161/STROKEAHA.108.531277 PMID:19095984

Wertheimer, A. (2008). *A dented image: Journeys of recovery from a subarachnoid haemorrhage*. London: Routledge.

WHO. (2013) *Annual mortality statistics*. Retrieved from http://www.who.int/healthinfo/statistics/mortality/en/

ADDITIONAL READING

Al-Khindi, T., Macdonald, R. L., & Schweizer, T. A. (2010). Cognitive and functional outcome after aneurysmal subarachnoid hemorrhage. *Stroke*, *41*(8), e519–e536. doi:10.1161/STROKEAHA.110.581975 PMID:20595669

Alonso, A., Logroscino, G., Jlick, S. S., & Hernan, M. A. (2009). Incidence and lifetime risk of motor neurone disease in the United Kingdom: A population based study. *European Journal of Neurology*, *16*(6), 745–751. doi:10.1111/j.1468-1331.2009.02586.x PMID:19475756

Baldi, I., Coureau, G., Jaffré, A., Gruber, A., Ducamp, S., & Provost, D. et al. (2011). Occupational and residential exposure to electromagnetic fields and risk of brain tumors in adults: A case–control study in Gironde, France. *International Journal of Cancer*, *129*(6), 1477–1484. doi:10.1002/ijc.25765 PMID:21792884

Berry, E. (1998). Post-traumatic stress disorder after subarachnoid haemorrhage. *The British Journal of Clinical Psychology*, *37*(3), 365–367. doi:10.1111/j.2044-8260.1998.tb01392.x PMID:9784890

Beseoglu, K., Pannes, S., Steiger, H. J., & Hänggi, D. (2010). Long-term outcome and quality of life after nonaneurysmal subarachnoid hemorrhage. *Acta Neurochirurgica, 152*(3), 409–416. doi:10.1007/s00701-009-0518-8 PMID:19784546

Chen, Y.-Y., Wu, K. C.-C., Yousuf, S., & Yip, P. S. F. (2012). Suicide in Asia: Opportunities and challenges. *Epidemiologic Reviews, 34*(1), 129–144. doi:10.1093/epirev/mxr025 PMID:22158651

Cook, C. C. (2014). Suicide and religion. *The British Journal of Psychiatry, 204*(4), 254–255. doi:10.1192/bjp.bp.113.136069 PMID:24692751

Covey, J., Noble, A. J., & Schenk, T. (2013). Family and friends' fears of recurrence: Impact on the patient's recovery after subarachnoid haemorrhage. *Journal of Neurosurgery, 119*(4), 948–954. doi:10.3171/2013.5.JNS121688 PMID:23876000

Day, T. G., Scott, M., Perring, R., & Doyle, P. (2007). Motor neurone disease mortality in Great Britain continues to rise: Examination of mortality rates 1975–2004. *Amyotrophic Lateral Sclerosis: Official Publication of the World Federation of Neurology Research Group on Motor Neuron Diseases, 8*(6), 337–342. doi:10.1080/17482960701725455 PMID:18033591

Gearing, R. E., & Lizardi, D. (2009). Religion and suicide. *Journal of Religion and Health, 48*(3), 332–341. doi:10.1007/s10943-008-9181-2 PMID:19639421

Goldacre, M. J., Duncan, M., Griffith, M., & Turner, M. R. (2010). Trends in death certification for multiple sclerosis, motor neurone disease, Parkinson's disease and epilepsy in English populations 1979–2006. *Journal of Neurology, 257*(5), 706–715. doi:10.1007/s00415-009-5392-z PMID:19946783

Heros, R. C. (2013). Fear of recurrence. *Journal of Neurosurgery, 119*(4), 943–945. doi:10.3171/2013.2.JNS13252 PMID:23875959

Katati, M. J., Santiago-Ramajo, S., Pérez-García, M., Meersmans-Sánchez Jofré, M., Vilar-Lopez, R., & Coín-Mejias, M. A. et al. (2007). Description of quality of life and its predictors in patients with aneurysmal subarachnoid haemorrhage. *Cerebrovascular Diseases, 24*(1), 66–73. doi:10.1159/000103118 PMID:17519546

Lodhi, L. M., & Shah, A. (2005). Factors associated with the recent decline in suicide rates in the elderly in England and Wales, 1985-1998. *Medicine, Science, and the Law, 45*(1), 31–38. doi:10.1258/rsmmsl.45.1.31 PMID:15745271

Marcilio, I., Gouveia, N., Pereira Filho, M. L., & Kheifets, L. (2011). Adult mortality from leukemia, brain cancer, amyotrophic lateral sclerosis and magnetic fields from power lines: A case-control study in Brazil. *Revista Brasileira de Epidemiologia, 14*(4), 580–588. doi:10.1590/S1415-790X2011000400005 PMID:22218657

Mercy, L., Hodges, J. R., Dawson, K., Baker, R. A., & Brayne, C. (2008). Incidence of early onset dementia in Cambridgeshire, United Kingdom. *Neurology, 71*(19), 1496–1499. doi:10.1212/01.wnl.0000334277.16896.fa PMID:18981371

Milner, A., Spittal, M. J., Pirkis, J., & LaMontagne, A. D. (2013). Suicide by occupation: Systematic review and meta-analysis. *The British Journal of Psychiatry, 203*(6), 409–416. doi:10.1192/bjp.bp.113.128405 PMID:24297788

Noble, A. J., & Schenk, T. (2008). Posttraumatic stress disorder in the family and friends of patients who have suffered spontaneous subarachnoid hemorrhage. *Journal of Neurosurgery, 109*(6), 1027–1033. doi:10.3171/JNS.2008.109.12.1027 PMID:19035715

Passier, P. E. C. A., Visser-Meily, J. M. A., Van Zandvoort, M. J. E., Post, M. W. M., Rinkel, G. J. E., & Van Heugten, C. (2010). Prevalence and determinants of cognitive complaints after aneurysmal subarachnoid hemorrhage. *Cerebrovascular Diseases*, *29*(6), 557–563. doi:10.1159/000306642 PMID:20375498

Powell, J., Kitchen, N., Heslin, J., & Greenwood, R. (2002). Psychosocial outcomes at three and nine months after good neurological recovery from aneurysmal subarachnoid haemorrhage: Predictors and prognosis. *Journal of Neurology, Neurosurgery, and Psychiatry*, *72*(6), 772–781. doi:10.1136/jnnp.72.6.772 PMID:12023423

Pritchard, C. (1988). Suicide, unemployment and gender in the British Isles and European Economic Community (1974-1985): A hidden epidemic? *Social Psychiatry and Psychiatric Epidemiology*, *23*(2), 85–89. doi:10.1007/BF01788426 PMID:3133784

Pritchard, C., Cox, M., Foulkes, L., & Lindsay, K. (2011). The patient's voice in neuro-surgery: Psycho-socio-economic benefits of a patient-designed versus standard service following treatment for a subarachnoid haemorrhage. *Social Care and Neurodisability*, *2*(2), 80–96. doi:10.1108/20420911111142759

Rinkel, G. J. E., & Algra, A. (2011). Long-term outcomes of patients with aneurysmal subarachnoid haemorrhage. *Lancet Neurology*, *10*(4), 349–356. doi:10.1016/S1474-4422(11)70017-5 PMID:21435599

Viner, R. M., Coffey, C., Mathers, C., Bloem, P., Costello, A., Santelli, J., & Patton, G. C. (2011). 50-year mortality trends in children and young people: A study of 50 low-income, middle-income, and high-income countries. *Lancet*, *377*(9772), 1162–1174. doi:10.1016/S0140-6736(11)60106-2 PMID:21450338

Wermer, M. J. H., Kool, H., Albrecht, K. W., & Rinkel, G. J. E. (2007). Subarachnoid hemorrhage treated with clipping: Long-term effects on employment, relationships, personality, and mood. *Neurosurgery*, *60*(1), 91–98. doi:10.1227/01.NEU.0000249215.19591.86 PMID:17228256

Wong, G. K. C., Poon, W. S., Boet, R., Chan, M. T. C., Gin, T., Ng, S. C. P., & Zee, B. C. Y. (2011). Health-related quality of life after aneurysmal subarachnoid hemorrhage: Profile and clinical factors. *Neurosurgery*, *68*(6), 1556–1561. doi:10.1227/NEU.0b013e31820cd40d PMID:21311383

KEY TERMS AND DEFINITIONS

Acoustic Neuroma (AN): A growth on the auditory (hearing nerve) usually benign but causing increasing deafness and affecting balance. The condition usually requires both an ear, nose, and throat surgeon's intervention as well as neurosurgical intervention through the performance of a craniotomy (surgery to the brain).

Post-Traumatic Stress Disorder (PTSD): A set of responses that often develop following a traumatic event, such as a life-threatening stroke. The disorder may involve re-living the traumatic event through recurring memories involving intrusive images and nightmares; physical symptoms, such as panic attacks and heart palpitations; increased startle response; emotional numbing; and avoidance behaviours.

Specialist Neurovascular Nurse (SNVN): A nurse who provides specialised psycho-social and psycho-education support to patients following sub-arachnoid haemorrhage. The nurse works systemically with patients and their partners, caregivers, and families.

Sub-Arachnoid Haemorrhage (SAH): An aneurysm on one of the major arteries of the brain. A type of stroke.

This work was previously published in Evidence Discovery and Assessment in Social Work Practice edited by Margaret Pack and Justin Cargill, pages 212-234 copyright year 2015 by Information Science Reference (an imprint of IGI Global).

Chapter 68

Participatory Mapping Approaches to Coordinate the Emergency Response of Spontaneous Volunteers after Hurricane Sandy

Pamela Wridt
City University of New York, USA

Scott Fisher
City University of New York, USA

John E. Seley
City University of New York, USA

Bryce DuBois
City University of New York, USA

ABSTRACT

This article demonstrates the potential of participatory mapping approaches to coordinate spontaneous volunteers and assist government agencies and humanitarian organizations in emergency contexts. The research focuses on one case study of a volunteer mapping project in the Rockaways in New York City to help communicate the needs reported by community members to outsiders after Hurricane Sandy. The map proved to be helpful in the coordination of relief efforts by volunteers and in understanding the variety of groups involved in emergency response. However, the map could not be sustained for long-term community recovery. The research offers new evidence of the potential contributions of spontaneous volunteers that can be leveraged, replicated and improved upon for future disaster planning and response. It also highlights the importance of volunteered geographic information in ensuring that emergency response is guided by the needs reported by citizens themselves, even if they do not have access to technology.

INTRODUCTION

This article provides an analysis of a participatory mapping approach to assist with emergency response after Hurricane Sandy. It focuses on one case in particular: a volunteer project in the Rockaways, Queens, one of the hardest hit areas in New York City. Hurricane Sandy formed on October 22, 2012 and subsided on October 31, 2012, causing over 315 million USD in damages

DOI: 10.4018/978-1-4666-8756-1.ch068

to the Caribbean and over 62 billion USD in damages to the United States, making it the second costliest hurricane in the history of the United States (Roca, 2012). Globally 285 people lost their lives, with at least 125 deaths in the United States (Roca, 2012).

Hurricane Sandy reached 725 kilometers beyond its core and affected 50 to 60 million people in the northeast region of the United States (Walsh, 2012). Sandy hit major urban centers such as Boston, New York City, and Atlantic City. During this time, over 7.5 million people were without power (Roca, 2012), which was not restored in some areas for several months. Blackout conditions made it unsafe to walk at night and in building hallways, and to enter and exit high-rise apartment buildings without working elevators. Portions of New York City were submerged under water, and many subway lines and regional trains cancelled service making the commute to Manhattan challenging for several weeks (McKenzie, 2012). Some subway lines, such as the A train which serves the Rockaways, were shut down all together with an estimated six months of repairs (Pereira, 2013). With wind speeds up to 145 kilometers per hour, trees were uprooted, roofs caved in, and some neighborhoods were flooded from a powerful storm surge (Silverman, 2012). Beach communities like the Rockaways were hit especially hard with waves over nine meters high that tore up boardwalks and eroded coastlines (Freedman, 2012).

Sandy prompted a substantial government response in the United States. For example, the Fire Department of New York (FDNY) had a major role in emergency response in New York City, building upon their experiences after 9/11 (2001), and Hurricanes Katrina (2005), Gustav (2008), and Irene (2011). However, the scale of need often overwhelmed their effective response because of the labor required for rescue operations. In one case during the peak of the storm, the FDNY was fighting the equivalent of three six-alarm fires simultaneously in Queens, one

of five boroughs in New York City (Daly, 2013; Esposito, 2013; Manahan, 2013). A typical six-alarm fire might consist of over 200 firefighters, including 25 engine companies, 13 ladder companies, nine Battalion Chiefs, two Deputy Chiefs, two Assistant Chiefs, the Chief of Operations, and a dozen or more special units for communication and injuries (Esposito, 2013). Despite these challenges, within three months after Hurricane Sandy, the FDNY and the National Guard had distributed approximately 6,400 blankets, 4,200 electric blankets, 3,300 cases of water, over 41,000 MREs (Meals Ready to Eat), 4,200 comfort kits (toothpaste, soap, etc.), 800 electric heaters, and inspected over 103,000 dwelling units (Daly, 2013; Esposito, 2013; Manahan, 2013).

Hurricane Sandy was an unprecedented event in New York City in terms of its environmental damage and regional economic impact. Media coverage of the event for those with power helped attract volunteers, and a surge of local residents began converging to help within the impacted regions. Although thousands of New York City residents assisted in a variety of ways, the lack of a coordinated volunteer response often led to a spatial mismatch between the needs reported by community residents and outsiders' perceptions of their needs in the impacted areas (Turk, 2012). For example, some organizations had to turn volunteers away because supplies were not available for them to distribute. In other cases, large numbers of volunteers went to serve in locations where there was no need for their response.

The emergency response to Hurricane Sandy was similar to other disaster situations, in which over stretched public services cannot adequately respond to the scale of need, and when a lack of coordination often hampers well-intentioned volunteer efforts (Fernandez et al., 2006a; *Managing Spontaneous Volunteers in Times of Disaster*, 2005; *Preventing a Disaster within the Disaster*, 2002). While research recognizes the important role of intra-governmental and volunteer coordination, it is less clear how these groups interact with one another during the emergency response phase (Fernandez et al., 2006a). This is particularly true for spontaneous volunteers who are not affiliated with any aid organization.

The different ways citizens self-mobilize and assist in emergencies are not well researched, although the findings reported in this article suggest it is an important area of inquiry, especially in poor communities. In particular, this study contributes to an emerging area of research in disaster planning and management that recognizes the importance of e-planning tools for emergency response (Klosterman, 2012) by examining how these tools can be leveraged in communities without access to technology. It does so by providing an analysis of the authors' own volunteer mapping efforts to raise awareness of the needs of community residents among outside volunteers who wanted to assist in the emergency response of the Rockaways.

While there was no initial goal of our volunteer activities, nor the intention of publishing the experience of our relief efforts, over time we began to realize the value of the volunteered geographic information we were gathering to critically analyze the emergency response in the Rockaways. Our approach might fit best with the idea of "citizens as sensors," or of "citizen scientists" who collect information about places and populate the data onto online maps for learning purposes (Chun & Artigas, 2012; Goodchild, 2007a). Therefore this research is unique because it was not based on a pre-determined research design, and it is not an objective assessment of someone else's use of volunteered geographic information for emergency response. Rather, it is a critical self-assessment of the potential and challenges of e-planning tools in the emergency response of poor and working class communities in large urban centers in the United States.

Through a case study approach, we explore how coordination and communication between government officials, volunteers, community groups, and affected citizens in emergency contexts can be enhanced through the participatory and hybrid use of paper-based and online mapping tools. This approach is needed in communities like the Rockaways that experience damage to their communication infrastructure after a disaster, have limited access to online technologies to report their needs, and a general lack of trust for government officials. This case study can therefore serve as a model to help others learn better ways to include spontaneous volunteers in disaster response and preparedness in marginalized communities. We conclude with a discussion on the untapped potential of citizen-led emergency response efforts, and suggest ways to integrate online mapping tools and the concept of volunteered geographic information into community and school based disaster preparation programs.

CITIZEN INVOLVEMENT IN EMERGENCY RESPONSE

There is a long history of citizen involvement in emergency response to disasters. Solnit (2009) documents many examples, including the San Francisco earthquake of 1906, the shipping explosion of 1917 in Halifax, Nova Scotia, the Mexico City earthquake in 1985, New York City after September 11, 2001, and New Orleans after Hurricane Katrina in 2005. Her research provides evidence that large groups of citizens without a pre-planned role come together to assist those in need after disasters. For example, after the Mexico City earthquake, some two million people (or 10 percent of the population) helped others. Similarly, after the Loma Prieta earthquake in California, 60 percent of the population of San Francisco, and 70 percent of the population of Santa Cruz helped others (Solnit, 2009). It is estimated that some 40,000 unsolicited volunteers helped at the World Trade Center site after 9/11 in New York City (Fernandez et al., 2006a).

According to researchers, there are two types of citizens who volunteer in emergency response: 1) affiliated volunteers, and 2) spontaneous (or unaffiliated) volunteers (Fernandez et al., 2006a; Fernandez et al., 2006b). Affiliated volunteers are associated with a government agency or non-governmental organization (such as Doctors Without Borders) and have been trained for a specific role or function in disaster response. Spontaneous volunteers are not initially affiliated with any group or agency, nor are they trained for specific roles in disaster relief. Depending on the particular context or situation, it is also possible for an individual to be both an affiliated and spontaneous volunteer. Thus the terms "affiliated" and "spontaneous" more accurately represent a continuum of volunteerism among individuals who may be more or less informed about emergency response.

The role and impact of spontaneous volunteers is not well understood, but one study suggests they often self-organize into small groups to achieve a common goal based on perceived needs in a disaster context (Fernandez et al., 2006a). Spontaneous volunteers may consist of adults who are anxious and want to help, the curious, returnees, or individuals who try to profit from the situation (Fritz & Mathewson, 1957). Children and youth also serve as spontaneous volunteers, and recent studies show they are capable of helping with disaster preparedness and recovery activities (Peek, 2008; UNICEF, 2007). For example, children and youth participated in emergency response activities after the Asian tsunami of 2004, providing psychosocial support to their peers, helping with community and school recovery efforts, and disseminating disaster risk information (Penrose & Takaki, 2006; UNICEF, 2007).

Aid organizations and government agencies often turn away spontaneous volunteers because they are not prepared for them, and because they are often not considered in disaster preparation and response planning (Fernandez et al., 2006a). The National Response Framework for emergencies in the United States recognizes state and local governments as having the primary responsibility for spontaneous volunteer management. It notes: "Volunteers and donors can support response efforts in many ways, and it is essential that governments at all levels plan ahead to effectively incorporate volunteers and donated goods into their response activities (U.S. Department of Homeland Security, 2008, p. 21). Only 30 out of 58 US states and territories address the role and management of spontaneous volunteers in their plans (Fernandez et al., 2006a). A large number of spontaneous volunteers can cause problems by overwhelming the capacity of organizations to effectively and safely engage them.

At the same time, spontaneous volunteers can solve problems that are not adequately addressed by formal response activities that are bound by legal policies and procedures. Spontaneous volunteers often have the ability to experiment with and improvise new strategies, tools, and technologies (both quantitatively and qualitatively) that formal responders may not be able to explore. For example, after 9/11, a group of telecommunications employees and companies joined together to create a "wireless emergency response team" which created a system and process to identify the location of mobile phones of missing people (Fernandez et al., 2006a). Given that spontaneous volunteers offer innovation in a time of crisis, more research needs to be conducted on these groups so they can be adequately integrated and linked to emergency management organizations.

Research has shown there is an "opportunity-bubble" for the government to enlist volunteers in emergencies as partners in response (Moghaddam & Breckenbridge, 2011). Taking better advantage of spontaneous volunteers during and after a disaster is one key suggestion for governments outlined in several emergency management manuals produced by the United States Federal Emergency Management Administration (FEMA) and other organizations (Fernandez et al., 2006b; *Preventing a Disaster Within the Disaster*, 2002).

This article demonstrates the potential assets of spontaneous volunteers to assist government agencies and humanitarian organizations through the use of online participatory mapping tools. In doing so, we offer new evidence on the innovation and contributions of spontaneous volunteers that can be leveraged, replicated and improved upon for future disaster planning and response.

THE GEOGRAPHY OF EMERGENCY RESPONSE

If appeals to the general public for emergency assistance lack specific details about what is needed and where, a large number of people will converge in areas that do not require help, or in locations that make volunteer management challenging or unsafe (Fernandez et al., 2006a; Fernandez et al., 2006b). This situation happened after Hurricane Sandy in New York City, and was further complicated by gasoline shortages and power outages that made communication among government agencies, aid organizations, and volunteers challenging. The result was a spatial mismatch between the needs reported by community residents and the actual services being offered to them by government agencies and relief groups.

Emergency response activities will vary by the type of disaster, the scale of impact, access to transportation and communication infrastructure, social class, and access to political networks and organizations (Archer & Booynyabancha, 2011; Wisner et al., 2005; Zoleta-Nantes, 2002). Therefore, emergency response is not linear (occurring as an evenly distributed sequence of events within the impacted region); it has spatial specificity (events that occur at varying times in different places within the impacted region). We therefore recognize that emergency response varies depending upon a wide range of social, political and environmental factors that interact with one another, and shape the overall landscape within which relief activities occur.

Recognizing spatial mismatch in emergency response means that governments and aid organizations should have better tools to help them understand the needs of communities in space and time, and mechanisms to help them better communicate with each other as they work in different impacted regions. A very logical tool is a map that can incorporate useful information about what is needed, where and when. While initially undervalued in emergency response because of their reliance on electricity and a functioning communication infrastructure, ICT and open source mapping programs are becoming increasingly recognized as important tools to gather and disseminate spatial information in emergency contexts (Klosterman, 2012; Mubaraka et al., 2005; Zook et al., 2010).

The participatory use of computerized geographic information systems (GIS) in emergency response is becoming more common and is part of a larger movement to democratize the creation of spatial information (Elwood, 2008). Traditionally, formal organizations such as the government were the most common creators of geospatial information (for example, see NYC Department of City Planning Bytes of the Big Apple http://www.nyc.gov/html/dcp/html/bytes/applbyte.shtml; and New York State GIS Clearinghouse gis.ny.gov/gisdata/). However, it is becoming more common to find volunteered geographic information (VGI) or spatial information that comes from unofficial sources being used to make decisions (Budhathoki et al., 2008). VGI is particularly important in emergency management because citizens and humanitarian organizations can share information the government may not have or be aware of and improve the timeliness of responses.

The quality of information shared and disseminated through VGI varies depending on its accessibility and inclusivity and often comes from multiple sources (Flanagin & Metzger, 2008; Goodchild, 2007b). Maps can be created remotely by crowd-sourcing data to cartographically visualize disparate data from multiple sources and news media outlets, such as those created after the 2010 Haitian Earthquake (Zook et al., 2010) and in post-conflict Iraq (Mubaraka et al., 2005). Information can also be collected from online social networks to compile maps. For example, citizens have contributed to emergency responses by uploading pictures, maintaining blogs, and facilitating communication among relief groups (Laituri & Kodrich, 2008).

After Hurricane Sandy, groups of spontaneous volunteers used social media and open source mapping tools to coordinate relief efforts via text messaging, using Twitter and Facebook. For example, Occupy Sandy, a local spinoff of the "Occupy Wall Street" social action network, created a New York City map of volunteer opportunities using the free "My Maps" program in Google (http://occupysandy.net/map/). Building upon its experience with Hurricane Katrina, Google began spearheading a "crisis map" for the larger region impacted by the storm to communicate recovery efforts working in partnership with local governments and private citizens (http://google. org/crisismap/2012-sandy). In Hoboken, New Jersey, a small group of citizens created a "power map" to track its restoration block-by-block that witnessed over 600,000 views during the five days the map was active after the event until power was restored (http://hobokensandymaps.com/). In another case, a group of local high school students partnered with an adult volunteer group to create a "gasoline map" of open filling stations by calling each location to determine its status and populating the data in "Mappler," which then fed into Google's Sandy Crisis Map (http://mappler. net/gasstation/).

These examples provide evidence of the power citizens now have to contribute to relief efforts after a disaster using a combination of low bandwidth platforms such as Facebook and Twitter as well as online mapping platforms such as Google and Mappler. While it is clear that these maps were viewed by large numbers of people to help them make informed decisions, it is less certain if these examples can serve as experiments to help disaster response and preparedness in poorer communities (Meier & Leaning, 2009). In the Rockaways, it was not possible for residents to use Facebook or other low bandwidth platforms to volunteer geographic information that would assist in their emergency response. In this article, we provide a detailed case study of a citizen-led emergency response effort after Hurricane Sandy using volunteered geographic information and a hybrid of paper-based and online mapping tools. The case examines how the authors of this article volunteered in the Rockaways in New York City to help communicate the needs reported by community members to outsiders and analyzes the impact of this effort.

Community Context

The Rockaways is a group of neighborhoods located on an 18-kilometer peninsula at the southern end of Queens in New York City (Figure 1). The Rockaways is comprised of communities that vary in income, housing density, racial and cultural groups, and land use. For example, at the western edge of the peninsula, The *New York Times* called the neighborhood of Breezy Point "the whitest neighborhood in the city" (Scott, 2001, June 18). A predominantly middle class Jewish population resides on the eastern edge of the peninsula in the neighborhood of Far Rockaway. In the center of the peninsula are many neighborhoods comprised of poor or working class African American, Asian and Hispanic families who reside in high-rise public housing developments, or subsidized private housing developments.

In 2010, the population of the Rockaways was 115,000 with no clear racial majority (42 percent white, 23 percent black, and 19 percent Hispanic), and 37 percent of the population was on income support (Infoshare, 2013).

In many ways the Rockaways is isolated from the rest of New York City because of its distance from Manhattan and its history as a relocation

Figure 1. Location map of the Rockaways

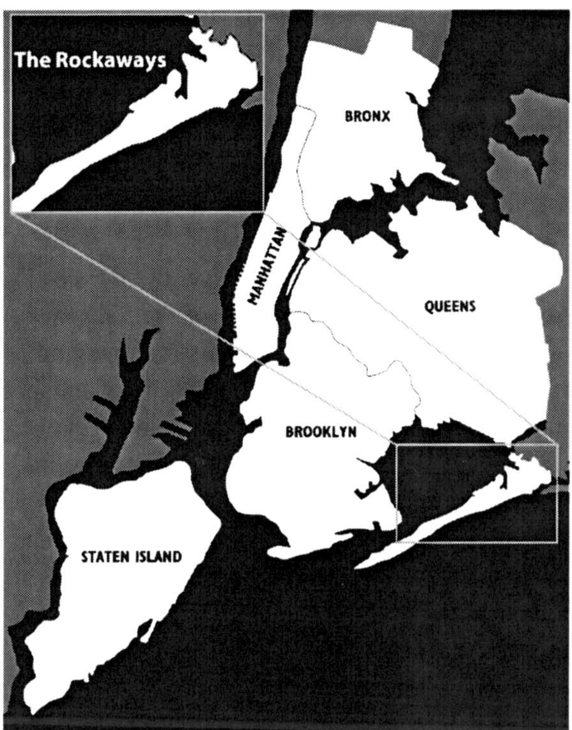

site for the poor. As Greenberg (2013, January 10) describes it, "The Rockaway public housing projects, many between 14 and 24 stories high, were isolated and self-contained, a separate, forgotten world, with some of the city's highest rates of infant mortality, infectious diseases, and unemployment" (n.p.). By 1975, 57 percent of all the low-income housing in Queens was located in the Rockaways. It was also the place where group homes for the mentally disabled and nursing homes for the poor elderly became more common than any other part of the city (Schwarzfeld, 2008). Commenting on the remains of many years of relocating the poor into massive housing projects, Miller (2012) writes:

Today, in the aftermath of the storm [Sandy], it is hard not to see the Rockaway projects as inherently flawed, doomed not only by their exposure to the storm-churned waters of the Atlantic, but

by their very design. Densely populated, without any retail space, and isolated from the rest of the city, the mostly poor residents have relied on help arriving from the outside. [Robert] Moses may have thought he was breaking up the city's ghettos; in fact, he was relocating them and setting them in concrete (n.p.).

In recent years, there have been attempts to create mixed-income housing developments as well as modern and expensive seaside developments for upwardly mobile young adults. These new housing developments have transformed resident demographics and land use. For example, after a six percent growth in population from 1990 to 2000, the Rockaways grew an additional 7.8 percent between 2000 and 2010. About 30 percent of the land use now consists of single- and two-family houses, while about 10.5 percent are multi-family units. Roughly 40 percent of the residents live in owner-occupied housing, but the large public housing developments remain (NYC Department of City Planning, 2013).

Research Design

Four days after Hurricane Sandy occurred, the authors of this article, who are researchers affiliated with a local university, traveled to the Rockaways. Our goal was to assess if we could help with relief efforts given our expertise in environmental studies and emergency planning. As mentioned in the introduction section, we had no intention of conducting research on Sandy's impact in the Rockaways, nor did we have a goal for the relief efforts we eventually conducted there. Initially we were simply among the many thousands of spontaneous volunteers to converge in areas impacted by Sandy to see how we could help. However, as researchers we did enter the situation with a critical lens to assess and evaluate the needs of community residents. In doing so, we implemented a participatory action research process to understand the situation and to develop an approach for our volunteer efforts.

Participant Observation

Our first interaction with community residents in the Rockaways was as participant observers. We drove along the peninsula and made observations of the type of damages we saw, taking photographs, and talking with groups of people who were gathering in different places outdoors. Initially we informally interviewed about a dozen community residents, volunteers and government officials. Community residents expressed concern for their safety at night given blackout conditions, and for residents living in high-rise apartment buildings without access to water and electricity. Most community residents also requested information about what was happening because residents could not use their mobile phones or listen to the news on television or radio. What we observed and discovered through our informal conversations with residents was troubling. Namely, there was a minimal emergency response by the government in the poorest and most densely populated neighborhoods of the Rockaways.

Four days after Sandy, the response by government officials included one City Council member who visited community groups on a frequent basis to assess the situation. In addition, several New York State Senate staff members and one National Guard unit were located in a neighborhood park distributing hot meals. But these public officials left the Rockaways by dusk each evening because there was no power, and admitted that they considered it unsafe to be there at night. Police officers were observed outside of their precinct reading newspapers, with only a handful of police stationed at specific intersections to direct traffic. These officers also left after dusk, leaving the Rockaway residents without any way to communicate with public officials given the blackout situation and damaged communications infrastructure.

Based on our observations and informal interviews, community residents and spontaneous volunteers were the primary first responders after Hurricane Sandy in the poorest neighborhoods of the Rockaways. For example, the Rockaway Youth Task Force, an existing youth-led group, mobilized emergency supplies with support from their members and conducted needs assessments with over 2,000 residents in high-rise residential developments, serving over 700 families within four days after the disaster (http://www.rytf. org). In addition, Occupy Sandy and Doctors Without Borders (an international aid agency) were observed providing emergency services in the area, along with a handful of church groups and individuals from other states in the region.

On several occasions we observed a mismatch between the emergency services being provided by relief workers from outside the community and the needs reported to us by community residents. For example, a representative from an international aid agency was seen trying to deliver blankets at one location in the community where none were needed. We also observed bags of clothing being dropped off on the front lawns of churches, going untouched by residents who actually needed hot meals, diapers, infant formula, transportation, money for rent from lost wages due to the storm, and electricity (a situation that was also reported by Turk, 2012). Participant observation led us to the conclusion that we needed to conduct a more comprehensive rapid community assessment of the situation to understand resident needs and the extent of existing relief efforts.

Rapid Community Assessment

We developed a rapid community assessment interview protocol to use with groups leading relief efforts in the poorest neighborhoods of the Rockaways, as well as with residents living in high-rise apartment buildings. The goal was to determine services being provided at the location, as well as resident reported needs. The protocol included a simple form (Figure 2) to indicate the name, organization and contact information of the person providing the information, the address or nearest intersection where the interview took place,

Figure 2. Rapid community assessment protocol

<table>
<tr><td>

Location Name:
Address:
Contact:
Group(s) Providing Services:

Services at Location:
- Food distribution
- Meal Service
- Clothing distribution
- Water distribution
- Other supply distribution (flashlights, batteries)
- Health center
- FEMA information center
- Police station
- Fire station
- Humanitarian Aid center
- Other ______________

Needs at Location:
- Food
- Clothing
- Water
- Other emergency supplies
- Infant supplies
- Health supplies
- Volunteers
- Information about recovery process
- Other ______________

</td><td>

Location Name:
Address:
Contact:
Group(s) Providing Services:

Services at Location:
- Food distribution
- Meal Service
- Clothing distribution
- Water distribution
- Other supply distribution (flashlights, batteries)
- Health center
- FEMA information center
- Police station
- Fire station
- Humanitarian Aid center
- Other ______________

Needs at Location:
- Food
- Clothing
- Water
- Other emergency supplies
- Infant supplies
- Health supplies
- Volunteers
- Information about recovery process
- Other ______________

</td></tr>
</table>

and a checklist of the likely needs and services at that location over the next week as identified by volunteers and residents.

After conducting a rapid assessment of the situation through interviews with over 25 volunteers and community residents, it was obvious that there was a lack of coordination and communication among the groups providing services in the area. At the same time, there was no way for residents to communicate their needs to willing volunteers outside of the community. We therefore decided to create an online public map of the emergency response efforts based on the data we collected through the rapid community assessment to ensure that individuals, groups and organizations who wanted to help were aware of the needs reported by community residents in specific locations along the peninsula.

Emergency Mapping Methodology

Google was selected as the social media platform to create this map because it provides an easy, intuitive way to manage information and to allow others to update the content themselves. However, due to the lack of power and access to technology, we understood that the map would be more effective for those outside of the Rockaways who wanted to help community members living there. Over time and with electricity restored, we hoped residents and groups such as the Rockaway Youth Task Force could take over the mapping process to ensure the community was involved in the long-term recovery process.

The map was created with a total of 11 volunteers: 4 researchers, 1 journalist, 1 social worker, 1 early childhood development specialist, 2 youth from the community, and 2 outside relief workers. Researchers mapped most of the data because of their access to technology, while other volunteers gathered information with different stakeholders and reported it directly to researchers. The map was updated on five different occasions at different time intervals ranging from one to six days. The map information was updated based on the repeated use of the rapid interview protocol with residents and volunteers to determine community needs and services at specific locations where activity was observed along the peninsula, as well as with paper maps to mark observation points. A spreadsheet including the rapid community assessment data associated with each mapped point was developed to keep track of the time sequence of events and information. Table 1 provides a comprehensive description of the mapped points.

The *Rockaway Emergency Response Map* initially contained very minimal information, as there were few emergency service providers or government agencies responding after the disaster (Figure 3). Over time, the items that were mapped changed, based on the growing needs expressed by community residents and relief workers. The map is not comprehensive, but contains information primarily along the major arterials within the poorest neighborhoods of the Rockaways because this is where emergency relief activities were concentrated.

Sharing and Validating the Emergency Map

The map was hosted on a blog that also contained information about the status of schooling and childcare centers, news articles about what was happening in the Rockaways, and recovery information (http://rockawayrecovery.wordpress. org). Users could click on each mapped point to

Table 1. Description of mapped points

Item	Description
Location Name	The name of the mapped point, such as "Conch Playground," if appropriate
Address	A street address or the nearest intersection of the mapped point
Organizer	The name and contact information of the individual or groups providing services at the location
Community Needs	A list of needs requested by residents or relief workers at the location
Community Services	A list of services being led by or provided to the community from individuals or groups at a specific location
Floodlights	The location of floodlights to help residents identify where they could walk safely at night
Traffic Police	The location of traffic police so residents could contact officials in the event of an emergency
Emergency Command Centers	The location of the National Guard, ambulances, the Office of Emergency Management (OEM) stations and other emergency services operated by the city, state and federal authorities
Recovery Information Centers	The location of FEMA, City Council representatives, and other groups offering assistance with social services and insurance claims
Phone Charging Stations	The location of mobile phone charging stations (generally provided by private corporations or citizens)
Food Trucks	The location of food trucks sponsored by private corporations, the City of New York, and local not-for-profit food truck associations
Medical Centers	The location of local and mobile medical centers and their hours of operation
Waste Removal	The location of the dumping site for all of the debris and waste caused by damage from the Hurricane
Transportation	The location of a temporary ferry going to Manhattan
Portable Toilets	The location of portable toilets available to relief workers

Figure 3. Snapshot of the Rockaway emergency response map

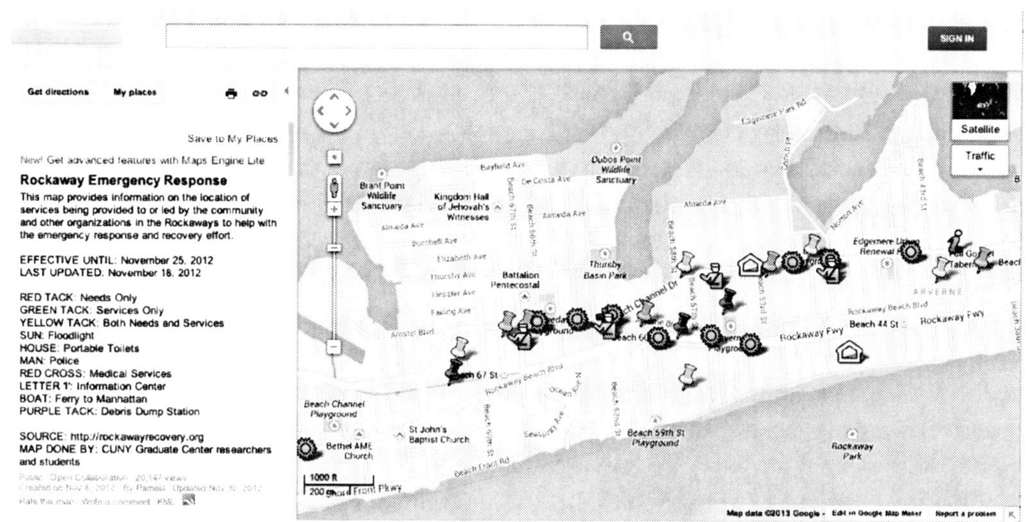

learn additional information that was gathered through the field research process (Figure 4). Users were also encouraged to add their own information to the map given its public nature, and a link to a mapping tutorial was provided so individuals without experience could participate in the process.

Information about the map and how to update it was also shared with every community group or public official providing services, and shared with other online networks and relief efforts such as Google's Sandy Crisis Map, Occupy Sandy Map, the Crisis Mappers Network, the New York Presbyterian Church, senior centers, government

Figure 4. Snapshot of information contained in a mapped point

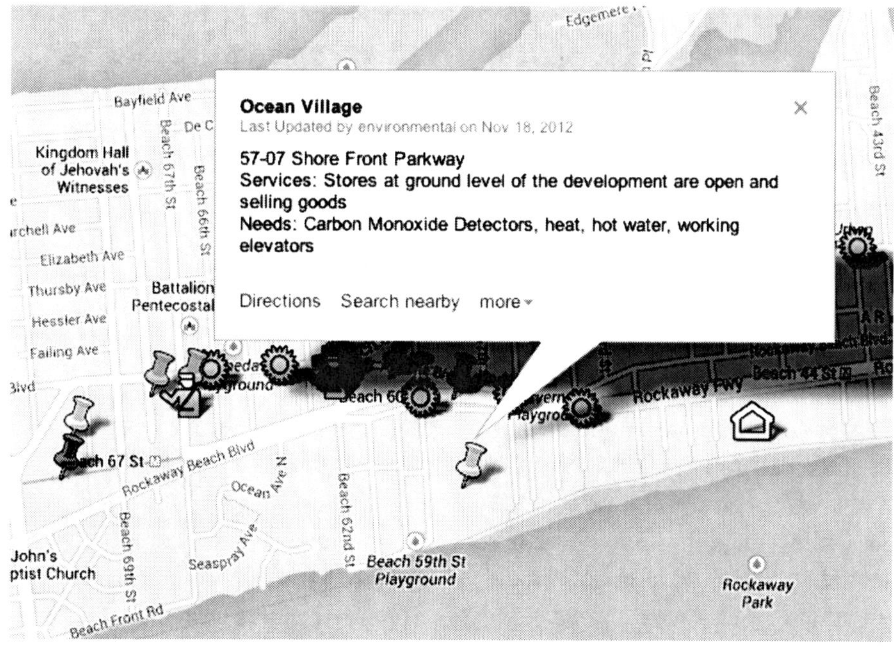

agencies (such as the FDNY, FEMA, OEM), the City of New York, City Council members, and Rockaway Facebook networks.

The map was active for a total of 20 days (from November 5 until November 25, 2012), during which time researchers conducted follow up interviews with community organizers and officials to determine if the map was working. The links to the Google Sandy Crisis Map and the Occupy Wall Street relief efforts gave it greater visibility in Internet searches about the event. In addition, local groups began linking the map to their respective organizational websites. Unfortunately, power was restored unevenly in different sections of the Rockaways, and some homes did not receive electricity for over a month. Therefore, access to the Internet and to technology that could have supported local residents to take over and continue using the map was limited.

Results of the Rockaway Emergency Map

Outsiders viewed the map more than community residents. During the 20 days the map was active, it was viewed a total of 18,260 times. Based on website statistics, most views (about 90%) came from online searches and via Google's Sandy Crisis map, with minimal views coming from the project blog (about 800 views). Our initial hypothesis that the map would be more useful for individuals and groups outside of the Rockaways proved to be true, in large part because of the long-term lack of electricity after the storm. Based on follow up interviews with relief workers, volunteers outside of the community who wanted to help the Rockaways recover viewed the map more than community residents. This finding suggests online maps can provide an effective way to share real time information with spontaneous volunteers who reside outside of an impacted area. Online mapping tools therefore have the potential to assist government agencies or humanitarian organizations in managing spontaneous external volunteers in emergency contexts to help avoid their convergence in areas where they are not needed.

The map worked to coordinate and match emergency services with needs, but it could not be sustained for long-term recovery efforts. Evidence from follow up interviews and observations suggest the map worked to better coordinate and match services and needs in the emergency response phase. For example, one key informant stated that his church received services they requested from volunteers who saw the map of their needs online. There is also evidence that relief workers updated the map on their own, so the public nature of the map worked in some ways to enhance their participation in providing emergency information. However, the map had to be monitored because sometimes individuals who volunteered geographic information moved or placed symbols in incorrect locations. Overall, given the sustained lack of electricity and entry errors, it was best to rely on researchers to populate a majority of the mapped points. Therefore, the number of stakeholders involved in updating the map was limited. Despite the usefulness of the map, no humanitarian aid agency, community group, or government entity was identified that was willing to maintain the map during the emergency phase or for the long-term recovery of the Rockaways. The reasons for this included a lack of resources or capacity to frequently and consistently update the information as well as the liability involved in endorsing and promoting volunteered geographic information that could not be verified by official sources. Finally, because there was no overall coordinating entity managing the response in the Rockaways, such as a federal or state emergency management agency, the map ceased to be populated with information approximately three weeks after the event.

The map helped keep track of a fluid situation of evolving needs, but a coordinating entity is needed to provide consistent, up-to-date information. By keeping a database of mapped points, we were able to analyze the different needs expressed by residents and relief workers over limited time and space. In general, the needs of the community shifted from emergency supplies (such as water, food, and flashlights) to long-term recovery issues (such as access to heat and hot water, carbon monoxide detectors, mental health support, public health issues associated with mold, and sink holes). Relief workers expressed the need to have information on the map updated more frequently as the situation would often change from hour to hour. A lack of electricity limited the ability of community groups to provide up-to-date information on the map on their own. Therefore, in these situations, a coordinating entity or group is needed to gather data through interviews before entering volunteered geographic information online. This does not mean a return to government-centric planning per say, but rather a participatory emergency planning framework that combines humans as sensors from within communities and online mappers outside the impacted region with access to technology to advocate for an improved response in poor communities (Chun & Artigas, 2012).

The map enabled the analysis of the different groups involved in the emergency response and suggests the need for collaborative disaster planning. Based on an analysis of the mapped points, we can conclude that volunteers and smaller community based organizations played a major role in providing immediate emergency relief services in the Rockaways (Figure 5). For example, a variety of religious groups with connections to the community through their members delivered food and emergency supplies after the disaster. Some of the larger emergency service organizations did not arrive to assist in the area for several weeks. The National Guard and other local, state and federal authorities were largely absent from immediate emergency response in the neighborhoods we mapped, with most services appearing ten days after the disaster and lasting for a period of one week. The lack of an immediate government or professional humanitarian response to Sandy in the Rockaways suggests an urgent need for citizens to be better prepared for disasters. It also suggests the continuing need for independent study that analyzes government relief efforts in

Figure 5. Number of relief services mapped over time, by group leading process

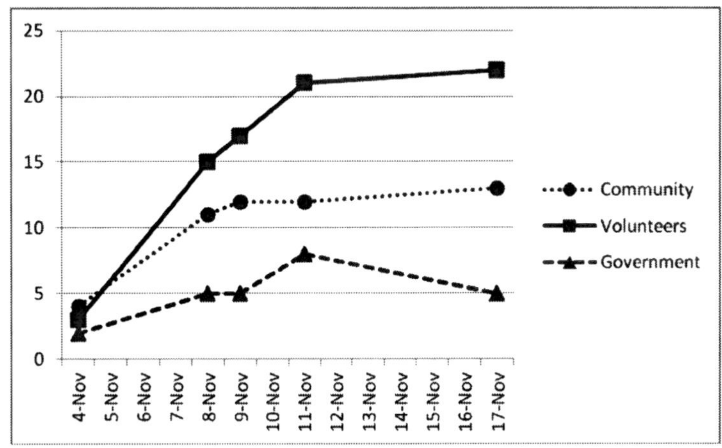

Group	5-Nov	9-Nov	10-Nov	12-Nov	18-Nov
Community	4	11	12	12	13
Volunteers	3	15	17	21	22
Government	2	5	5	8	5
Total Mapped Points	9	31	34	41	40

impacted regions to determine if additional steps can be taken to improve emergency response in poor communities.

The map integrated the emergency response efforts across multiple sectors, such as health, public safety, and social services. The *Rockaway Emergency Response Map* was unique among other Sandy crisis maps mentioned previously because it offered a cross-sector perspective on the emergency response process. It did this by integrating the efforts of public health officials, police, transportation officials, and community groups in a defined geographic area. This enabled map users to understand the different roles that citizens, humanitarian organizations, and government agencies had in the relief process, and areas that need to be improved. A community map that integrates information and communication among different government sectors, volunteers and aid agencies enables groups to respond to the needs reported by citizens. The map can enable all stakeholders to avoid the duplication, spatial mismatch, or unnecessary convergence of relief efforts in the impacted region.

The map highlighted the important role and needs of young people in emergency response and recovery after a disaster. Youth aged 15 to 24 played an important role in the emergency response efforts in the Rockaways, especially in assisting immobile seniors in high-rise housing developments. The needs of younger children were consistently a concern of residents, such as access to childcare, infant formula and pampers. Older youth were concerned about their safety due to a lack of lighting on the streets and they began avoiding going out after dark all together. The lack of electricity and access to battery powered radios in the Rockaways made it difficult for children, youth and families to obtain information about the status of their schools. For those dependent on public transport, public buses shut down at dark (around 17:00 hours) and the subway line serving the Rockaways was canceled for six months. New York City Public Schools were overwhelmed by the number of displaced students and could only provide alternative transportation options to a portion of elementary school children. As a result of these safety and transportation issues, many young people were unable to travel to school for several weeks, denying them a right to education.

CONCLUSION

The *Rockaway Emergency Response Map* was developed after Hurricane Sandy because no coordinating entity was managing the disaster response in the area, even though national policies suggest the local government should have this role (Fernandez et al., 2006a). Despite a directive from the U.S. Department of Homeland Security to state and local agencies, the role of governments, private companies, and citizens is not clearly delineated in emergency response. Government services were largely absent until ten days after the storm, and as a result, everyday citizens served as first responders in the Rockaways, including youth from community based organizations and religious groups of all denominations. With many different types of stakeholders involved in emergency response, it is not uncommon for confusion to occur. The responsibility for the on-site coordination of unaffiliated volunteers needs to be clearly designated by state and local leadership prior to an incident or event.

This research provides evidence that the coordination of relief efforts by government officials, volunteers, and community groups in emergency contexts can be enhanced through the use of participatory mapping tools. Volunteered geographic information from citizens was found to be useful in informing outside volunteers what was needed, where, and when based on the needs reported by community members in the Rockaways. Instead of relying on volunteer-based coordination efforts like this in future disasters, we believe that there needs to be a functioning information management system for coordinating unaffiliated volunteers in response operations that is clearly designated by state and local leadership. Be it a central phone bank that will combine with a web-portal to provide the public with access to information on volunteer opportunities and provide coordinators with the capacity to match volunteers skills with opportunities, or some other proposal, we believe such a system is necessary in New York City. Such a system would allow volunteer managers to redirect individuals to places with ongoing needs in the community through the use of various ITC mediums.

It is plausible that our map could have had long-term use beyond the emergency response period. Unfortunately, without an organization committed to maintaining the map, it was not possible to document the evolving needs and services of the Rockaway community after the emergency response period ended. But there are a number of possible ways to use maps for long-term recovery planning after the emergency response period is over. One possibility is to train active local groups like the Rockaway Youth Task Force (RYTF) to lead a post-disaster community needs assessment with the results shared on a public map. For instance, the RYTF could identify the location of childcare services that are open and list the status of schools, playgrounds and other places important for children, youth and their families. Another suggestion is to raise awareness about the utility of volunteered geographic information and online mapping in disaster situations. This could be done through community workshops and after school programs that focus on disaster preparedness and building the capacity of citizens to respond in emergencies.

Yet, there is a paradox of a wired society in disaster situations. On the one hand, many people own cell phones and smart phones as well as computers of varying kinds (desktop, laptop, tablet). Online mapping platforms and social networking sites can be major assets in communicating needs and services in a coordinated way as long as access is available. On the other hand, even if electronic signals remain available during or after a disaster, low-income groups often do not have access to this technology. The Pew Research Center's "Internet and American Life Project" (2013) studied usage by income and found that, although cell phone ownership was high among all income groups (91 percent), smart phone usage was much less for low-income populations. Whereas 56 percent of Americans have smart phones and use them for Internet access, only 43 percent of individuals with incomes below $30,000 USD per year own smart phones (Brenner, 2013). Therefore, we need to think of new ways to gather, input and use volunteered geographic information in disaster contexts through a hybrid of online and face-to-face methods, especially in poorer communities.

More research is needed to analyze the many aspects of disaster preparedness in marginalized communities within large urban centers like New York City, including the utility and validity of volunteered geographic information. For example, studies that examine the effectiveness of volunteers from many perspectives, including inter-agency coordination, placement, safety, and management through ICT are required. While this project was wholly about attempting to facilitate the recovery of one section of New York City, we chose to write about this project because we hope the findings add to the academic conversation around VGI in emergency response. We believe that academic institutions should support disaster mitigation by increasing applied research to study the effectiveness of volunteers in emergency situations and in delineating the role of technical assistance to relevant agencies or organizations.

Our research suggests spontaneous volunteers offer innovation in a time of crisis, and their roles need to be better understood, leveraged and adequately integrated into emergency management planning. In particular, we suggest that citizen use of participatory mapping tools can prove a timely and valuable asset in emergency response and recovery.

ACKNOWLEDGMENT

The authors would like to thank citizens of the Rockaways, Hella Winston and Briana Baxter for their support and contributions to this publication.

REFERENCES

Archer, D., & Boonyabancha, S. (2011). Seeing a disaster as an opportunity: Harnessing the energy of disaster survivors for change. *Environment and Urbanization, 23*(2), 351–364. doi:10.1177/0956247811410011

Brenner, S. (2013). Pew Internet: Mobile. *Pew Internet & American Life*. Pew Research Center. Retrieved August 26, 2013 from, http://pewinternet.org/Commentary/2012/February/Pew-Internet-Mobile.aspx

Budhathoki, N. R., Bruce, B., & Nedovic-Budic, Z. (2008). Reconceptualizing the role of the user of spatial data infrastructure. *GeoJournal, 72*(3-4), 149–160. doi:10.1007/s10708-008-9189-x

Chun, S. A., & Artigas, F. (2012). Sensors and crowdsourcing for environmental awareness and emergency planning. *International Journal of E-Planning Research, 1*(1), 56–74. doi:10.4018/ijepr.2012010106

Daly, J. D. Assistant Chief of Operations, FDNY (2013). FDNY response to Hurricane Sandy. Presentation to the Fire Bell Club of New York, New York, NY.

Elwood, S. (2008). Volunteered geographic information: Future research directions motivated by critical, participatory, and feminist GIS. *GeoJournal, 72*(3-4), 173–183. doi:10.1007/s10708-008-9186-0

Esposito, J. E. Chief of Operations, FDNY. (2013). FDNY response to Hurricane Sandy. Presentation to the Fire Bell Club of New York, New York, NY.

Fernandez, L., Barbera, J., & van Dorp, J. (2006a). Spontaneous volunteer response to disasters: The benefits and consequences of good intentions. *Journal of Emergency Management, 4*(5), 57–68.

Fernandez, L., Barbera, J. & van Dorp, J. (2006b). Strategies for managing volunteers during incident response: A systems approach. *Homeland Security Affairs, 2*(3).

Flanagin, A. J., & Metzger, M. J. (2008). The credibility of volunteered geographic information. *GeoJournal, 72*(3-4), 137–148. doi:10.1007/s10708-008-9188-y

Freedman, A. (2012). 32-foot-plus waves from Hurricane Sandy topple records. *Climate Central*. Retrieved on August 26, 2013, from http://www.climatecentral.org/news/32-foot-wave-from-hurricane-sandy-topples-records-noaa-finds-15241

Fritz, C., & Mathewson, J. H. (1957). *Convergence behavior in disasters: A problem in social control.* Washington, DC: National Academy of Sciences/ National Research Council.

Goodchild, M. (2007a). Citizens as voluntary sensors: Spatial data infrastructure in the world of Web 2.0. *International Journal of Spatial Data Infrastructures Research, 2*, 24–32.

Goodchild, M. (2007b). Citizens as sensors: The world of volunteered geography. *GeoJournal, 69*(4), 211–221. doi:10.1007/s10708-007-9111-y

Greenberg, M. (2013). Occupy the Rockaways! *New York Review of Books*. Retrieved on January 10, 2013 from, http://www.nybooks.com/articles/archives/2013/jan/10/occupy-rockaways/?pagination=false

Infoshare. (2013). *Infoshare online*. Retrieved August 26, 2013 from, http://infoshare.org/main/public.aspx

Klosterman, R. (2012). E-planning: Retrospect and prospect. *International Journal of E-Planning Research*, *1*(1), 1–4. doi:10.4018/ijepr.2012010101

Laituri, M., & Kodrich, K. (2008). On line disaster response community: People as sensors of high magnitude disasters using internet GIS. *Sensors (Basel, Switzerland)*, *8*(5), 3037–3055. doi:10.3390/s8053037

Managing spontaneous volunteers in times of disaster: The synergy of structure and good intentions. (2005). Monograph of the Points of Light Foundation, NVOAD, and UPS Foundation. Retrieved on August 1, 2013, from http://www.fema.gov/pdf/donations/ManagingSpontaneous-Volunteers.pdf

Manahan, J. (2013). FDNY post-Hurricane Sandy analysis. Presentation to the Fire Bell Club of New York, New York, NY.

McKenzie, T. (2012). *NYC evacuation zones: Bloomberg orders 'zone A' residents to evacuate*. All Media NY. Retrieved August 26, 2013 from, http://www.allmediany.com/news/6316-nyc-evacuation-zones-bloomberg-orders-zone-a-residents-to-evacuate

Meier, P., & Leaning, J. (2009). *Applying technology to crisis mapping and early warning in humanitarian settings*. Working Paper Series. Cambridge, MA: Harvard Humanitarian Initiative.

Miller, J. (2012). How the coastline became a place to put the poor. *New York Times*, December 12. Retrieved August 1, 2012, from http://www.nytimes.com/2012/12/04/nyregion/how-new-york-citys-coastline-became-home-to-the-poor.html?pagewanted=all

Moghaddam, F. & Breckenbridge, J. (2011). The post-tragedy 'opportunity-bubble' and the prospect of citizen engagement. *Homeland Security Affairs, 7*.

Mubaraka, S., Khudhairy, D., Bonn, F., & Aoun, S. (2005). Standardizing and mapping open-source information for regions in crises. Case study: Post-conflict Iraq. *Disasters*, *29*(3), 237–254. doi:10.1111/j.0361-3666.2005.00289.x PMID:16108990

NYC Department of City Planning. (2013). *Community district needs*. Retrieved August 26, 2013, from http://www.nyc.gov/html/dcp/

Peek, L. (2008). Children and disasters: Understanding vulnerability, developing capacities, and promoting resilience. *Children, Youth and Environments*, *18*(1), 1–29.

Penrose, A., & Takaki, M. (2006). Children's rights in emergencies and disasters. *Lancet*, *367*(9511), 698–699. doi:10.1016/S0140-6736(06)68272-X PMID:16503472

Pereira, I. (2013). Six months later, New York still recovering from Sandy's wrath. *AM New York*. Retrieved August 26, 2013 from, http://www.amny.com/urbanite-1.812039/six-months-later-new-york-still-recovering-from-sandy-s-wrath-1.5157662

Preventing a disaster within the disaster: The effective use and management of unaffiliated volunteers. (2002). Monograph of the Points of Light Foundation and Volunteer Center National Network. Retrieved on August 13, 2013, from https://www.nationalserviceresources.org/online-library/items/m3248

Roca, T. (2012). 11 facts about Hurricane Sandy. *Do Something*. Retrieved August 26, 2013, from http://www.dosomething.org/tipsandtools/11-facts-about-hurricane-sandy

Schwarzfeld, M. (2008). In far Rockaway, pretty beach meets housing bust. *City Limits*. Retrieved August 1, 2013 from, http://www.citylimits.org/articles/3568

Scott, J. (2001). The census: A region of enclaves; Amid a sea of faces, islands of segregation. *The New York Times*. Retrieved August 21, 2013 from, http://www.nytimes.com/2001/06/18/nyregion/the-census-a-region-of-enclaves-amid-a-sea-of-faces-islands-of-segregation.html

Silverman, R. (2012). Why New York City is the worst place for a hurricane. *National Geographic Daily News*. Retrieved August 26, 2013 from, http://news.nationalgeographic.com/news/2012/11/121101-new-york-city-sandy-hurricane-bight-science-environment-nation/

Solnit, R. (2009). *A paradise built in hell*. New York, NY: Penguin Books.

Turk, B. (2012). Far Rockaway non-profits speak out on post-hurricane needs. *Community Resource Exchange News*. Retrieved August 13, 2013, from http://www.crenyc.org/_blog/News_and_Views/post/Far_Rockaway_Nonprofits_Speak_Out_on_Post-Hurricane_Needs/

UNICEF. (2007). *The participation of children and young people in emergencies: A guide for relief agencies*. New York, NY: UNICEF.

United States Department of Homeland Security. (2008). *National response framework*. Washington, DC.

Walsh, B. (2012). Frankenstorm: Why Hurricane Sandy will be historic. *Time (Science & Space)*. Retrieved August 26, 2013, from http://science.time.com/2012/10/29/frankenstorm-why-hurricane-sandy-will-be-historic/

Wisner, B., Blaikie, P., Cannon, T., & Davis, I. (2005). *At risk: Natural hazards, people's vulnerability and disasters*. New York, NY: Routledge. doi:10.4324/9780203428764

Zoleta-Nantes, D. (2002). Differential impacts of flood hazards among the street children, the urban poor and residents of wealthy neighborhoods in metro Manila, Philippines. *Mitigation and Adaptation Strategies for Global Change*, 7(3), 239–266. doi:10.1023/A:1024471412686

Zook, M., Graham, M., Shelton, T., & Gorman, S. (2010). Volunteered geographic information and crowdsourcing disaster relief: A case study of the Haitian earthquake. *World Medical & Health Policy*, 27(2), 123–141.

This work was previously published in the International Journal of E-Planning Research (IJEPR), 3(3); edited by Carlos Nunes Silva, pages 1-19 copyright year 2014 by IGI Publishing (an imprint of IGI Global).

Chapter 69
Operative Role Management in Information Systems

Taina Kurki
University of Eastern Finland, Finland

Hanna-Miina Sihvonen
Emergency Services College, Finland

ABSTRACT

Operative role management relates to the commanding officers' work of managing their resources dealing with emergency situations. It concerns assigning and delegating the right roles to the right resources at a specific moment. Role management is commonly understood as system role management, relating to access control and administrative role management. Operative role management is in turn the practical daily work of emergency organizations' personnel and relates to overall resource management. In-depth ethnographic research has been carried out, and the difference between operative and system role management has been distinguished in this chapter. The research concentrates both on the practical work processes of the emergency management staff and on the information systems and their functionalities. Through this two-folded approach, role management approach has been divided into three domains: administrative management domain, operative domain, and their common domain. The chapter focuses on describing the interdependencies between the role management approaches with examples from field studies and findings from literature.

INTRODUCTION AND BACKGROUND

Commonly, role management refers to an organization's capability to manage the roles in which each employee performs as part of his or her job functions. In technological terms, role management relates to managing access control/authorization and specifying the resources the users are allowed to access in an application or computer system (Aedo, Diaz & Sanz, 2006; Al-Kahtani & Sandhu, 2002; Ferraiolo, Kuhn & Chandramouli, 2007). RBAC (Role-Based Access Control) regulates the access to resources and computer system objects based on the roles defined in an organization (Sanz, Aedo, Diaz & de Castro, 2006; Ferraiolo, Kuhn & Chandramouli, 2007). The key RBAC hypothesis is that roles and related responsibilities are much more persistent than users (Sanz et al.,

DOI: 10.4018/978-1-4666-8756-1.ch069

2006; Aedo et al., 2006). After the responsibilities of an organization are defined, they rarely change. Usually, what changes is the user or users that work with a specific responsibility in a specific situation. Much of the previous research in this field is based on RBAC, its mechanisms and extensions (Sanz, Gómez Bello, Díaz, Sainz & Aedo, 2007; Haibin & MengChu, 2006; Aedo & al., 2006; Tahir, 2007), such as context-aware dynamic access control (Kim et al., 2005; Zhang & Parashar, 2004) or attribute-based user-role assignment (Al-Kahtani & Sandhu, 2002).

In multi-authority emergency situations where collaboration between authorities emerges, it is often necessary to share information within or between organizations. The organizations have implemented various information and communication systems to support the activities in the command and control rooms as well as in-the-field actions (Mehrotra, Butss, Klashnikov & Venkatasubramanian, 2004; Sanz & al., 2007; Smirnov, Pashkin, Levashova, Shilov & Kashevnik, 2007). The information technology challenges focus on the systems and procedures to get the right information to the right person at the right time (Sanz & al., 2007; Ianella & Henricksen, 2007). RBAC can be used to control information sharing in the systems and to solve some of the information sharing obstacles. However, RBAC still requires improvements to function in a dynamic environment. Moreover, challenges are caused by relatively low integration of information and communication technologies in the emergency management field (Wybo & Lonka, 2002).

According to Haibin and MengChu (2006), role-based collaboration is a recent innovation, which pays attention to how productive collaborations can be maximized by manipulating role assignments and the configuration of teams. It is a new methodology for organizing collaboration by providing role specification, assignment, transition, and negotiation mechanisms. With these mechanisms, people in collaboration know their roles, thereby making collaboration more productive. Operative role management focuses in particular on the command and control activities of an emergency organization (Kurki & Sihvonen, 2012; Sihvonen & Kurki, 2010). It refers to managing the different roles that personnel can dynamically assume during an emergency situation. In emergency organizations, roles vary from operative field roles to tactical and strategic command, control and coordination roles and to administrative roles. Role transfers take place dynamically several times during emergency situations and shifts, and are largely based on verbal communications and face-to-face briefings. Even though a human user in collaboration cannot be physically changed, his/her role in collaboration may be changed (Sanz & al., 2006). In their work, Ianella and Henricksen (2007) describe how in a small incident one person could undertake the role of incident controller as well as the tasks of planning, operations, and logistics; in a medium-sized incident a person can be required in each of the four roles; and in a major incident dozens of people may be required to handle the various management functions. Role management is challenging, as a change in one role can initiate a series of role changes within and across organizational boundaries when forming situation-organizations (Zhu & Zhou, 2006).

Operative role management in information systems denotes management of real-world roles with integrated information system support. Operative work planning, command and control as well as field activities affect both information system role management and access control. This research concentrates on the practical work processes of the emergency management staff and not merely on information systems and their functionalities. This research illustrates how operative role management in information systems combines both technological and operative work approaches.

RESEARCH METHOD AND SETTINGS

Research Context and Objectives

Social science and information technology approaches provide a multidisciplinary approach to studying the operational and system role management issues in real-life emergency operations (Wybo & Latiers, 2006; Mehrotra & al., 2004). In their research, Wybo and Latiers (2006) have presented a theoretical approach to studying emergency situations. The approach is multidisciplinary. Emergency situations can be studied as complex and collective work situations. First, the socio-organizational dimension should be noted, covering organizational structures, distribution of roles and the social interactions. Second, the spatial dimension should be taken into account, as emergency actors often go to places they do not know beforehand. It affects the tactics, the way in which management personnel are deployed, and how distant communications, coordination and commands are dealt with. Third, the temporal dimension of how time constraints are dealt with needs to be noted. The research has been conducted as multiple case studies using ethnographic research method in Finnish emergency organizations. The overall study covers the following emergency domain organizations: an emergency response center, a rescue department and emergency medical services, a police department, a social and crisis emergency center, a rescue helicopter and a university hospital. Yin (2009) suggests that a case study like this is an empirical inquiry that investigates a contemporary phenomenon within its real life context using multiple sources of evidence. Case study research is characterized by a search for similarities in seemingly different cases (Yin, 2009). A case study enables the researcher to gain a holistic view of a certain phenomenon or series of events and can contribute to a more complete picture since many sources of evidence are used (Eisenhardt,

1989). In this study, findings are presented using a rescue department as an example organization, while the findings apply to all of the previously mentioned organizations. The objective of the research presented is to address how operative role management in information systems combines both technological and operative work approaches.

Data Collection

The data collection was conducted between 2009 and 2013. Data was collected by extended periods of field observations with field notes of observations on who used what information and to what purpose. The observations were performed in actual real-world field cases and exercises in different types of emergency scenarios varying from small daily incidents to larger emergencies. These observations were carried out by making field notes and using recording, videotaping, and photographing. Data gathering included reading reports and different manuals, such as preparedness and response plans, information system manuals, development discussions templates, process guides, legislative documents and log files. Emergency management domain training, education, conferences and seminars have been participated in. One valuable information source was coffee room discussions where people were more relaxed and the researcher could get a more extensive and in-depth view of operations analyzed out of the box. Over a hundred half-structured theme interviews have been done using the ethnography method, where previous interview results can change the structure of the next interview. By using this iterative approach, a strong expert participation and perspective to findings has been obtained during the data collection and validation phase, as opposed to following the original interview structure throughout the research process.

Since 2011, the data collection has been on monitoring status, and system and legislation reforms have been followed on as new information has been reported. There are extensive reforms

Figure 1. Examples of applied business process and use case models used for analysis in this research work

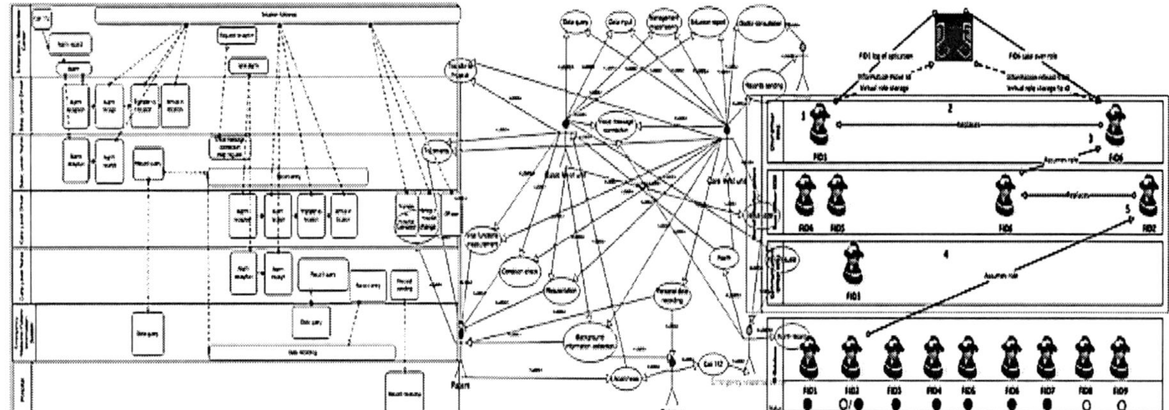

ongoing in Finland in the public safety domain, relating to both information systems and operative/administrative environments. These projects have given new information to this research, e.g. updates on what is planned to be implemented or is on implementation phase. This information has provided grounds to reflect research findings to actual implementations.

Data Analysis and Validation Process

Case study research is often characterized by an overlap between data collection and analysis stages. Overlapping data analysis with data collection gives the researcher a head start in analysis and allows him or her to take advantage of flexible data collection and making adjustments during the data collection process (Eisenhardt, 1989). Comparisons of interactions in emergency operations have been done a priori, in real time, and a posteriori. Within-case and cross-case analysis of data were selected as analysis techniques.

For data analysis, use cases and process descriptions were built concurrently, which were initially based on the observations and field notes. Examples of different process and use cases are presented in Figure 1. The process phase and

use case descriptions were defined according to emergency scenarios from which the data was acquired. As notation for descriptions, business process model notation (BPMN) with role pools to get process views of emergency scenario phases was used (White & Miers, 2008). BPMN is a commonly-used process notation for emergency services and governmental organizations in Finland (Wiikinkoski & Rantanen, 2010).

The use cases and business processes have been used to analyze

- What information triggers a function/process phase
- What actors are involved and what they do
- What roles are involved and what they do
- What information has been communicated between whom/what
- Why a certain function has been assigned to a certain identity
- What really happened as opposed to what was described, and
- Whether or not the function/situation triggers another function/s.

Interviews have been built upon the use case and business process findings to get a more in-depth view and details of the events. Other materials such as reports, manuals, and videotapes of events were used to refine the use cases and process descriptions. Based on the overall findings, model descriptions of role management in emergency organizations were constructed iteratively.

Data was categorized and put into comparable forms. The combination of within-case and cross-case analysis reduces the risks of inferential errors that emerge from using either method alone. For the ethnographic method, iterative interviewing reflecting findings from previous ones were found suitable for analysis. The analysis was built on comparing ideas and data using validation interviews. After the analysis the findings were validated using reflective interviews with the previously mentioned organizations' key informants who have experience of the processes and technologies in their respective organizations (Yin, 2009; Hammersley & Atkinson, 1996). Based on the formed categories, other data (e.g. reports, manuals) was used to support findings on actions taken and information needs. Those use cases are

validated by end users at different organizational levels. The validation process of this research work is described in Figure 2.

The research applies case study techniques using construct validity. In this research, multiple sources of evidence have been used. During the research chain of evidence was established and case study reports were reviewed (Yin, 2009) with case organizations' representatives. To increase the validity of research, three types of triangulation, proposed by Denzin (1989) were used and extended with methodological triangulation (Meadows & Morse, 2001) as follows: 1) data triangulation including time, space, and person: using several data sources, studying emergency situations in different conditions, a priori, in real time during emergencies, and a posteriori, 2) investigator triangulation: involving two investigators in the research process, comparing the results throughout the data analysis and 3) methodological triangulation combining analytic approaches and analyzing the same data with two

Figure 2. Validation process of this research

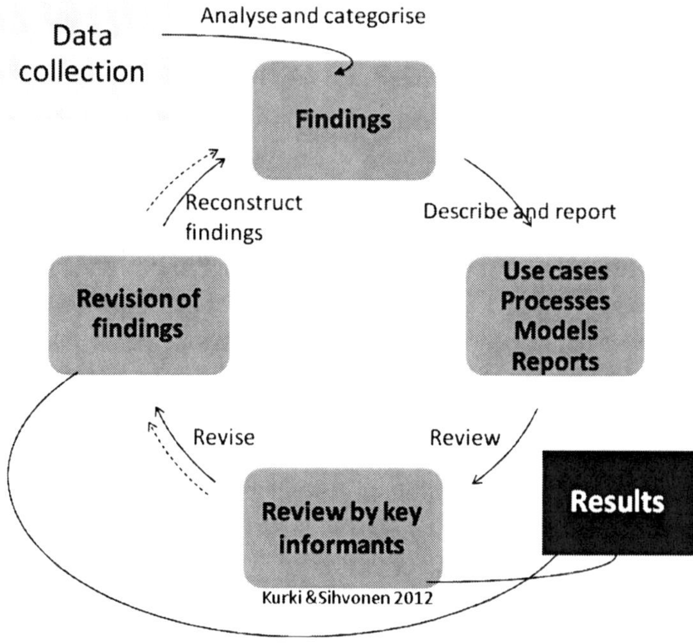

different methodological approaches. The use of appropriate multiple methods has resulted in more valid research findings.

OPERATIVE ROLE MANAGEMENT IN INFORMATION SYSTEMS

Relations of Information System and Operative Role Management

In technological terms, role management relates to managing access control/authorization and specifying the resources the users in an application or computer system are allowed to access (Aedo & al., 2006; Al-Kahtani & Sandhu, 2002; Ferraiolo & al., 2007). In operative role management, the identities in commanding officer and field officer roles are allowed to use the resources and applications that support their current role's operative functions for example in a forest/building fire, traffic accident, or chemical spill, among others.

Officers in emergency organizations perform operative work planning, command and control functions and mobilize emergency units to carry out operative functions in the field. A function can be a practical task relating to operative work or a system operation performed in an information system. Examples of function as a practical task could be in rescue services "extinguish fire", "smoke dive" or "rescue". Examples of function as a system operation could be "read", having access to read a specific document, "write", "delete", "update", having rights to modify a specific document, or "accept", having rights for example to approve persons' work leave.

In an emergency organization:

- An identity has a position,
- The position has many roles,
- A role has many functions,
- The same function can belong to different roles,

- The functions and identity are connected to one another by capabilities of an identity,
- The capability of an identity to perform a function can be valid or invalid.

Functions are performed by specific roles. The roles are occupied by identities who are in a position to assume the role of e.g., senior executive fire officer, executive fire officer, fire foreman, fireman, as well as capabilities, e.g. education, license, or skill, to perform function(s). Capabilities can be temporarily or permanently invalid. Temporary invalidity can be revoked, e.g. person can acquire/get back a certain capability, e.g. license, physical condition. Permanent invalidity can be for example a change in health condition, which disables performing some functions, e.g. smoke diving function is impossible due to asthma. Each person has an identity, which individualizes him/her. Each identity has a position in an organization. The position is comprised of several roles. A role defines what rights and responsibilities each identity has while performing functions of a specific role. In a technical system sense, RBAC in contrast regulates the access to resources and computer system objects based on the roles defined in an organization (Sanz et al., 2006; Ferraiolo et al., 2007)

The operative actions in the field as well as the command and control actions have an impact in two different ways: 1) how the operative actions affect the identity's access rights and 2) what roles an identity can be assigned to through command and control. Figure 3 illustrates how an identity has its operative role as "fireman", who uses various information and communications systems during emergency operations, and how the field actions taken affect the database values related to the identity. The database structure in Figure 3 is merely used to illustrate a few data structures and values.

When an identity has the same role, which affects both the information system level and operative functions, the operative functions that are

Figure 3. Operative role and related database information

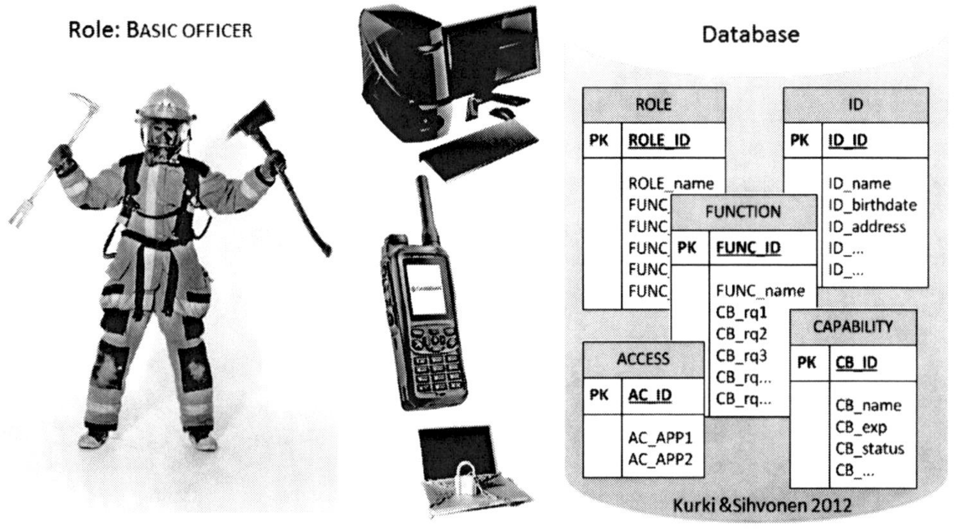

taken affect the information system values. These changes can thus affect access control aspects. The identity's role can change when command and control structures change in an emergency situation. The access control and operative functions of the role can be reduced or extended.

A function which an identity has carried out can affect his/her capabilities to function during a certain period. Some functions can conflict with each other and are not allowed to be done by the same identity, even though the role and capabilities would allow it. For example, if an officer planned his/her own vacation, he/she cannot approve it even if he/she normally had the right to perform this function. On the other hand, some field functions are not allowed to be performed at the same time, e.g. smoke diving and commanding.

Managing Operative Human Resources

The commanding officers use both administrative and operative resource management information to management of emergency situations. In command and control situation, the required information is often stored in the administrative systems as opposed to the operative systems. However, accessing both types of information is required to allocate resources effectively. The administrative systems are separate from the operative systems and integration/interfacing of the two types of systems would be both justified and necessary.

In a hierarchical emergency organization, command and control are clear and structured, and orders come from an identity in an upper hierarchy level to a lower hierarchy level identity or identities (Figure 4).

In this type of organization, the command and control hierarchy structure has similarities with the access control hierarchy structure (Figure 5). The command and control functions require that both the operative roles of the officers and the system roles in the information system need to be taken into account. For example, in a commanding situation the commanding officer should be able to view the current role of each resource, to which other roles it can be assigned, and with what capabilities it can perform the functions of these roles. Additionally, it is necessary to see the resource pool from which the needed resources can be alerted. The purpose of Figure 5 is to demonstrate the interdependencies of the opera-

Figure 4. Fire and rescue department organizational hierarchy

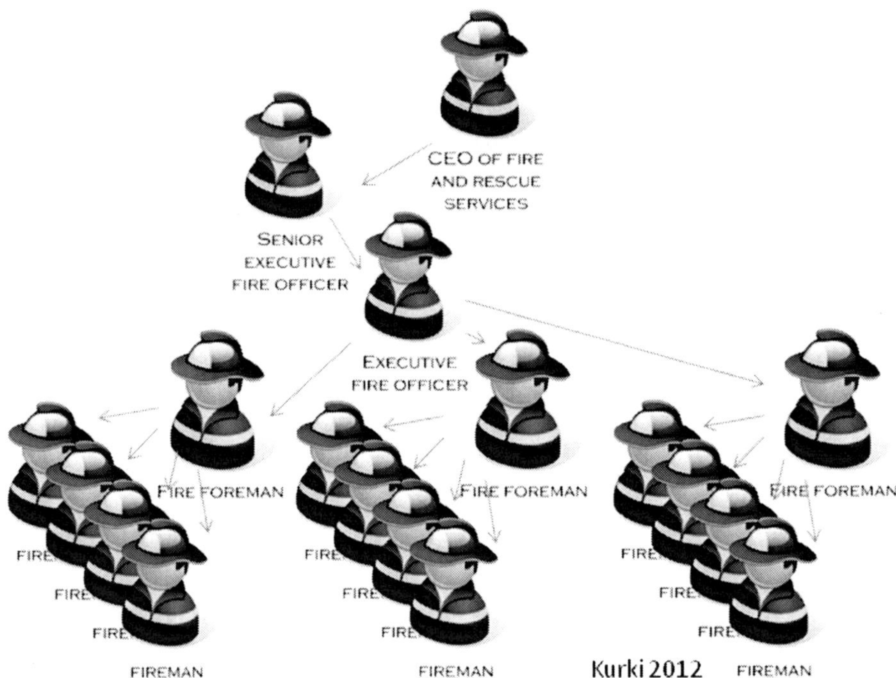

tive and system role. Naturally, there are more or less and different operative and system roles than presented in Figure 5, but those roles correspond to each other at every level of the role hierarchy.

Information System Views: Operative and Administrative Views

In information systems three different domains exist: administrative management domain, operative domain, and common domain. Administrative management domain and operative domain provide different views to the system user and common domain consists of information that the two previous synthesize according to user's role. In this study, system view refers to user interface. As an identity (user) logs into the information system, the system identifies all the roles this identity is allowed to assume, both the command and control and the administrative roles. The identity can choose the role which he/she needs and is allowed to from the role list provided by the information system. Changing the role in the information system, either because one is assigned to or one needs to, should not be bound to the login/logout procedure in the information system. This is time-consuming in emergency situations, in which the role changes often take place in an ad-hoc and time-critical manner. Changing the role should be a rapid and simple procedure, for example merely by choosing the role from the role list. In this context it is crucial to recognize the escalation of the emergency situations, which can initiate the process where role changes follow one another. In these situations, an identity can be assigned with a role by a commanding officer. The role assignment comes from higher up the role hierarchy, potentially via an information system and via data/voice messaging. This initiates the changes of the identity's operative role and its access control rights. These changes are updated in real time to the information system and the role list of the assigned identity will be automatically updated to include the new role(s).

Figure 5. Hierarchical organization model and hierarchical role model

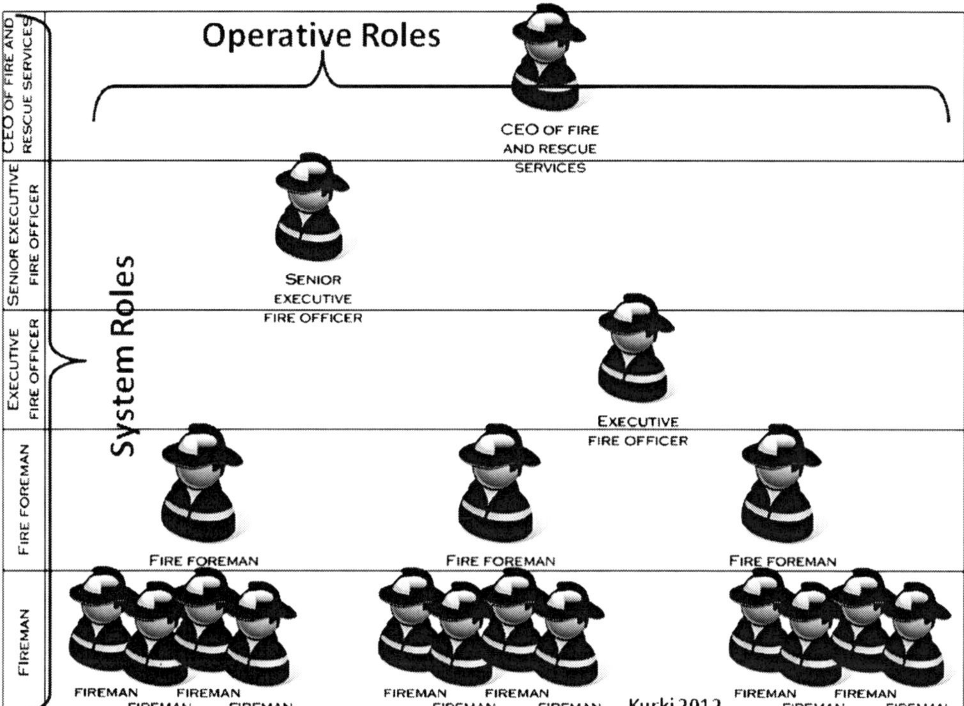

Thus, the required role can be easily taken into use from the role list.

The role change should also filter the information system view according to information and function needs of the specific role. This enables each role to have the necessary information and functions for performing their respective work. Filtering the view based on the active role can be used to constrain the user to access information which is not allowed in that role, e.g., it is not allowed to see the information which is preserved for the higher hierarchy roles. For example, if a fireman is assigned to fire foreman, he/she will need a more extensive view than being in the role of a fireman. The same applies if the fire foreman assumes a role in the higher hierarchy and will again need extended view and resource management rights. Depending on the role level, the need to view resource information varies, e.g. a fire foreman needs more detailed capability information about the resources but the deputy

chief fire officer needs task force views rather than details. The information system views of the roles (administrative management domain and operative domain) could be also filtered using capability information, e.g. whether an identity has the valid capability to perform a function or not. If the view needs to be partially constrained, it can be done using an identity's capability information by checking capability validities and only allowing functions for which the identity's capabilities are valid.

The officers should be able to perform both operative functions as well as administrative functions with operative systems. The two types of functions affect both the resources and their roles. When a user logs on to the information system and chooses a role, the user should also choose whether to work with an operative or administrative view.

In the operative domain view one can see and optionally manage several pieces of information that are maintained by the functionalities in the administrative management domain. The information related to the operative domain view can also be updated from the administrative management domain view by using information of common domain. The administrative functions cover for example preparedness planning, risk analysis, response planning, human resource management, shift planning, education and training planning, payroll and vacation information management, development discussion information management, identities' capability information management, reporting, work load management, and history data follow-up. The operative functions cover for example resource management, task follow-up, GIS updates, search functionalities, report and log follow-up, which are used for managing the emergency operations. Currently the systems for administration and operative work are separate. Both systems lack real-time information from one another and are updated as separate entities. The integration of the two types of system would support overall knowledge management in the organization.

Viewpoints to Operative Role Management in Information Systems

In initial state before the shift begins, the commanding officer has logged into the information system through access control. He/she gets view based on his/her role. At this point the resources are displayed to the commanding officer in offline state (Figure 6). He/she has knowledge at that point about capabilities and permissions (role permissions) of the resources. However, the resources have not yet been assigned in the system in available state. Resources become active in the information system upon their arrival to work and signing into the system. In the initial state, if a larger scale emergency occurs and the strength of the current shift is not adequate to response, additional resources can be alerted from the pool and moved to available state more easily. Commanding officers can pick and alert needed resources from resource pool, because system offers only those resources that are alertable and capable.

In the beginning of the shift each resource has been assigned/delegated a role by the com-

Figure 6. Initial information system view for commanding officer role

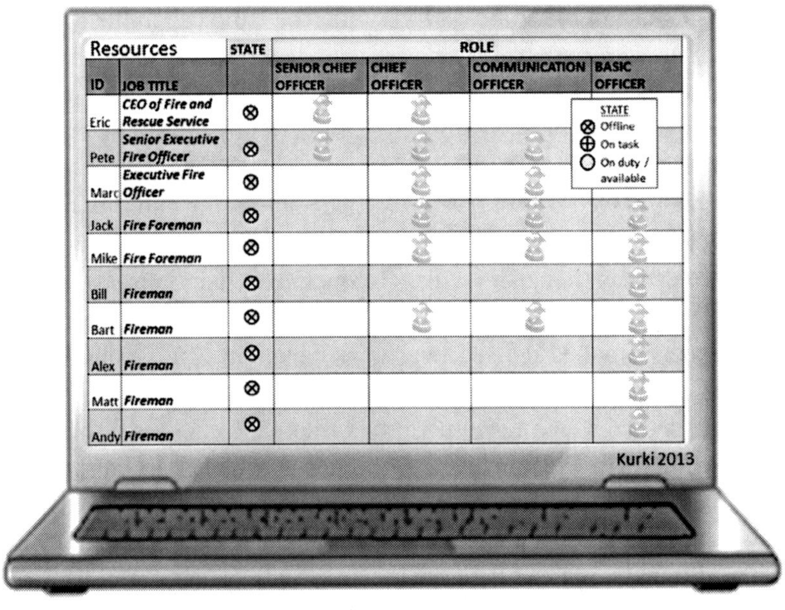

manding officer. State information is visible for the commanding officer, whether the resource is attached to a task (On task) or available for a task (On duty/available) during shift execution (Figure 7). When incidents take place these resources are alerted and assigned for various tasks, and this changes their state in information system.

During a shift situation in the field varies, depending on the number of tasks and scales of the incidents. Thus, also resourcing needs change; number of resources may reduce or increase, and the resources can be re-assigned with other roles or roles can be revoked by the commanding office. The role management performed by the commanding officer also changes the resource state information system view, comparing Figure 7 and 8.

Table 1 presents a summary of the viewpoints on operative role management in information systems. Different viewpoints to operative command and control work and its integration to access control and role management are introduced. Figures 6-8 have illustrated operative role management in information system using rescue services as

Figure 7. Role assignments / delegations by the commanding officer

Shift execution		STATE	ROLE			
ID	JOB TITLE		SENIOR CHIEF OFFICER	CHIEF OFFICER	COMMUNICATION OFFICER	BASIC OFFICER
Eric	CEO of Fire and Rescue Service	⊕				
Pete	Senior Executive Fire Officer	⊕				
Marc	Executive Fire Officer	⊕				
Jack	Fire Foreman	⊕				
Mike	Fire Foreman	O				
Bill	Fireman	O				
Bart	Fireman	⊕				
Alex	Fireman	O				
Matt	Fireman	O				
Andy	Fireman	O				

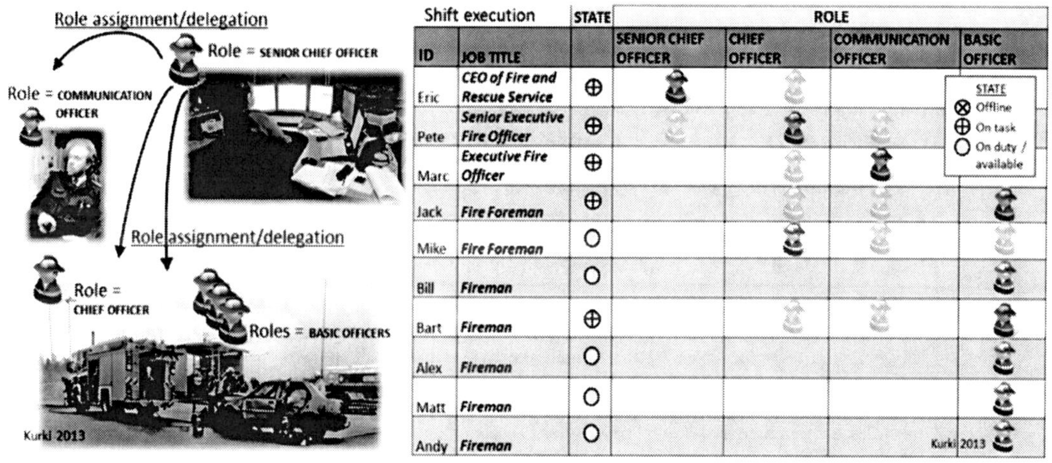

Figure 8. Role state changes of resource during a shift

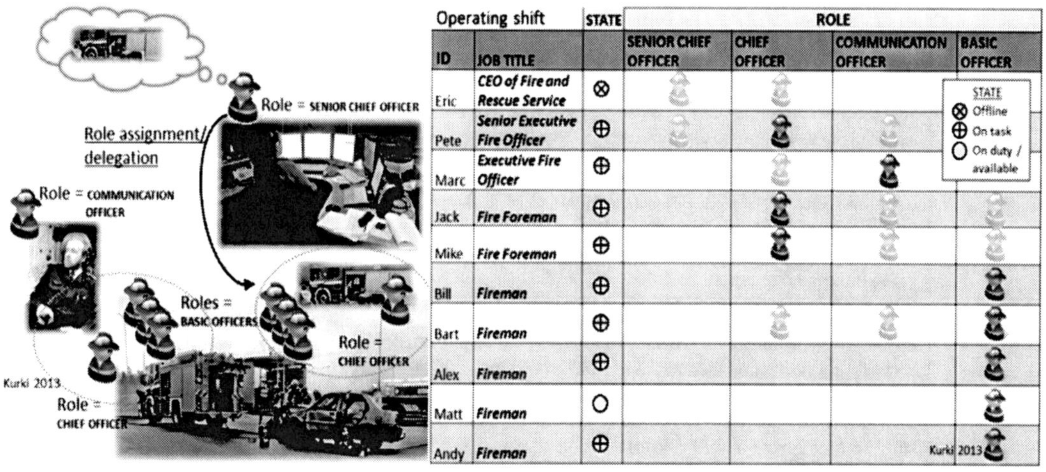

Operating shift		STATE	ROLE			
ID	JOB TITLE		SENIOR CHIEF OFFICER	CHIEF OFFICER	COMMUNICATION OFFICER	BASIC OFFICER
Eric	CEO of Fire and Rescue Service	⊗				
Pete	Senior Executive Fire Officer	⊕				
Marc	Executive Fire Officer	⊕				
Jack	Fire Foreman	⊕				
Mike	Fire Foreman	⊕				
Bill	Fireman	⊕				
Bart	Fireman	⊕				
Alex	Fireman	⊕				
Matt	Fireman	O				
Andy	Fireman	⊕				

an example. Table 1 gives more specific descriptions of the previous, bearing in mind the rescue services context.

CONCLUSION

As pointed out in this research, the operative actions in the field as well as the command and control actions can have an impact in two different ways: 1) how the operative actions affect the identity's access rights, and 2) to what roles an identity can be assigned through command and control by commanding officer. Therefore, both approaches should be taken into account in information system design. In an operative command and control situation, the needed information to manage the resources and their roles is often stored in the administrative systems as opposed to the operative systems. However, accessing both types of information is required in order to manage resources effectively. The administrative systems are separate from the operative systems and integration/interfacing of the two types of systems would be justified and necessary. The command and control hierarchy structure in emer-

Table 1. Summary of the viewpoints on operative role management in information systems

Viewpoint	Operative Role Management in Information Systems
Purpose of roles	Operative roles consist of operative functions. A role affects individual resource in both operative work and information system. Role gives to commanding officer information about resources and their capabilities. A commanding officer grants a role to a resource (identity), which gives in operative sense an individual the right to carry out the role's functions in his/her work. Role also gives specific information to role holder on information system level role rights. In an information system a role is used to define a set or group of privileges. These privileges are transferred from one user to another user with the role. The role concept in information systems is used to manage access control/authorization and to specify the resources the users in an application or computer system are allowed to access. A role determines the allowed information system functions.
Role permissions	Role permissions are related to the identity's job description and to what functions (operations) the identity is capable of performing at a specific moment. The types of functions (operations) an identity can perform can be e.g. shift planning, alert, locate, extinguish fire, smoke dive, and report. The types of operations (functions) that can be controlled depend on the system to which access control is applied to. The operations (functions) can be e.g. read, write, execute, insert, delete, append, update. Various types of operations in the information systems relate to these functions, as presented in technical description. To obtain permissions to any role in the specific organization, an identity must have a valid capability, e.g. in order to get any roles, you have to be on shift.
Role revocation	Commanding officer revokes the identity's right to perform in a certain role and the identity is not allowed to perform the operative functions of the role. Information system administrator revokes the role from a user, which only affects information system use, not on operative work. Performing of certain role can be removed from a person by administrator or commanding officer.
Role assignment/ delegation	Commanding officers in a hierarchical structure order resources to take over a specific role. Hence, identities in commanding officer roles have a right to delegate roles to other identities. A person can be delegated to take over a role, which another person is attending to. The user delegates his/her assigned role to the other user in order for him/ her to perform the functions permitted by the role. For example during a holiday of leave of absence an identity can request role delegation to another identity from information system administrator to take over role's permissions.
Access control	The functions that an identity in a role performs can lead to a situation whereby an identity is not allowed to perform some functions of the role. These functions can be both operative and system level functions. E.g. some operative function can temporarily remove an identity's rights to perform it for a certain period. Role grants permissions to do both operative and system functions. Role grants rights and permission to access applications, files, objects, and data in the information system.
Role management	Commanding officer manages resources, to which he/she can assign/delegate/revoke roles during the emergency operations via commanding orders. In Finnish context an officer in duty has to give and take over roles personally, because an information system alone cannot do such "commanding duty", it can only assist and propose. In technological terms, role management relates to managing access control/authorization and specifying the resources the users in an application or computer system are allowed to access. This information system approach alone is not sufficient for command and control.

gency organizations has similarities to the access control hierarchy structure. The command and control functions require that both the operative roles of the officers and the system roles in the information system need to be taken into account.

Changing the role in the information system, either because one is assigned to or one needs to, should not be bound to the login/logout procedure of the information system. Changing the role should be a rapid and simple procedure in information system for both commanding officer assigning and delegating roles and officer taking over a role. In this context it is crucial to recognize the escalation of the emergency situations, which can initiate the process where role changes follow one another. In these situations, an identity can be assigned with a role from above in the role hierarchy, which he/she may not usually work with. Role assignment comes from higher up in the role hierarchy, potentially via an information system and via data/voice messaging. This initiates the changes in the identity's operative role and its access control rights. The officers should be able to perform both command and control functions as well as administrative functions with the command and control system. The two types of functions affect both the resources and their roles. Although the interdependencies between the system and operative role management can be addressed, the potential of integrating the two approaches is ongoing work in information systems development projects.

FUTURE RESEARCH DIRECTIONS

Some findings from the research work accomplished are exploited also while elaborating the ProntoX report (Kortelainen & Ketola, 2012), which describes the development needs for the rescue services future centralized data storage for personnel registers and the common system service layer. The future storage system also enables a structured way to store and utilize information related to role management, e.g. information on personnel resources, equipment and capabilities (Sipilä, 2013). Other system development projects ongoing in Finland, e.g. emergency response centre system (Ministry of the Interior, 2013) and field command information system (Pelastuslaitosten kumppanuusverkosto, 2013; Saarinen, 2013), which also deal with the topics of role management, can utilize the results from the research work. There are other types of organizations too, which are dynamic hierarchical and need operative resource management support. Thus, in future research implementing this approach to other contexts could be researched.

ACKNOWLEDGMENT

We would like to acknowledge our authority partners from the North Savo Emergency Response Center, North Savo Rescue Department, North Savo Police Department, Ilmari Rescue Helicopter, Kuopio University Hospital, Vantaa Social and Crisis Emergency Services, and Emergency Services College for enabling and supporting in the research. Many of the ideas presented in this paper have evolved from the discussions and field work with them. The work presented in this publication builds upon the research work reported at the Hawaii International Conference on System Sciences 2012 in the paper "Kurki, T.A. & Sihvonen, H.-M., 2012. A Role-Based Resource Management Approach for Emergency Organizations".

REFERENCES

Aedo, I., Diaz, P., & Sanz, D. (2006). An RBAC model-based approach to specify the access policies of web-based emergency information systems. *International Journal of Intelligent Control and Systems, 11*(4), 272–283.

Al-Kahtani, M. A., & Sandhu, R. S. (2002). A model for attribute-based user role assignment. In *Proceedings of 18th Annual Computer Security Applications Conference* (ACSAC 2002). Las Vegas, NV: IEEE Computer Society.

Eisenhardt, K. (1989). Building theories from case study research. *Academy of Management Review, 14*, 532–550.

Ferraiolo, D. F., Kuhn, D. R., & Chandramouli, R. (2007). *Role-based access control*. Norwood, MA: Artech House, Inc.

Haibin, Z., & MengChu, Z. (2006). Role-based collaboration and its kernel mechanisms. *IEEE Transactions on Systems, Man and Cybernetics. Part C, Applications and Reviews, 36*(4), 578–589. doi:10.1109/TSMCC.2006.875726

Hammersley, M., & Atkinson, P. (1996). *Ethnography: Principles in practice*. London: Routledge.

Ianella, R., & Henricksen, K. (2007). Managing information in the disaster coordination centre: Lessons and opportunities. In *Proceedings of International Community on Information Systems for Crisis Response and Management* (ISCRAM 2007). Delft, The Netherlands: International Community on Information Systems for Crisis Response and Management.

Kim, Y. G., Mon, C. J., Jeong, D., Lee, J. O., Song, C. Y., & Baik, D. K. (2005). Context-aware access control mechanism for ubiquitous applications. In P. S. Szczepaniak, J. Kacprzyk, & A. Niewiadomski (Eds.), *Advances in web intelligence (LNCS)* (Vol. 3528, pp. 932–935). Berlin: Springer. doi:10.1007/11495772_37

Kortelainen, P., & Ketola, J. (2012). *Pelastustoimen rekisteri- ja tilastointijärjestelmien tarpeet ja toteutus malli: ProntoX - hankkeen loppuraportti*. Kuopio: Pelastusopisto.

Kurki, T., & Sihvonen, H.-M. (2012). A role-based resource management approach for emergency organizations. In *Proceedings of Hawaii International Conference on System Sciences*. Maui, HI: IEEE Computer Society.

Meadows, M. L., & Morse, J. M. (2001). *Constructing evidence within the qualitative project*. Thousand Oaks, CA: Sage.

Mehrotra, S., Butss, C. T., Klashnikov, D., & Venkatasubramanian, V. (2004). Project RESCUE: Challenges in responding to the unexpected. In *Proceedings of IS&T/SPIE International Conference on Internet Imaging*. DSM Publications.

Ministry of the Interior. (2013). *Hätäkeskusuudistuksen toteutuminen*. Retrieved October 27, 2013, from http://www.intermin.fi/download/44557_102013.pdf

Pelastuslaitosten kumppanuusverkosto. (2013, May 15). *KEJO-tietojärjestelmähankinta käynnistyy*. Retrieved October 27, 2013, from http://www.pelastuslaitokset.fi/index.php?p=Ajankohtaista&id=50

Saarinen, M. (2013). *Viranomaisten yhteinen kenttäjärjestelmähanke KEJO -hanke*. Retrieved October 27, 2013, from http://www.kunnat.net/fi/tietopankit/tapahtumat/aineisto/atk-paivat/2013-05-29/Documents/2013-05-29-09-02-saarinen.pdf

Sanz, D., Adeo, I., Diaz, M., & de Castro, J. (2006). Modelling emergency response communities using RBAC principles. In *Proceedings of International Community on Information Systems for Crisis Response and Management* (ISCRAM 2006). Newark, NJ: International Community on Information Systems for Crisis Response and Management.

Sanz, D., Gómez Bello, P., Díaz, P., Sainz, F. J., & Aedo, I. (2007). Supporting physical and logical communication in emergency management virtual distributed teams. In *Proceedings of Intelligent Human Computer Systems for Crisis Response and Management* (ISCRAM 2007) (pp. 439-448). Delft, The Netherlands: International Community on Information Systems for Crisis Response and Management.

Sihvonen, H.-M., & Kurki, T. (2010). Role management diversity in emergency situations. In *Proceedings of IEEE International Conference on Technologies for Homeland Security (HST'10)*. Boston, MA: IEEE Computer Society.

Sipilä, M. (2013). *VARANTO pelastustoimen tietovaranto ja järjestelmät 2013-2014*. Retrieved October 27, 2013, from http://www.cmcfinland. fi/pelastus/home.nsf/pages/F1C7C0CAFF39F4 9CC2257B17002C0B48/$file/VARANTO%20 15052013%20Tutkimushautomo.pdf

Smirnov, A. V., Pashkin, M., Levashova, T., Shilov, N., & Kashevnik, A. (2007). Role-based decision mining for multiagent emergency response management. In V. Gorodetsky, C. Zhang, V. Skormin, & L. Cao (Eds.), *Autonomous intelligent systems: Multi-agents and data mining (LNCS)* (Vol. 4476, pp. 178–191). Berlin: Springer. doi:10.1007/978-3-540-72839-9_15

Tahir, M. N. (2007). C-RBAC: Contextual role-based access control model. *Ubiquitous Computing and Communication Journal, 2*(3).

White, S. A., & Miers, D. (2008). *BPMN modeling and reference guide*. Future Strategies Inc.

Wiikinkoski, T., & Rantanen, H. (2010). *Erityistilanne prosessina - Formaalin kuvausmenetelmän käyttökelpoisuus moniviranomaistilanteen yhteistoiminnan kehittämisessä*. Pelastusopisto.

Wybo, J.-L., & Latiers, M. (2006). Exploring complex emergency situations' dynamic: Theoretical, epistemological and methodological proposals. *International Journal of Emergency Management, 3*(1), 40–51.

Wybo, J.-L., & Lonka, H. (2002). *Emergency management and information society how to improve the synergy? Workshop Emergency Telecommunications*. ETSI.

Yin, R. (2009). *Case study research design and methods* (4th ed.). Thousand Oaks, CA: SAGE Publications.

Zhang, G., & Parashar, M. (2004). *Context-aware dynamic access control for pervasive applications*. Paper presented at the Communication Networks and Distributed Systems Modeling and Simulation Conference. San Diego, CA.

Zhu, H., & Zhou, M. C. (2006). The role transferability in emergency management systems. In *Proceedings of International Conference on Information Systems for Crisis Response and Management* (ISCRAM 2006). Newark, NJ: International Community on Information Systems for Crisis Response and Management.

KEY TERMS AND DEFINITIONS

Access Control: Refers to any means of controlling access to any resource. Access control refers to security features that control who can access resources in the operating system. Applications call access control functions to set who can access specific resources or control access to resources provided by the application.

Command and Control: Refers to the exercise of authority and direction by a properly designated commander over assigned and attached forces in the accomplishment of the mission. Command and control functions are performed through an arrangement of personnel, equipment, communications, facilities, and procedures employed by a commander in planning, directing, coordinating, and controlling forces and operations in the accomplishment of the mission. Also called C2.

Emergency Organization: Refers to an organization that operates in the field of emergency management in planning, response and coordination of activities in emergencies and crisis.

Information System: Refers to a combination of hardware, software, infrastructure and trained personnel organized to facilitate planning, control, coordination, and decision making in an organization.

Operative Role Management: Refers to assigning, delegating and changing the roles of identities performing operative work in emergency organizations.

Role: Used to define a set or group of privileges. It also refers to persons role in operative work.

Role Management: Refers to an organization's capability to manage the roles in which each employee performs as part of his or her job functions. Role management relates to managing access control/authorization and specifying the resources the users are allowed to access in an application or computer system.

This work was previously published in IT in the Public Sphere edited by Zaigham Mahmood, pages 1-17 copyright year 2014 by Information Science Reference (an imprint of IGI Global).

Chapter 70
Mobile Health Systems for Bipolar Disorder:
The Relevance of Non–Functional Requirements in MONARCA Project

Oscar Mayora
CREATE-NET, Italy

Mads Frost
ITU Copenhagen, Denmark

Bert Arnrich
ETH Zurich, Switzerland

Franz Gravenhorst
ETH Zurich, Switzerland

Agnes Grunerbl
TU Kaiserslautern, Germany

Amir Muaremi
ETH Zurich, Switzerland

Venet Osmani
CREATE-NET, Italy

Alessandro Puiatti
SUPSI, Switzerland

Nina Reichwaldt
PLRI-BITZ, Germany

Corinna Scharnweber
PLRI-BITZ, Germany

Gerhard Troster
ETH Zurich, Switzerland

ABSTRACT

This paper presents a series of challenges for developing mobile health solutions for mental health as a result of MONARCA project three-year activities. The lessons learnt on the design, development and evaluation of a mobile health system for supporting the treatment of bipolar disorder. The findings presented here are the result of over 3 years of activity within the MONARCA EU project. The challenges listed and detailed in this paper may be used in future research as a starting point for identifying important non-functional requirements involved in mobile health provisioning that are fundamental for the successful implementation of mobile health services in real life contexts.

DOI: 10.4018/978-1-4666-8756-1.ch070

INTRODUCTION

When designing mobile health systems the focal point of research is frequently concentrated on the design of innovative developments for improving the practice of healthcare and increase of wellbeing with a strong focus on functional requirements. On this regard, the aspects related to definition of non-functional requirements of mobile health provisioning are often underestimated or left as a secondary item to take into consideration by researchers. However only through a thorough consideration of potential implications on design of non-functional requirements, the mobile health innovations can find an opportunity to transform into sustainable solutions that can be applied in real life contexts. These kinds of requirements comprise all the practical aspects of healthcare provisioning that are necessary to implement mobile health services ranging from human factors to important medical and technological issues.

In this paper we introduce the experiences learnt in MONARCA project for developing a mobile monitoring system for better handling the treatment of bipolar disorder and the challenges found related to its implementation in a real life context. The main contribution of this paper focus not only on the innovative mobile health solution proposed by MONARCA but also on the technological and clinical aspects that were necessary for conducting multidisciplinary research in the context of such project and on other non-functional requirements that are key in the development of technological solutions for the design, development and evaluation of mobile health systems. Such requirements include aspects related to technology, human factors, medical practice, regulatory aspects and other practical issues that are identified in this paper as key challenges in the development of future mobile personal health systems and services (See Figure 1).

MOBILE TECHNOLOGY AND BIPOLAR DISORDER TREATMENT

Current medical practice of bipolar disorder treatment is based on identification and analysis of

Figure 1. Relevant aspects in multidisciplinary IT-based clinical research

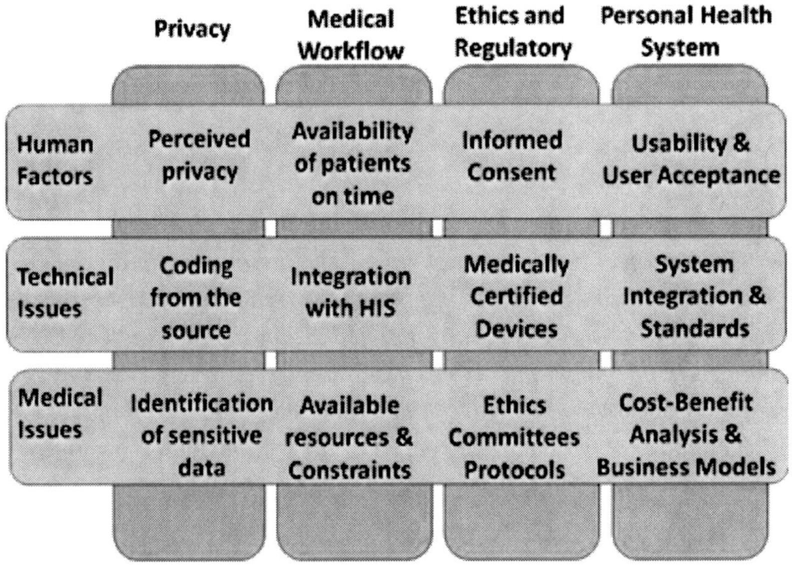

	Privacy	Medical Workflow	Ethics and Regulatory	Personal Health System
Human Factors	Perceived privacy	Availability of patients on time	Informed Consent	Usability & User Acceptance
Technical Issues	Coding from the source	Integration with HIS	Medically Certified Devices	System Integration & Standards
Medical Issues	Identification of sensitive data	Available resources & Constraints	Ethics Committees Protocols	Cost-Benefit Analysis & Business Models

mood instability episodes at different intervals of time without possibility of continuous monitoring in a practical way. On this regard, with the use of currently available technology and innovative processes proposed by recent research approaches (Mayora, 2011) it is envisioned in the short term a new generation of services to improve healthcare provisioning in the treatment of mental health diseases (Arnrich et al., 2010; Arnrich et al., 2013). In particular due to the wide acceptability of mobile devices and the growing interest in the development of healthcare-related apps, there is a clear trend on the use of mobile phones as a key enabler of new wellbeing/healthcare services. In fact, some of these new developments are already going in the direction of using mobile phone-based sensing for monitoring conditions related to specific mental diseases such as bipolar disorder (Puiatti et al., 2011). In such kind of applications, the mobile-phone-based sensing architecture integrates the set of novel services and supports key functionalities on sensing and data analysis, patients interfaces (client side) and hospital and health information systems (server side) as in MONARCA system in Figure 2 (Mayora, 2011).

Regarding the specific treatment of bipolar disorder, during the past years, as well as in other healthcare domains, there has been a major organizational switch in paradigm from inpatient treatment to outpatient treatment. On this regard, there is currently a scientific switch going on in the paradigm of treatment in bipolar disorder from focus on the mood episodes to focus on the inter-episodic mood instability (Bonsall, 2012) (See Figure 3).

The role of mobile phones in continuous monitoring of personal health condition for bipolar disorder patients implies a novel way to include objective data regarding patients activity and behavioral conduct while allowing also for more subjective input based on self-assessment (as in traditional bipolar disorder therapy). In this way, the information received by clinicians is complemented for a better decision support while defining the patients' therapy. In fact the ability of subjective measures such as self-assessment to detect prodromal symptoms of depression and mania may be not be sufficient compared to objective measures such as speech, social and physical activity that is indeed achievable with the use of

Figure 2. MONARCA system basic components

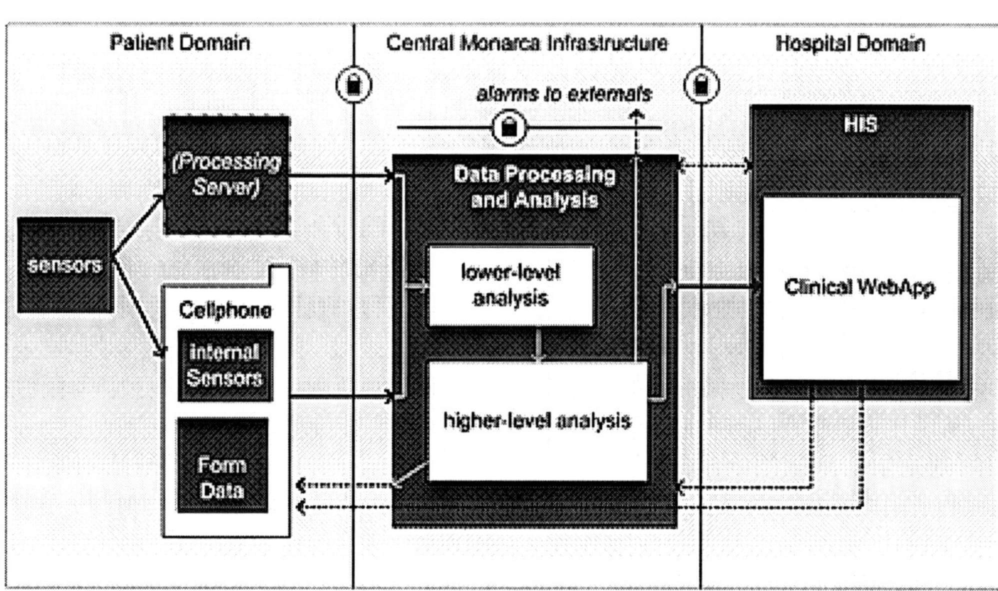

Figure 3. Inter-episodic mood instability from Bonsall et al. (2012)

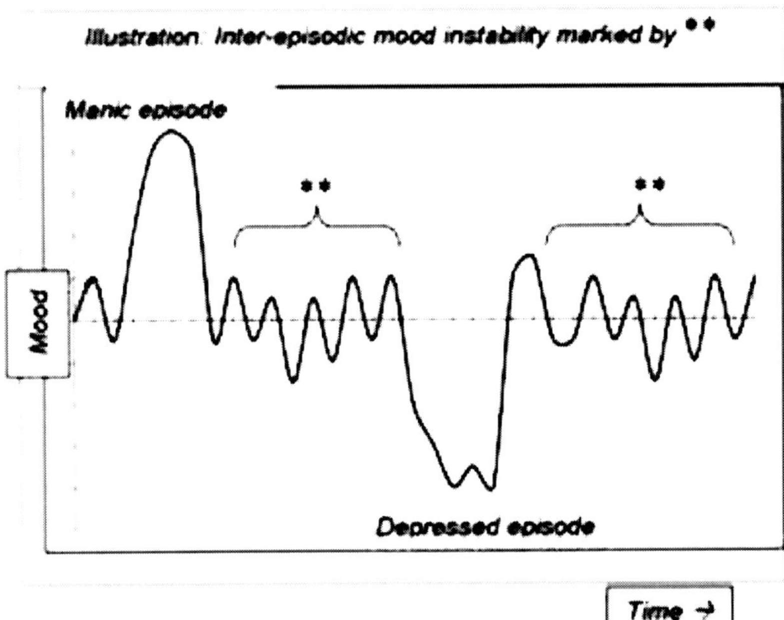

mobile eHealth technology (Sobin et al., 1997; Benazzi, 2009; Weinstock et al., 2008; Kuhs et al., 1992). However, all these behavior-related features that are actually obtainable as objective measurements with current technology, pose a series of challenges and open research questions on translating them into meaningful information for physicians and patients.

It is important to consider that the utilization of technical monitoring systems in the field of mental health inevitably causes several challenges on the patients' sphere. On this regard, mobile sensing systems have to be suitable for the daily use and need to incorporate adaptive user-friendly strategies regardless of whether the patient is depressive or manic. The design needs to consider that the use of the system should impact on the patients' mental state because any technical issue that may be cause of additional stress. In addition, future personal health systems should enable agreement (concordance) between patient, relatives and clinicians, which is highly important for treatment outcome. It is very often

a crucial problem that patients, relatives and clinicians comprehend the patient condition in different ways and consequently they will each aim for different (treatment) methods and goals.

The following sections provide a series of requirements that have to be taken into consideration when designing mobile health applications in the field of mental health. The proposed requirements are the result of the experiences and reflections on MONARCA three-year project and constitute a series of recommendations to take into consideration in future mental health developments.

HUMAN FACTORS IN MEDICAL HEALTH RESEARCH

Conducting research in healthcare domain that involves humans either if they are clinicians, patients or caregivers is notably different from other domains and presents special challenges to researchers. There is a very high focus on ethics and patient safety, and there are challenges in maintaining confidentiality high while operating in very private spheres. In these contexts, if not treated carefully, there is a high risk that the researcher may be considered an intruder. In addition, there are difficulties in establishing a common language between medical practitioners and technologists, and a high risk of the potential impact in patient treatment that the developed systems may produce. Through our work with patients and clinicians in the MONARCA project, many interesting questions arose, many thoughtful moments occurred, many considerations were done, and many lessons were learnt, and thus, we have tried to summarize some of the key human factors we have encountered during our work:

Exposure To Patients

Emotions among patients with mood disorders are intense and can be twisted. Experiencing patients crying, shouting, wanting to die, strapped to their beds, etc., can be a disturbing experiences for non-clinical researchers. It is hard to prepare for this, but at least you should be aware of it.

Functional vs. Non-Functional

Often HCI researchers are very focused on the functionality of the systems, but there are a lot of non-functional aspects that have to be in place for the technology to work. For instance, we encountered examples of ensuring patients having a data plan for their 3G connection, enabling them to transmit their data from the phone to the hospitals server. The need for teaching the clinicians how to operate the system, to be able to access the data, and prepare user guides as well as a hotline for technical assistance for when they encounter issues they cannot solve. For a project to be successful, it is important to pay attention to non-functional aspects, as they can become showstoppers if not taken into consideration. This is a highly difficult and exhausting task, especially with elaborate and multi-user systems, but it must not be neglected.

Trust and Transparency

Trust or the lack there of, is a foundational part of any relationship. In particular it is critical to relationships in the realm of healthcare. The patient trusts that their team of healthcare professionals is going to manage their wellness appropriately. When introducing a new technology, like the MONARCA system, it is important to build a trustworthy relationship with the patients, ensuring their commitment and willingness to provide intimate health care data, which is maintained by a transparency in both systems and actions. If it fails, the patients will stop to use the system and the value of the system supporting the treatment is lost.

Usability and Acceptance Issues in Real-Life Conditions

Conducting a real-life study including people suffering from a mental illness who are not necessarily trained in using technology can arise issues of human nature.

1. **MONARCA Mobile Phone-Based Approach:** Using familiar devices in these kind of studies such as mobile phones, and base the monitor platform on them could eliminate the main obstacles posed for example in requiring the use of external sensors (i.e. wearable devices) which people may not be so familiar with and that may stigmatize users. On this regard, MONARCA approach was that of proposing a mobile phone sensing approach under the hypothesis that people have a large acceptance of such devices and normally are not afraid to get in touch with them. Nevertheless a certain attraction of test-subjects and patients to modern technology turned out to be a necessary precondition for a successful deployment of this study. In fact, in some cases we came across this issue especially with the first patients, who

even though were very eager to participate in the study, eventually were overwhelmed by the various unfamiliar functionalities the smart-phone provided and therefore dropped out.

2. **Users Perception of System Usefulness:** To our surprise, most patients were not much concerned about privacy as long as it was guaranteed to them a sensitive and anonymized treatment of their data. Bipolar patients, when they start to realize and accept their disorder, are aware that they need help, because they do not want to experience extreme episodes. Therefore, a lot of them were willing to try new ways, especially if those ways might help them to reduce the amount of anti-depressant or mood stabilizing medicine, as these medications normally cause unwanted side effects. Therefore, when they were asked to participate in a study, which might help them in the future to deal with their disease, a sufficient number of patients were willing to participate. So with the help of the psychiatrists who established the contact to the patients, the recruitment of patients was easier than expected.

TECHNOLOGICAL CHALLENGES IN MENTAL HEALTH RESEARCH

When deploying a real-life study in health care and especially in a psychiatric environment a number of challenges have to be faced (Gruenerbl, 2012). Very often these challenges are a mix of regulatory and human requirements that have a strong implication in the technical solution to be implemented. In particular, these requirements pose a series of restrictions that have to be addressed from a technical viewpoint including privacy constraints, security aspects, battery limitations and in general a series of non-functional needs that if not addressed properly during the solution design, can jeopardize the successful adoption of the proposed system.. On this regard, a series of technical challenges faced during the development of MONARCA project were identified as follows:

Need to Technically-Obscuring Sensitive Data

Being a project relying on identifying high-level behavioral information from patients' activity, MONARCA used a number of different sensors acquiring sensitive data. On this regard, a very important requirement was that all the sensor readings had to be anonymized before analyzing them to guarantee the privacy of the participants. This meant that different precautions should have been taken right after the data acquisition to avoid reconstructing signals that could be related to specific patients as follows:

1. Location parameters such as GPS coordinates, extracted from the mobile phone had to transferred into a neutral coordination system before processing them. In addition Wi-Fi and Bluetooth signals were used for establishing presence in certain areas and proximity to other users without necessarily establishing a clear correspondence to whom and where in particular.

2. In order to perform frequency-analysis on voice during phone calls, the respective algorithms for speech acquisition had to be developed in a way that scrambled the actual signal to avoid its original reconstruction while keeping the required properties for analyzing the voice. The scrambling mechanisms work in a way that the voice was sliced into small chunks and these slices were randomly permuted within each second, resulting in a negligible speech intelligibility. In this way, the speech of the person become not understandable, while at the same time the performance of the acoustic analysis of the speech was not degraded.

3. In addition to codifying the speech signal, the recorded scrambled conversations were anonymized before stored on the smart phone.
4. Data security was achieved by encrypting all the acquired data directly inside the smartphone memory with the Advanced Encryption Standard (AES) and the communication between the smartphone and the server was done via HTTPS, resulting in an additional security layer in the data transfer process.

Flexible Strategies for Data Transmission

Personal health systems collecting patients' information for further processing need to establish a clear strategy for secure data transmission from the monitoring device to the server. The original set-up in MONARCA project for data transmission was designed to automatically transmit the data. All data would have been transmitted to a secure server belonging to the psychiatric hospital facilities via a secure connection at least once a day. Even though the infrastructure was already set up in this way (and worked properly in Copenhagen trial), in one of the trials in Austria it had to be changed before the study started as it turned out that most of the possible participants neither owned an appropriate wireless Internet connection at home, nor full 3G Network and DSL coverage was guaranteed. To overcome this issue, the set-up was changed to internal storage of all sensor readings using SD Card, which were transferred every 2-3 weeks into the server during the appointment of the patients at the psychiatric hospital facilities. d Even using the external SD Card, it was a challenge to store data in different ASCII format files for more than a couple of weeks. Therefore, we serialized all the data being collected using the Google Protocol Buffers. This resulted in a 70% reduction in size of data stored in the SD Card.

Software Stability and OS Versions

Another technical issue consisted in finding an appropriate Android operating system in which implement MONARCA solution. In general, one of the big advantages of the Android system is, that it is not limited to one specific smart phone brand but is available for various different cell phone types from different smart phone producers. Yet this advantage turnout to be a big limitation we had to deal with because the Android OS is partially adapted for different producers. The main issue here was, to find an Android based smart phone with an OS, which allowed accessing the sensors even though having the display turned off. Not all OS variances permitted this by the time the study was conducted. In later updated versions of the operating system this feature came per default and thereby eliminated this issue later. However a relevant aspect to consider in further developments is the extend in which different versions of operating systems may work in different devices and therefore a good strategy has to be defined to overcome this kind of issues.

Devices Performance Limitations

When involving different types of monitoring devices, it is not granted that all devices will have the expected performance in real life as in ideal conditions. In particular in MONARCA, the first tests of the running smart-phone application revealed that the smart-phone tended to get rather hot for some specific set-ups. This was especially true when no Wi-Fi signal was available, because this set-up triggered the Wi-Fi port to increase the scan-frequency by default of the OS. Next to increasing the smart-phone's temperature it decreased the battery-life tremendously. This brings us to another technical issue that is the battery life itself. As in numerous other technical applications, the main critical part in using a smart phone for data recording is the phone's battery life. Constant operating of all sensors in a high-resolution mode reduces the battery life to few hours making some applications unusable in real-life conditions. To overcome these issues of battery usage, the design of the system was optimized as follows:

1. The acceleration sensor was used to trigger most other sensors. This was feasible as for example on unmoved cell-phones (that will not change their position), therefore GPS/Wi-Fi sensing was reduced to a minimum while the cell-phone was identified as not moving.
2. Furthermore, as long as a person stays inside of a building GPS is only of little use, while Wi-Fi if available would provide the needed position information. Therefore, the usage of GPS, which itself is highly power consuming, was turned off indoors while Wi-Fi was available.

Physiological Monitoring Constraints

Besides the mobile phone with its incorporated sensors the MONARCA system consists of two further sensing modalities: A wrist-worn activity monitor and a mobile electro-dermal activity (EDA) sensor. The two major technical challenges faced concerning the requirements of these continuous measurements were the mobility and the unobtrusiveness. To ensure the mobility of the system, the sensors have to be lightweight, small and offer an acceptable battery lifetime. Incorporating the wrist-worn activity sensor in an unsuspicious watch and hiding the EDA electrodes under the socks reached the unobtrusiveness aimed for. Since in state-of-the-art EDA systems, the signals are recorded at the fingers and under lab conditions, studies had to be performed to prove the value of EDA signals obtained at the feet during every-day activities (Setz, 2013). Besides these technical challenges, the system has to be certified for clinical use. The Ethical committee issued this legal requirement. Facing limited resources and time,

this basically prevented us from developing own custom-designed sensor modules, and we opted for off-the-shelf certified devices.

Integration Issues

A multi-component project like MONARCA typically needs to integrate multi-parametric data with origin in different sources such as sensing devices, mobile technologies, medical records, data repositories, etc. This is a challenging task that has to be clear well in advance of the development of single components. The definition of input and output data formats, communication protocols and synchronization parameters is of utmost importance for a proper integration. Moreover, due to the usually high complexity of heterogeneous clinical IT environments, particular focus should be put on robust, flexible, scalable and secure system architecture. MONARCA platform utilized an approach based on a flexible technology (CouchDB) for storing and rendering multi-parametric data accessible from the different modules of the system.

ETHICS, REGULATORY AND INTEGRATION IN MEDICAL WORKFLOWS AND TRIALS

Ethics and Regulations

While conducting experimentations involving clinical trials, it is necessary to be compliant with ethical and regulatory constraints. In fact, it is necessary to get the approval of an Ethical Committee before starting any data collection with patients. Moreover, the regulations in each Country (and occasionally in different states of the same Country), very often are different and in general are complicated and time consuming. Because of this, it is crucial to contact very early in the process the respective Ethic Commissions and to get a clear knowledge of the regulatory framework and potential limitations to the expected trials. In fact, during MONARCA we were required to work at several ethic approvals. First of all the approval for the acceptance of conducting clinical trials for a project with the conceptual framework of continuous monitoring like MONARCA and second an approval for each single trial during the project including in detail the scope of the trial, the policy for users consent and the specific devices to be utilized. This process is a time consuming one and if not done in an opportune way can slow-down and jeopardize the timeline of the project. Moreover, the use of medically certified devices in clinical trials is mandatory and very often this situation constrains researchers to utilize off-the-shelf certified devices to avoid delays. On this regard, special attention has to be put to specific state-of-the-art devices that still don't have a general regulatory framework regarding their potential use as medical devices (i.e. mobile phones and mobile e-health apps).

Integration in Clinical/ Medical Workflows

Clinical workflows describe the processes a clinician is working in with patients towards provisioning the required healthcare services. On this regard, in order to implement an accurate working plan towards the development, testing and validating of a PHS, the single steps required to build a continuous healthcare services workflow have to be modeled in a coordinated way between clinicians and technologists. Secondly, the integration of extra working steps for a clinical trial and later for the use of the PHS has to be discussed and modeled into the existing workflow in a way that does not disrupt the healthcare service provisioning plan but instead improve it. Moreover, it remains a significant challenge to fit the workflow into clinical routine since patients or existing resources may not be available as planned for specific trials.

Trials Constraints

The entire study was conducted in a real-life deployment. In order to avoid difficulties in following deployments an important part was to learn every possible lesson: The first big issue we came across was obtaining the approval of the ethics committee. Not every parameter can be influenced here yet the better one is prepared the less surprises will come along. As long as authorities (specifically in health care) do not approve a study the hands are tied and this can turn down or cut in a study or cause severe delays. Therefore it is important to carefully examine and understand local and countrywide laws and regulations in order to design equipment to be as fitting to the regulations as possible. More over in real-life deployments in health care it is inevitable to use certified equipment. If sensors used, are in-house productions they should be certified beforehand. Otherwise the study might run into trouble. Here it can help a lot to have a back-up solution available and ready.

As part of the trials, the appropriate rewards and compensations for motivating patients to take part should be considered. While conducting MONARCA studies it turned out that an appropriate beneficiary/compensation system was useful for motivating participation. This is particularly relevant specifically in the studies where the pool of possible test subjects is limited. In our study the practice of letting the test subject keep the smart phone after the trial proved to be an additional motivation for some of the participants.

CONCLUDING REMARKS

This paper presented a series of challenges for developing mobile health solutions for mental health. The proposed challenges can be codified as a set of non-functional requirements that are relevant in the design, development and evaluation of mobile monitoring systems. In fact the general requirements presented here are a collection of recommendations from the lessons learnt after three years of the MONARCA EU Project on supporting the treatment of bipolar disorder with mobile technologies. The challenges discussed in this paper may be used in future research as a set of relevant guidelines in the development of innovative solutions for mental health treatment and in a broader way for future research on personal health systems.

ACKNOWLEDGMENT

This work has been partially funded by the EU Contract N. 248545-MONARCA under the 7th FP. Moreover, we would like to thank all patients involved in the project for their contributions and enthusiasm during our research work.

REFERENCES

Arnrich, B., Mayora, O., Bardram, J., & Tröster, G. (2010). Pervasive healthcare - Paving the way for a pervasive, user-centered and preventive health-care model. *Journal of Methods of Information in Medicine*, *1*, 67–73. PMID:20011810

Arnrich, B., Osmani, V., & Bardram, J. (2013). Mental health and the impact of ubiquitous technologies. *Personal and Ubiquitous Computing*, *17*(2), 211–213. doi:10.1007/s00779-011-0464-3

Benazzi, F. (2009). What is hypomania? Tetrachoric factor analysis and kernel estimation of DSM-IV hypomanic symptoms. *The Journal of Clinical Psychiatry*, *70*, 1514–1521. doi:10.4088/JCP.09m05090 PMID:19744407

Bonsall, M. B., Wallace-Hadrill, S. M., Geddes, J. R., Goodwin, G. M., & Holmes, E. A. (2012). Nonlinear time-series approaches in characterizing mood stability and mood instability in bipolar disorder. *Proceedings. Biological Sciences*, *279*, 916–924. doi:10.1098/rspb.2011.1246 PMID:21849316

Cornelia, S., Gravenhorst, F., Schumm, J., Arnrich, B., & Tröster, G. (2013). *Towards long term monitoring of electrodermal activity in daily life*. Personal and Ubiquitous Computing Journal.

Gruenerbl, A., Bahle, G., Weppner, J., & Lukowcz, P. (2012). Towards smart-phone based monitoring of bipolar disorder. In *Proceedings of the Second ACM Workshop on Mobile Systems, Applications, and Services for Healthcare, (SenSys-2012)*, Toronto, Canada. ACM.

Kuhs, H., & Reschke, D. (1992). Psychomotor activity in unipolar and bipolar depressive patients. *Psychopathology*, *25*, 109–116. doi:10.1159/000284760 PMID:1502292

Mayora, O. (2011). The MONARCA project for bipolar disorder treatment. *Journal of Cyber-Therapy & Rehabilitation, 1*.

Puiatti, A., Mudda, S., Giordano, S., & Mayora, O. (2011). Smartphone-centred wearable sensors network for monitoring patients with bipolar disorder. In Conf Proc IEEE Eng Med Biol Soc. (pp. 3644-7). doi:. doi:10.1109/IEMBS.2011.6090613

Sobin, C., & Sackeim, H. A. (1997). Psychomotor symptoms of depression. *The American Journal of Psychiatry, 154*, 4–17. PMID:8988952

Weinstock, L. M., & Miller, I. W. (2008). Functional impairment as a predictor of short-term symptom course in bipolar I disorder. *Bipolar Disorders, 10*, 437–442. doi:10.1111/j.1399-5618.2007.00551.x PMID:18402632

Chapter 71
CoSeMed:
Cooperative and Secure Medical Device Sharing

Andreas Kliem
Technische Universität Berlin, Germany

ABSTRACT

E-health systems need to dynamically integrate heterogeneous types of medical sensors and provide access to streams of sensed medical data in order to properly support patient treatment. Treatment processes usually include several steps and medical departments, which means that sensors could be moved between networks of Care Delivery Operators instead of being reattached every time. Therefore, the authors propose a novel approach that allows sharing medical devices among different operators in this chapter. This means that each operator books a medical device as long as it delivers required data and is present in the operator's network, which the authors call the medical device cloud. Besides cost effectiveness, this approach can extend traditional cloud-based e-health systems, usually designed to share Electronic Health Records, by sharing the devices that emit the data. This mitigates judicial constraints because only the data sources and not the data itself are shared, and allows for more real-time access to mission-critical data.

INTRODUCTION

The evolution of Information and Communication Technology (ICT) in the healthcare domain is heavily influenced by upcoming distributed architectures that integrate and facilitate medical sensors in a ubiquitous fashion (Varshney, 2007). Streams of medical data emitted by integrated medical devices can support physicians in their decision-making process. However, a huge variety of heterogeneous sensors has to be considered in order to get a meaningful survey of a patient's condition. Treatment decisions often have to be made under time constraints, which require an aggregated view of the available data streams. Each stream utilized may differ regarding its specific characteristics, which might include real time requirements, used data formats and nomenclatures or, the communication protocol used by the medical device that provides the stream.

DOI: 10.4018/978-1-4666-8756-1.ch071

The resulting device integration and data aggregation problems often lead to proprietary solutions. Medical device vendors gain flexibility in handling specific hardware requirements, protecting innovations or optimizing their products towards their design preferences. Additionally, market exclusivity can be achieved, which often forces Care Delivery Operators (CDOs) to be dependent on a vendor (i.e. vendor lock-in). However, proprietary solutions hinder the development of open and fully integrated e-health systems, which are required to efficiently deliver cost-effective health services. Moreover, the vendor lock-in problem is intensified, if the movement of medical devices is considered. Since each operator might rely on different solutions, interoperability cannot be achieved. Due to the aforementioned variety, interoperability in the e-health domain can only be achieved, if medical devices can be integrated at any required location regardless of the protocol (proprietary or standard-based) they are based on.

This leads to two options to design medical device integration systems. Either, try to implement all required protocols into one system or rely on standardization. Both options underlie serious obstacles. Although appropriate standards like ISO/IEEE 11073 (ISO/IEEE, 2004) or the Bluetooth Health Device Profile (Bluetooth SIG [BSIG], 2013) exist, the variety of medical devices and regarding requirements makes it difficult to achieve a widespread standardization in a reasonable time span (Buxmann, Weitzel, von Westarp & König, 1999). Moreover, even a lot of standards allow for vendor defined extensions, which again introduces proprietary parts. And, most standards rely on the definition of device profiles to express functionality needed for a certain kind of device. Due to the decreasing time to market, these profiles are changed or added rapidly, which requires to adapt the device integration system too. Implementing all required protocols into one system does not scale, since compute nodes, like smartphones or other embedded systems that are usually used as medical device integration systems underlie resource constraints and often do not allow to implement several protocol stacks in parallel. This raises the question, how a middleware for medical device integration systems can be designed, to achieve interoperability among several protocols, to fit to the rapidly changing requirements and, to be deployable on mobile embedded systems.

Apart from integrating medical devices, data availability has to be considered. Nowadays, treatment processes usually include several steps and institutions (i.e. CDOs), ranging from monitoring at home, emergency transportation or different hospitals, whereat each location might be managed by a different operator. If we assume that a patient is already equipped with a set of wearable medical devices that are organized in a Body Area Network (BAN), real time access to the emitted data could provide better knowledge to physicians. At each location the BAN can grow or shrink (i.e. new medical devices are integrated), in order to fit the set of medical devices to the current treatment situation. However, to prevent reattachment or replacement of the already given medical devices, it is required that the data streams can be accessed by every CDO that is involved in the treatment process. This means that handover processes and some kind of device access management have to be introduced, in order to share the medical devices among different networks and operators.

Based on these problem definitions, the major challenges for middleware architectures in the e-health domain are:

- **Medical Device Integration:** The process of medical device integration shall be organized in an autonomous and dynamic way. In order to integrate unknown or new medical devices in a Plug and Play fashion, the middleware shall allow for reconfiguration at runtime and hide the heterogeneity and complexity of transport protocols from the application layer.

- **Data Aggregation:** Proper data aggregation heavily depends on the characteristics and the semantic interoperability of the incoming data streams. Therefore, the middleware shall provide capabilities to achieve semantic interoperability among heterogeneous data formats and to dynamically deploy and (re)orchestrate data utilization modules along streams of medical data.
- **Data Availability and Mobility:** Seamless monitoring of vital signs relies on the availability of the medical data streams. Since medical devices might be mobile and interconnected using wireless transports, the middleware has to cope with handover processes between different networks and aggregators, while application layer transparency shall be preserved.
- **Security and Privacy:** Due to the requirements of the application domain, data security and privacy has to be preserved. Vulnerabilities that arise out of the dynamically organized system design and the

medical device mobility have to be analyzed and covered properly.

As shown in Figure 1, the approach I will present, extends the traditional way cloud computing concepts are adopted to the e-Health domain. Instead of sharing the data by using cloud computing in the sense of a shared data store for Electronic Health Records (EHR), I try to establish a cloud of medical devices, where the data sources are shared. The data availability and mobility problem are targeted by enabling each CDO along the treatment path of a patient to access the medical devices. A device integration middleware, that allows for dynamic reconfiguration during runtime and provides concepts to handle unknown or new device types, targets the underlying integration and interoperability problem.

BACKGROUND

As a result of the problem definition, the device integration middleware acts as a core enabler for

Figure 1. The Medical Device Cloud approach

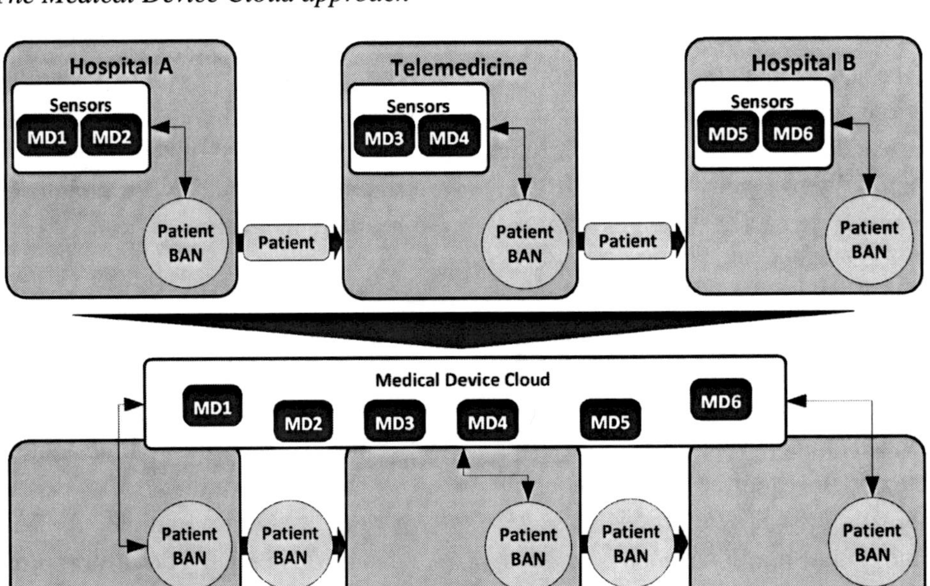

the Medical Device Cloud features, because it ensures interoperability among participating Care Delivery Operators. Therefore it is necessary to discuss general concepts of device integration architectures. As the approach allows to integrate devices based on different protocols and data formats, hiding the variety from the application layer is required. This refers to semantic interoperability and common data formats, which I will discuss briefly.

Following this description, I will introduce basic Cloud concepts related to the Medical Device Cloud approach. The analysis of the interaction of ubiquitous devices and Cloud Computing can be referred to as Cyber Physical or Vehicular Cloud approaches. Additionally, as the presented system is an extension to EHR Cloud Applications, sharing medical data via Cloud infrastructures will be discussed.

Device Integration

Integrating (mobile) embedded devices and sensors involves several steps, like data transmission, data aggregation and processing as well as storage or visualization. Streams of data thereby follow a dynamic path where the sensor can be considered as the source and some storage or end user application as the sink. Each step in the integration path can be realized by different types of devices, where the position in the path basically depends on two important properties: the offered mobility and the offered resources. The mobility property usually decreases towards the sink, whereas the offered resources like processing power or storage capabilities increase. As shown in Figure 2, this leads to a generic three layered model of device integration architectures, where the three layers can be defined as:

- **Devices:** A set of (wearable) devices offering (standard-based) data transmission and location-independent operation to allow for seamless monitoring. The devices (i.e. sensors) are usually highly resource constrained and do not offer any capabilities to execute custom components. Their main purpose is to sense the environment and transmit the results to higher layers.

- **Aggregation:** One or more (wearable) devices that offer higher functionality in order to manage and integrate devices, aggregate data and transmit results to a backend. Devices in this layer (e.g. smartphones or routers) provide an operating system; offer several communication links and allow to execute custom components (e.g. parts of the integration middleware). The main

Figure 2. Generic layered model for ubiquitous device integration architectures

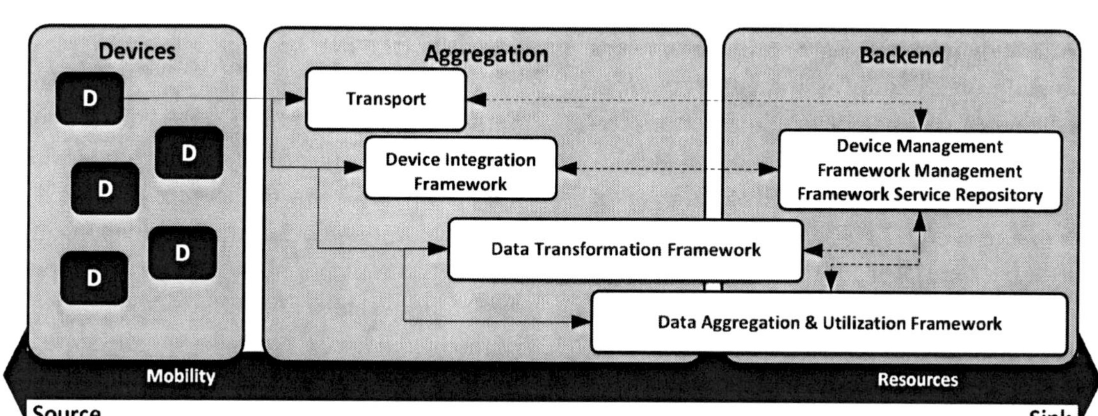

purpose of aggregation devices is to integrate sensing devices into a network and collect data from them. Dependent on the application domain, pre-processing or application layer components, like visualization, can also be placed at this layer.

- **Backend:** A backend primarily used by operating staff, offering persistent storage, monitoring and configuration capabilities, interfaces to higher level information systems (e.g. Hospital Information Systems for medical applications) as well as acting as an enabler (due to resource constraints in the device and aggregation layer) for security, mobility and interoperability enhancements. Components in the backend can be used to control and configure the behavior of aggregation layer devices (e.g. provide data collection plans or additional modules required to integrate a certain device).

In contrast to the OSI (ISO/IEC, 1994) layer model, the given layers are related to the devices and systems found at the respective position in the data path. This view allows for a more precise distinction between components related to the integration middleware and components related to data processing (i.e. application layer). However, this implies that the application layer can cross different layers of the given model. Based on the use case, application layer components might be present at both, the aggregation and the backend layer. I define application layer components as data utilization modules, where utilization refers to evaluation, presentation or storage for instance. Since the focus is on the device integration, utilization modules are treated as black boxes. A utilization module offers some kind of aggregation or processing service. These services are stored within the backend layer and the middleware shall provide a uniform execution framework that allows executing such a service where it is required (i.e. at the aggregation or backend layer) and where the resource constraints are fulfilled.

Since device integration architectures deal with several diverse data sources, the architectural model is somehow related to the ETL (Extract, Transform, Load) or Data Integration process. This is reflected by several mandatory components. The aggregation layer integrates the sensing devices and therefore is required to host a transport and a device integration component, that allow to establish a connection to required devices and collect data from them, which refers to the extract process. The load process is related to store the data into the end target (e.g. a database) and therefore refers to the data utilization part at the backend, which as mentioned deals with storage and interfaces to information systems. Similar to the application layer components, the transformation component can cross both, the aggregation and backend layer. This is due to the fact, that transformation at the aggregation layer is only required, if a utilization module is deployed at this layer too. Otherwise, transformation at the aggregation layer would introduce unnecessary overhead. Finally, device management and a framework management component provides knowledge about the sensing devices and allows to configure the aggregation layer in order to fit to the current requirements.

In the following section I will have a deeper look at the transformation component and its theoretical basis, which can be referred to as semantic interoperability.

Semantic Interoperability - ISO/IEEE 11073

Semantic interoperability refers to a common understanding of the incoming data streams among all actors in the system (Heiler, 1995). A common nomenclature and a canonical data format give the opportunity for interoperable applications that are not affected by replacement of medical devices. Nowadays, replacement of a medical device often leads to adaption processes of an interface application (e.g. GUI) for instance, because in most cases the interface developer has to build directly upon the incoming data format. To bear on standardization and common nomenclatures at the application interface layer is no opposition to the already mentioned obstacles regarding standards at the device integration layer. While it is difficult to achieve interoperability at the device integration layer by constraining each vendor towards one standard, the benefits of semantic interoperability at the data processing or application layer can still be achieved by using data transformation approaches.

The canonical data format and the underlying nomenclature have to be chosen carefully. Important requirements are a sufficient coverage over the domain of context, the possibility to rapidly adopt user defined types (i.e. mechanisms for terminology management) and, a data exchange format suitable for mobile environments. Therefore we decided to rely on the ISO/IEEE 11073 family of standards, which is also promoted by the Continua Health Alliance (Continua Health Alliance [CHA], 2013). It not only provides a huge nomenclature, but also allows to model medical devices with an object oriented Domain Information Model (DIM) approach. This is an important capability, because it allows to store and share medical device configurations and functionalities among Care Delivery Operators (CDOs) participating in the Medical Device Cloud. This common way of describing a device, enables our middleware to automatically integrate and handle new device types. The extensibility of the nomenclature given by already established terminology management mechanisms, allows to model a huge variety of different medical devices, even if for instance a proprietary device is not completely covered by the nomenclature.

Development of the ISO/IEEE 11073 family of standards (x73) started in 1982 in order to provide interoperability and Plug and Play functionality for medical devices. The main application domains of the first versions were hospital and clinical environments. Due to the dissemination of mobile and wearable medical devices, effort was made on improving the original standard towards Telemedicine and Personal Health Device (PHD) environments (Yao & Warren, 2005), (ISO/IEC/ IEEE, 2010). The following parts out of the x73 standard family are important for our approach:

- **11073-10101 Nomenclature:** A basic nomenclature to enhance semantic interoperability by providing a common meaning of numeric values throughout components in the system.
- **11073-10201 Domain Information Model (DIM):** Describes an object-oriented self-descriptive approach to model medical devices, their configuration and, capabilities.
- **11073-20601 Optimized Exchange Protocol:** Defines the transformation of a x73-DIM to an interoperable transmission format optimized for PHD environments.
- **11073-104xx:** Device specializations composed of a subset of available classes and services in the Domain Information Model. Each medical device in the Cloud has to be described by such a specialization. If a proprietary device is not covered with the existing specializations, a new one can be defined.

In terms of x73, medical devices are called agents and devices in the aggregation layer (e.g. a smartphone) are called managers. The basic concept of medical data exchange is to establish a connection between an agent and a manager and to create a local copy of the agent's DIM at manager side by using a service and communication model. The invocation of defined services allows the manager to keep its local copy up-to-date, if new measurements are provided by the agent. The manager provides the recorded data to higher application layers (e.g. GUI components). However, as we only rely on x73 towards the application layer, the main task is to transform the incoming data streams into the x73 format. This means that for each integrated medical device, a kind of virtual manager has to be created by the integration middleware.

The nomenclature defined in ISO/IEEE 11073-10101 (ISO/IEEE, 2004) (i.e. medical data information base (MDIB)) provides a common data dictionary applicable to a broad range of vital signs ranging from intensive care (e.g. ECG) over laboratory to common parameters, like weight or blood pressure. In x73 the nomenclature is primarily used to specify attributes that can appear in data streams (i.e. protocol data units) and are not statically defined. This allows communication partners to get a common semantic understanding of the exchanged data. An entry (i.e. term) in the nomenclature basically consists of a term code and a human readable reference identifier. For efficiency reasons, all nomenclature terms are organized in partitions (e.g. dimensions), where each partition has a set of private term codes that allow for vendor specific extensions. Using terminology management concepts like the Rosetta Terminology Management (RTM) (IHE International [IHE], 2013b), project started by the IHE (IHE International [IHE], 2013a), allows us to extend the nomenclature in case of proprietary devices that are not completely covered.

Besides the nomenclature, x73 defines a Domain Information Model (DIM), which consists of several classes and attributes that are used to model medical devices in an object-oriented fashion. Each class and attribute is referenced using nomenclature codes, thus interoperability is ensured through preserving the same semantic meaning among different implementations. A model of a medical device (i.e. agent) is composed of a set of objects that refer to the data sources accessible by manager devices. The set of objects and corresponding attributes is usually defined by device specializations that correlate to an actual medical device (e.g. blood pressure monitor). Each specialization picks out a defined set of objects and attributes available in the DIM to realize its

intended functionality. Important for the approach to be presented is, that specializations define a static (e.g. system type) and dynamic (e.g. measurement value) set of attributes. If an aggregating device has predefined knowledge about the DIM of a specialization, only the dynamic attributes have to be exchanged and can be merged into the existing static part of the DIM later. Therefore each incoming proprietary data stream to be transformed has to be matched against a device specialization available in x73 or subsequently added to our system. Measurements encoded in the stream have to be translated by a transformation module to x73 attributes and merged into the DIM as dynamic attributes.

CLOUD COMPUTING IN E-HEALTH

The adoption of Cloud Computing concepts for the e-Health domain both raises opportunities and challenges. Evolving concepts like Electronic Health Record (EHR) Clouds, that allow to share patient data and help making the data available, or governmental initiatives and research funding for Cloud based e-Health services (EU, 2013), show that Cloud Computing already found its way into the healthcare domain and is not just a concept under discussion any more. Apart from the serious privacy and security issues related to sharing health records in clouds (Löhr, Sadeghi & Winandy, 2010), the availability of the data is of crucial importance. The data distributed by EHR Clouds usually was recorded in the past, which means that the history of a patient is reflected. However, as our approach just covers the real time data (i.e. the data currently emitted by the patients sensors), a hybrid architecture composed out of both, cloud based EHR sharing and medical device sharing, is required to allow for proper treatment decisions. Therefore I will shortly discuss the fundamentals of EHR cloud approaches.

As mentioned in the introduction, patient treatment nowadays is organized in a multi-tenant fashion, where multiple operators have to collaborate. Each participant in the treatment process must take knowledge about the patient's history and past treatments into consideration, while making own decisions. Knowledge about a patient is stored in patient records, where according to the HIMSS definitions (Garets & Davis, 2006) one has to distinguish between Personal Health Records (PHRs), Electronic Medical Records (EMRs) and Electronic Health Records (EHRs). A PHR should provide a complete summary of the health status and the medical history by gathering information from various sources, like EMRs or EHRs. These records are usually maintained by an individual (i.e. the patient) and allow to make the health status information available for those who are involved in the treatment process. EMRs are maintained by Care Delivery Organizations (CDOs) and are used to represent and document the health care services delivered to a patient by the maintaining CDO. In most cases each CDO hosts its own database to store EMRs. In order to share this knowledge between CDOs involved in a treatment process, EHRs can be used. An EHR is a subset of the knowledge maintained within the EMRs of the involved CDOs. This means an EHR is used to provide the knowledge required for present and future health care decisions and to exchange this knowledge between participating CDOs. Based on the EMR definition, the primary purpose of an EHR Cloud Application is to obtain relevant knowledge from the EMRs located at different CDOs and to distribute it among involved health care providers. Therefore the main challenges for EHR Cloud Applications are related to security and privacy (Lounis, Hadjidj, Bouabdalla & Challal, 2012).

As most EHR Cloud Applications are organized in a patient-centric fashion and are based on community cloud service models, like the Microsoft HealthVault (Microsoft Corporation [MS], 2013), the security and privacy challenges seen from the patient perspective are reviewed first. As the content of an EHR usually is collected from

several EMRs, it has to be defined how access to EMRs from inside the EHR application can be managed. In concerns of privacy, it has to be considered that a patient might only want to make parts of the EHR available to physicians that for instance are only involved in a specific subset of the overall healthcare services delivered during the treatment process. Another crucial requirement is the authenticity of the data represented by EHRs. It has to be ensured that the author (i.e. a physician or a CDO) can be verified, which basically refers to the process of data authentication (Devanbu, Gertz, Martel & Stubblebine, 2002). Treatment decisions based on altered or unauthentic data can cause serious damage to the healthiness of a patient. Seen from a physician's point of view, the capability to collect data from multiple EMR/EHR repositories in a scalable and secure way is important, since a physician might have to handle patients that are present in different EMR systems. This is somehow related to the EMR access management challenge. Moreover, gathering access to patient data stored in multiple CDOs, requires an access control model that involves multiple entities, since both the patient's as well as the respective CDO's authorization is required. Finally, ensuring the data integrity is important, since undesired changes to the data or any loss of information have to be avoided. This is a critical issue when considering multiple CDOs that are updating an EHR, as knowledge might get lost or loose accuracy, if update processes are not properly managed.

EHR Cloud Applications have to cope with the given challenges, in order to provide proper and accepted patient record sharing solutions and to benefit from the cost-effectiveness and availability offered by Cloud based systems. As proposed by Zhang and Liu (2010), the security and privacy challenges can be mapped to three core problems. Secure EHR collection and integration refers to the process of gathering all required knowledge to properly handle the current treatment situation, which also involves that only data related to the current problem is disclosed. Secure storage and access management of EHRs is related to the data authenticity challenge, since the collection of relevant EMRs requires that the resulting EHR is authentic and access can be granted properly. Finally, secure EHR usage models refer to trust between the involved CDOs and physicians (i.e. the consumers of the data), because each involved entity has to ensure that the source of the data can be verified. The main challenge in the next years will be to verify and implement such security models, in order to boost the widespread adoption of EHR Cloud Applications as one building block for the overall information dissemination problem in the healthcare domain.

In order to extend the EHR Cloud capabilities with access to real time data emitted by moving medical sensors, our approach assumes, that medical devices can be shared among CDOs. Therefore we treat medical devices as resources of data. A data resource is considered to be required, if it becomes visible to a CDOs network and emits data. A required resource can be booked and integrated, which refers to the Pay-as-you-go usage model common to Cloud Computing environments. The Medical Device Cloud can either be operated by a third party, a health insurance for instance, or it can be operated in a federated fashion, which means that each participating CDO deploys its own medical devices to the Cloud and allows other CDOs to book them. Treating medical devices as resources of data can be referred to as Information-Acquisition-as-a-Service, which basically was introduced by upcoming concepts like Cyber-Physical Clouds (Craciunas, Haas, Kirsch, Payer, Röck, Rottmann, Sokolova & Trummer, 2010), Vehicular Clouds or Mobile Cloud Computing (Gerla, 2012) respectively.

Cyber-Physical Clouds are based on a sensor virtualization approach. This means that each mobile sensor does not directly execute any application code, but rather hosts a virtualization engine that allows deploying virtual sensors to it. Physical sensors basically act as servers that move in space and execute virtual sensors (Kirsch, Pereira, Sengupta, Chen, Hansen, Huan & Vizzini, 2012). Virtual sensors can migrate between physical ones, which is referred to as cyber-mobility (i.e. moving between sensors hosts). Additionally, virtual sensors can move with their sensor host, which is referred to as physical mobility. Similar to regular Cloud Computing, this allows for efficient resource utilization and enables robust and safe execution of virtual sensors, since each virtual sensor can be isolated from each other. However, as sensors (i.e. medical devices) in the health domain are still very resource constrained, sensor virtualization is not suitable at the moment. Therefore, our approach defines a one-to-one mapping between a physical and a virtual sensor. If a CDO successfully booked and integrated a sensor from a different CDO, a kind of a virtual sensor exists in our backend architecture, which simply refers to a binding inside the device control component. This notion of a virtual sensor allows the application layer to treat the sensor as a regular one, which means that the origin, the owner, the vendor and even the concrete data protocol (semantic interoperability) are hidden by our middleware and the system just interacts with a virtual sensor of a defined type that emits data currently required.

Device Integration Architecture

In order to provide an overall understanding of the required components, I introduce the basic concepts of our architecture for a single operator environment first. I explain how to extend the approach towards the Medical Device Cloud in the next section.

As already introduced, the approach is based on the assumption, that each participating patient is monitored by a Body Area Network (BAN) composed of medical devices with at least one device acting as an aggregator (i.e. smartphone) present. The aggregating device hosts the device integration middleware. The BAN is organized in a fully dynamic fashion, which means that devices can enter or exit at any time without the need for manual reconfiguration. As shown in Figure 3, the architecture aligns to the general model discussed in the background section. In the following I will discuss the backend and the aggregation layer. As the devices layer just consists of a set of medical devices and we do not make any assumptions regarding the device properties (protocol, data format, etc.), no further explanation is required for this layer. A measurement profile to be defined by a physician describes which device types shall be used at which time. After the aggregating device is bound to a patient, the corresponding measurement profile is loaded from the backend and the device integration process is started.

Backend Layer: Apart from general capabilities like patient management, monitoring, persistent storage or interfaces to Hospital Information Systems (HIS), that refer to the Data Utilization Layer, the backend layer primarily offers a Device Control Layer that is related to the device management component introduced in the background section. All devices currently used or known by an operator are registered in the Device Directory (DD). This means the DD is the central control point for distributing medical devices among the aggregators the operator is responsible for. Therefore, the DD offers two main services. First, it provides knowledge about a medical device, which allows each aggregator device to query all information required to integrate and handle a probably unknown device. Second, a device locking mechanism, that allows to dynamically bind a medical device to an aggregator, is implemented.

Each medical device entry in the DD contains some general information like the vendor, device type or state (e.g. location, time last connected). To support dynamic integration of unknown devices, the general information is extended by supporting modules and the device configuration. A supporting module can be either a device driver,

Figure 3. Overview of the general system architecture in a single operator environment

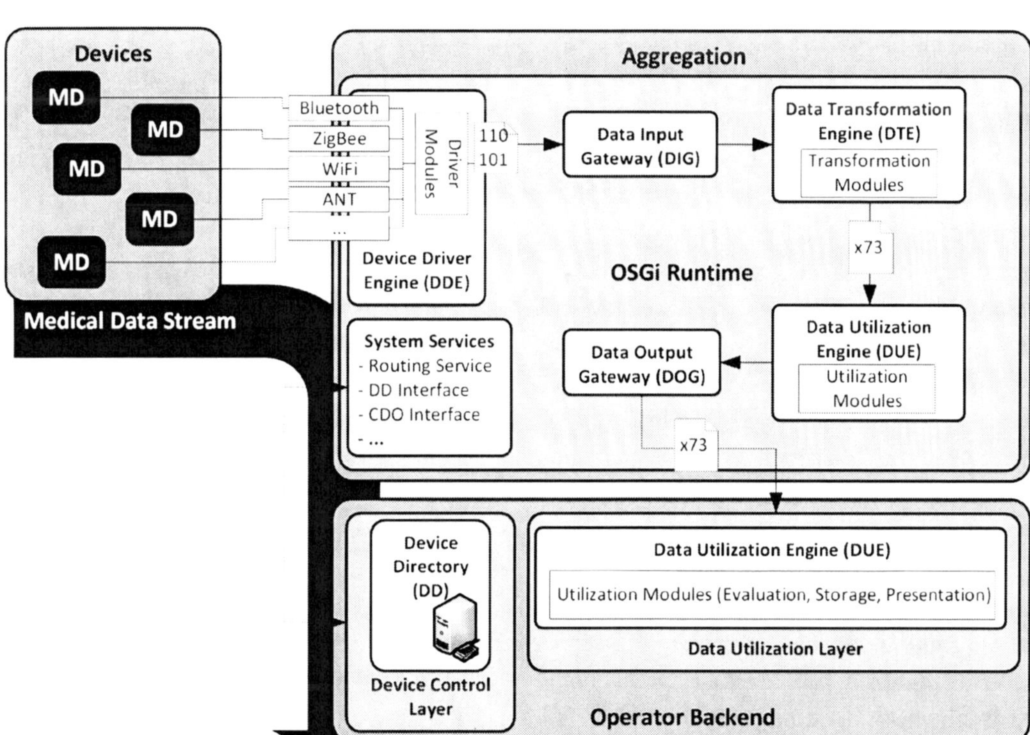

a transformation module or a data utilization module. The integration middleware is able to load these modules during runtime, which means the middleware dynamically reconfigures itself to fit the current requirements. A device driver module refers to the transport component of the integration middleware and allows establishing a connection to a medical device. The resulting data stream might be in any (proprietary) format. Therefore, a transformation module can be loaded and deployed into the data transformation component. If required, the middleware can deploy data utilization modules too. However, as the main purpose is to integrate medical devices and provide the corresponding data streams, deployment and design of data processing or visualization modules is not in scope of this work. Besides the supporting modules, the device configuration is stored. The configuration basically refers to the static part of a x73 Domain Information Model (DIM) as introduced in the background section. Since the DIM is designed in a self-descriptive way, data utilization modules can properly process incoming data streams. If measurements are recorded from a medical device, the values are mapped to the dynamic attributes of the DIM and merged into the static part, that is loaded from the Device Directory. Besides general attributes like the system type, the static part of the DIM provides the semantics that allow to correctly understand and interpret the dynamic measurement attributes.

The second service offered by the Device Directory is a locking mechanism, that allows to bind a medical device to an aggregator (i.e. the patient the aggregator belongs to). This allows the system to dynamically distribute available medical devices among the patients. The effort required to deploy the system is reduced, since no manual interaction is needed if a device is added, replaced or, the measurement configuration is changed. If medical devices are considered as resources, the utilization is optimized, because sharing between patients is allowed. If an aggregator discovers a required medical device, it has to request an

exclusive lock for this device from the directory prior to integrating it. A succeeded lock attempt results in a temporary binding between the medical and the aggregating device. The medical device only can be locked by another aggregator, if the current owner frees the lock or the lock timed out.

As the system manages concrete devices, a mechanism to uniquely identify them is required. Medical devices based on x73 already provide such a globally unique identifier, which is based on IEEE EUI-64. Medical devices not based on x73 have to provide an equivalent ID, which could be a concatenation of vendor and serial number. Which concrete values are used, depends on the device discovery process, since the aggregator must be able to extract the ID prior to actually integrating it.

Aggregation Layer: Aggregator devices like smartphones or routers are responsible to integrate medical devices and provide the data streams to the application layer (i.e. data utilization modules). Therefore, they host an OSGi (OSGi Alliance [OA], 2013) based middleware as shown in Figure 3. Because each component is designed as an OSGi bundle, the middleware can be reconfigured during runtime (i.e. device drivers or transformation modules can be reloaded). I will first discuss some general issues regarding aggregators and then introduce the main components of our middleware solution.

The given approach makes a clear distinction between medical and aggregator devices. This is because we do not allow to share aggregators among operators, which means that one aggregator always belongs to one operator, even if it is moved together with the devices it integrates (e.g. in case of a smartphone). Due to security reasons, most operators of medical IT-Networks cannot allow to dynamically integrate such aggregator devices, because they are not as resource constrained as medical devices, usually execute a complete operating system and are often targets of malicious attacks. Moreover, relying on shared aggregators to provide real time access to the medical data streams does not fit for every situation, since we cannot assume that a patient always carries his aggregator with one (e.g. emergency scenarios). Therefore an aggregator always transmits the data it records to the operator it belongs to.

Another important question is how to establish a relation between medical devices and patients. If a patient equipped with a medical device BAN enters a hospital for instance, it is unclear how the aggregator device in the hospital is able to identify, that all medical devices belong to the patient. Obviously, the aggregator is able to discover the medical devices, but cannot make any assumptions about the fact that they all belong to the same BAN or even more important that the medical devices belong to the patient. The hospital staff could equip each new patient with its own private aggregator that again loads the measurement profile and reintegrates all the medical devices based on that profile. However, this does not scale and intensifies possible conflicts, since the medical devices could be discovered by other aggregators and no relation between patient and medical device exists. This means that sharing medical devices is based on establishing new relations between medical devices, aggregators and patients. Therefore, we define two types of aggregator devices, bound and unbound ones:

- **Bound Aggregator:** These aggregators are manually bound to one patient, which means they are able to query the measurement profile from the operator's backend and can establish initial pairings between medical devices and patients.
- **Unbound Aggregator:** Unbound aggregators can handle medical devices from different patients at the same time (e.g. to be used in environments with multiple patients present). To preserve a valid mapping between patient and medical device, unbound aggregators can only connect to sensors that are already bound to a patient (i.e. a lock exists in the Device Directory).

If an aggregator acts as a bound or unbound one has to be decided by the operator. In case a sensor moves between aggregators belonging to the same operator, the DD provides knowledge about active relations and allows integrating the sensor. But if the sensor moves between networks of different operators, a higher-level instance is required to allow for coordination between operators, which is discussed in the Medical Device Cloud section.

The integration of medical devices is handled by the Device Driver Engine (DDE) module. The basic idea of the DDE is to provide a framework for device driver execution that can be implemented on different platforms. Thus, every device vendor just provides one device driver module that complies to the specification of the DDE and therefore can be executed by each DDE implementation. Drivers are stored as supporting modules in the Device Directory and are loaded dynamically if a medical device is discovered. This allows the DDE to handle both proprietary and standard based devices while preserving resources, as only currently required drivers have to be loaded in the system. The DDE specification basically consists of three layers. A hardware abstraction layer hides the complexity of different transport protocols from the device drivers and allows for platform independence, because the driver modules only interact with well defined interfaces provided by the DDE and not with the actual transport protocol stack, that can differ from platform to platform. A discovery layer provides modules that allow discovering devices available through different transport protocols. This layer again consists of several modules that can be loaded during runtime. This is because some proprietary medical devices might rely on proprietary discovery mechanisms (e.g. broadcasts with special magic packets) and cannot be covered with general discovery modules (e.g. in case of Bluetooth). A session layer provides interfaces to the application layer, manages concrete device sessions (i.e. an established connection to a medical device) and reloading of required modules from the DD. If a medical device is discovered by the DDE, an event is generated and the application layer decides based on the measurement profile if the medical device is required. If this is the case, the DDE tries to acquire a lock from the DD. If the lock request succeeded, a session ID, which corresponds to the lock, is generated and the medical device is integrated by loading and instantiating the driver (if required).

The DDE wraps the recorded data and the session ID, into a data container that is forwarded to the Data Input Gateway (DIG). The session ID enables the DIG to identify the device type and configuration and to query the DD for required transformation or utilization modules to load. If a module has to be loaded depends on the configuration of the application layer (e.g. an app executed on the smartphone to display intermediate results) and on dependencies between the modules. A utilization module might depend on the respective transformation module, if the incoming data stream is not aligned according to x73. Based on the loaded modules the DIG performs the actual routing of the incoming data containers. Therefore it uses the routing system service that provides knowledge about the loaded modules as well as the required input streams and produced output streams. A common setup would be to first execute the transformation module and then forward the resulting x73 data containers to all registered data utilization modules.

Transformation modules are hosted inside the Data Transformation Engine (DTE). As mentioned in the Background section, the DTE allows us to achieve semantic interoperability at the application layer. Similar to the DDE, the DTE is able to dynamically load required transformation modules from the Device Directory. As shown in Figure 4, the approach behind the transformation modules can be referred to as template mapping (Sani, Polack & Paige, 2010). Compared to ontology mapping approaches, for instance, template mapping requires providing multiple pairs of templates and their mappings. However, as outlined in Ivanov, Kliem & Kao (2013), the approach is more lightweight and allows for better modularity and it fits to our device driver model. If a device driver module is provided by a vendor, a mapping module can be added easily. Ontology mapping would be the preferred approach, if an openly disclosed and documented abstract meta-model for each incoming data stream (proprietary or standard based) would exist, which is not the case for every vendor. Moreover, adoption of required technologies like the Web Ontology Language (W3C, 2012) or the Resource Description Framework is only partially supported or nonexistent for mobile and embedded systems usually, because of the required resources. The template mapping approach, therefore, fits to our general system model, because it allows to split the overall problem in a lot of lightweight modules and to deploy them if required.

After all registered utilization modules that perform manipulation on the incoming data stream were executed, the stream can be forwarded to the Data Output Gateway (DOG). The DOG then utilizes the CDO interface to transmit the stream to the backend. Communication between the aggregator and the backend is currently realized with Restful Web Services, because the required libraries are very lightweight and available for most mobile embedded systems.

Depending on the type of the medical device, the measurement profile and, the locking rules defined in the DD, the device might be unlocked if the measurement was completed. This allows to bind the device to a new aggregator (i.e. patient). Another instance of the aggregation middleware might be hosted at the backend, if further utilization modules have to be executed. This can happen, if two or more aggregators transmit data of one patient or complex algorithms are required to process the data.

In summary, the aggregator provides a lightweight middleware that is able to be reconfigured during runtime without any manual interaction. Therefore the middleware uses the knowledge

Figure 4. Template Mapping example from a binary input stream to a x73 aligned output stream

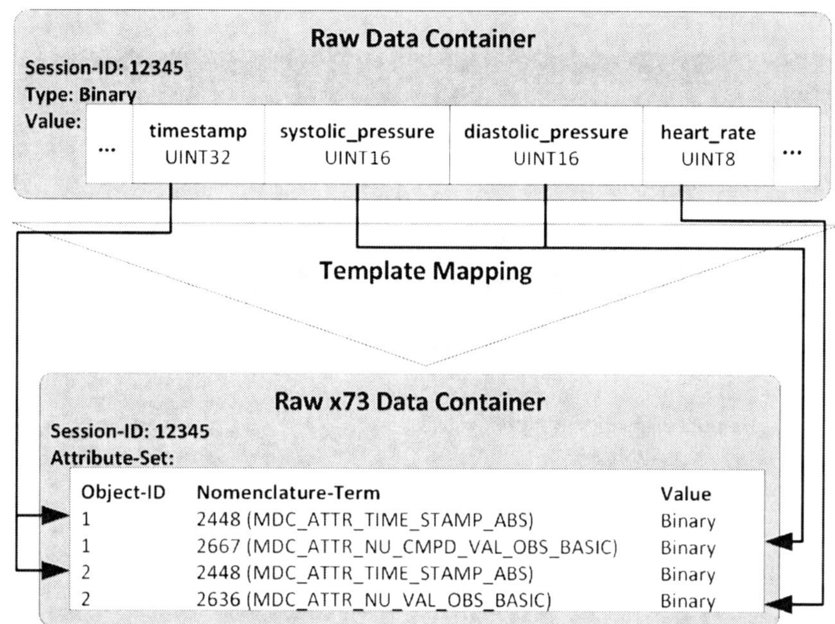

about the available medical devices provided by the backend (i.e. the Device Directory). The next subsection will briefly discuss, how medical data streams are modeled.

Data Stream Representation

In order to model medical data streams, a data container format is introduced. Each component and module in the system expects a data container that provides a session ID. As already mentioned, the session ID generated by the Device Directory during the lock process allows to identify the corresponding medical device and to load additional modules from the backend, that are required to process the stream. Three types of data containers are defined:

- **Raw Data Container:** Contains the session ID, a type flag and a field with raw (proprietary) data emitted by the device driver. The type flag denotes the type of the raw data (e.g. binary, XML or text).

- **Raw x73 Data Container:** Contains the session ID, a timestamp denoting when the transformed values were recorded and a set of transformed data values aligned to fit the x73 model. This means that, as shown in Figure 4, every entry is of the shape {object-ID - nomenclature-term - value}, where object-ID refers to the unique identifier of an object in the corresponding DIM and the value is aligned according to the x73 definitions.

- **DIM x73 Data Container:** Contains the session ID, an order ID and a set of data values aligned to fit the x73 model. In addition to the entry shape of the raw x73 data container, a timestamp and a Boolean flag, denoting whether the entry refers to a static or dynamic attribute in the DIM, is used. The order ID enables the data utilization layer to preserve the correct order of incoming containers. For efficiency reasons, only the first container of one session contains the complete static attribute set.

Figure 5. Medical Data Stream representation with a generic container format

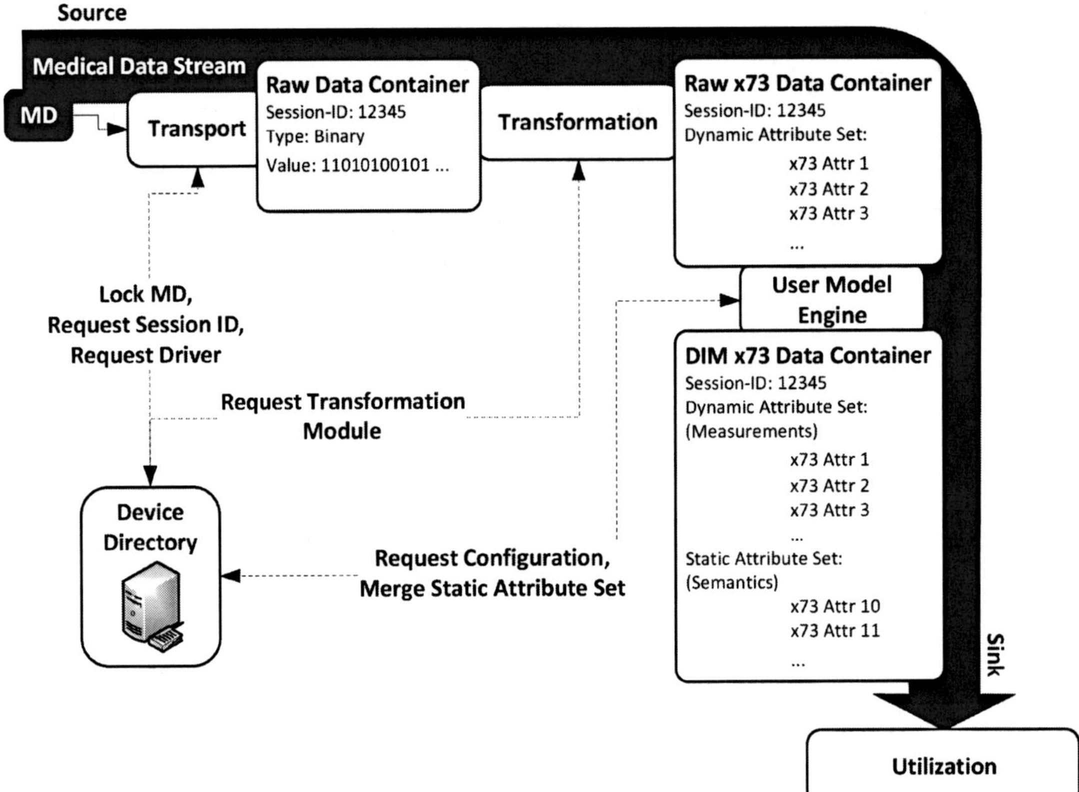

A raw data container is emitted by the Device Driver Engine every time a new measurement is recorded from the medical device identified by the session ID. The included raw data field can be in any format as defined by the protocol spoken by the medical device. The Data Input Gateway acts as a dispatcher that redirects incoming data containers to the corresponding transformation or utilization module. Therefore it maintains a mapping table and has knowledge about all already loaded transformation or utilization modules. If the required transformation module is loaded, the raw data container is forwarded.

As described in the last section, transformation could be realized through ontology mapping. However, we decided to use an approach based on specific modules (i.e. template mapping) for each medical sensor or group of sensors that refer to one standard (e.g. ANT+) (DII, 2013)

instead of using a uniform transformation engine. This is because the medical data streams emitted by the transport layer can heavily differ. Some sensors produce pure binary values in a very efficient format (e.g. only a small set of ASN.1 encoded integers). Other sensors might produce only text formatted values. In case of a uniform transformation engine, these values first must be transformed to a format expected by the engine (usually XML), which would be very inefficient. The transformation module takes the incoming raw data container and transforms it to a raw x73 container. This is done by extracting the measurement values encoded in the incoming container (i.e. the raw data field) and mapping them to the dynamic attribute set of the corresponding x73 Domain Information Model (DIM), as already explained in the Background section. Because the static part of the DIM is missing at this step, the container is called raw x73. Without the static part that provides the semantics required to understand the measurement values, data utilization modules are not able to process the data. As it is unclear if any utilization module is already required at the aggregation layer, it would be unnecessary overhead to create the complete DIM at this step (if no module is loaded, the complete DIM can be generated at the backend).

However, if any utilization module is loaded, the complete DIM has to be provided. This means that the dynamic and the static part of the DIM have to be merged together. The static part is saved as the medical device configuration at the backend. Merging means that the dynamic attributes just have to be added to the static ones, which results in a DIM x73 data container. One possible approach to supply the merged DIM is to exploit the object-oriented model provided by our x73 stack implementation. This layout directly refers to the standard's recommendations and is very easy to process. However, as the DIM x73 Data Container format is organized in an incremental fashion (only the first container includes the static DIM attributes) and the transmission of the whole object tree is rather expensive, we decided to use a table based representation similar to the Raw x73 Data container instead. Every row includes the x73 aligned attribute itself, the object-ID the attribute belongs to and a timestamp reporting when the attribute entry was changed. This way, each client (i.e. data utilization module) is able to restore the complete state of a DIM at any time of a valid session. Moreover, this table based approach makes it easier to transmit the DIM to remote utilization models (e.g. at the backend) or to store it to a database.

MEDICAL DEVICE CLOUD

The device integration middleware presented in the last section already allows sharing medical devices among patients that belong to one opera-

tor. However, most treatment scenarios require introducing different medical institutions that often belong to different operators. Therefore, this section explains how the Device Directory (DD) approach can be extended in order to share medical devices among different operators and to treat them in a Cloud like fashion as pure resources of data. Related to the introduction of Cloud Computing for E-Health, the approach is based on a federated architecture, which means that each participating Care Delivery Operator (CDO) deploys his own devices into the Cloud and allows other CDOs to book them.

The main prerequisite of a medical device cloud is the capability to uniquely identify a medical device among all participating operators. Therefore, we simply extend the Device Directory by implementing a Global Device Directory (GDD). As shown in Figure 6, the GDD acts as a negotiator between different operators and provides a global registry of all devices available in the Medical Device Cloud. If a medical device is discovered inside a CDOs network and the respective aggregator decides to integrate the device, a lock request is sent to the CDOs local DD. If the operator does not find the medical device in his local DD, the GDD has to be queried. The GDD then provides all necessary modules (e.g. device driver, transformation module) required to integrate the device. A medical device not registered in the local DD, implies that a different CDO owns the device. Each operator participating in the Medical Device Cloud acts as the device master for the medical devices he owns. In order to temporally transfer the access rights, the discovering operator has to enter a negotiation phase with the device master. The GDD maintains a master entry for every device known, which allows to identify the master for each medical device. The negotiation phase is similar to the device locking process described in the previous section. Instead of granting the lock to an aggregator, the master grants the lock to another operator (i.e. a local DD). According to the sensor virtualization definition in the background section, a succeeded lock request results in a temporally binding of a physical medical device to virtual one present in the local device directory of the CDO. This notion of a virtual medical device hides the Cloud complexity from the using CDO, since it is not important who owns the physical device and which concrete device type is used, as long as the resulting data streams aligns to the definitions in the local Device Directory and the expected format. The virtual device entry in the directory provides all necessary knowledge (x73 configuration, device driver, transformation module) to properly handle the integration and the resulting stream.

Besides granting access rights, withdrawal has to be considered. If the medical device is moved to another aggregator, the protocol described leads to an access request at the master. One could assume that the medical device already left the network of the previous CDO and therefore can be integrated without any conflicts. But this assumption does not hold in case of nearby located or overlapping operator networks. A typical scenario for overlapping networks is a mobile aggregator (e.g. smartphone) that belongs to the Telemedicine operator and is carried into the range of a hospital operator network. The mobile aggregator still holds an active connection to the medical devices (i.e. the BAN or the patient), but the hospital physician needs access to the data streams. As a result, the master is always required to withdraw active locks prior to granting access to new operators.

The problem of overlapping networks results in a decision making process. The owning CDO needs to decide when to withdraw and grant locks. One approach is to simply rate participating CDOs according to their criticality. A hospital for instance, would get a higher rating than a Telemedicine-provider for instance and therefore be allowed to take the lock. This approach involves a lot of manual configuration and might not be fine grained enough (e.g. in case of a transition between the Telemedicine-provider and a practitioner). Another approach is to introduce a state model for medical devices. A medical device in the Cloud can be represented by global parameters (device owner and lock owner) and CDO dependent parameters (Location, Visibility, Collecting Data). Global parameters are unambiguous among the whole cloud whereas each CDO can have a differ-

Figure 6. Medical Device Cloud infrastructure

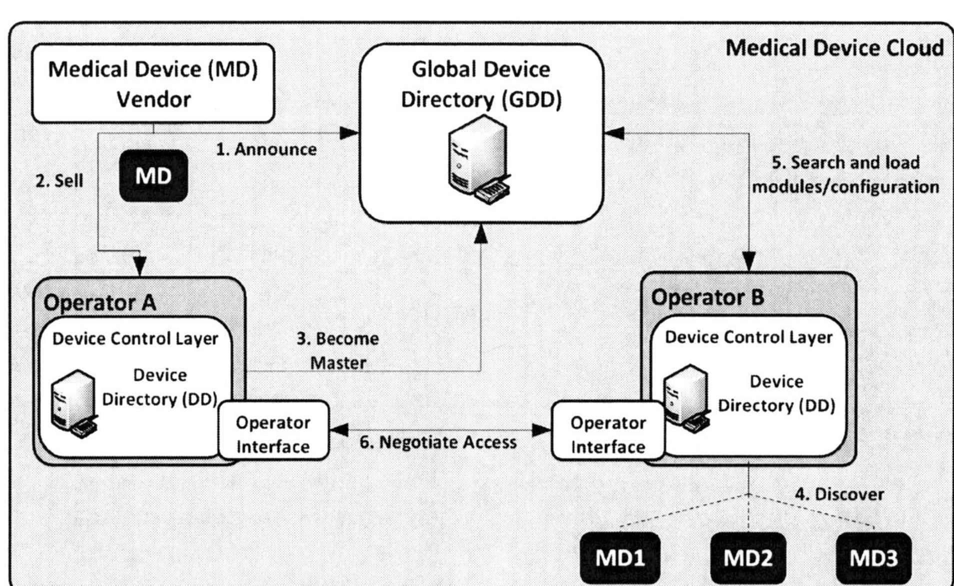

ent observation of the dependent parameters. The visibility for instance defines whether a medical device is visible to a CDOs network. These variant observations lead to ambivalent states, that refer to a transition between CDOs and can be used during the decision making process. However, especially the visibility parameter is difficult to handle in case of mobile aggregators that are able to span their own network inside the one of another CDO (as described above). Therefore the decision making process has to be covered in more detail in future work.

As explained in the previous section, the interoperability challenge, as the core requirement in order to allow CDOs to share medical devices independent from the model or vendor, is covered with distributing knowledge about a device through the Device Directory structure. Every CDO in the medical device Cloud is therefore enabled, to reconfigure its aggregation layer middleware according to the current needs. I will briefly explain how devices can be deployed to the Cloud in the next section.

Medical Device Deployment

Deployment of a medical device to the Cloud takes two steps. First the device has to be announced to the Global Device Directory. In case of a new device type or model, the supporting modules (device driver and transformation module) and the x73 aligned configuration have to be supplied. The second step is to define the device owner (i.e. the master). If the device was already announced by the owning CDO, this step is unnecessary. Otherwise, if the device was announced by the device vendor, for instance, taking the ownership can be protected by a predefined token, shared between the vendor and the CDO that bought the device. This model of vendor based device deployment, allows for a Plug and Play integration of medical devices, without any need for manual set-up procedures.

The x73 based configuration stored in the directory enables utilization modules to correctly understand and interpret an incoming data stream. As explained in the Background section, the configuration consists of the static attributes

Figure 7. Deployment of medical devices and corresponding supporting modules

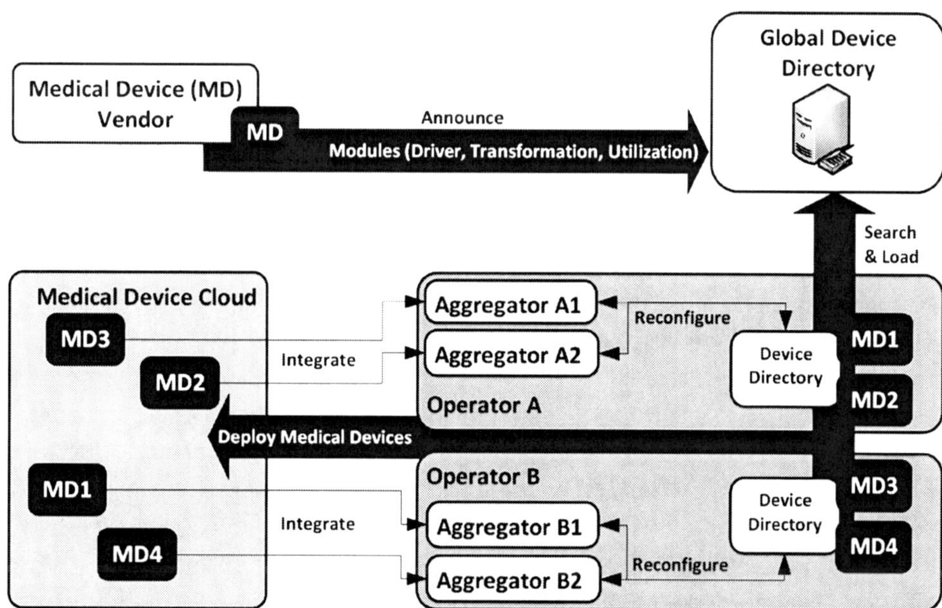

of a x73 Domain Information Model. The static attribute set is defined by device specializations (e.g. blood-pressure-monitor, weighing-scale). If no fitting specialization is available for a new medical device, it has to be created by the deploying entity. Two cases have to be considered:

If all required nomenclature terms to describe the device exist, one simply has to create a specialization for the sensor by defining the static and dynamic attribute set. This is possible because x73 DIMs are self-descriptive. Most attributes used do not represent measured values. Rather they are used as a semantic description of the actual measurement attributes. This is underlined by the fact, that x73 compliant managers are able to operate with an agent (i.e. medical device) without having predefined knowledge about the DIM. Instead the DIM is exchanged during a configuration phase in this case. Therefore, data utilization modules can be designed in a generic fashion and deal with unknown specializations.

In the second case, if required terms are missing and cannot be composed of several existing ones (e.g. a missing Dimension), the required terms have to be added to private areas (i.e. vendor defined) in the available x73 partitions. This would allow for a uniform understanding within the medical institution that hosts one instance of the drafted architecture. Data exchange between medical institutions can be realized through transformation from x73 to HL7 (Health Level Seven [HL7], 2013) for instance. However, adding nomenclature terms involves adapting data utilization modules, which want to process data from the new sensor. Terminology management as described in the background section could then be used to take the new terms to standardization.

SECURITY AND PRIVACY ISSUES

Privacy and security are core requirements in the healthcare domain. Therefore, common threats and possible attacks, especially the ones related to wireless sensor networks (e.g. Denial of Service, location tracking, eavesdropping or modification of medical data), have been discussed in several publications (Ko, Lu, Srivastava, Stankovic, Terzis, & Welsh, 2010;Ng, Sim & Tan, 2006). Besides threats related to the system performance and availability, a common classification can be found based on the principles confidentiality, integrity and authenticity (Marti, Delgado & Perramon, 2004).

Attacks related to confidentiality include eavesdropping, for instance, and basically are intended to get access to some kind of private information. This can be achieved by either intercepting the communication links or accessing stored data (i.e. attacking Hospital Information Systems). Eavesdropping of communication links is related to the entire data transmission chain. Regarding the device integration architecture, this includes the links between the devices and the aggregation layer as well as the links between the aggregation and the backend layer. Partala et al., (2013) analyzed threats related to the transmission chain. Their classification is based on a three tier model, that easily can be mapped to the three layered architecture defined in the Background section. Based on the possible threats and the distributed, multiple tier architecture of mobile e-health systems, they concluded that end-to-end security from the source to the sink of a medical data flow is not possible at the moment. Therefore, the vulnerability of tier 2 devices (i.e. aggregation layer) has to be further investigated in future work, since especially devices like smartphones are more frequently attacked in recent years. Because the device integration architecture allows for bound aggregators, that represent a concrete relation to a patient, data anonymization could be intercepted throughout the transmission chain. However, the security of our transmission chain is based on the protocols used. Since one of the main requirements was to provide interoperability among the Medical Device Cloud participants and allow to integrate sensors without restriction of used transport protocols, the system has to rely on the given security models provided by these transports (e.g. Bluetooth or Zigbee). The goal is, that the Device Driver Engine always enforces the usage of the highest level available for a certain transport. The transmission between aggregators and the backend layer is based on RESTful Web Services that can be encrypted using SSL. Since aggregators are bound to a CDO and not shared, the key distribution can be managed easily. A possible approach is to use PAKE (Password authenticated key exchange) protocols (Bellare, Pointcheval & Rogaway, 1992) during initialization of an aggregator, where the password could be an internal patient ID assigned by the CDO. Apart from the bound aggregator issue mentioned, eavesdropping attacks are mitigated due to anonymization, since each medical stream is only identified by the session ID generated during the device lock process. A mapping between patient and medical data streams first happens at the CDOs backend. Confidentiality threats related to unauthorized access of stored data, are not in scope or this work, since the middleware just forwards the data to the information systems of a CDO and do not persist it at any step. However, if an application layer module (i.e. data utilization module) executed at the aggregation layer (e.g. a GUI application on the smartphone) temporally stores intermediate data, this issue has to be further investigated.

The second principle, integrity, is related to attacks that intercept the transmission or access stored data in order to modify the content. Even if the transmission chain is protected against eavesdropping, by encryption for instance, an attacker might still modify the data blindly. Therefore, mechanisms like redundancy codes, checksums or, message signatures are required. At the moment the middleware relies on the integrity mechanisms provided by the transports and the data stream representation does not include any application layer mechanisms that allow signing the contents. However, I plan to integrate this feature in the future. It is planned that the device directory component provides capabilities for key distribution and message signatures, since it already generates the session ID, which identifies a medical data stream.

The third principle, authenticity, can be covered with shared secrets, because an attacker usually tries to make the recipient believe, that the data comes from an authentic source. With regard to the devices layer, it has to be ensured, that no malicious device is injected (e.g. an attacker could emulate a device of a certain type) into the Cloud. The only requirement for an attacker is to guess a valid pair of medical device ID and medical device type, which can be achieved rather easily. However, since the architecture has to rely on the capabilities of the transport protocols used and cannot modify the application layer protocol (i.e. inject shared secrets) used by a medical device, it is difficult to achieve authenticity among the devices layer. The problem could be mitigated by heuristic approaches that for instance observe the movement and the emitted data of a medical device, which would increase the effort required to guess a valid sensor ID and type pair at the estimated location. Authenticity regarding the aggregation layer is related to the already mentioned key distribution and PAKE protocols used during the initialization of an aggregator.

An issue specifically related to the Medical Device Cloud approach is the federated structure and the resulting device sharing problem. As mentioned in the Medical Device Cloud section, reliable granting and withdrawal of device access rights is required. Reliable granting and withdrawal of access rights relies on trusted relationships between the participating CDOs as well as between a CDO and its corresponding aggregators. Trusted relationships between operators have to be established on the basis of contracts between the CDOs participating in the Medical Device Cloud. This can be either organized by a third party (e.g. governmental health ministry) or on a peer to peer basis. Since a medical device owner can always reject incoming device access requests, CDOs with unconfirmed identity can be handled properly. Trusted relationships between CDOs and aggregators are related to the authenticity principle discussed above.

If the chain of trusted participants is intercepted, by a malicious aggregator for instance, especially the withdrawal process of access rights could be damaged, because medical device release requests can be rejected unexpectedly or without any acknowledgement. With regard to the authenticity principle definition, we developed a security protocol based on a Public-Key-Infrastructure (PKI) and shared secrets (Kliem, Hovestadt & Kao, 2012). The protocol allows for reliable granting and withdrawal of device access rights even if a compromised CDO or aggregator does not release a revoked device. However, the protocol involves adaption of the communication protocols used by medical devices and the medical devices itself, which is difficult to achieve and contradicts our interoperability requirement. Therefore it has to be analyzed how such a global concept can be properly mapped to the actual communication protocol capabilities used in the system (e.g. Bluetooth provides PIN based models).

As mitigation to this problem, code signing concepts provided by the OSGi security layer can be used. Because each device driver module is an OSGi bundle, it can be signed and verified prior to be executed. Therefore, we integrate the medical device locking and unlocking process into the device driver bundles. We only allow bundles that are signed by the Global Device Directory operator to be executed. This means that only bundles that are signed and verified are involved in the medical device integration process.

FUTURE RESEARCH DIRECTIONS

Currently the proposed device integration architecture and the device deployment model is applied to a broader range of application domains. In the scope of the - Forschungscampus: Connected Technologies - project (Forschungscampus Connected Technologies [FCT], 2013) parts of the system are used to integrate devices in the Smart Home and Ambient Assisted Living (AAL) domain.

Related to the Medical Device Cloud application, future work primarily targets the decision models used to negotiate device access requests and the security issues mentioned. Especially scenarios where CDO networks are located nearby or overlap need to be investigated. Smooth handover processes are required to allow seamless monitoring if a medical device is moved between different aggregators, even in case the aggregators belong to the same CDO (e.g. in case of separated clinical wards). It has to be further investigated, how the authenticity principle can be properly reflected by the protocol agnostic system architecture.

Regarding the medical data stream processing, the dynamic placement of data utilization as well as transformation modules has to be analyzed. It is not necessarily required to host the transformation module at the aggregation layer, if no utilization is performed here. Moreover, based on the data input and output format description introduced by the generic container format and the knowledge provided by the device directory, utilization and transformation modules could be orchestrated dynamically along the data path. This also includes to consider multiple transformation modules that for instance allow to transform the stream to formats used inside clinical or EHR Cloud environments (e.g. HL7).

Finally, with respect to the increasing resources of embedded mobile devices, the system architecture can be extended towards hybrid devices, that both allow for data sensing and aggregation. This also involves network structures, where multiple aggregators or hierarchies of aggregators can be used to collect and pre-process the medical data streams.

CONCLUSION

I presented an approach for E-Health systems that allows for Plug and Play integration of medical devices in a protocol and vendor agnostic fashion. The fundamental basis is a middleware solution that can be reconfigured dynamically during runtime. This is achieved by maintaining a global registry of devices and providing knowledge (i.e. modules), that is deployed to the middleware if required.

The overall architecture allows sharing medical devices among different networks and Care Delivery Operators, which I defined as the Medical Device Cloud. Due to the movement of a patient and the resulting treatment process that can be composed out of different involved institutions (CDOs), the architecture might fit the requirements of current e-health systems in a more suitable way. Compared to common knowledge dissemination approaches in the E-Health domain (e.g. EHR Clouds), the presented approach is about sharing the devices (i.e. the data sources) instead of sharing the data themselves. Sharing data often underlies several judicial restrictions. Sharing devices can mitigate this problem and allow for further treatment process optimizations.

The presented approach aims to increase resource utilization and cost-effectiveness as well as data availability by applying the popular Cloud Computing Pay-as-you-go model to a set of medical devices that are able to move in space. Medical devices are considered as resources of data that can be booked by a CDO as long as they are visible and the CDO considers them to be required. Therefore, the system is an extension to the upcoming Electronic Health Record Cloud Applications. EHR Clouds provide the history of a patient by gathering patient records from several institutions that were involved in the treatment, whereas the Medical Device Cloud allows for real-time access to the data emitted by the patient's sensors.

REFERENCES

Bellare, M., Pointcheval, D., & Rogaway, P. (2000). Authenticated key exchange secure against dictionary attacks. In *Proceedings of Advances in Cryptology–Eurocrypt 2000* (pp. 139–155). Bruges, Belgium: Springer. doi:10.1007/3-540-45539-6_11

Bluetooth, S. I. G. (BSIG). (2013). Health Device Profile. *Health Device Profile - Bluetooth Technology Special Interest Group*. Retrieved October 23, 2013, from https://www.bluetooth.org/en-us/specification/assigned-numbers/health-device-profile

Buxmann, P., Weitzel, T., von Westarp, F., & König, W. (1999). The standardization problem: An economic analysis of standards in information systems. In *Proceedings of the 1st IEEE Conference on Standardisation and Innovation in Information Technology SIIT '99* (pp. 57-162). IEEE.

Continua Health Alliance (CHA). (2013). About the Alliance. *About the Alliance - Continua Health Alliance*. Retrieved October 23, 2013, from http://www.continuaalliance.org/about-the-alliance

Craciunas, S. S., Haas, A., Kirsch, C. M., Payer, H., Röck, H., Rottmann, A., et al. (2010). Information-acquisition-as-a-service for cyber-physical cloud computing. In *Proceedings of the 2nd USENIX conference on Hot topics in cloud computing* (pp. 14-14). USENIX Association.

Devanbu, P., Gertz, M., Martel, C., & Stubblebine, S. G. (2002). Authentic third-party data publication. In *Data and Application Security* (pp. 101–112). Schoorl, The Netherlands: Springer US. doi:10.1007/0-306-47008-X_9

Dynastream Innovations Inc. (DII). (2013). ANT+. *ANT+ Vision*. Retrieved October 24, 2013, from http://www.thisisant.com/company/

European Commission (EU). (2013). Living Healthy, Ageing Well. *Digital Agenda for Europe*. Retrieved October 24, 2013, from http://ec.europa.eu/digital-agenda/en/life-and-work/living-healthy-ageing-well

Forschungscampus Connected Technologies (FCT). (2013). Forschnungscampus Connected Technologies. In *Connected Living e.v.: Forschnungscampus*. Retrieved October 23, 2013, from http://www.connected-living.org/projekte/forschnungscampus

Garets, D., & Davis, M. (2006). *Electronic medical records vs. electronic health records: Yes, there is a difference* (policy white paper). Chicago: HIMSS Analytics.

Gerla, M. (2012). Vehicular Cloud Computing. In *Proceedings of Ad Hoc Networking Workshop (Med-Hoc-Net),* (pp. 152-155). IEEE.

Health Level Seven International (HL7). (2013). About HL7. *About Health Level Seven International.* Retrieved October 23, 2013, from http://www.hl7.org/about/index.cfm?ref=nav

Heiler, S. (1995). Semantic interoperability. *ACM Computing Surveys*, *27*(2), 271–273. doi:10.1145/210376.210392

International, I. H. E. (IHE). (2013a). Integrating the Healthcare Enterprise. *IHE - Integrating the Healthcare Enterprise* Retrieved October 23, 2013, from http://www.ihe.net/

International, I. H. E. (IHE). (2013b). PCD Profile Rosetta Terminology Mapping. *PCD Profile Rosetta Terminology Mapping - IHE wiki*. Retrieved October 23, 2013, from http://http://wiki.ihe.net/index.php?title=PCD_Profile_Rosetta_Terminology_Mapping

ISO/IEC. (1994). Information technology - Open Systems Interconnection - Basic Reference Model: The Basic Model. In ISO/IEC 7498.1:1994(E) (pp. 1-68). ISO/IEC.

ISO/IEC/IEEE. (2010). ISO/IEC/IEEE Health Informatics–Personal Health Device Communication–Part 20601: Application Profile–Optimized Exchange Protocol. In ISO/IEEE 11073-20601:2010(E) (pp. 1-208). IEEE.

ISO/IEEE. (2004). ISO/IEEE Health Informatics–Point-Of-Care Medical Device Communication–Part 10101. In ISO/IEEE 11073-10101:2004(E) (pp. 0-492). IEEE.

Ivanov, D., Kliem, A., & Kao, O. (2013). Transformation Middleware for Heterogeneous Healthcare Data in Mobile E-health Environments. In *Proceedings of the 2013 IEEE Second International Conference on Mobile Services* (pp. 39-46). IEEE Computer Society.

Kirsch, C., Pereira, E., Sengupta, R., Chen, H., Hansen, R., Huang, J., et al. (2012). Cyber-physical cloud computing: The binding and migration problem. In *Proceedings of the Conference on Design, Automation and Test in Europe* (pp. 1425-1428). EDA Consortium.

Kliem, A., Hovestadt, M., & Kao, O. (2012). Security and Communication Architecture for Networked Medical Devices in Mobility-Aware eHealth Environments. In *Proceedings of the 2012 IEEE First International Conference on Mobile Services* (pp. 112-114). IEEE.

Ko, J., Lu, C., Srivastava, M. B., Stankovic, J. A., Terzis, A., & Welsh, M. (2010). Wireless sensor networks for healthcare. *Proceedings of the IEEE*, *98*(11), 1947–1960. doi:10.1109/JPROC.2010.2065210

Löhr, H., Sadeghi, A. R., & Winandy, M. (2010). Securing the e-health cloud. In *Proceedings of the 1st ACM International Health Informatics Symposium* (pp. 220-229). ACM.

Lounis, A., Hadjidj, A., Bouabdallah, A., & Challal, Y. (2012). Secure and Scalable Cloud-based Architecture for e-Health Wireless sensor networks. In Proceedings of Computer Communications and Networks (ICCCN), (pp. 1-7). IEEE.

Martí, R., Delgado, J., & Perramon, X. (2004). Security specification and implementation for mobile e-health services. In *Proceedings of e-Technology, e-Commerce and e-Service* (pp. 241–248). IEEE. doi:10.1109/EEE.2004.1287316

Microsoft Corporation (MS). (2013). Explore HealthVault. *HealthVault - Overview*. Retrieved October 23, 2013, from http://www.healthvault.com/us/en/overview

Ng, H. S., Sim, M. L., & Tan, C. M. (2006). Security issues of wireless sensor networks in healthcare applications. *BT Technology Journal*, *24*(2), 138–144. doi:10.1007/s10550-006-0051-8

OSGi Alliance (OA). (2013). About the OSGi Alliance. *OSGi Alliance*. Retrieved October 23, 2013, from http://www.osgi.org/About/HomePage

Partala, J., Keränen, N., Särestöniemi, M., Hämäläinen, M., Iinatti, J., Jämsä, T., et al. (2013). Security threats against the transmission chain of a medical health monitoring system. In *Proceedings of the 2013 IEEE 15th International Conference on e-Health Networking, Applications and Services* (pp. 218-223). IEEE.

Sani, A. A., Polack, F., & Paige, R. (2010). Generating Formal Model Transformation Specification Using a Template-based Approach. In *Proceedings of the 3rd York Doctoral Symposium on Computing* (pp. 11-18). York, UK: University of York.

Varshney, U. (2007). Pervasive healthcare and wireless health monitoring. *Mobile Networks and Applications*, *12*(2-3), 113–127. doi:10.1007/s11036-007-0017-1

W3C. (2012). OWL 2 Web Ontology Language Document Overview (2nd Ed.). *W3C Recommendation*. Retrieved October 24, 2013, from http://www.w3.org/TR/owl2-overview/

Yao, J., & Warren, S. (2005). Applying the ISO/IEEE 11073 standards to wearable home health monitoring systems. *Journal of Clinical Monitoring and Computing*, *19*(6), 427–436. doi:10.1007/s10877-005-2033-7 PMID:16437294

Zhang, R., & Liu, L. (2010). Security models and requirements for healthcare application clouds. In Proceedings of Cloud Computing (CLOUD), (pp. 268-275). IEEE.

ADDITIONAL READING

Armbrust, M., Fox, A., Griffith, R., Joseph, A. D., Katz, H. R., & Konwinski, A. et al. (2010). A View of Cloud Computing. *Communications of the ACM*, *53*(4), 50–58. doi:10.1145/1721654.1721672

Asare, P., Cong, D., Vattam, S. G., Kim, B., King, A., Sokolsky, O., & Mullen-Fortino, M. (2012, January). The medical device dongle: an open-source standards-based platform for interoperable medical device connectivity. In *Proceedings of the 2nd ACM SIGHIT International Health Informatics Symposium* (pp. 667-672). ACM.

Bicer, V., Laleci, G. B., Dogac, A., & Kabak, Y. (2005). Artemis message exchange framework: semantic interoperability of exchanged messages in the healthcare domain. *SIGMOD Record*, *34*(3), 71–76. doi:10.1145/1084805.1084819

Boulos, M. N., Wheeler, S., Tavares, C., & Jones, R. (2011). How smartphones are changing the face of mobile and participatory healthcare: an overview, with example from eCAALYX. *Biomedical Engineering Online*, *10*(1), 24. doi:10.1186/1475-925X-10-24 PMID:21466669

Brito, M., Vale, L., Carvalho, P., & Henriques, J. (2010, August). A sensor middleware for integration of heterogeneous medical devices. In *Engineering in Medicine and Biology Society (EMBC), 2010 Annual International Conference of the IEEE* (pp. 5189-5192). IEEE.

Cayirci, E., & Rong, C. (2008). *Security in wireless ad hoc and sensor networks*. John Wiley & Sons.

Dagtas, S., Natchetoi, Y., & Wu, H. (2007, June). An integrated wireless sensing and mobile processing architecture for assisted living and healthcare applications. In *Proceedings of the 1st ACM SIG-MOBILE international workshop on Systems and networking support for healthcare and assisted living environments* (pp. 70-72). ACM.

Fan, L., Buchanan, W., Thummler, C., Lo, O., Khedim, A., Uthmani, O., & Bell, D. (2011, July). Dacar platform for ehealth services cloud. In *Cloud Computing (CLOUD), 2011 IEEE International Conference on* (pp. 219-226). IEEE.

Hassan, M. M., Song, B., & Huh, E. N. (2009, February). A framework of sensor-cloud integration opportunities and challenges. In *Proceedings of the 3rd international conference on Ubiquitous information management and communication* (pp. 618-626). ACM.

Kindberg, T., & Fox, A. (2002). System software for ubiquitous computing. *Pervasive Computing, IEEE, 1*(1), 70–81. doi:10.1109/MPRV.2002.993146

King, A., Procter, S., Andresen, D., Hatcliff, J., Warren, S., Spees, W., & Weininger, S. (2009, May). An open test bed for medical device integration and coordination. In *Software Engineering-Companion Volume, 2009. ICSE-Companion 2009. 31st International Conference on* (pp. 141-151). IEEE.

Kirn, S. (2003). Ubiquitous healthcare: The onkonet mobile agents architecture. In *Objects, Components, Architectures, Services, and Applications for a Networked World* (pp. 265–277). Springer Berlin Heidelberg. doi:10.1007/3-540-36557-5_20

Krumm, J. (Ed.). (2009). *Ubiquitous computing fundamentals*. CRC Press. doi:10.1201/9781420093612

Laukkarinen, T., Suhonen, J., & Hännikäinen, M. (2013). An Embedded Cloud Design for Internet-of-Things. *International Journal of Distributed Sensor Networks, 2013*. (pp. 13). Hindawi Publishing Corporation.

Yuriyama, M., & Kushida, T. (2010, September). Sensor-cloud infrastructure-physical sensor management with virtualized sensors on cloud computing. In *Network-Based Information Systems (NBiS), 2010 13th International Conference on* (pp. 1-8). IEEE.

KEY TERMS AND DEFINITIONS

Cloud Computing: Cloud allows to consume large amounts of resources, like computing, storage, or, software, over the Internet without the need for any long term contracts. Consumers do not have to be aware of the actual physical location or the physical system that provides the service. Cloud Computing is based on virtual infrastructures that allow to share physical infrastructures among several customers. This leads to a high degree of resource utilization and reduces costs. Customers rent and pay for virtual resources as long as they require them.

Electronic Health Record (EHR): A collection of health information or information about health services a patient received. It is associated with one individual (i.e. a patient). The purpose of an EHR is to share the health information among actors involved in the treatment process of a patient. Therefore, the necessary data is collected from Care delivery Operators that were involved in a patient's treatment process and maintain health information about this patient in their private information systems.

Interoperability: Allows actors in distributed systems to work together by providing a common understanding of the exchanged information. The general definition not only applies to information in the sense of data. It also includes components (e.g. devices) that can be integrated among different actors or replaced.

Mobile: Cloud Computing: An upcoming family of applications, where (embedded) mobile devices can be Cloud users and Cloud service providers at the same time. This on one hand refers to on-demand and real-time information dissemination and processing in peer-to-peer networks of mobile devices. On the other hand this can be considered as mobile resources that move in space and can be booked by consumers. The Cyber Physical Cloud approach extends this notion by adding virtualization to the mobile device domain. Physical mobile devices are servers that move in space and allow hosting virtual mobile devices.

Pay-as-You-Go: A popular billing model in the Cloud Computing domain. Related to Cloud Computing definition, it refers to the fact that customers just rent required resources as long as they consider them to be required, which means they just pay for the time they rented the infrastructure. Customers are not required to rely on long term contracts in order to access the resources they need.

Semantic Interoperability: A specialization of the general definition that is related to the understanding and interpretation of data that is exchanged for different actors of a system. Semantic interoperability provides a common understanding of the data, by using common nomenclatures and data formats. It targets the meaning of the data and not the packaging (i.e. syntax).

Template Mapping: An approach for data transformation between a source and a target model in order to achieve semantic interoperability. Template mapping assumes that for both the source and the target model instances exist (e.g. concrete medical device specializations). The predefined target instance then acts as a template, which is filled with dynamic values from the source instance (e.g. measurements).

This work was previously published in Cloud Computing Applications for Quality Health Care Delivery edited by Anastasius Moumtzoglou and Anastasia N. Kastania, pages 201-227 copyright year 2014 by Medical Information Science Reference (an imprint of IGI Global).

Chapter 72
Legal and Ethical Considerations in the Implementation of Electronic Health Records

Karen Ervin
Pennsylvania Hospital Librarian, USA

ABSTRACT

This chapter examines the literature of healthcare in the United States during the transitioning to electronic records. Key government legislation, such as the Health Insurance Portability and Accountability Act (HIPAA) and the Health Information Technology for Economic and Clinical Health Act (HITECH), which were part of the American Recovery and Reinvestment Act (ARRA) and the Affordable Health Care Act, are reviewed. The review concentrates on patient privacy issues, how they have been addressed in these acts, and what recommendations for improvement have been found in the literature. A comparison of the adoption of electronic health records on a nationwide scale in three countries is included. England, Australia, and the United States are all embarking in and are at different stages of implementing nationwide electronic health database systems. The resources used in locating relevant literature were PubMed, Medline, Highwire Press, State Library of Pennsylvania, and Google Scholar databases.

ORGANIZATION BACKGROUND

Legal and ethical issues regarding patient confidentiality in the adoption of electronic health records in the United States are the focus of this paper. The Privacy Rule, which protects all "individually identifiable health information" held in any form, is one of the most central and well known parts of the HIPAA Act (U.S. DHHS, 1996, p.1). Also, important are both the Affordable Care Act and the HITECH Act that deal with Medicare and Medicaid expansion ("HITECH," 2009). Additionally, the first phase of the Obama Administration's HITECH Act, which provides financial incentives to health care organizations that adopt and use electronic health records by the end of 2012, was put into law, effective in February 2009. The goal of obtaining over 100,000

DOI: 10.4018/978-1-4666-8756-1.ch072

health care providers using electronic health records (EHRs) by the end of 2012 has already been exceeded (Centers, 2012). Consequently, many hospitals and medical practices across the nation are confronted with the proper handling of electronic records to ensure patient confidentiality even before the legal and ethical ramifications have been critically discussed.

SETTING THE STAGE

The literature that investigates the process of automating patient records and confidentiality, as defined in the HIPAA Act, must be explored in order to address questions of legal and ethical aspects involved. In order to address the confidentiality concerns one needs to understand the similarities and differences between electronic and paper records and to define exactly what is contained in each type. According to the Council on Ethical and Judicial Affairs (CEJA) of the American Medical Association (AMA), electronic medical records, also called electronic health records (and referred to as EHR hereafter), "are not merely digitized versions of paper records" (Sade, 2010, p. 40). Electronic records contain "large amounts of highly detailed clinical information," they are extremely compact, can be easily stored and rapidly transmitted between healthcare professionals and institutions (Sade, 2010, p. 40). Paper medical records do not present these characteristics; they are usually official forms and charts found in one central location, limited to each institution housing its own set of records for each individual served by the organization. Breaches of paper records usually do not occur outside of or beyond the individual organization. The potential for breaches of electronic records is much greater due to their inherent vulnerability. The characteristics which make them so attractive (ease of use, rapid transmission between providers, etc.) also make them potentially vulnerable. The USA Patriot Act of 2001 and the renewal of the law in 2006, made it

legal for the FBI to search confidential medical records as part of counterterrorism efforts (Landa, 2006). The HIPAA Privacy Rule does not restrict disclosure of de-identified health information, which may be used by law enforcement officials, making it easier for these officials to have access to private health information, without the knowledge or consent of the patient. The AMA Council on Ethical and Judicial Affairs does not address this concern at all (Sade, 2010).

In order to fully appreciate what is considered protected health information, one must read the statement on confidentiality or at least the Summary of the HIPAA Privacy Rule (U.S. DHHS, 1996). Protected health information refers to the protection of all "individually identifiable health information" held or transmitted by a covered entity or its business associates. This includes all forms: paper, electronic, and oral.

Individually identifiable health information is information, including demographics, that relates to:

1. The individual's past, present or future physical or mental health or condition.
2. The provision of health care to the individual.
3. The past, present or future payment for the provision of health care to the individual (U.S. DHHS, 1996, p. 1).

This information either identifies the individual or can be used to identify them. It includes common identifiers such as name, address, date of birth, and social security number. Excluded from protection are employment records that a covered entity (employer, insurance company) maintains in its capacity as employer, and "certain other records…defined in the Family Educational Rights and Privacy Act" (U.S. DHHS, 1996, p. 1). There are no restrictions on the use or disclosure of de-identified health information. De-identified information refers to health information that has been de-identified either by a formal determination by a qualified statistician, or by the removal of specified identifiers of the individual, their relatives, household members, and employment history, and is only used when the covered entity has no knowledge that the information could be used to identify the individual (U.S. DHHS, 1996). As mentioned in another article, de-identified health information may not be as protected or secure in the online environment as once thought (Sittig & Singh, 2011).

CASE DESCRIPTION

Protected Use of Private Health Information

The United States permits the sale of consumer health data that has been de-identified to private data collection industries for analysis, which is something that is severely restricted in most European countries (Anderson, 2007). Security of EHR's in the U. S. is, therefore, at greater risk than in other countries. A comparison of the United Kingdom's (UK) and Australia's systems, along with that of the U. S., will point out some of the differences involved in the implementation of nation-wide electronic health information databases. A review of protected uses of private health information in the U.S., followed by uses of Personal Health Records and social networking sites, is presented. An overview of psychiatric concerns is also discussed.

Among the ethical dilemmas posed by widespread use and implementation of electronic health records are questions about the ownership of protected health information. As stated earlier, HIPAA does not protect personal health information once it has become de-identified, but in the electronic environment, what protections exist to prevent this information from becoming re-identified? Several EHR vendors, including GE Healthcare and Allscripts, have sold de-identified copies of patient databases to pharmaceutical companies, medical device-makers, and medical researchers.

Furthermore, de-identified data "can often be re-identified using publically available external data sources" (Sittig & Singh, 2011, p. e1044). So the question of what role does research play in the use of electronic records must be considered. If de-identified information can be used in medical research, without protection or patient consent, how does this affect the integrity of the research? The Common Rule, the Federal Policy for the Protection of Human Subjects, which predates HIPAA, allows de-identification of data for current and future studies where patients have given their consent. The HIPAA Privacy Rule prohibits patients' consent for future studies, but provides no safeguards unless the organization is a 'covered entity,' meaning data held by health plans, clearinghouses, or health care providers. All other information held by non-covered entities (data management and pharmaceutical companies) remains unregulated. The Institute of Medicine recently determined that the HIPAA Privacy Rule does not adequately safeguard patient privacy and can seriously impede quality medical research (Gostin & Nass, 2009). Due to the stringent consent features in the HIPAA Privacy Rule, more terminally ill patients are missing out of potential life-saving opportunities through participation in clinical trials. In the United States, medical research carried out by government agencies is subject to more strict regulatory oversight than is research carried out by private corporations, causing additional inconsistencies. Most other countries do not make this distinction (Gostin & Nass, 2009).

Health care service providers agree that EHRs will improve a caregiver's decision making and a patient's outcomes, but to achieve the potential value of using EHRs, they need to be administered in a meaningful way. The Centers for Medicare and Medicaid Services (CMS) and the Department of Health and Human Services (DHHS) are charged with developing specific "meaningful use" objectives as part of the HITECH Act of 2009. The purpose of "meaningful use" objectives is to achieve significant improvements and advancements in healthcare by implementing use of EHRs. Meaningful use objectives will be tied to payments to health care providers by the Centers for Medicare and Medicaid Services (Blumenthal &Tavenner, 2010; "HITECH," 2009). With the meaningful use rule in place, DHHS hopes that it will create a private and secure electronic health information system for the 21st century. It still remains to be seen, however, if the CMS is ready to oversee the collection, aggregation, verification, and analysis of the data needed for this secure and private system.

The widespread adoption of EHRs, as outlined in the HITECH Act, will allow for improvements in medical research by giving researchers access to "real-time population data" (Pearson, Brownstein & Brownstein, 2011, p. 199) by including such descriptive information as Body/Mass Index (BMI), smoking status, and alcohol use. Administrative databases, such as insurance company databases, have been using electronic billing of prescriptions for years in the U.S., but this hasn't previously been linked with physician-oriented medical records that can provide co-existing conditions, ethnicity, health behaviors, and other important conditions (Pearson et al., 2011). Combining these existing records into one electronic record can greatly improve the potential for better healthcare monitoring and collection of research. Adding the patient-controlled Personal Health Record (PHR) will allow patients to have better access and control over their health information and thus, increase participation in their own care (Halamka, Mandl & Tang, 2008; Pearson et al., 2011). The authors of both these studies also believe that access through patient consent, even for de-identified or aggregated data, will allay concern of data privacy and confidentiality, while empowering and engaging patients (Halamka et al., 2008; Pearson et al., 2011).

Personal Health Records, Social Network Health Sites, Health Record Trusts

The Personal Health Record (PHR) and social networking sites have been used to advance medical research. Unlike those who are concerned about their private, previously identified health information that may have the potential for being re-identified by third parties, there are those who are advocating for, even advertising, their own private health information to be used for medical research. Social networking sites, such as TuDiabetes or PatientsLikeMe, enable patients to monitor their symptoms and therapy regimens (Pearson et al., 2011). Information at these sites is shared with other users, seemingly without much regard to their own privacy. The ability to conduct research into patient behaviors is greatly expanded. Information generated by these sites is "already of great interest to pharmaceutical companies and public health researchers" (Pearson et al., 2011, p. 197). What is not mentioned is: are there currently any guidelines set at these sites to address potential litigation? If so, are the Web sites in charge of monitoring their own adherence to their stated acceptable-use policies (Pearson et al., 2011; Ray & Wimilasiri, 2006)? Social networking health sites present a good way for patients to share experiences with others who have the same diagnoses, but they currently do not provide a great deal of privacy.

De-identified health information is something that is currently legally attainable via the Privacy Rule in the HIPAA law, so if this is amended, as suggested by researchers, it can affect medical research (Gostin & Nass, 2009). Among the benefits of expanding access to de-identified health information is having patients set up their own Personal Health Records, as part of their electronic health record. It is thought that access to this information "will increase the ability of health researchers to perform translational research, better understand clinical effectiveness of therapeutics, and open doors to increased understanding of environmental behavioral influences on diseases" (Pearson et al., 2011, p.197). Large databases, such as national EHRs, Medicaid, and HMO databases provide diverse populations for researchers to study a specific disease while comparing drug efficacy and its impact on ethnicity, age, location, and duration of use. Specifically mentioned is the large-scale use of EHRs in diabetes research in the United Kingdom and Canada (Pearson et al., 2011).

Personally controlled health records have been implemented in Australia's national healthcare system. The Personally Controlled Electronic Health Record (PCEHR) is a new initiative in Australia's National E-Health Transition Authority (NEHTA), and presents a new challenge to the traditional structure of health care (Spriggs, Arnold, Pearce, & Fry, 2012). PCEHRs shift control of personal health information from the provider to the patient, yet ethical questions surrounding this shift remain unanswered. MyChart is an electronic health record product that allows patients to review most of the contents of their medical records. MyChart has been used at the Palo Alto Medical Foundation in the U.S. since 2000 (Halamka et al., 2008). There has been some debate over specific information that should or should not be available for patient view or patient input. Some studies have indicated that allowing for greater patient involvement in electronic health records will solve many of the problems with patient privacy and confidentiality since the responsibility will now be with the patients themselves (Halamka et al., 2008; Spriggs et al., 2012).

Health Record Trusts present another way for patients to have a greater role in their personal health information. A health record trust or bank would give patients control over how broadly their health information is distributed and to whom. The health record trust is a way to provide additional privacy of health information that HIPAA fails to provide (Kendall, 2009). The idea that patients will be more confident that privacy will not be violated if they have more control over what information is being transmitted is reiterated in this study. Using patient health record trusts with patient privacy preferences will give patients the option to customize their health records, similar to that of a Web browser's settings. For added security, patients would be able to set up a health record trust account in a way comparable to some communities that have developed a regional health information organization (RHIO). Giving patients a default option that allows a balance between disclosing too much information and of not sharing relevant information, will, in the author's opinion, encourage more patient involvement with their healthcare (Kendall, 2009). A patient may choose to block transmission of information on an abortion, for example, to certain providers. Of course, there could be potential harm in not making all information available. A patient may choose not to disclose information on an infectious disease that may prove to have dire consequences in the future. This sort of picking and choosing on the part of patients could interfere with the integrity of the electronic health record if providers are not given the full complete medical record. A national effort to make electronic health systems interoperable would centralize this process and alleviate some of the guesswork involving which practitioner or clinician knows what – unless a patient chooses to edit certain information from certain providers. The amount of access patients have to the information available in their own health records remains to be determined.

Psychiatric Concerns of Electronic Health Records

Among the different types of physician specialists polled regarding use of electronic health records, psychiatrists and other mental health professionals weighed in with the greatest hesitation. "In a survey of outpatient physicians, psychiatrists were the least likely to use EHRs" (Salomon, et.al, 2009, p.55). The perception of risks from breaches in data security is greater in the psychiatric setting among not only patients, but psychiatrists as well. Interestingly, when psychiatrists were asked about having their own psychiatric record included with the general medical record and made available to other providers, 50% of those surveyed "strongly" stated they did not want their own personal psychiatric record included while another 20% "disagreed" with its inclusion (Salomon et al., 2009). Among the reasons given for their concerns was that the information would be misunderstood by non-mental health providers. Overall, though, use of electronic health records is seen as helpful to the patient/psychiatrist relationship. They caution that, although the records may seem to be more complete, they may also be less factual. They argue that the records "may be getting more of the non-sensitive data… without an increase in clinically important but more sensitive detail" (Salomon et al., 2009, p. 59).

The sensitive nature of the psychiatric record is discussed. It is noted that data pertaining to the subjective narrative of progress notes, when electronic, "heighten risks from diverse threats, ranging from breaches in data security to unintentional data misuse or misinterpretation by non-psychiatric clinicians and other professionals" (Salomon et al., 2009, p. 54). Subjective progress notes often contain extremely personal information such as life histories, perceptions, experiences, and thoughts, which can be of a highly sensitive nature (Salomon et al., 2009; Stewart, Kroth, Schuyler, & Bailey, 2010). Regarding the security of electronic records, the administrators of clinics using EHRs need to establish who will have access to these records, based on their qualifications. The authors identify issues such as whether employees of hospitals and clinics, who are not involved directly with psychiatric patients, should have access to the EHR. Rules regarding the release of an individual EHR to third party payers (such as insurance companies) need to be investigated,

along with the transition from paper to electronic format. Patients may also choose to find mental health providers who are not part of their primary care networks (Salomon et al., 2009).

The patient/psychiatrist relationship is more concerned with privacy and confidentiality issues than other types of medical research due to the continued stigma placed on those with mental illness (Salomon et al., 2009; Stewart et al., 2010). A survey involving adult outpatients with chronic mental illness was conducted. Patients were asked to volunteer to participate in a before and after satisfaction survey on the implementation of electronic health records at a university medical clinic. The survey used a modified Rand Corporation previously validated Patient Satisfaction Questionnaire -18 (PSQ-18) as the starting point. The survey questions include areas such as: general satisfaction, technical quality, interpersonal manner, communication, time spent with psychiatrist, anxiety, computer use, and confidentiality. The pre- and post-test questionnaires were the same. There were 149 pre-EHR implementation surveys and 137 post-implementation surveys completed. Contrary to what the authors expected, they found no negative reactions to the use of EHRs: "we found no change in patient satisfaction in the Communication and Education, Confidentiality, Anxiety, or any other satisfaction subscales" (Stewart et al., 2010, p. 5). However, the findings could indicate that EHR use truly has no negative impact on the patient/psychiatrist relationship, or it could be due to limitations of the study (Stewart et al., 2010).

The study was approached with an awareness of the stigma of mental illness, believing that this would influence and "magnify" (Stewart et al., 2010, p. 2) patient concerns about confidentiality, which could lead to less truthful communication between patient and psychiatrist. There were concerns that anxiety about the use of EHRs could exacerbate anxiety-related illnesses, such as depression, bipolar disorder, schizophrenia, and post-traumatic stress disorder. It was even "hypothesized that EHR use would decrease patient satisfaction scores" (Stewart et al., 2010, p. 2), which were not found. The conclusion the researchers made was that while communication is a top priority in the patient/psychiatrist relationship, electronic health record adoption, in and of itself, is not likely to present a disruption to patient satisfaction (Salomon et al., 2009; Stewart et al., 2010).

CURRENT CHALLENGES

Among the challenges to implementing a nationwide electronic health records database in the U. S. are patient access to medical records, meaningful use laws, and concerns of privacy and confidentiality. Regarding patient access, HIPAA mandates patients have access to their medical records, but it does not state how that access should be given (Halamka et al., 2008; U.S. DHHS, 1996). One suggested way is the Personal Health Record, easily created as part of the electronic health record and a goal of the HITECH Act that will be nationally implemented. However, this access raises questions such as to what information should be shared, how should patients be "authenticated," and how privacy will be protected (Halamka et al., 2008).

Several challenges shared among various healthcare organizations during the implementation phase of electronic health records include: (1) the sharing of the entire problem list, or medical record of diagnoses; (2) the sharing of the entire medication and allergy list; (3) the sharing of laboratory and diagnostic test results; (4) the sharing of clinical notes; (5) the authentication or verification of patients to access the Personal Health Record (PHR); (6) the creation of PHRs for minors establishing shared access via proxies; and (7) the capacity for secure clinician/patient messaging. These challenges were presented by clinicians and researchers at the Beth Israel Deaconess Medical Center and the Children's Hospital in Boston, Massachusetts and the Palo

Alto Medical Foundation in Palo Alto, California during the adoption and implementation phase of Personal Health Records (Children's Hospital Informatics Program, 2007; Halamka et al., 2008). The following information presents each issue with preliminary resolutions:

- Challenge number one regards the sharing of the complete list of medical problems and diagnoses. The sharing of psychiatric records was specifically debated, questioning if sharing would "impede patient therapy or erode trust in clinicians" (Halamka et al., 2008, p. 3). It was decided to share the entire record of diagnoses, but not to divulge the full psychiatric notes with the patient, hoping this would lead to helpful discussions among providers and patients.
- Challenge number two concerned access to the entire medication and allergy list. In Massachusetts, one of the states involved in the case studies, there are laws that prevent sharing of restricted drugs, such as HIV drugs, substance abuse treatment, and psychiatric disorder treatments from health plan databases. The laws do not restrict sharing provider or retail pharmacy data with patients, so it was decided to share the entire medication list with patients (Halamka et al., 2008).
- Challenge number three involved disclosing all laboratory and diagnostic test results. It was agreed that even though sharing this may sometimes bring negative news, all lab and test results, except those restricted by state laws, should be released. It was also noted that preference is given to the provider to review results prior to the information becoming available to the patient. Ideally, the provider would be able to "annotate, explain, or deliver the result verbally," to the patient (Halamka et al., 2008, p. 4).

- Challenge number four focused on releasing clinical notes to the patient. It was agreed among the three institutions surveyed in this case study not to share progress notes since a certain level of explanation is required for patients to understand their contents. Some clinicians also stated that the intent purpose of the progress note is not always meant to be shared.

- Challenge number five was concerned with authentication issues in order for patients to access the PHR. It was agreed that a username and password generated by each providing institution should be implemented since the U.S. does not have a national identifier system.

- Challenge number six involved the creation of private PHRs for minors and whether patients can share access via proxies. The three cases involved in this review chose to develop standard policies to address the issue of minors. At Children's Hospital Boston, where most patients are minors, the policy was divided by age groups. For patients under 12, the primary guardians have full access while patients themselves have limited or no access to the information. For those between 12 and 18 years old, both guardians and patients have access, but specific content may be restricted to either group. For those over 18 years, patients have complete access and control to their PHR, although they can still allow guardian access during the transition to adulthood (Children's Hospital Informatics Program, 2007; Halamka et al., 2008).

- Challenge number seven focused on allowing secure clinician/patient messaging. It was decided to enable clinician/patient secure messaging as part of the Personal Health Record. By restricting enrollment to patients who established physician/patient relationships, it was determined that "legal liability risk is minimal" (Halamka et al., 2008, p. 5).

The authors state that providing patient control of healthcare information is appealing because "it solves many of the privacy and consent issues faced by organizations" by putting the control in the patients' hands (Halamka et al., 2008, p. 7). Their experience with the three institutions presented, thus far, shows that personal health records that share data between provider and patient can be used successfully, but attention must be paid to privacy and security issues, data stewardship, and personal control.

Another study suggested that the problems of security and privacy could be solved by technical applications. Ray and Wimalasiri (2006) concentrate on privacy issues for EHR based on case studies in different parts of the world. Specifically, two cases were studied: HealthLink in Australia and HIPAA in the U. S. The HealthLink began in 2006 as a trial system in parts of Australia for people over 65 years old while simultaneously in another part of the country for people under 15 years old.

In the U. S., the study focused on the Privacy Rule of HIPAA. The authors' primary interest concerned the rules that "standardize the communication of electronic health information between healthcare providers and health insurers" (Ray & Wimalasiri, 2006, p. 4686). These communication applications have been electronic since the rules went into effect, while individual health records are still new to the electronic scene in the U. S. The rules in the Privacy Rule of HIPAA are intended to protect the privacy and security of individually identifiable health information (Ray & Wimalasiri, 2006; U.S.DHHS, 1996). The rules govern the use and disclosure of collected and protected health information.

Ray and Wimalasiri (2006) apply seven categories regarding privacy. They use their experience in e-business and apply this research to the medical model. The seven categories of privacy issues are: consent, transparency, control over record, collection limitation, data security, accuracy, and identifiers. A brief summary of the U.

Table 1. A summary of privacy issues in the United States and Australia

Consent	This category in the Australian model has an "opt-out" clause, which includes all medical information available on patients until the patient opts out of the electronic health record.
	HIPAA's Privacy Rule prohibits providers from disclosing information to healthcare administrators, but does not require consent for treatment; therefore, emergency care will be provided and no consent is required for transmission of electronic records from one provider to another.
Transparency	Transparency in Australia's system involves access to the EHR and disclosure of how the system works over the Internet.
	U. S. system states that healthcare providers can request full transcripts of EHR from other providers, but may not be aware of other requests.
Control	Control over Record involves controlling visibility of part of the record. Australia's model allows any participating provider to see the whole record. This also allows any healthcare provider access to any patient regardless if they are their providing physician.
	The U. S. model gives the individual the right to request an amendment or correction to the record, although they may not know how many copies exist.
Collection Limitation	Collection Limitation involves restricting the collection of some information. Australia's model does not allow the user the ability to select.
	In the U. S. model, users have no control over which parts of the record are visible to which providers.
Data Security	Any provider has access rights to any patient electronic health record. In Australia, this can mean that privacy breaches cannot be detected automatically.
	In the U. S., numerous HIPAA compliant organizations show a lack of training, education, and technical standard to privacy requirements, which lead to security and privacy breaches.
Accuracy	In Australia's HealthLink, users (patients) are allowed to access and verify contents of the electronic health record, and to modify information if necessary.
	In the U. S., HIPAA currently has no component to allow patients to access, verify, or modify.
Identifiers	Australia's HealthLink unambiguously links a person's medical information to that person.
	The U. S.'s Employer Identifier Rule of 2002 establishes a unique employer identifier.

S. and Australia's systems follows in Table 1. This summary compares how each country currently addresses the seven privacy issues.

One of the challenges when considering electronic records in the use of medical research is "when it is ethically acceptable to use private health information for public purposes" (Spriggs et al., 2012, p. 3). Several issues regarding the legitimate uses of personally controlled electronic health records (PCEHRs) are:

1. The acceptable secondary uses need to be defined in the domains of policy, research, audit, and public health.
2. The ways in which data will be used, stored, passed on, or sold to third parties need to be explored.

3. Guidelines will need to be developed for researchers and Human Research Ethics Committees to ensure ethical practices in using information from PCEHR's.

Additional issues regarding personal control, privacy, and consent are:

1. What constitutes informed consent and what is relevant information regarding advantages and disadvantages of having a PCEHR need to be identified.
2. How consent will be negotiated and recorded in virtual space needs to be addressed.
3. The issue of minors' access to PHRs and parent control to lock off information for or from their children need to be investigated.

4. Challenges of privacy and trust must be addressed to 'avoid deterring young people from seeking necessary healthcare.'
5. Research studies that collect biological samples and other data from children linked to continuously updated EHR's need to be explored (Spriggs et al., 2012, p. 4).

One of the strongest criticisms of the National Healthcare Services (NHS) Care Records Service, the national electronic health record system of the UK, has been its focus on technical issues and its "failure to adequately consider ethics" (Spriggs et al., 2012, p. 4). The authors of one study found that while acknowledging their strength in the technical and business end, the system does not address "specific ethical questions" that wide-spread use of electronic health records may encompass (Spriggs et al., 2012). They state that ethics and values have been cited as key factors in the failure of the UK health record system, listing several similarities and differences between the UK system and the proposed PCEHR system in Australia. Both systems include a health care summary that contains information such as current medications, adverse reactions, allergies, and immunizations. Both systems raise questions regarding transparency of how health data will be used, stored, or passed on, or sold to third parties.

Several key themes found in the UK system of electronic records, and highlighted in a study conducted by Robertson et al. (2010), need to be addressed:

- How the NHS Care Records Service has evolved.
- Hospital staff consensus on the type of electronic record or scale of data sharing.
- Increasing uncertainties on the future of the current program.
- Adverse consequences of centrally negotiated contracts.

- Tailored systems to meet needs of particular organizations rather than standardized systems.
- The preference for community level implementation of EHR's and data sharing.

The authors of several studies agree that the original plan for the adoption of a large scale national electronic health records database in England "has faltered" (Robertson et al., 2010; Spriggs et al., 2012). The original plan in the UK was to use a "top-down" approach to administering the national database. This approach had to evolve, for reasons stated above, "into an approach that is more responsive to the circumstances… of individual health trusts" (Robertson et al., 2010, p. 9).

In contrast, the U. S. was a "bottom-up" approach that could "preserve existing local systems [and] interoperability standards" (Robertson et al., 2010, p. 10), which the top-down approach falls short. They argue, however, that conforming to the U. S. government's meaningful use clause may not allow for as much local control as suggested. The authors also feel that the bottom-up approach will not provide enough detail for any single, shared electronic record. The Australian model uses a "middle-out" approach, balancing central support for national goals with incentives that can be used as encouragements to implement compliance in incremental steps with standards at the local level (Robertson et al., 2010). A number of recommendations are proposed to other countries looking to adopt national electronic health record databases, based on the experiences of those in the three countries studied. Among their recommendations are to adopt a "middle-out" approach that allows for a "balance between local level freedoms and constraints" (Robertson et al., 2010, p. 10) within the national requirements. They encourage public debate, flexibility, local adaptability, and warn that creating a national health care database is best when conceived in incremental stages that will take many years to complete.

SOLUTIONS AND RECOMMENDATIONS

The proposed solutions to unintended privacy breaches of electronic health records include World Wide Web services securities and Extensible Markup Language (XML)-based securities. Since the American model uses a provider-driven electronic health record, Ray and Wimalasiri (2006) recommend the Web services "Service Orientated Architecture" technology and security features that "provides additional support for its use within a healthcare architecture" (p. 4688). The Service Orientated Architecture involves breaking down the EHR into individual business functions and extending the functionality of specifications to meet requirements of the healthcare industry. In other words, they suggest molding the software to fit the provider-based healthcare model currently in operation in the U. S. via HIPAA. The XML-based security standards include:

1. XML Key Management Services, which use digital signatures to authenticate sources.
2. XML Encryption, which protects privacy of the message.
3. XML Key Management Services, representing key registration and validation (Ray & Wimalasiri, 2006, p. 4689).

The electronic health record will be in the form of an XML document, which can be transmitted allowing for additional security measures in the form of encryption, if needed. The encrypted elements within the XML document will be readable and accessed only by providers with the appropriate key or access rights. This type of encryption and transmission of sensitive medical information will be able to keep semantic information intact, which is beneficial, especially in a psychiatric environment.

However, an over-reliance on electronic solutions will not work without making some changes to specific wording in some existing contracts with Health Information Technology (HIT) vendors. For some physician practices that have already set up electronic health records, they found a "hold harmless" clause existed in their contracts. "Vendors shifted liability to users and inserted other contractual language that effectively concealed from users the fuller knowledge of serious faults in their HIT systems" (Koppel & Kreda, 2009, p. 1278). They found that this "hold harmless" clause included not only mistakes that were not the fault of the vendors, but also serious patient safety errors that should have been addressed by their software programs (Koppel & Kreda, 2009).

Platform for Privacy Preferences (P3P) is another privacy option that consumers have. Patients who access healthcare-related sites over the Web will often run into this privacy statement. P3P was developed as a Web industry standard "to provide an automated way for users to gain more control over the use of personal information on the Website they visit" (Ray & Wimalasiri, 2006, p. 4689). However, it was not designed to protect privacy of health information in healthcare. The software does not have the capability to monitor whether Web sites adhere to their own stated policies (Ray & Wimalasiri, 2006). The authors conclude that although there are some promising beginnings with technical applications to address privacy issues of personal health information, a more comprehensive solution is required. A solution that can encompass various technological, legal, and social factors is needed; one that would have the ability to verify and enforce privacy policies stated by the Web site would be most beneficial.

This analysis of the literature of the legal and ethical considerations in the adoption of electronic health record databases concludes with several recommendations. Care needs to be given to choice of vendor who will carry out the transference from paper to electronic format. A thorough investigation into each vendor's policies relating to patient confidentiality, security, and safety should be undertaken before any agreements are signed. The electronic healthcare environment is not just the same as paper-based. Vendors who do not adhere to local and national laws, even unwittingly, regarding patient privacy should not be "held harmless" (Koppel & Kreda, 2009) due to software limitations, but instead the software must be written so that it conforms to requirements of the healthcare industry (Ray & Wimilasiri, 2006). Rules and standards should be implemented to address the unique problems that will arise in the adoption of a national health record database system. Finally, sharing experiences with other countries, especially similar countries to the UK and Australia, could alleviate some of the common problems inherent in the electronic healthcare environment.

REFERENCES

Act Enforcement Interim Final Rule, H. I. T. E. C. H. (2009, October 30)... *Federal Register, 74*(209). Retrieved from http://www.hhs.gov/ocr/privacy/hipaa/administrative/enforcementrule/enfifr.pdf

Anderson, J. G. (2007). Social, ethical and legal barriers to e-health. *International Journal of Medical Informatics, 76,* 480–483. doi:10.1016/j.ijmedinf.2006.09.016 PMID:17064955

Blumenthal, D., & Tavenner, M. (2010). The "meaningful use" regulation for electronic health records. *The New England Journal of Medicine, 363*(6), 501–504. doi:10.1056/NEJMp1006114 PMID:20647183

Centers for Medicare & Medicaid Services. (2012, June 19). *Press release.* Retrieved from http://cms.gov/pf/

Children's Hospital Informatics Program. (2007). *Indivo.* Retrieved from chip.org

Gostin, L. O., & Nass, S. (2009). Reforming the HIPAA privacy rule: Safeguarding privacy and promoting research. *Journal of the American Medical Association, 301*(13), 1373–1375. doi:10.1001/jama.2009.424 PMID:19336713

Halamka, J. D., Mandl, K. D., & Tang, P. G. (2008). Early experiences with personal health records. *Journal of the American Medical Informatics Association, 15*(1), 1–7. doi:10.1197/jamia.M2562 PMID:17947615

Kendall, D. B. (2009). Protecting patient privacy through health record trusts. *Health Affairs, 28*(2), 444–446. Retrieved from content.healthaffairs.org doi:10.1377/hlthaff.28.2.444 PMID:19276001

Koppel, R., & Kreda, D. (2009). Health care information technology vendors' "hold harmless" clause: Implications for patients and clinicians. *Journal of the American Medical Association, 301*(12), 1276–1278. doi:10.1001/jama.2009.398 PMID:19318655

Landa, A. S. (2006, March 27). FBI retains access to medical records under the newly reauthorized patriot act. *American Medical News.* Retrieved from amednews.com

Pearson, J. F., Brownstein, C. A., & Brownstein, J. S. (2011). Potential for electronic health records and online social networking to redefine medical research. *Clinical Chemistry, 57*(2), 196–204. doi:10.1373/clinchem.2010.148668 PMID:21159898

Ray, P., & Wimalasiri, J. (2006, August). *The need for technical solutions for maintaining the privacy of EHR.* Paper presented at the 28th IEEE EMBS Annual International Conference. New York, NY. Retrieved from www.ieee.org/about/index

Robertson, A., Cresswell, K., Takian, A., Petrakaki, D., Crowe, S., & Cornford, T. et al. (2010). Implementation and adoption of nationwide electronic health records in secondary care in England. *British Medical Journal, 341*(4564), 1–12. PMID:20813822

Sade, R. M. (2010). Breaches of health information: Are electronic records different from paper records? *The Journal of Clinical Ethics, 21*(1), 39–41. PMID:20465074

Salomon, R. M., Blackford, J. U., Rosenbloom, S. T., Seidel, S., Clayton, E. W., Dilts, D. M., & Finder, S. G. (2009). Openness of patients' reporting with use of electronic records: Psychiatric clinicians' views. *Journal of the American Informatics Association, 17,* 54–60. doi:10.1197/jamia.M3341 PMID:20064802

Sittig, D. F., & Singh, H. (2011). Legal, ethical, and financial dilemmas in electronic health record adoption and use. *Pediatrics, 127,* e1042–e1047. Retrieved from pediatrics.aappublications.org doi:10.1542/peds.2010-2184 PMID:21422090

Spriggs, M., Arnold, M. V., Pearce, C. M., & Fry, C. (2012). Ethical questions must be considered for electronic health records. *Journal of Medical Ethics, 38*(9), 1–5. doi:10.1136/medethics-2011-100413 PMID:22573881

Stewart, R. F., Kroth, P. J., Schuyler, M., & Bailey, R. (2010). Do electronic health records affect the patient-psychiatrist relationship? A before & after study of psychiatric outpatients. *BioMedCentral Psychiatry, 10*(3), 1–9.

U.S. Department of Health and Humann Services (DHHS). (1996). *OCR privacy brief: Summary of the HIPAA privacy rule.* Retrieved from http://www.hhs.gov/ocr/privacy/hipaa/understanding/summary/privacysummary.pdf

KEY TERMS AND DEFINITIONS

Electronic Health Record: A collection of health information in electronic format, for individual patients or groups of patients, and also known as an Electronic Medical Record (EMR). It has the potential for storing large amounts of data and for being shared among many providers and networks.

Extensible Markup Language: A Web language that defines a set of rules for encoding documents for human and machine reading. XML encryption is a secure way of transmitting data over the Internet since it requires a validated signature and decrypting data to read.

Health Information Technology: Computer technology that provides the framework for the delivery and management of electronic health systems across many spectrums.

Health Information Technology for Economic and Clinical Health: Part of the American Recovery and Reinvestment Act of 2009, HITECH includes the nationwide transition to electronic health records in the U.S.

Health Insurance Portability and Accountability Act of 1996: This established provisions for the Department of Health and Human Services to adopt national standards of healthcare and serves as the main protection of patient privacy of healthcare in the U. S. via the Privacy Rule.

National Electronic-Health Transition Authority: The Australian agency in charge of their national transition to electronic health record format.

National Health System: The United Kingdom's agency that oversees all health care in the UK, including the transition to electronic health records.

Personal Health Record: An electronic health record that patients can access.

Personally Controlled Electronic Health Record: An electronic health record that is fully controlled by the patient, currently used in Australia as a component of their electronic health system.

Platform for Privacy Preferences: A Web protocol that informs users of a particular Web site's data management practices. Users who register their personal information will be prompted by the Web site to allow for the collection of certain privacy information.

This work was previously published in Cases on Electronic Records and Resource Management Implementation in Diverse Environments edited by Janice Krueger, pages 193-210 copyright year 2014 by Information Science Reference (an imprint of IGI Global).

Chapter 73
A Pharmaco–Cybernetics Approach to Patient Safety:
Identifying Adverse Drug Reactions through Unsupervised Machine Learning

Kevin Yi-Lwern Yap
National University of Singapore, Singapore

ABSTRACT

Pharmaco-cybernetics is an upcoming interdisciplinary field that supports our use of medicines and drugs through the combined use of computational technologies and techniques with human-computer-environment interactions to reduce or prevent drug-related problems. The advent of pharmaco-cybernetics has led to the development of various software, tools, and Internet applications that can be used by healthcare practitioners to deliver optimum pharmaceutical care and health-related outcomes. Patients are becoming more informed through health information on the Internet, which empowers them to better participate in the management of their own conditions. Focusing on patients with cancer, this chapter describes the use of a pharmaco-cybernetics approach to identify clinically relevant predictors of two debilitating adverse drug reactions, which are a cause of patient safety – chemotherapy-induced nausea and vomiting and febrile neutropenia. The early identification of such clinical predictors enables clinicians to prevent or reduce the occurrence of adverse drug reactions in cancer patients undergoing chemotherapy through appropriate management strategies. The computational methods used in this approach involve two unsupervised machine-learning techniques – principal component and multiple correspondence analyses. Using two case examples, this chapter shows the potential of machine-learning techniques for identifying patients who are at greater risks of these adverse drug reactions, thus enhancing patient safety. This chapter also aims to increase the awareness among healthcare professionals and clinician-scientists about the usefulness of such techniques in clinical patient populations, so that these can be considered as part of clinical care pathways to enhance patient safety and effectively manage cancer patients on chemotherapy.

DOI: 10.4018/978-1-4666-8756-1.ch073

INTRODUCTION

Pharmaceutical care is critical for improving medication management in patients, particularly those with chronic diseases. The practice of pharmaceutical care is the basis of clinical pharmacy and it involves identifying, preventing and solving drug-related problems with regards to patients' drug therapies (American Society of Hospital Pharmacists, 1993; Westerlund, Almarsdóttir, & Melander, 1999). Simply put, it helps patients make the best use of their medications. Drug-related problems exist in many forms, but essentially, they are events or circumstances involving drug therapies that can actually or potentially interfere with desired health outcomes (American Society of Hospital Pharmacists, 1993; van Mil, Westerlund, Hersberger, & Schaefer, 2004). Drug-related problems impact medication safety, and as a consequence, patient safety as well. The Pharmaceutical Care Network Europe Foundation categorizes drug-related problems in terms of problems and causes (Pharmaceutical Care Network Europe, 2010), while the American Society of Health-System Pharmacists classifies drug-related problems into eight main categories - see Figure 1. Drug-related problems can result due to a lack of knowledge or misinterpretation of drug information, which can compromise patients' safety and quality of life if not treated effectively and appropriately.

Cancer is a highly prevalent health problem with increasing incidence worldwide. In 2007, one in 8 deaths was due to cancer (Garcia et al., 2007). The global burden of cancer is also expected to grow to 27 million new cancer cases and 17.5 million cancer deaths by 2050 (Garcia et al., 2007). The rapid growth of informatics technologies and the World Wide Web in the last decade has enabled the development of many applications that can assist clinicians in delivering optimum pharmaceutical care and health-related outcomes. Patients with cancer are becoming more well informed through online health information that is readily accessible, and they can better participate in the management of their own conditions through knowledge obtained from the Internet. However, despite the advancement of informatics technologies, little has been done in clinical oncology practice to leverage on the use of these

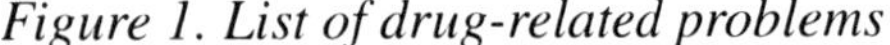

Figure 1. List of drug-related problems

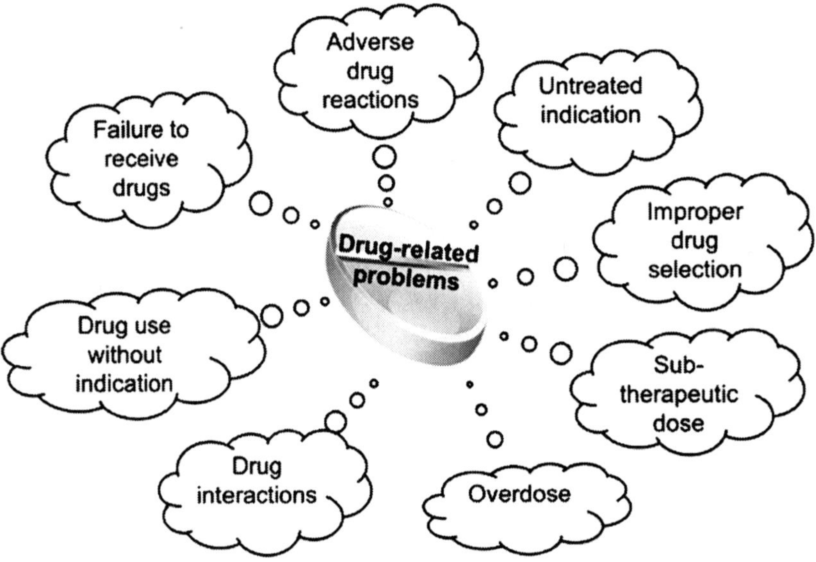

technologies to improve the pharmaceutical care of patients with cancer.

The advancement of informatics technologies has led to the development of various software, tools, and Internet applications that can be used by healthcare practitioners to deliver optimum pharmaceutical care and health-related outcomes. Pharmaco-informatics - the use of informatics and internet technologies to target drug-related problems - has changed the way in which healthcare is practiced (Yap, Chan, & Chui, 2009). Pharmaco-cybernetics, an upcoming interdisciplinary field, involves advanced skills and expertise to deal with technologies and human-computer-environment interactions in relation to the management of medicines and drugs (Yap et al., 2009). The term 'pharmaco' is derived from the Greek term 'pharmakon' meaning drugs or poisons, and 'cybernetics' comes from the Greek term 'kubernetes', which means 'the art of steering'. Cybernetics is a multi-disciplinary area that applies the principles of regulation and communication in the science of discovery and design, and has been applied in healthcare since the 1970s. However, the traditional concept of cybernetics has evolved into a modern theory known as 'new cybernetics', in which individuals build new knowledge through interactions with their environment. Thus, 'pharmaco-cybernetics' (also known as 'cybernetic pharmacy') aptly describes the science of supporting our use of medicines or drugs through the application of computational technologies and techniques, combined with the principles of human-computer-environment interaction, to reduce or prevent drug-related problems. This chapter illustrates how a pharmaco-cybernetics approach can be used to enhance the pharmaceutical care of patients with cancer using chemotherapy-related adverse drug reactions as its focus. The chapter will incorporate two case examples that have been carried out to illustrate how this approach can be applied in clinical practice. Although this chapter specifically targets clinical oncology practices, its concepts can be applied

to various healthcare fields, and would relevant to healthcare professionals and students/trainees in any field of the medical and health sciences.

BACKGROUND

Patients who are on certain chemotherapies tend to suffer from certain adverse drug reactions, of which chemotherapy-induced nausea and vomiting (CINV) is one of the most distressing (Rhodes & McDaniel, 2001; Stieler, Reichardt, Riess, & Oettle, 2003). The prevalence of CINV ranges from 13-58% for acute nausea and vomiting (NV lasting up to 24 hours after chemotherapy) and 15-75% for delayed nausea and vomiting (NV occurring after 24 hours and lasting up to 5 to 7 days) (Booth et al., 2007; Cohen, de Moor, Eisenberg, Ming, & Hu, 2007; Erazo Valle, Wisniewski, Figueroa Vadillo, Burke, & Martinez Corona, 2006; Grunberg et al., 2004; Liau et al., 2005; Molassiotis et al., 2008). CINV not only causes extreme discomfort in cancer patients, but it also impairs their quality of life (Bloechl-Daum, Deuson, Mavros, Hansen, & Herrstedt, 2006; Lindley et al., 1992; Roscoe et al., 2010; Schnell, 2003). Uncontrolled CINV can lead to metabolic imbalances and nutrient depletion in patients, as well as injury to the oesophageal tract (Bender et al., 2002; Cohen, et al., 2007; DiVall & Cersosimo, 2007). In addition, patients' fear of developing CINV can also de-motivate them to follow recommended treatment regimens, resulting in potential cessation of chemotherapy. On the other hand, patients who are non-adherent to their antiemetics may experience suboptimal CINV control (Chan, Low, & Yap, 2012). The uncontrolled CINV can cause patient safety issues and an increased risk of patient deterioration, as well as potentially increase the total direct and indirect costs of cancer treatments because of the use of additional antiemetics, hospitalisations and loss of productivity (Ballatori et al., 2007; Neymark & Crott, 2005). Effective management of CINV can prevent patients from unnecessary hospitalisations and expenditures (Wu, Graff, & Yuen, 2005). Thus, it is crucial that healthcare professionals manage CINV appropriately to prevent other complications.

There are multiple risk factors for CINV. These include the emesis potentials of chemotherapy regimens and patient-related factors - e.g. young age, females, prior CINV experiences, histories of morning and motion sickness, low alcohol use, presence of anxiety, fatigue and labyrinthitis (Hesketh, 1999; Lohr, 2008; Molassiotis, Yam, Yung, Chan, & Mok, 2002; National Comprehensive Cancer Network, 2011; Pollera & Giannarelli, 1989; Roscoe et al., 2010; Shih, Hee, & Chan, 2009). Some risk factors, such as anxiety and fatigue, are subjective in nature and difficult to quantify. Moreover, the methods of assessing certain risk factors have not been consistent in the literature. For example, studies assessing alcohol intake and CINV improvement have used different parameters for analysis, such as the quantities of alcohol consumed (more than 100g of ethanol per day or 5 mixed drinks per week) (Gralla et al., 1999; Hesketh, Aapro, Street, & Carides, 2010), or the use of alcohol-drinking categories (current versus non-current drinkers) (Needles et al., 1999). Methods of evaluating anxiety as a predictor of CINV have also ranged from a simple query to patients (Shih et al., 2009), to semi-structured interviews (Bergkvist & Wengström, 2006) and a combination of study scales and interviews (Molassiotis et al., 2002). Conflicting results have appeared in the literature. For example, anxiety has been reported to increase the intensity of nausea and vomiting, as well as the duration of delayed nausea in patients receiving emetogenic chemotherapy (Molassiotis, et al., 2002). On the other hand, studies have also suggested that patients with anxiety were less likely to experience acute nausea (Shih et al., 2009).

Objective instruments for assessing CINV risk factors, such as anxiety (Shek, 1993; Spielberger, Gorsuch, 1983) and fatigue (Mendoza et al., 1999; Minton & Stone, 2009), are not commonly used in the clinical setting to prescribe antiemetics due to time constraints during consultations, as well as the inconvenience of using the instruments. Oncology practitioners tend to prescribe antiemetics based on established clinical guidelines (ASHP Commission on Therapeutics, 1999; Kris et al., 2006; National Comprehensive Cancer Network, 2011; Roila, Hesketh, & Herrstedt, 2006), along with their clinical experience and professional judgement. Hence, clinicians need appropriate measures to better assess their patients' risks of CINV in daily practice.

Febrile neutropenia (FN, also known as neutropenic fever) is a serious complication of chemotherapy, especially in patients who receive myelosuppressive chemotherapy (National Comprehensive Cancer Network, 2012). Its incidence ranges from 6.3-25.0% in breast and lymphoma patients receiving myelosuppressive chemotherapies (Chan, Chen, Chiang, Tan, & Ng, 2011 August 5; Chan, Fu, et al., 2011; Chan, Leng, et al., 2011; Ng et al., 2011). The occurrence of FN may lead to undesired dose reductions of chemotherapies and treatment delays, which may compromise cancer treatment outcomes (Heuser & Ganser, 2005). Furthermore, events resulting from FN may also be associated with an increased financial burden and risk of mortality (Kuderer, Dale, Crawford, Cosler, & Lyman, 2006). Management of chemotherapy-induced FN generally involves the prophylactic use of granulocyte colony-stimulating factors (G-CSFs) in patients who are at risk (Aapro et al., 2006; National Comprehensive Cancer Network, 2012; Smith et al., 2006). However, patient-specific risk factors (e.g. advanced age, previous episodes of FN, bone marrow involvement with tumour), disease-related and chemotherapy-related characteristics affect its clinical outcome and should be considered during clinical management in patients. The multiple risk factors of FN tend to vary among different patients and in different populations. As with CINV, it is also not practical to obtain every risk factor for each patient in clinical practices. Hence, it is essential that clinically-relevant risk factors are identified for specific cancer populations.

The studies that are presented in this chapter relate to using a pharmaco-cybernetics approach to identify clinically-relevant predictors of CINV and FN through the use of computational modelling techniques (Chen, Chan, & Yap, 2013; Yap, Low, & Chan, 2012; Yap, Low, Chui, & Chan, 2012). The models used are based on unsupervised machine learning, mainly principal component analysis (PCA) and multiple correspondence analysis (MCA). Through a discussion of its concepts and applications in clinical oncology practice, this chapter aims to provide an awareness of the usefulness of such techniques among healthcare professionals for clinical patient populations. Readers are referred to these studies for further details.

MACHINE LEARNING AS A PHARMACO-CYBERNETICS TECHNIQUE IN PATIENTS WITH CANCER

Statistical learning theory characterizes the performance of learning machines based on their ability to predict future data (Evgeniou & Pontil, 2001). Machine learning is a field in artificial intelligence, originally conceived in the early 1960s, to design computational algorithms and techniques capable of inducing knowledge from data (Data Mining Articles). In general, there are two main types of machine learning techniques – supervised and unsupervised. In supervised learning, there is a set of training data (input objects) which predict a set of desired outputs. The output of the function can either be a continuous value (i.e. regression) or a class label of the input object (i.e. classification). In simple terms, based on a set of training examples (input and output data), the 'supervised learner' is able to predict the output value of any valid input object. On the other hand, unsupervised learning typically involves a model that is generated to fit observations. Unlike the former method, there is no a priori output for unsupervised machine learning. Therefore, interesting characteristics about the data set can be described from the observations without any predefined target.

This chapter focuses on the application of two unsupervised machine learning methods known as principal component analysis (PCA) and multiple correspondence analysis (MCA) in cancer patients. It also illustrates how such machine learning techniques may reduce patient safety risk and related incidents by investigating a combination of patient-related risk factors that can potentially predict whether patients will experience adverse drug reactions, such as CINV and FN, in the clinical setting. PCA is a multivariate projection technique that can investigate relationships among multiple variables and explain the causes of variance in a data set (Dunteman, 1989). The concept of PCA is to linearly transform an original set of variables (which translate to the risk factors of CINV and FN in the presented cases) into a substantially smaller set of uncorrelated variables known as principal components (PCs), which represent most of the information in the original set of data. Two correlated variables can be combined into 1 PC which maximizes the rotation of the original variable spaces. This process runs consecutively, resulting in a number of consecutive PCs that are independent and maximizes the remaining variability that is not captured by the preceding component (Cengiz & Kuruoğlu, 2006). In essence, the data is 'simplified' in PCA so that the data can be classified, and relationships and/ or similarities among the variables can be found.

The data for PCA can be represented by a data matrix (R) for a set of "P" variables as a function of the eigenvalues (λ) and eigenvectors (a), shown by the following equation:

$$R = \sum_{i=1}^{p} \lambda_i a_i a'_i \qquad (1)$$

In the equation, the eigenvalues and eigenvectors explain the variation and the weighting of the variables in the data set. The amount of variance explained by a PC is the ratio of its eigenvalue over the number of variables, expressed as a percentage. The number of PCs to represent the variation in the data set is usually determined using Jolliffe's eigenvalue cut-off criteria of either 0.7 or 0.7 of the average eigenvalue for correlation and covariance matrices respectively, Catell's scree plot principle, or an 80% variance cut-off (Dunteman, 1989).

Figure 2 shows an illustration of how PCA can be applied to a set of data. For 'n' variables, every variable (e.g. risk factors for CINV or FN) can be plotted for each patient in 'n-dimensional' space. PCA reduces the data into a smaller subset of variables that can represent majority of the variation in the whole data set. Let's simplify matters by considering 3 variables to represent the overall risks of patients experiencing an adverse drug reaction. Each patient can be plotted in 3-dimensional space based on the PC scores of the variables. The plotted data is centred to vary around zero and a hypothetical line of best fit (PC) can be drawn in the 3-dimensional space to explain the variation in the whole data set. PC1 (dotted and dashed line) gives the direction of maximum variance, while PC2 (dashed line) is at right angles to PC1 and oriented to the direction which gives the maximum remaining variability. Similarly, PC3 (solid line) can be drawn at right angles to both PCs 1 and 2. This process repeats for the remaining PCs until the rest of the variability in the data set is explained. As shown in the figure, all the PCs have a common origin of centred data. Furthermore, since the PCs are perpendicular to each other, the variables are uncorrelated. The eigenvalues (variation) or the eigenvectors (weighting) of the variables can then be used to interpret the PC data.

In recent years, PCA has been an upcoming technique in the field of oncology. For example, this method has been used to evaluate symptom clusters in patients suffering from bone and brain metastases (Chow et al., 2008; Hadi et al., 2008). Another similar method, known as factor analysis, has also been used to identify symptom clusters in lung cancer patients (Gift, Jablonski, Stommel, & Given, 2004; Wang, Tsai, Chen, Lin, & Lin, 2008). Albeit the fact that both methods try to explain the variation in an observed variable set there are important differences between them. Factor analysis separates the total variance into a common and unique variance based on an underlying statistical model. It focuses on explaining the common variance in the observed variables based on a few underlying factors (Dunteman, 1989; Floyd & Widaman, 1995). In contrast, PCA does not assume an underlying statistical model and it focuses on explaining the total variation in the set of observed variables.

Multiple correspondence analysis (MCA), another multivariate technique for exploring data, is similar to PCA but is catered towards discretized categorical data. It allows the analysis of data matrices with non-negative values, and usually involves frequency tables or counts (M. Greenacre & Blasius, 2006). Cross tables of multiple sets of variables are assembled into a supermatrix called the Burt matrix. On the other hand, the original data can also be used to construct an indicator matrix. MCA involves the correspondence analysis algorithm applied to the Burt or indicator matrix. This technique examines the relationships within a set of variables and converts the data matrix into a graphical representation whereby the rows (i.e. patients in the case examples) and columns (variables) are depicted as points (M. Greenacre & Hastie, 1987; M. J. Greenacre, 1991). For more details on this technique, readers are referred to the concepts and examples provided by Greenacre and Blasius (M. Greenacre & Blasius, 2006).

Figure 2. Concept of PCA

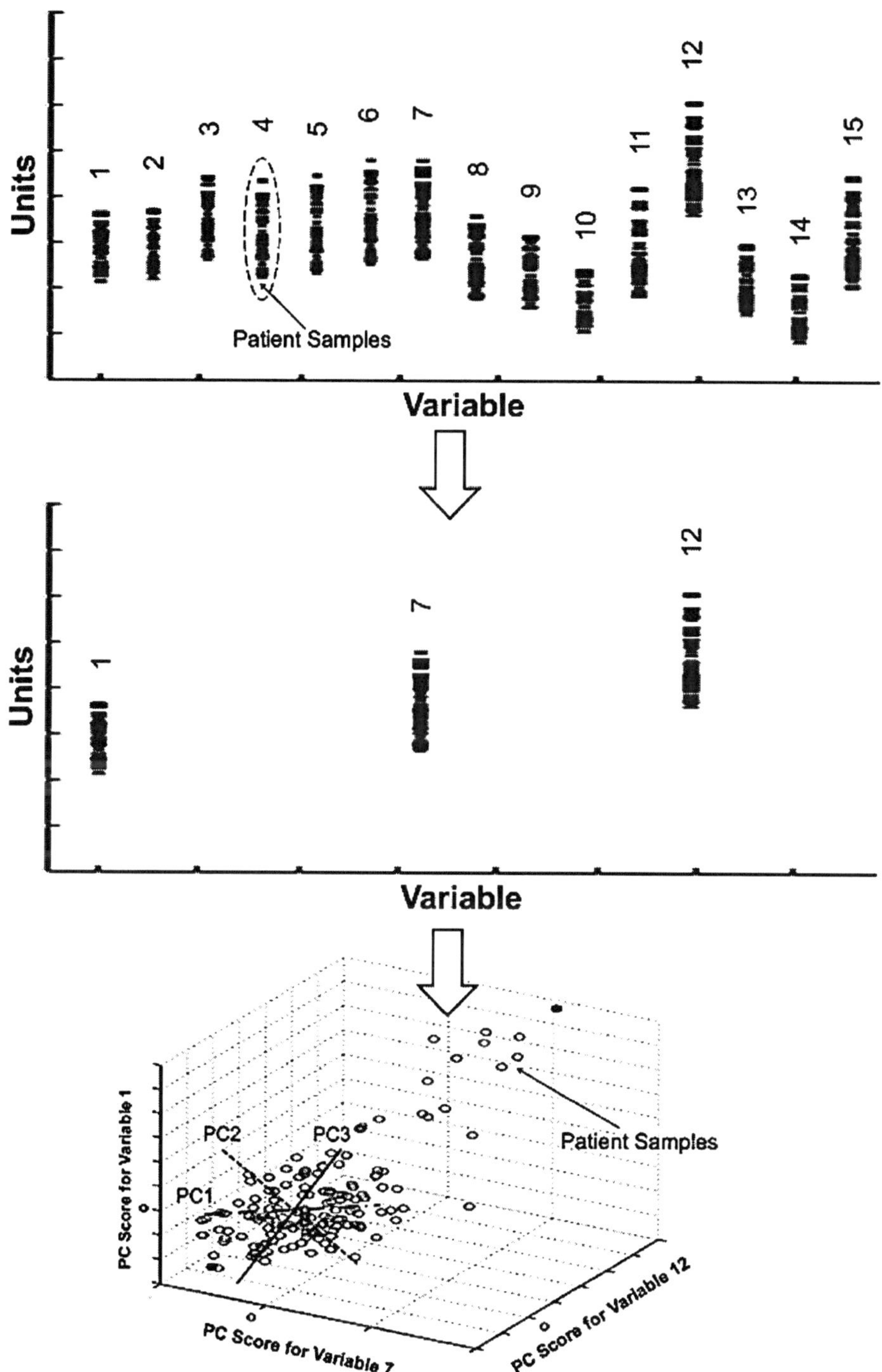

APPLICATION OF PHARMACO-CYBERNETICS IN THE PREDICTION OF ADVERSE DRUG REACTIONS

Case Example: Prediction of CINV

In a clinical study of over 700 cancer patients receiving a variety of chemotherapy regimen cocktails with different emetic potentials, PCA was used to identify the risk factors that could potentially predict patients' risks of CINV with regards to various clinical CINV endpoints involving vomiting and nausea responses (Yap, Low, & Chan, 2012; Yap, Low, Chui, et al., 2012). Five out of 12 risk factors were identified to played important roles in terms of distinguishing the clinical endpoints for patients on chemotherapy regimens with high or moderate emetic (i.e. vomiting) potentials – history of alcohol drinking, history of chemotherapy-induced nausea, history of chemotherapy-induced vomiting, fatigue and female gender (Yap, Low, & Chan, 2012). The period of drinking (classified as ex-/current drinkers) managed to differentiate CINV in patients on highly emetic regimens, while the frequency of drinking (social/ current drinkers) accounted for regimens that were moderately emetogenic.

In addition, PCA was also used to assess anxiety in these patients through a clinical instrument (i.e. the Beck anxiety inventory) (Yap, Low, Chui, et al., 2012). Among 21 anxiety symptoms categorized into 4 main domains (autonomic, neuro-physiological, panic and subjective), 7 symptoms were identified as potential predictors of CINV. Generally, symptoms that belonged to the panic and subjective domains were more able to differentiate cancer patients with and without the CINV endpoints. In particular, the 7 symptoms identified were feeling faint, having a fear of dying, fear of the worst, hot/cold sweats, nervousness, numbness, and being unable to relax.

According to the authors, there were no studies that had compared CINV risk factors in much detail, both in terms of breath and depth, prior to

their study. Other studies have generally concentrated on analysing individual risk factors or a variety of separate risk factors (George Dranitsaris et al., 2009; P. J. Hesketh, et al., 2010; Molassiotis, et al., 2002; Osoba et al., 1997; Petrella et al., 2009; Roscoe, et al., 2010; Warr, Street, & Carides, 2011), but their study managed to analyse a combination of 12 risk factors in a variety of chemotherapy regimens with different emetic potentials, all through the use of unsupervised machine learning. In the literature, some authors have suggested that data is usually not collected without an a priori idea on the relationship among the variables (Floyd & Widaman, 1995). However, in this case, the evidences for some of the risk factors identified in previous studies assessing CINV have been sparse. Moreover, the results of studies that have analysed anxiety as a risk factor have been inconsistent (Bergkvist & Wengström, 2006; Molassiotis, et al., 2002; Shih, et al., 2009). Without having an idea on whether these factors (e.g. anxiety) were positively or negatively correlated with CINV, PCA was potentially a useful technique to 'visualise' the data of these cancer patients for CINV risks. The results presented by the authors not only contributed to the current CINV literature, but also gave an insight to oncology clinicians regarding the specific risk factors that could potentially be used for the assessment of CINV risk in cancer patients in their clinical practices. Effective management strategies (e.g. prescribing appropriate antiemetics) can then be taken to prevent or reduce the occurrence of uncontrolled CINV in patients at high risk, thereby improving their safety profiles.

Case Example: Prediction of Febrile Neutropenia

In another study which pooled data from 4 cancer registries, PCA and MCA were utilised to identify the risk factors of FN occurrence in over 500 patients with different cancers receiving a variety of chemotherapy regimens (Chen, et al.,

2013). Based on 28 variables that included demographics, medical histories, disease-related and chemotherapy-related parameters, as well as the haematological, hepatic and renal characteristics of the patients, those that were clinically predictive of FN included the cancer type, chemotherapy regimen, liver and kidney function tests, prior use of G-CSFs and the presence of diabetes mellitus. In terms of chemotherapy regimens, those that were anthracycline-based or taxane-based were more predictive of FN occurrence. In relation to the types of cancer, lymphomas were more predictive than breast cancers. With regards to the liver and kidney characteristics of patients, the clinically-relevant parameters were levels of alanine transaminase, alkaline phosphatase and serum creatinine. The PCA results showed that liver impairment explained a higher proportion of the variation for FN occurrence than kidney impairment in the cancer patients. Patients with poor hepatic functions who were on anthracycline-based or taxane-based regimens could have been at a higher risk of experiencing FN due to the higher exposure of the chemotherapy agents. Extrapolating this scenario to clinical oncology practices, if clinicians are aware of these risk factors in their patients, appropriate management plans such as dosage adjustments of the chemotherapy agents can be taken.

The results of this study supported several recent risk models that have been developed for predicting chemotherapy-induced FN (G. Dranitsaris et al., 2008; Pettengell et al., 2009; Ziepert, Schmits, Trumper, Pfreundschuh, & Loeffler, 2008), even though conflict may exist with regards to certain characteristics. The use of PCA and MCA also allowed the identification of other risk factors that were predictive of patients with FN risks, such as diabetes and prior G-CSF use. In the PCA technique for this study, a subset of the variables, called principal variables, was used to represent the data variation. These principal variables were represented by the risk factors that had the highest loadings on their corresponding PCs. Principal variables that were unique to the FN positive group were identified as potential clinical predictors. Additionally, principal variables that were identified in both the positive and negative FN groups were further 'visualised' by MCA using a joint plot. Essentially, principal variables that were grouped within the vicinity of the FN endpoints (with and without FN) were more likely to be predictors of FN and non-FN respectively. Readers are referred to the study for further details about the visual plot (Chen, et al., 2013).

The predictors identified in this study through the PCA and MCA approaches are clinically significant due to the fact that it can compromise the safety of cancer patients. Besides identifying predictors that were consistent with the literature (e.g. types of cancers) (Pettengell, et al., 2009; Pettengell et al., 2008; Ziepert, et al., 2008), these techniques also managed to identify other predictors such as liver and kidney dysfunctions, and other chronic conditions such as diabetes mellitus, all of which can affect patient safety. Many anticancer drugs are metabolised by the liver and excreted by the kidneys. As such, dose reductions may be needed to avoid increased drug toxicities due to delayed drug clearances. For example, the anticancer agent etoposide may prone patients with kidney dysfunctions to an increased risk of haematologic toxicities (Joel, Shah, Clark, & Slevin, 1996). On the other hand, anthracycline-based or taxane-based regimens can also pose a greater risk of systemic toxicities to patients with liver dysfunctions (Chen, et al., 2013). Furthermore, the presence of uncontrolled diabetes in patients may lead to poorly resolved infections or unhealed wounds, which may further increase their risks for FN (Srokowski, Fang, Hortobagyi, & Giordano, 2009). Identification of such predictors through PCA and MCA not only contributes to the sparse literature on the modelling of FN predictors, but also provides a basis for clinicians to optimise their G-CSF therapies in appropriate patients.

IMPLICATIONS TO PATIENT SAFETY

Adverse drug reactions play a role in medication safety, which can consequently impact patient safety. Medication safety is an international concern and increased attention has been focused on patient safety in recent years (Carayon & Wood, 2010). However, the paucity of reliable data, challenges in improving electronic healthcare systems, and difficulty in engaging clinicians to participate in patient safety efforts have hindered the progress of enhancing patient safety in various organisations and at the national level (Carayon & Wood, 2010). The paradigm shift towards patient-centred care has changed the safety climate of healthcare institutions, and increased the awareness among healthcare professionals regarding the need to target both patient care and safety. Studies have suggested that even though patients themselves have the potential to improve safety, several barriers exist. These include their lack of health-related knowledge and confidence, sociodemographic factors and inertia to accept the new patient role (Ward et al., 2011). Oncology clinicians can work together with patients to enhance the safety culture in the field if they keep abreast with upcoming interventions that can target the underlying causes of patient safety, of which PCA and MCA are examples. Based on the Eindhoven Classification Model (Smits, Groenewegen, Timmermans, van der Wal, & Wagner, 2009), these methods of data reduction can identify and streamline the relevant characteristics that predispose cancer patients to adverse drug reactions such as CINV and FN. Working in multidisciplinary teams also allows the facilitation of knowledge transfer through the sharing of information regarding the applicability and usefulness of these methods in clinical oncology practices. As exemplified by the case examples described in this chapter, the incorporation of machine learning techniques as part of clinical management pathways is definitely attractive and can potentially provide a "slice" to the Swiss cheese model of safety incidents (Perneger, 2005), so that patient safety can be enhanced.

FUTURE DIRECTIONS

Supervised machine learning (e.g. linear discriminate analysis, k nearest neighbours, decision trees, neural networks, etc) is becoming popular in the development of classification and regression models in healthcare (Burges, 1998; Cortes & Vapnik, 1995; Evgeniou & Pontil, 2001). Among them, support vector machines (SVMs) are useful as generalized linear classifiers for the prediction of future data (Evgeniou & Pontil, 2001). Through the solving of constrained quadratic optimisation problems, SVMs can be applied in clinical practices to predict certain health-related outcomes based on various patient parameters.

In SVMs, the data of interest in a training set is mapped into higher dimensional space. A hyperplane which separates the positive and negative data is constructed (Figure 3). On each side of the separating hyperplane, parallel hyperplanes are constructed and these are based on the support vectors (dark circles and triangles in the figure). The resultant optimal margin defines the largest separation between the 2 classes of data. Thus an unknown test pattern can be classified once the SVM is applied, depending on the side of the separating hyperplane in which it lies.

The advantage of SVMs is their relatively low sensitivities to overfitting of data, even when a large number of redundant and overlapping descriptors are used. This advantage makes this method particularly useful for prediction of adverse drug reactions since some of patient risk factors that have been reported are scarce in the literature. However, large numbers of samples are required for the classification system to be developed and irrelevant descriptors may reduce the accuracy of the prediction algorithm, thereby limiting the usefulness of this method in datasets which have small patient numbers. It has been suggested that suitable sample sizes for such techniques should be of a subject-to-variable ratio of approximately 5:1 to 10:1 (Osborne & Costello, 2004). Nevertheless, machine learn-

Figure 3. Concept of SVM

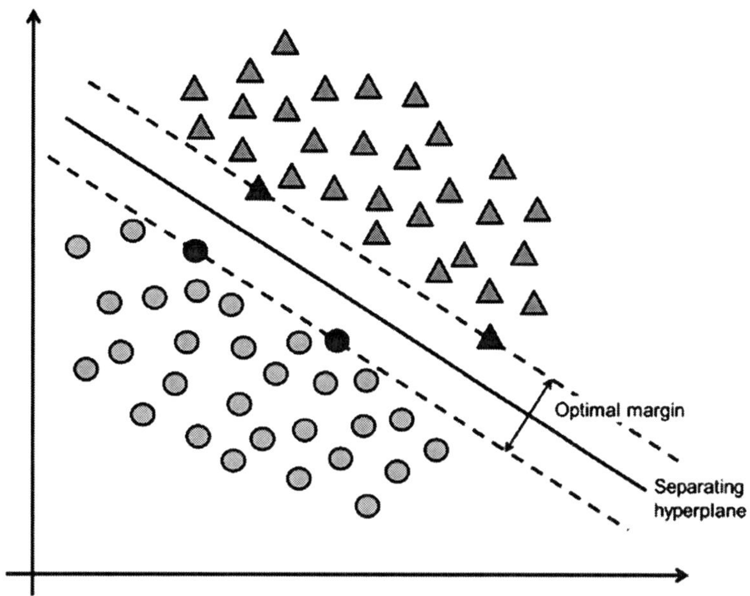

ing techniques, such as SVMs, are attractive for determining clinical predictors of health-related outcomes in various chronic diseases; and can potentially be powerful methods of analysis when combined with prospective collection of patient data through large-scale clinical studies or trials.

CONCLUSION

This chapter has demonstrated how a pharmaco-cybernetics approach can fill the 'gap' in clinical practice as an aid to healthcare professionals for improving the pharmaceutical care and safety of patients. The concepts of unsupervised machine learning as a pharmaco-cybernetics technique are illustrated through the identification of risk factors that can potentially predict chemotherapy-induced adverse drug reactions in clinical patient populations. Even though the studies presented in this chapter are exploratory in nature, they demonstrate the utility of such multivariate projection techniques for the prevention and management of drug-related problems, as well as improvements in patient safety by reducing the probability of adverse drug reactions and a reduction in the amount and frequency of clinical interventions that can result as a consequence, which may predispose the patient to other medical errors. I hope that these case examples will increase the awareness among clinicians and clinician-scientists regarding the importance of identifying clinically-relevant predictors in patients suffering from debilitating side-effects, such as CINV and FN. By knowing these predictors, patients who are at greater risks of these adverse effects can be identified, thereby allowing clinicians to effectively plan their management strategies for these patients. Furthermore, these case examples can provide a foundation for future research to be carried out so that the roles of these predictors can be better established.

There is a huge potential for healthcare technologies and informatics techniques to change healthcare practices in the near future. Advancement in informatics and cybernetics has led to the 'computerised tailoring' of health information in the attempt to cater towards individualised healthcare (Park, McDaniel, & Jung, 2009). With upcoming specialised fields in genomics, epigenetics and metabolomics, among others, tailorised care will likely be a better fit to the patients' physiology and care needs. The health information generated from these domains will also improve the patients' safety profiles. However, many of these technologies and techniques are still in its infancy and more detailed analysis is required to ensure that the PCA and MCA approaches do not introduce new patient safety risks and unforeseen events that may reduce patient safety. Therefore there is a need for effective collaborations among institutional and research organizations and support from major stakeholders, so that these pharmaco-cybernetic approaches can be brought to maturity. As medication therapies and management strategies continue to evolve in this digital age, will a new form of alternative therapy – 'e-therapy' – emerge? The answer is not clearly obvious. Nonetheless, pharmaco-cybernetics will elevate the processes of drugs and medications management to a whole new level and will be the driving force for healthcare professionals to improve the pharmaceutical care and safety of their patients. The 'Generation C' healthcare professionals who are digitally connected to their devices (e.g. computers/laptops, iPads/tablets and mobile/smartphones) are already starting to emerge (Fox, 2012; Scher, 2012). Through interdisciplinary training, this new breed of healthcare professionals will not only have the knowledge and skills to develop usable tools for clinical practices, but they will pave the way for new and improved technologies in the near future.

REFERENCES

Aapro, M. S., Cameron, D. A., Pettengell, R., Bohlius, J., Crawford, J., Ellis, M., & Zielinski, C. (2006). EORTC guidelines for the use of granulocyte-colony stimulating factor to reduce the incidence of chemotherapy-induced febrile neutropenia in adult patients with lymphomas and solid tumours. *European Journal of Cancer*, *42*(15), 2433–2453. doi:10.1016/j.ejca.2006.05.002 PMID:16750358

American Society of Hospital Pharmacists. (1993). ASHP statement on pharmaceutical care. *American Journal of Hospital Pharmacy*, *50*, 1720–1723.

ASHP Commission on Therapeutics. (1999). ASHP therapeutic guidelines on the pharmacologic management of nausea and vomiting in adult and pediatric patients receiving chemotherapy or radiation therapy or undergoing surgery. *American Journal of Health-System Pharmacy*, *56*(8), 729–764. PMID:10326616

Ballatori, E., Roila, F., Ruggeri, B., Betti, M., Sarti, S., Soru, G., & Deuson, R. R. (2007). The impact of chemotherapy-induced nausea and vomiting on health-related quality of life. *Supportive Care in Cancer*, *15*(2), 179–185. doi:10.1007/s00520-006-0109-7 PMID:16941136

Bender, C. M., McDaniel, R. W., Murphy-Ende, K., Pickett, M., Rittenberg, C. N., Rogers, M. P., & Schwartz, R. N. (2002). Chemotherapy-induced nausea and vomiting. *Clinical Journal of Oncology Nursing*, *6*(2), 94–102. doi:10.1188/02.CJON.94-102 PMID:11889684

Bergkvist, K., & Wengström, Y. (2006). Symptom experiences during chemotherapy treatment - with focus on nausea and vomiting. *European Journal of Oncology Nursing, 10*(1), 21–29. doi:10.1016/j.ejon.2005.03.007 PMID:15908274

Bloechl-Daum, B., Deuson, R. R., Mavros, P., Hansen, M., & Herrstedt, J. (2006). Delayed nausea and vomiting continue to reduce patients' quality of life after highly and moderately emetogenic chemotherapy despite antiemetic treatment. *Journal of Clinical Oncology, 24*(27), 4472–4478. doi:10.1200/JCO.2006.05.6382 PMID:16983116

Booth, C. M., Clemons, M., Dranitsaris, G., Joy, A., Young, S., Callaghan, W., & Petrella, T. (2007). Chemotherapy-induced nausea and vomiting in breast cancer patients: A prospective observational study. *The Journal of Supportive Oncology, 5*(8), 374–380. PMID:17944146

Burges, C. J. C. (1998). A tutorial on support vector machines for pattern recognition. *Data Mining and Knowledge Discovery, 2*(2), 121–167. doi:10.1023/A:1009715923555

Carayon, P., & Wood, K. E. (2010). Patient safety - The role of human factors and systems engineering. *Studies in Health Technology and Informatics, 153*, 23–46. PMID:20543237

Cengiz, B., & Kuruoğlu, H. R. (2006). Interpretation of the repetitive nerve stimulation test results using principal component analysis. *Clinical Neurophysiology, 117*(9), 2073–2078. doi:10.1016/j.clinph.2006.05.023 PMID:16890013

Chan, A., Chen, C., Chiang, J., Tan, S. H., & Ng, R. (2011, August 5). Incidence of febrile neutropenia among early-stage breast cancer patients receiving anthracycline-based chemotherapy. *Supportive Care in Cancer*. doi:10.1007/s00520-011-1241-6 PMID:21818641

Chan, A., Fu, W. H., Shih, V., Coyuco, J. C., Tan, S. H., & Ng, R. (2011). Impact of colony-stimulating factors to reduce febrile neutropenic events in breast cancer patients receiving docetaxel plus cyclophosphamide chemotherapy. *Supportive Care in Cancer, 19*(4), 497–504. doi:10.1007/s00520-010-0843-8 PMID:20232087

Chan, A., Leng, X. Z., Chiang, J. Y., Tao, M., Quek, R., Tay, K., & Lim, S. T. (2011). Comparison of daily filgrastim and pegfilgrastim to prevent febrile neutropenia in Asian lymphoma patients. *Asia Pacific Journal of Clinical Oncology, 7*(1), 75–81. doi:10.1111/j.1743-7563.2010.01355.x PMID:21332654

Chan, A., Low, X. H., & Yap, K. Y. (2012). Assessment of the relationship between adherence with antiemetic drug therapy and control of nausea and vomiting in breast cancer patients receiving anthracycline-based chemotherapy. *Journal of Managed Care Pharmacy, 18*(5), 385–394. PMID:22663171

Chen, C., Chan, A., & Yap, K. (2013). Visualizing clinical predictors of febrile neutropenia in Asian cancer patients receiving myelosuppressive chemotherapy. *Journal of Oncology Pharmacy Practice, 19*(2), 111–120. doi:10.1177/1078155212457806 PMID:23014897

Chow, E., Fan, G., Hadi, S., Wong, J., Kirou-Mauro, A., & Filipczak, L. (2008). Symptom clusters in cancer patients with brain metastases. *Clinical Oncology, 20*(1), 76–82. doi:10.1016/j.clon.2007.09.007 PMID:17981447

Cohen, L., de Moor, C. A., Eisenberg, P., Ming, E. E., & Hu, H. (2007). Chemotherapy-induced nausea and vomiting: incidence and impact on patient quality of life at community oncology settings. *Supportive Care in Cancer, 15*(5), 497–503. doi:10.1007/s00520-006-0173-z PMID:17103197

Cortes, C., & Vapnik, V. (1995). Support-vector networks. *Machine Learning, 20*(3), 273–297. doi:10.1007/BF00994018

Data Mining Articles. (n.d.). *Data mining definition and origins.* Retrieved 9 November, 2012, from http://www.dataminingarticles.com/data-mining-introduction.html

DiVall, M. V., & Cersosimo, R. J. (2007). Prevention and treatment of chemotherapy-induced nausea and vomiting: A review. *Formulary (Cleveland, Ohio), 42*(6), 378–388.

Dranitsaris, G., Joy, A., Young, S., Clemons, M., Callaghan, W., & Petrella, T. (2009). Identifying patients at high risk for nausea and vomiting after chemotherapy: The development of a practical prediction tool: Acute nausea and vomiting. *The Journal of Supportive Oncology, 7*(4), W1–W8.

Dranitsaris, G., Rayson, D., Vincent, M., Chang, J., Gelmon, K., Sandor, D., & Reardon, G. (2008). Identifying patients at high risk for neutropenic complications during chemotherapy for metastatic breast cancer with doxorubicin or pegylated liposomal doxorubicin: The development of a prediction model. *American Journal of Clinical Oncology, 31*(4), 369–374. doi:10.1097/COC.0b013e318165c01d PMID:18845996

Dunteman, G. H. (1989). *Principal components analysis.* Newbury Park, CA: Sage Publications, Inc.

Erazo Valle, A., Wisniewski, T., Figueroa Vadillo, J. I., Burke, T. A., & Martinez Corona, R. (2006). Incidence of chemotherapy-induced nausea and vomiting in Mexico: Healthcare provider predictions versus observed. *Current Medical Research and Opinion, 22*(12), 2403–2410. doi:10.1185/030079906X154033 PMID:17257454

Evgeniou, T., & Pontil, M. (2001). Support vector machines: Theory and applications. *Lecture Notes in Computer Science, 2049,* 249–257. doi:10.1007/3-540-44673-7_12

Floyd, F. J., & Widaman, K. F. (1995). Factor analysis in the development and refinement of clinical assessment instruments. *Psychological Assessment, 7*(3), 286–299. doi:10.1037/1040-3590.7.3.286

Fox, Z. (2012, February 23). Forget generation Y: 18- to 34-year-olds are now 'generation c', online news. *Mashable.* Retrieved from http://mashable.com/2012/02/23/generation-c/?utm_source=feedburner&utm_medium=feed&utm_campaign=Feed%3A+Mashable+%28Mashable%29

Garcia, M., Jemal, A., Ward, E. M., Center, M. M., Hao, Y., & Siegel, R. L., & the American Cancer Society. (2007). *Global cancer facts and figures 2007.* Retrieved 9 November, 2012, from http://www.cancer.org/Research/CancerFactsFigures/GlobalCancerFactsFigures/global-cancer-facts-figures-2007

Gift, A. G., Jablonski, A., Stommel, M., & Given, C. W. (2004). Symptom clusters in elderly patients with lung cancer. *Oncology Nursing Forum, 31*(2), 202–212. doi:10.1188/04.ONF.203-212 PMID:15017438

Gralla, R. J., Osoba, D., Kris, M. G., Kirkbride, P., Hesketh, P. J., Chinnery, L. W., & Pfister, D. G. (1999). Recommendations for the use of antiemetics: Evidence-based, clinical practice guidelines. *Journal of Clinical Oncology, 17*(9), 2971–2994. PMID:10561376

Greenacre, M., & Blasius, J. (2006). *Multiple correspondence analysis and related methods.* Boca Raton, FL: CRC Press. doi:10.1201/9781420011319

Greenacre, M., & Hastie, T. (1987). The geometric interpretation of correspondence analysis. *Journal of the American Statistical Association, 82*(398), 437–447. doi:10.1080/01621459.1987.10478446

Greenacre, M. J. (1991). Interpreting multiple correspondence analysis. *Applied Stochastic Models in Business and Industry, 7*(2), 195–210. doi:10.1002/asm.3150070208

Grunberg, S. M., Deuson, R. R., Mavros, P., Geling, O., Hansen, M., Cruciani, G., & Daugaard, G. (2004). Incidence of chemotherapy-induced nausea and emesis after modern antiemetics: Perception versus reality. *Cancer, 100*(10), 2261–2268. doi:10.1002/cncr.20230 PMID:15139073

Hadi, S., Fan, G., Hird, A. E., Kirou-Mauro, A., Filipczak, L. A., & Chow, E. (2008). Symptom clusters in patients with cancer with metastatic bone pain. *Journal of Palliative Medicine, 11*(4), 591–600. doi:10.1089/jpm.2007.0145 PMID:18454612

Hesketh, P. J. (1999). Defining the emetogenicity of cancer chemotherapy regimens: Relevance to clinical practice. *The Oncologist, 4*(3), 191–196. PMID:10394587

Hesketh, P. J., Aapro, M., Street, J. C., & Carides, A. D. (2010). Evaluation of risk factors predictive of nausea and vomiting with current standard-of-care antiemetic treatment: analysis of two phase III trials of aprepitant in patients receiving cisplatin-based chemotherapy. *Supportive Care in Cancer, 18*(9), 1171–1177. doi:10.1007/s00520-009-0737-9 PMID:19756774

Heuser, M., & Ganser, A. (2005). Colony-stimulating factors in the management of neutropenia and its complications. *Annals of Hematology, 84*(11), 697–708. doi:10.1007/s00277-005-1087-4 PMID:16047204

Joel, S. P., Shah, R., Clark, P. I., & Slevin, M. L. (1996). Predicting etoposide toxicity: Relationship to organ function and protein binding. *Journal of Clinical Oncology, 14*(1), 257–267. PMID:8558207

Kris, M. G., Hesketh, P. J., Somerfield, M. R., Feyer, P., Clark-Snow, R., Koeller, J. M., & Grunberg, S. M. (2006). American society of clinical oncology guideline for antiemetics in oncology: Update 2006. *Journal of Clinical Oncology, 24*(18), 2932–2947. doi:10.1200/JCO.2006.06.9591 PMID:16717289

Kuderer, N. M., Dale, D. C., Crawford, J., Cosler, L. E., & Lyman, G. H. (2006). Mortality, morbidity, and cost associated with febrile neutropenia in adult cancer patients. *Cancer, 106*(10), 2258–2266. doi:10.1002/cncr.21847 PMID:16575919

Liau, C. T., Chu, N. M., Liu, H. E., Deuson, R., Lien, J., & Chen, J. S. (2005). Incidence of chemotherapy-induced nausea and vomiting in Taiwan: Physicians' and nurses' estimation vs. patients' reported outcomes. *Supportive Care in Cancer, 13*(5), 277–286. doi:10.1007/s00520-005-0788-5 PMID:15770489

Lindley, C. M., Hirsch, J. D., O'Neill, C. V., Transau, M. C., Gilbert, C. S., & Osterhaus, J. T. (1992). Quality of life consequences of chemotherapy-induced emesis. *Quality of Life Research, 1*(5), 331–340. doi:10.1007/BF00434947 PMID:1299465

Lohr, L. (2008). Chemotherapy-induced nausea and vomiting. *Cancer Journal (Sudbury, Mass.), 14*(2), 85–93. doi:10.1097/PPO.0b013e31816a0f07 PMID:18391612

Mendoza, T. R., Wang, X. S., Cleeland, C. S., Morrissey, M., Johnson, B. A., Wendt, J. K., & Huber, S. L. (1999). The rapid assessment of fatigue severity in cancer patients: Use of the brief fatigue inventory. *Cancer, 85*(5), 1186–1196. doi:10.1002/(SICI)1097-0142(19990301)85:5<1186::AID-CNCR24>3.0.CO;2-N PMID:10091805

Minton, O., & Stone, P. (2009). A systematic review of the scales used for the measurement of cancer-related fatigue (CRF). *Annals of Oncology, 20*(1), 17–25. doi:10.1093/annonc/mdn537 PMID:18678767

Molassiotis, A., Saunders, M. P., Valle, J., Wilson, G., Lorigan, P., Wardley, A., & Rittenberg, C. (2008). A prospective observational study of chemotherapy-related nausea and vomiting in routine practice in a UK cancer centre. *Supportive Care in Cancer, 16*(2), 201–208. doi:10.1007/s00520-007-0343-7 PMID:17926070

Molassiotis, A., Yam, B. M. C., Yung, H., Chan, F. Y. S., & Mok, T. S. K. (2002). Pretreatment factors predicting the development of postchemotherapy nausea and vomiting in Chinese breast cancer patients. *Supportive Care in Cancer, 10*(2), 139–145. doi:10.1007/s00520-001-0321-4 PMID:11862503

National Comprehensive Cancer Network. (2011, July 20). *NCCN clinical practice guidelines in Oncology™ Antiemesis v.1.2012.* Retrieved 9 November, 2012, from http://www.nccn.org/professionals/physician_gls/PDF/antiemesis.pdf

National Comprehensive Cancer Network. (2012, February 22). *NCCN clinical practice guidelines in oncology - Myeloid growth factors version 1.2012.* Retrieved 9 November, 2012, from http://www.nccn.org/professionals/physician_gls/pdf/myeloid_growth.pdf

Needles, B., Miranda, E., Garcia Rodriguez, F. M., Diaz, L. B., Spector, J., & Craig, J., S3AA3012 Study Group. (1999). A multicenter, double-blind, randomized comparison of oral ondansetron 8 mg b.i.d., 24 mg q.d., & 32 mg q.d. in the prevention of nausea and vomiting associated with highly emetogenic chemotherapy. *Supportive Care in Cancer, 7*(5), 347–353. doi:10.1007/s005200050274 PMID:10483821

Neymark, N., & Crott, R. (2005). Impact of emesis on clinical and economic outcomes of cancer therapy with highly emetogenic chemotherapy regimens: A retrospective analysis of three clinical trials. *Supportive Care in Cancer, 13*(10), 812–818. doi:10.1007/s00520-005-0803-x PMID:15834590

Ng, J. H., Ang, X. Y., Tan, S. H., Tao, M., Lim, S. T., & Chan, A. (2011). Breakthrough febrile neutropenia and associated complications in non-Hodgkin's lymphoma patients receiving pegfilgrastim. *Acta Haematologica, 125*(3), 107–114. doi:10.1159/000321545 PMID:21109731

Osborne, J. W., & Costello, A. B. (2004). Sample size and subject to item ratio in principal components analysis. *Practical Assessment, Research & Evaluation, 9*(11).

Osoba, D., Zee, B., Pater, J., Warr, D., Latreille, J., & Kaizer, L. (1997). Determinants of postchemotherapy nausea and vomiting in patients with cancer. *Journal of Clinical Oncology, 15*(1), 116–123. PMID:8996132

Park, E. J., McDaniel, A., & Jung, M. S. (2009). Computerized tailoring of health information. *Computers, Informatics, Nursing, 27*(1), 34–43. doi:10.1097/NCN.0b013e31818dd396 PMID:19060620

Perneger, T. V. (2005). The Swiss cheese model of safety incidents: Are there holes in the metaphor? *BMC Health Services Research, 5,* 71. doi:10.1186/1472-6963-5-71 PMID:16280077

Petrella, T., Clemons, M., Joy, A., Young, S., Callaghan, W., & Dranitsaris, G. (2009). Identifying patients at high risk for nausea and vomiting after chemotherapy: The development of a practical prediction tool: Delayed nausea and vomiting. *The Journal of Supportive Oncology, 7*(4), W9–W16.

Pettengell, R., Bosly, A., Szucs, T. D., Jackisch, C., Leonard, R., Paridaens, R., & Schwenkglenks, M. (2009). Multivariate analysis of febrile neutropenia occurrence in patients with non-Hodgkin lymphoma: Data from the INC-EU prospective observational European neutropenia study. *British Journal of Haematology, 144*(5), 677–685. doi:10.1111/j.1365-2141.2008.07514.x PMID:19055662

Pettengell, R., Schwenkglenks, M., Leonard, R., Bosly, A., Paridaens, R., Constenla, M., & Jackisch, C. (2008). Neutropenia occurrence and predictors of reduced chemotherapy delivery: Results from the INC-EU prospective observational European neutropenia study. *Supportive Care in Cancer, 16*(11), 1299–1309. doi:10.1007/s00520-008-0430-4 PMID:18351398

Pharmaceutical Care Network Europe. (2010, January 14). *PCNE classification for drug-related problems v6.2.* Retrieved 9 November, 2012, from http://www.pcne.org/sig/drp/documents/PCNE%20classification%20V6-2.pdf

Pollera, C. F., & Giannarelli, D. (1989). Prognostic factors influencing cisplatin-induced emesis: Definition and validation of a predictive logistic model. *Cancer, 64*(5), 1117–1122. doi:10.1002/1097-0142(19890901)64:5<1117::AID-CNCR2820640525>3.0.CO;2-R PMID:2667749

Rhodes, V. A., & McDaniel, R. W. (2001). Nausea, vomiting, and retching: complex problems in palliative care. *CA: a Cancer Journal for Clinicians, 51*(4), 232–248. doi:10.3322/canjclin.51.4.232 PMID:11577489

Roila, F., Hesketh, P. J., & Herrstedt, J. (2006). Prevention of chemotherapy- and radiotherapy-induced emesis: Results of the 2004 Perugia international antiemetic consensus conference. *Annals of Oncology, 17*(1), 20–28. doi:10.1093/annonc/mdj078 PMID:16314401

Roscoe, J. A., Morrow, G. R., Colagiuri, B., Heckler, C. E., Pudlo, B. D., Colman, L., & Jacobs, A. (2010). Insight in the prediction of chemotherapy-induced nausea. *Supportive Care in Cancer, 18*(7), 869–876. doi:10.1007/s00520-009-0723-2 PMID:19701781

Scher, D. L. (2012, May 30). *Young physicians will become the champions of technology.* Retrieved 9 November, 2012, from http://www.kevinmd.com/blog/2012/05/young-physicians-champions-technology.html

Schnell, F. M. (2003). Chemotherapy-induced nausea and vomiting: the importance of acute antiemetic control. *The Oncologist, 8*(2), 187–198. doi:10.1634/theoncologist.8-2-187 PMID:12697943

Shek, D. T. (1993). The Chinese version of the state-trait anxiety inventory: Its relationship to different measures of psychological well-being. *Journal of Clinical Psychology, 49*(3), 349–358. doi:10.1002/1097-4679(199305)49:3<349::AID-JCLP2270490308>3.0.CO;2-J PMID:8315037

Shih, V., Hee, S. W., & Chan, A. (2009). Clinical predictors of chemotherapy-induced nausea and vomiting in breast cancer patients receiving adjuvant doxorubicin and cyclophosphamide. *The Annals of Pharmacotherapy, 43*(3), 444–452. doi:10.1345/aph.1L437 PMID:19193584

Smith, T. J., Khatcheressian, J., Lyman, G. H., Ozer, H., Armitage, J. O., Balducci, L., & Wolff, A. C. (2006). 2006 update of recommendations for the use of white blood cell growth factors: An evidence-based clinical practice guideline. *Journal of Clinical Oncology, 24*(19), 3187–3205. doi:10.1200/JCO.2006.06.4451 PMID:16682719

Smits, M., Groenewegen, P. P., Timmermans, D. R., van der Wal, G., & Wagner, C. (2009). The nature and causes of unintended events reported at ten emergency departments. *BMC Emergency Medicine, 9,* 16. doi:10.1186/1471-227X-9-16 PMID:19765275

Spielberger, C. D., Gorsuch, R. L., & R.E., L. (1983). *State-trait anxiety inventory for adults.* Palo Alto, CA: Mind Garden.

Srokowski, T. P., Fang, S., Hortobagyi, G. N., & Giordano, S. H. (2009). Impact of diabetes mellitus on complications and outcomes of adjuvant chemotherapy in older patients with breast cancer. *Journal of Clinical Oncology, 27*(13), 2170–2176. doi:10.1200/JCO.2008.17.5935 PMID:19307509

Stieler, J. M., Reichardt, P., Riess, H., & Oettle, H. (2003). Treatment options for chemotherapy-induced nausea and vomiting: Current and future. *The American Journal of Cancer, 2*(1), 15–26. doi:10.2165/00024669-200302010-00002

van Mil, J. W. F., Westerlund, L. O. T., Hersberger, K. E., & Schaefer, M. A. (2004). Drug-related problem classification systems. *The Annals of Pharmacotherapy, 38*(5), 859–867. doi:10.1345/aph.1D182 PMID:15054145

Wang, S. Y., Tsai, C. M., Chen, B. C., Lin, C. H., & Lin, C. C. (2008). Symptom clusters and relationships to symptom interference with daily life in Taiwanese lung cancer patients. *Journal of Pain and Symptom Management, 35*(3), 258–266. doi:10.1016/j.jpainsymman.2007.03.017 PMID:18201865

Ward, J. K., McEachan, R. R., Lawton, R., Armitage, G., Watt, I., & Wright, J. (2011). Patient involvement in patient safety: Protocol for developing an intervention using patient reports of organisational safety and patient incident reporting. *BMC Health Services Research, 11*, 130. doi:10.1186/1472-6963-11-130 PMID:21619575

Warr, D. G., Street, J. C., & Carides, A. D. (2011). Evaluation of risk factors predictive of nausea and vomiting with current standard-of-care antiemetic treatment: Analysis of phase 3 trial of aprepitant in patients receiving adriamycin-cyclophosphamide-based chemotherapy. *Supportive Care in Cancer, 19*(6), 807–813. doi:10.1007/s00520-010-0899-5 PMID:20461438

Westerlund, T., Almarsdóttir, A. B., & Melander, A. (1999). Factors influencing the detection rate of drug-related problems in community pharmacy. *Pharmacy World & Science, 21*(6), 245–250. doi:10.1023/A:1008767406692 PMID:10658231

Wu, H. T., Graff, L. R., & Yuen, C. W. (2005). Clinical pharmacy in an inpatient leukemia and bone marrow transplant service. *American Journal of Health-System Pharmacy, 62*(7), 744–747. PMID:15790803

Yap, K. Y., Chan, A., & Chui, W. K. (2009). Improving pharmaceutical care in oncology by pharmacoinformatics: The evolving role of informatics and the internet for drug therapy. *The Lancet Oncology, 10*(10), 1011–1019. doi:10.1016/S1470-2045(09)70104-4 PMID:19796753

Yap, K. Y., Chuang, X., Lee, A. J. M., Lee, R. Z., Lim, L., Lim, J. J., & Nimesha, R. (2009). Pharmaco-cybernetics as an interactive component of pharma-culture: Empowering drug knowledge through user-, experience- and activity-centered designs. *International Journal of Computer Science Issues, 3*, 1–13.

Yap, K. Y., Low, X. H., & Chan, A. (2012). Exploring chemotherapy-induced toxicities through multivariate projection of risk factors: Prediction of nausea and vomiting. *Toxicological Reviews, 28*(2), 81–91. doi:10.5487/TR.2012.28.2.081 PMID:24278593

Yap, K. Y., Low, X. H., Chui, W. K., & Chan, A. (2012). Computational prediction of state anxiety in Asian patients with cancer susceptible to chemotherapy-induced nausea and vomiting. *Journal of Clinical Psychopharmacology, 32*(2), 207–217. doi:10.1097/JCP.0b013e31824888a1 PMID:22367655

Ziepert, M., Schmits, R., Trumper, L., Pfreund-schuh, M., & Loeffler, M. (2008). Prognostic factors for hematotoxicity of chemotherapy in aggressive non-Hodgkin's lymphoma. *Annals of Oncology, 19*(4), 752–762. doi:10.1093/annonc/mdm541 PMID:18048382

KEY TERMS AND DEFINITIONS

Adverse Drug Reaction: A condition experienced by patients characterised by injury or harm associated with the use of drugs/medications (e.g. chemotherapies) at normal dosages during normal use.

Chemotherapy-Induced Nausea And Vomiting: An adverse drug reaction characterised by nausea and vomiting experienced by patients with cancer receiving emetogenic chemotherapies. Acute nausea and vomiting usually lasts up to 24 hours after chemotherapy; while delayed nausea and vomiting usually occurs after 24 hours and lasts up to 5 to 7 days.

Drug-Related Problem: An event or circumstance which involves drug therapies that can actually or potentially interfere with the desired health outcome for patients.

Febrile Neutropenia: An adverse drug reaction that is usually a serious complication of chemotherapy, particularly in cancer patients who receive myelosuppressive chemotherapies. This condition is characterised by a fever and a significant reduction in their white blood cells.

Machine Learning: A field in artificial intelligence which designs computational algorithms and techniques capable of inducing knowledge from data. Generally, there are two main types: supervised and unsupervised learning.

Multiple Correspondence Analysis: A multivariate technique within unsupervised machine learning for exploring data. It is similar to PCA but is catered towards discretized categorical data and usually involves frequency tables or counts.

Pharmaceutical Care: A concept involving identifying, solving and preventing potential or actual drug-related problems with regards to a patient's drug therapy.

Pharmaco-Cybernetics: An upcoming interdisciplinary field that describes the science of supporting medicines or drugs use through the application of computational technologies and techniques, combined with the principles of human-computer-environment interaction, to reduce or prevent drug-related problems. Also known as cybernetic pharmacy.

Pharmaco-Informatics: A field of pharmacy which involves the use of informatics and internet technologies to target drug-related problems. It is focused on the acquisition, dissemination, storage, analysis and use of medication-related knowledge and data within the continuum of healthcare systems.

Principal Component Analysis: A multivariate projection technique within unsupervised machine learning that can investigate relationships among multiple variables and explain the causes of variance in a data set. This technique linearly transforms an original set of variables into a substantially smaller set of uncorrelated variables called principal components, which represent most of the information in the original data set.

Supervised Machine Learning: A computational method that is able to predict the output value of an unknown object based on the training of a set of training examples (input and output data).

Unsupervised Machine Learning: A computational method that typically involves a model that is generated to fit observations. Unlike supervised learning, there is no a priori output, therefore characteristics about the data set can be described from the observations without any predefined target.

This work was previously published in the Handbook of Research on Patient Safety and Quality Care through Health Informatics edited by Vaughan Michell, Deborah J. Rosenorn-Lanng, Stephen R. Gulliver, and Wendy Currie, pages 179-197 copyright year 2014 by Medical Information Science Reference (an imprint of IGI Global).

Chapter 74
Auditing Privacy for Cloud–Based EHR Systems

Jonathan Sinclair
RepKnight Ltd., UK

Benoit Hudzia
Stratoscale Ltd., UK

Alan Stewart
Queen's University Belfast, UK

ABSTRACT

An EHR is a modern specialisation of a Customer Relationship Management that specifically focuses on the collection and exchange of electronic health information about individual patients between healthcare organisations. Electronic Heath Records systems hold personally identifiable information, especially that which falls under the category of sensitive personal data. As with all industries, the eHealth industry sees potential in cloud-based service offerings and the reduced infrastructure cost they imply, whilst realising the issues regarding security and privacy that may be encountered from outsourcing processing and storage to untrustworthy Cloud Service Providers (CSPs). In this chapter, the authors propose an approach to handle and audit data privacy requirements by leveraging a carefully designed architecture deployed for auditing data privacy in cloud ecosystems.

INTRODUCTION

Most organisations manage their customer data through a Customer Relationship Management (CRM) system. CRM is a widely adopted strategy for enhancing and maintaining customer relationships and the information that pertains to the customer through the phases of administration, marketing, sales and support. Most commercial CRM offerings didn't provide the support and services required for the health industry and, therefore, a specialised form of CRM, the Electronic Health Record (EHR) system was developed. An EHR is a modern specialisation of a CRM which specifically focuses on the collection and exchange of electronic health information about individual patients between healthcare organisations. EHR systems hold personally identifiable

DOI: 10.4018/978-1-4666-8756-1.ch074

information especially that which falls under the category of sensitive personal data. As with all industries the eHealth industry sees potential in cloud-based service offerings and the reduced infrastructure cost they imply, whilst realising the issues regarding security and privacy that may be encountered from outsourcing processing and storage to untrustworthy CSPs. The loss of control has been highlighted as a concern in regards to the compliance of privacy laws and is required in order to control and enforce the access to records by third parties.

In this chapter, we first propose an approach to defining data privacy requirements. Second, we present an architecture deployed for auditing data privacy. Third we present the validation and verification of a data locality results and finally propose a pragmatic approach to breach of compliance prediction in the light of analysis.

BACKGROUND

E-Health

E-Health refers to the utilisation of information systems within the healthcare industry (I.T. Union 2008). Two goals of e-Health as mentioned by Edworthy (2001) are:

1. To provide greater efficiency; and
2. To scale patient services.

Moreover, the World Health Organisation (WHO) defined e-Health in 2005 as:

Use of information and communications technologies (ICT) in support of health and health-related fields, including health-care services, health surveillance, health literature, health education, knowledge and research.

The E-Health domain is heavily regulated, and Figure 1 shows important healthcare laws taken from the EU, UK and US. Current laws highlighted in red; superseded laws are displayed in black. These laws typically address electronic healthcare considerations but do not extend to issues arising from the use of cloud and virtualisation technologies. Revisions of current laws to address issues arising from technological advances are pending.

E-Health Technologies

Various E-Health related technologies have been developed. They aim to provide a unified platform for processing health records, which delivers services to a variety of types of user. But also, enable access to health records from a range of platforms and devices while providing integration of health records across different health-care domains and deliver an efficient health management and administration process.

The recent development and evolution of e-Health systems needs address the economies of scale while providing efficient data management

Figure 1. Timeline for healthcare privacy laws

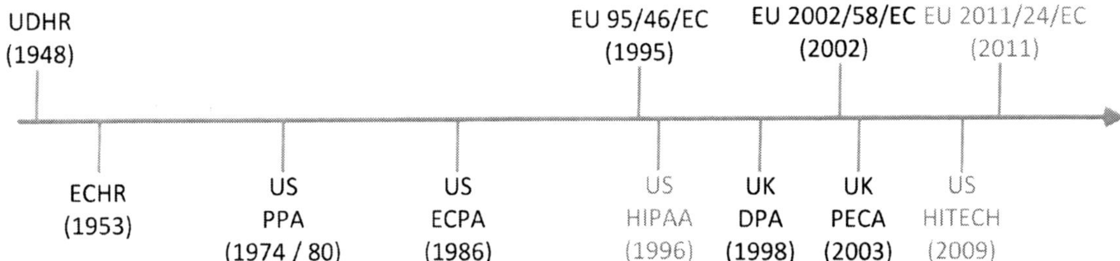

processes which operate across cross-jurisdictional boundaries without compromising patients' data privacy rights. It has been identified that, despite the development of laws in some jurisdictions to deal with privacy in EHR's, many in the field argue that regulation is providing an insufficient level of granularity regarding the use of EHR's in the context of the technology stack (WHO, 2005).

Electronic Medical Record (EMR), Electronic Health Record (EHR)

Often the terms electronic medical record (EMR), electronic health record (EHR) and personal health record (PHR) are used interchangeably. However, there is a clear difference between the three kinds of record in both their content and in the underlying technology. EMRs were the first mainstream system that medical professionals used to record the diagnosis and treatment of medical conditions for patients. EHRs were derived from EMRs and record information about all aspects of patient health, not just medical conditions. Figure 2 shows how the technology supporting EHRs allows different departments, sites and organisations to share patient information. Finally, PHRs are derived from an EHR and allow patients to view and administer aspects of their healthcare records.

Many implementations of EMR, EHR and PHR systems exist with different architectures, communication standards and deployment methods. Here we consider the OpenVistA project in a virtualised context. OpenVistA is an open source implementation of an EHR system, VistA. An existing deployment of VistA in the US supports 8 million patients, 180,000 health professionals in 163 hospitals, 800 clinics and 135 nursing homes.

Cloud Supply Chains

Cloud supply chains are a new field of research driven by an evolution of supply chains through

Figure 2. Source composition for EHRs

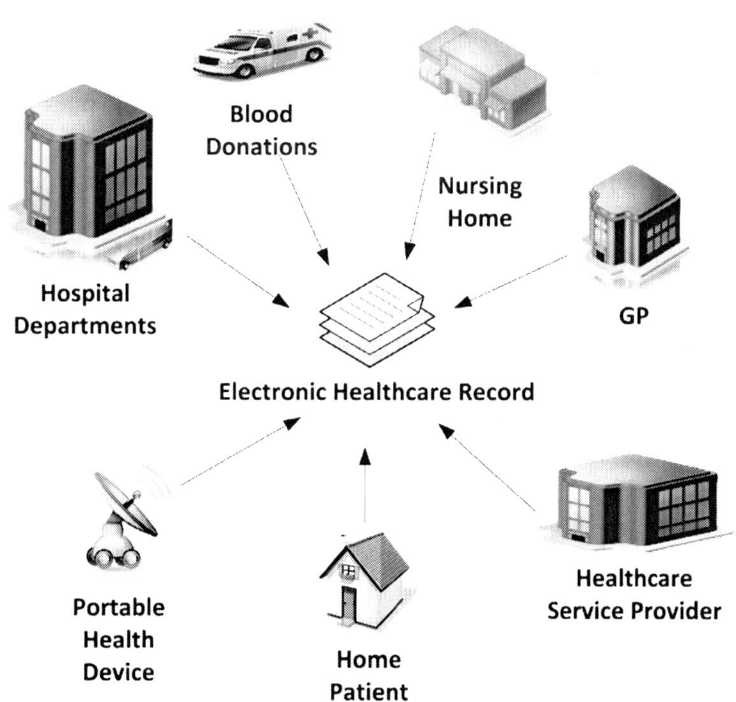

the adoption of cloud computing as described by Lindner et al., (2010) and Zhou et al., (2012). The concept of the cloud supply chain is a convergence of existing of different business models as depicted by Kijl (2005), Bouwman (2006), and Porter (1980). These models cover all aspects of the supply chain and business lifecycle acknowledging regulations as an influencing factor of dynamic business models such as that involving cloud computing. Lindner et al., (2010) describe how Cloud supply chains are defined as two or more parties linked by the provision of Cloud services, related information and funds.

eHealth Cloud Supply Chain

The e-Health Cloud supply chain shown in Figure 3 is a concept used to describe the different actors and parts involved throughout the end-to-end life cycle of health care related Cloud services. As a result, the eHealth Cloud supply chain is a system of business processes that are executed in order to satisfy the demands of Cloud consumers as described by Lindner et al., (2010,2011), in this case health care providers. This concept is similar to a typical supply chain where a product/service exists at the beginning of the chain and a customer at the end. However, within the context of Cloud computing, the product/service would be a Cloud offering in the form of Software as a Service (SaaS), Platform as a Service (PaaS), Infrastructure as a Service (IaaS) or a combination of these. Lindner et al., (2011a) present how these can be combined to offer an aggregated service to consumers providing them with value-adding services. There can be a number of actors and components involved in the Cloud supply chain such as the Cloud service provider, the Cloud consumer and possibly a Cloud broker. The Cloud broker's role is to establish a relationship with various Cloud providers to find the best offering to suit the consumer's needs. As well as a number of components existing within a Cloud, consumers can utilise more than one type of cloud,

however this causes complexities throughout the supply chain, because of the various clouds and the different components in each of these (Lindner et al., 2011a). Other components that are passed through the Cloud supply chain include information and funds. Cloud services are traditionally consumed through a pay-per-use model, where the consumer only pays for how much they use. However, other methods of payment include pay monthly (subscription-based method) or fixed price. E.g., if a Cloud consumer uses more than one cloud to fulfil a service, each cloud may have its own payment model and the cloud consumer may pay monthly for one cloud and pay-per-use for another cloud. As a result, this can increase significantly the complexity of the EHR supply chain. Stewart (2009) present how this make it more difficult to ensure compliance and carry out the process of auditing which is critical when it comes to health information of patients.

EHR SCENARIO

We consider a scenario that requires the monitoring of data protection requirements for EHR in a cloud environment. This use case highlights the contrast between the traditional and cloud-based EHR scenarios and the interactions between both the public and private sector.

Data Protection Compliance for EHR Systems

The challenges of assessing the data privacy compliance of cloud-based EHR systems are complex. Interactions between multiple parties and devices occur in real-time. Individuals have the ability to access their medical records; held by third-party healthcare service providers, using a range of wireless devices. Services that utilise stored information about a patient's diet, medication and location access sensitive personal information (subject to privacy legislation). An individual

Figure 3. Audit supply chain

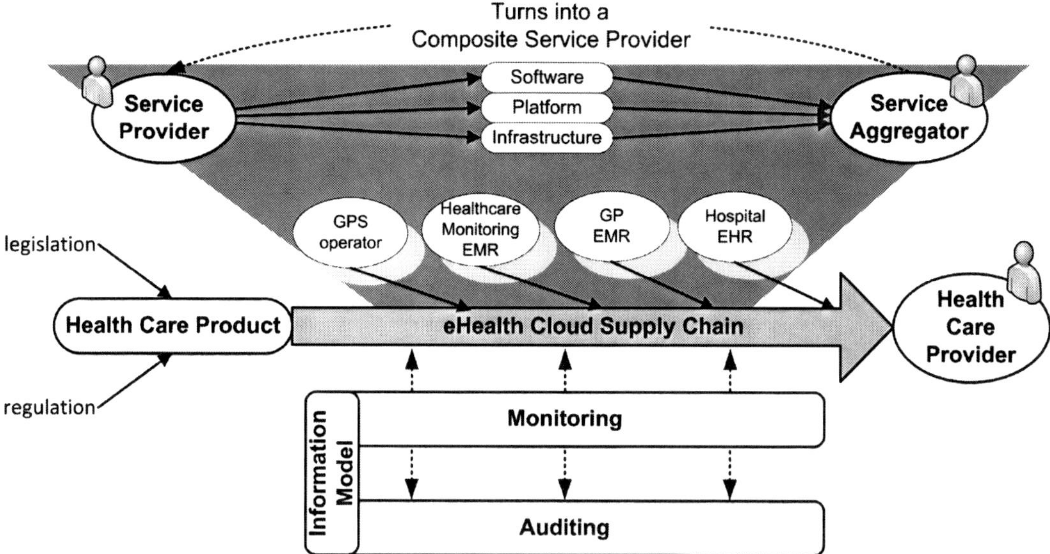

should be provided with guarantees about how their personal data is managed. Health institutions store details in addition to an individual's medical history. A patient should be able to monitor who has access to their personal information. Figure 4 shows an EHR system composed of an EHR Database, EHR Client, Patient WebPortal and EHR Imaging services.

DEFINING EHR DATA PRIVACY REQUIREMENT

In order to define international, national or local privacy constraints it is necessary to take into account the diversity of data privacy legislation relating to healthcare. Some requirements of data protection laws involve:

1. Backup of data;
2. Managing passwords;
3. Controlling the location of the system and system access;
4. Properly erase media that runs the system;
5. Encrypting system processes when appropriate; and
6. Recording and auditing system usage.

It should be noted that the various laws are inconsistent with respect to:

1. Retention duration;
2. Encryption standards;
3. Locality restrictions; and
4. Audit frequencies.

One way to represent variations in privacy laws is to parameterise requirements (see Figure 5).

EHR Service Level Agreements

In the remainder of this chapter, we will focus attention on location constraints that arise from data privacy laws (e.g. running services within a specific geographic region, or preventing access and data transfer to/from different geographies). An SLA template for geolocation constraints for an OpenVistA EHR service is shown in Listing 1. In line 2 the name of the agreement, EHRAgree-

Figure 4. EHR system as a service

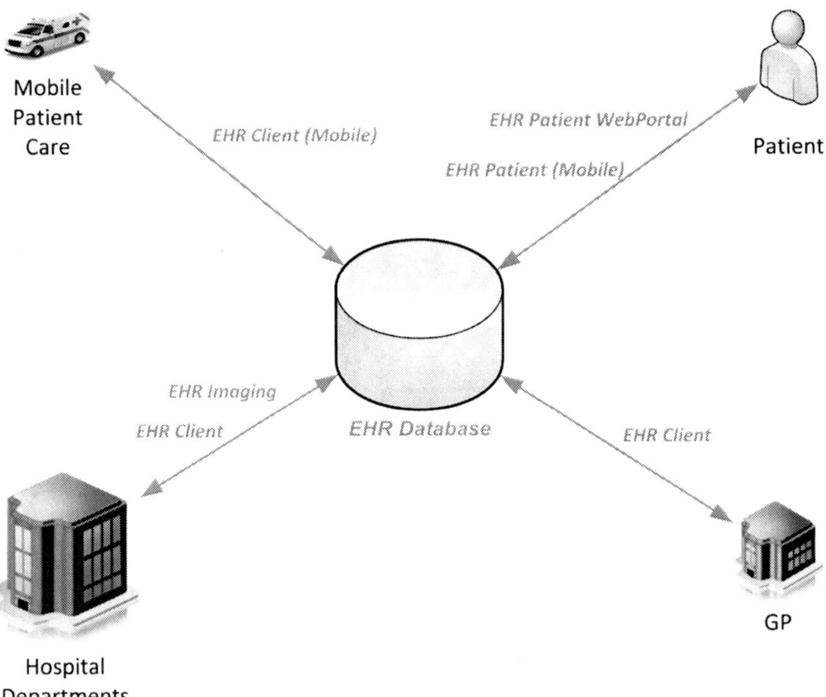

ment, is defined. Following this lines 3 through 10 describe the context for the agreement in terms of expiration and the template used for definition. The remainder of the agreement focuses on the terms; Service-based, GuaranteeTerms and AuditTerms.

The ServiceDescriptionTerms, ServiceProperties and ServiceReferences describe different aspects of a service referring to the service name, openVistA EHR. The ServiceProperties defines a location property, locationProp in line 16 which has a variable set, lines 18-21, used to measure the location in terms of IP with a metric range of countries. The GuaranteeTerms section provides the monitoring conditions for the ipLocation variable of the service property, locationProp.

The condition on line 30 states the ipLocation variable should be a country within the predefined set of countries which represent the

Figure 5. Compliance WS-agreement structure

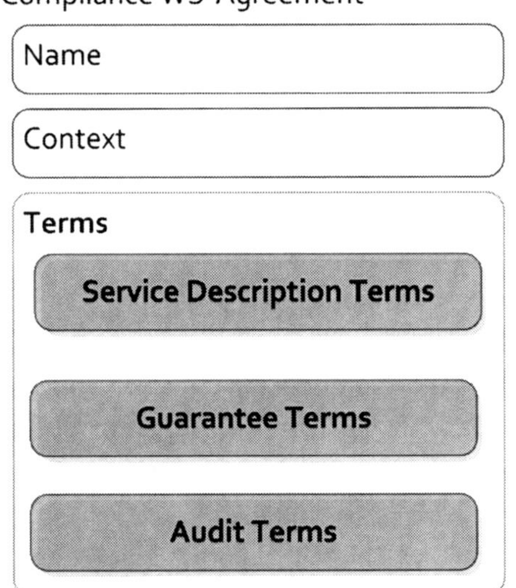

EU. Finally lines 33-57 describe the extended audit terms section. It refers to the ServiceDescriptionTerm, named geoLocation in line 13 and associates it with a compliance law, UK DPA, indicating that it should be continuously monitored. Lines 36-44 defined the scope for the audit in terms of the proposed novel framework. Finally lines 45-50 define the conditions of the compliance audit.

CONTINUOUS COMPLIANCE AUDITING SERVICE (CCAS) SYSTEM LANDSCAPE FOR EHR

The CCAS system has been customised for the OpenVistA EHR example. The OpenVistA services have been deployed on an OpenNebula Cloud Infrastructure (see Figure 6). The Cloud architecture consists of a management machine which hosts the OpenNebula Cloud Manager, a Service Broker and a Service Hoster which execute the service lifecycle and five cloud machines which are used to host OpenVistA services and the service auditor.

Specification of System Architecture

The specifications of the machines used in the cloud ecosystem are detailed in Table 1

EHR CLOUD ECOSYSTEM

An EHR Cloud ecosystem is the evolution of an EHR system which incorporates distributed and mobile sources (see Figure 7). The cloud supply chain, for the OpenVistA EHR cloud system is shown in Figure 3. EHR cloud supply chains utilise a number of virtualised services (deployed within

Table 1. System specification

	BW 1	BW 2	BW 3	BW 4	BW 5	BW 6
CPU (Cores/Threads)	8/16	4/8	4/8	4/8	12/24	4/8
Memory	8 Gb	16 Gb	16 Gb	16 GB	128 Gb	6 Gb
Hard Disk	300 Gb	500 Gb	500 Gb	500 Gb	1 Tb	300 Gb
Network Interfaces	3	2	2	2	2	2

Figure 6. CCAS system landscape

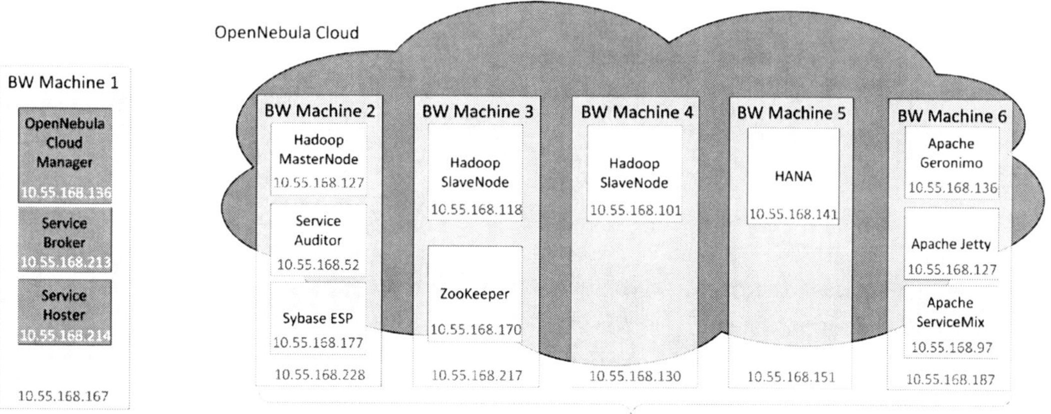

Listing1. Example EHR SLA,frame

```
1  <wsag:Agreement AgreementId=``AGSV2032">
2      <wsag:Name> EHRAgreement </wsag:Name>
3      <wsag:AgreementContext>
4          <wsag:AgreementInitiator>uuid:d9769f3d-0ab0-4fb8-803b-0d1120ffcf54</wsag:AgreementInitiator>
5          <wsag:AgreementResponder>medsphere.com</wsag:AgreementResponder>
6          <wsag:ServiceProvider>AgreementResponder</wsag:ServiceProvider>
7          <wsag:ExpirationTime>1396674000</wsag:ExpirationTime>
8          <wsag:TemplateId>3287</wsag:TemplateId>
9          <wsag:TemplateName>EHRTemplate</wsag:TemplateName>
10     </wsag:AgreementContext>
11     <wsag:Terms>
12         <wsag:All>
13             <wsag:ServiceDescriptionTerm wsag:Name=``geoLocation"
14                     wsag:ServiceName="openVistA EHR">
15         </wsag:ServiceDescriptionTerm>
16         <wsag:ServiceProperties wsag:Name=``locationProp"
17                 wsag:ServiceName="EHR">
18             <wsag:VariableSet>
19                 <wsag:Variable wsag:Name=``ipLocation"
20                     wsag:Metric="country">
21                 </wsag:Variable>
22             </wsag:VariableSet>
23         </wsag:ServiceProperties>
24         <wsag:ServiceReference wsag:Name=``locationRef"
25             wsag:ServiceName="EHR">
26         </wsag:ServiceReference>
27         <wsag:GuaranteeTerm wsag:Name=``validLocations"
28             Monitored="True">
29             <wsag:ServiceLevelObjective>
30                 ipLocation IS_WITHIN EU
31             </wsag:ServiceLevelObjective>
32         </wsag:GuaranteeTerm>
33         <wsag:AuditTerm wsag:Name=``geoLocation"
34                     ComplianceName=``UK DPA"
35                     Continuous=``True">
36             <wsag:AuditScope>
37                 <wsag:Audit>...</wsag:Audit>*
38                 <wsag:AccessControl>...</wsag:AccessControl>*
39                 <wsag:DataSource>...</wsag:DataSource>*
40                 <wsag:DataPersistence>...</wsag:DataPersistence>*
41                 <wsag:DataTransport>...</wsag:DataTransport>*
42                 <wsag:DataConsumer>...</wsag:DataConsumer>*
43                 <wsag:RiskManagement>...</wsag:RiskManagement>*
44             </wsag:AuditScope>
45             <wsag:AuditCondition>
46                 <wsag:GuaranteeName>...</wsag:GuaranteeName>
47                 <wsag:RequiredValue>...</wsag:RequiredValue>
48                 <wsag:PreferredValue>...</wsag:PreferredValue>
49                 <wsag:Restrictions>...</wsag:Restrictions>
50             </wsag:AuditCondition>*
51             <wsag:ServiceLevelObjective Type=``xs:string">
52                 ...
53             </wsag:ServiceLevelObjective>*
54             <wsag:BusinessValueList>
55                 ...
56             </wsag:BusinessValueList>
57         </wsag:AuditTerm>
58         </wsag:All>
59     </wsag:Terms>
60 </wsag:Agreement>
61
```

the cloud environment). In Figure 6 we show how the CCAS is deployed alongside an EHR system (as described in Figure 7) in the cloud. Each EHR service has an audit probe that interacts with it and provides auditing data.

EHR Events

A patient's medical record can be updated following the trigger of a variety of events:

Figure 7. EHR use case architecture

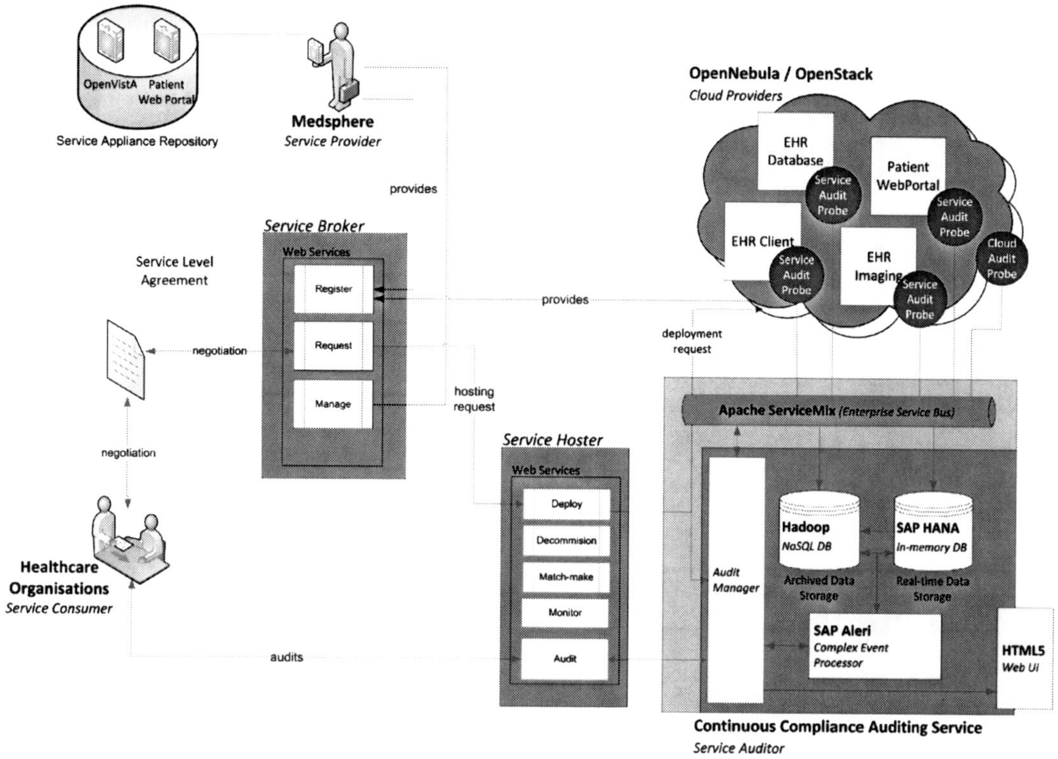

1. Medical sensors e.g. pulse or blood sugar;
2. Location sensors e.g. global positioning;
3. Medical tests e.g. x-ray or blood results; and
4. Prescribed care, medical or diet e.g. medication.

Each of these events may be atomic or consist of multiple sub-events which occurred over a time period. An EHR system allows medical practitioners and healthcare professionals to be able to gain a broader and more detailed view of a patient's health over the duration of their lifetime. It is very important in EHR systems that each event recorded is given an accurate time-stamp as this determines further diagnosis and treatment.

EHR Logs

There are two common types of log / messaging formats used within EHR systems; HL7 used to store details of a patient's diagnosis, care and treat-ment to include medical history such as known allergies (shown in Figure 8 and CCR used to store detailed information regarding prescribed care, medication or diet over a continuous period (as per example in Listing 2). The HL7 example in Figure 8 shows that an event took place at 11.23 18/08/1988 for a patient PATID1234, William Jones; who has an allergy to penicillin which brings him out in hives, the event had a diagnosis of primary malignant neoplasm of liver. The CCR example in Listing 2 details the prescription of medication to patient 001 of 90 doses of 0.125mg of Digoxin. Each of these formats is normalised using adapters in the messaging bus defining standard parsing methods to conform to the CCAS logging format in Figure 9.

EHR Complex Event Processing

In order to assess the overall compliance of business processes against a given principle (i.e.

Figure 8. HL7 log format

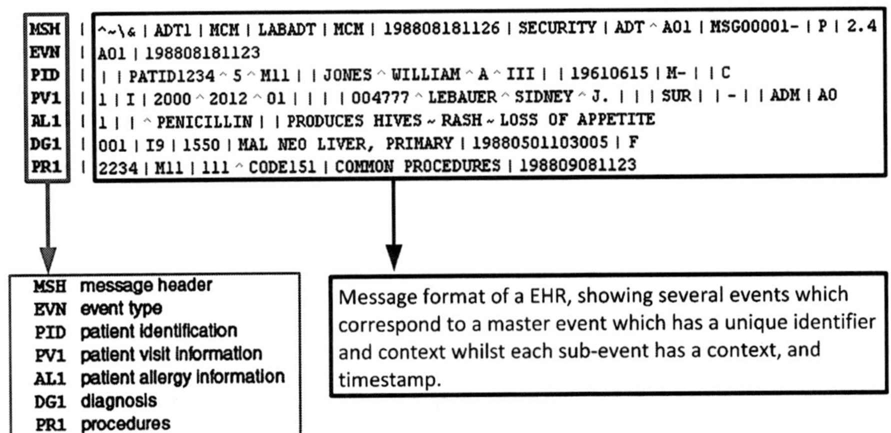

Figure 9. Event log format

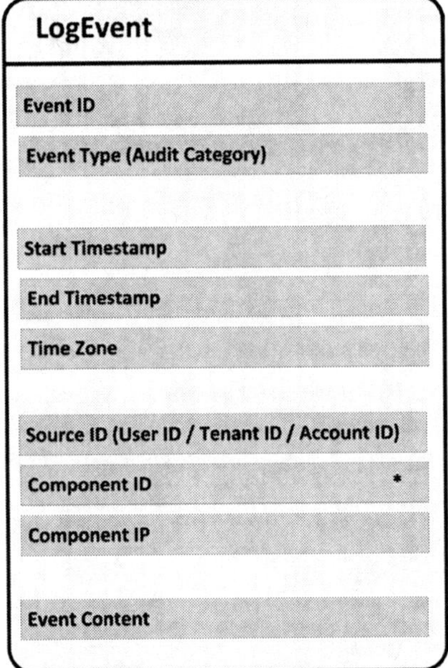

* not required for physical device logs

locality) an event processing network (EPN) is generated from the relevant input sources, requirements and measurement databases in order to determine an output, this approach was previously used by Rozsnyai et al., (2007) to cope with the deluge of data.

The Event Processing Network for locality (Figure 10) consists of input windows for HANA, Hadoop and SQL Anywhere (SQA) databases. The information for location of relevant services is then aggregated from both the HANA and Hadoop databases into a `ServiceLocations' input stream whilst the confidence values for relevant services are mapped to a `ServiceConfidence' input stream. Each of these streams along with the locality requirements from a `ServiceRequirements' input stream (determined at service deployment) and Locations input stream (sourced from an IP database) are all fed into an output window `CurrentLocation'. This output window is the trigger to run an assessment of each service by the `NonCompliant' output stream, which in turn is initiated by the `Location10' flex stream.

In the Figure you can see the event processing agent (EPA) query for the flex stream written in Continuous Computation Language (CCL). This EPA query calculates the time window for checking non-compliance every 10s. The resultant output of the non-compliance check is fed back to a HANA database.

Once triggered the output window compares the IP of a service with the IP database in order to determine a location and furthermore compares this location with the given ipLocation requirement to produce a compliance result which is stored in the Hadoop database. If non-compliant an alert is

Listing 2. An example Continuity Care Record (CCR)

```
1  <?xml version=``1.0" encoding=` `utf-8"?>
2  <ContinuityOfCareRecord xmlns='urn:astm-org:CCR'>
3      <CCRDocumentObjectID>MedDoc</CCRDocumentObjectID>
4      <Language>
5          <Text>English</Text>
6      </Language>
7      <Version>1.0</Version>
8      <DateTime>
9          <ExactDateTime>1374598308</ExactDateTime>
10     </DateTime>
11     <Patient>
12         <ID>001</ID>
13     </Patient>
14     <Medications>
15         <Medication>
16             <Description>
17                 <Text>Digoxin 0.125mg, 1 qDay, #90</Text>
18             </Description>
19             <Product>
20                 <ProductName>Digoxin</ProductName>
21                 <Strength>
22                     <Value>0.125</Value>
23                     <Units>mg</Units>
24                 </Strength>
25             </Product>
26             <Quantity>
27                 <Value>90</Value>
28             </Quantity>
29             <Directions>
30                 <Direction>
31                     <Dose>
32                         <Value>1</Value>
33                     </Dose>
34                     <Frequency>
35                         <Value>qd</Value>
36                     </Frequency>
37                 </Direction>
38             </Directions>
39         </Medication>
40 </ContinuityOfCareRecord>
41
```

produced and sent to the HANA database to be visualised on the dashboard in real-time.

EHR Audit

CCAS provides the audit results by means of a Web portal. This allows data to be visualised and presented to the consumer in different forms depending on the context of the data.

Initially the consumer would be presented with a services tab (Figure 11) listing all their services, active or inactive, that have been registered with the CCAS system to be audit assessed. Information such as ID, name and active status are provided by the service broker, whilst provider and rating are from the service registry. From this screen the auditor provides integration with the service marketplace allowing easy access to create services. Whilst on this screen if a compliance breach is detected for an active service the consumer is informed by way of a pop-up announcement upon which they can click to investigate further. These alerts are also able to be navigated in audit alerts tab of the service audit section (Figure 12). This page presents the user with an inbox of alerts, giving a title of each compliance breach, its occurrence data, other information such as status and priority may supplement this. On clicking an audit alert,

Figure 10. EHR locality complex event process

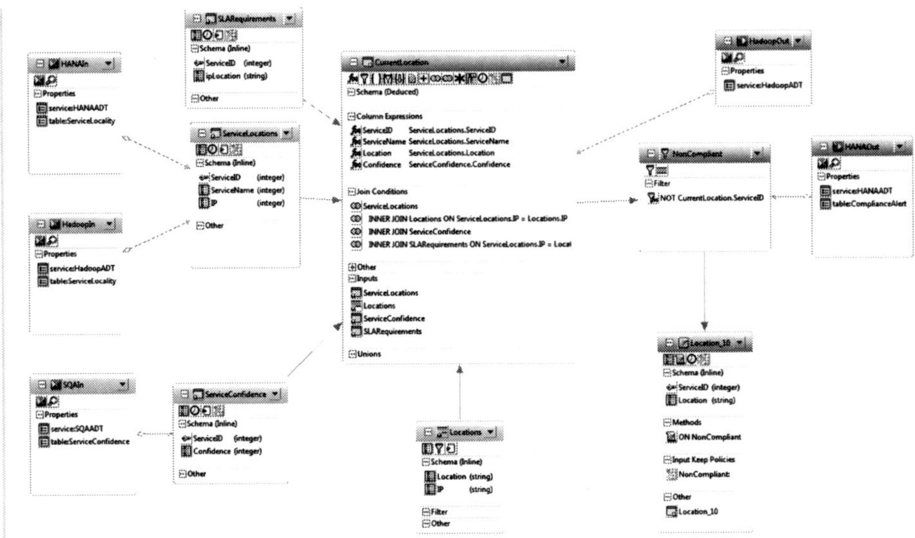

either on the services pop-up or the audit alert page, a window will be presented describing the detail of the compliance breach. In the case of a geo-location breach the window presented (Figure 13) shows a map of the service components and their location indicating compliance using the traffic light system (green for compliant, orange for compliant risk, red for non-compliant). This window also shows a summarised view of the audit alerts table which allows the user quickly to scroll through and change the content of the window to show details of a different alert.

Most importantly the audit portal allows the consumer to select a service and open an audit report. This report (Figure 14) shows a breakdown of the laws and their corresponding principles presenting a table of the service components and the test they have undergone to prove the principle stating the compliance for each, although we don't go as far as implementing confidence we provide a visualisation of how this could be presented

Figure 11. Audit portal - EHR consumer

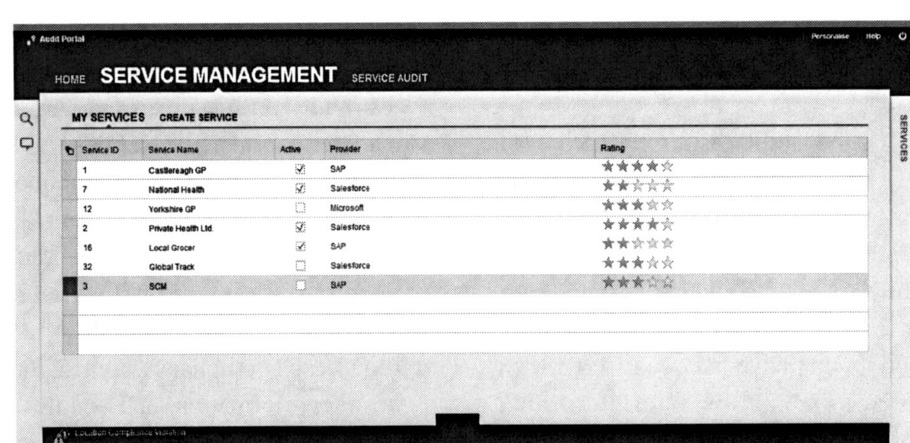

Figure 12. Audit alerts dashboard

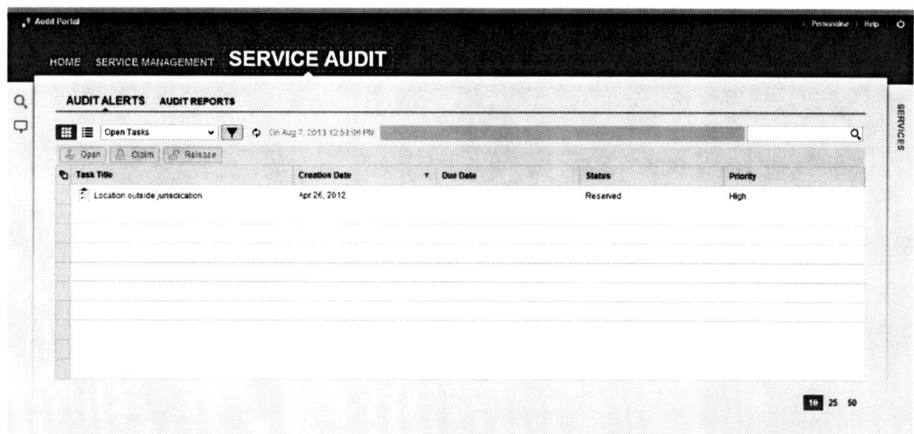

Figure 13. Location audit alert map

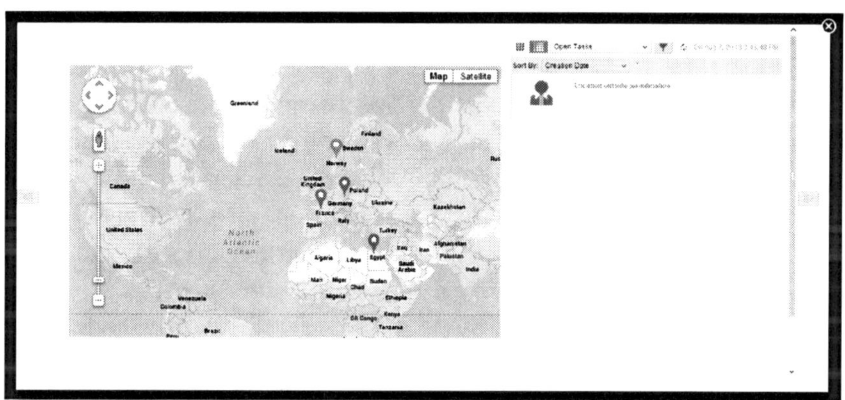

alongside each result. The corresponding service SLA can also be displayed alongside the report in order for the consumer to cross-reference the requirements that were defined.

AUDITING EHR DATA LOCALITY

In order to be compliant with particular legislation, consumers may only store data within certain geographical locations as described by Peterson (2011) Whilst it was possible for the consumer to enforce their own security measures for on-premise solutions, the cloud computing model makes them reliant upon the service providers to implement the required measures. Therefore a degree of trust is necessary between the consumer and service providers in the context of managing the geographic deployment and storage of services and data.

The SLA extensions implemented and the CCAS and corresponding distributed architecture implemented are utilised to provide an audit of geo-location compliance of EHR systems for privacy legislation.

The locality of services (virtual instances), and hosts (physical devices) can be determined by several approaches; IP databases, GPS (global positioning systems) and TPM (trusted platform modules).

Figure 14. Audit report - EHR service

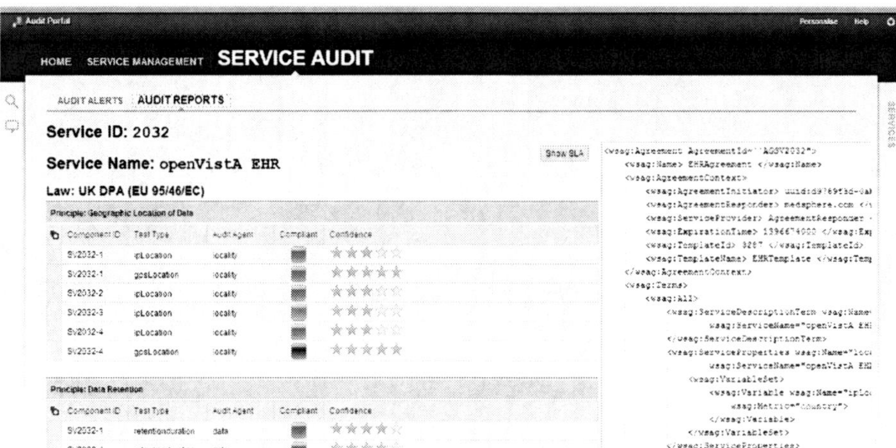

Host Geo-Location

The discovery of physical locality of a host on the Internet is a widely known problem. Geo-location approaches are widely used to limit services (i.e. gambling and television) to geographic regions. IP databases used for geo-location are setup using various evidence gathering techniques from DNS and Internet topology mapping, through to traceroutes and latency measurement. Whilst it is said that the accuracy of these databases is questionable as demonstrated by Huffaker et al., (2011) and Poese et al., (2011), Siwpersad (2008) found that the two most popular commercial databases only differ by 100km, which is well within satisfactory bounds for this research.

Service Geo-Location

The geo-location of a service is much harder to determine and can only be relied upon when it is cross-referenced with the location of the physical host upon which the service resides. IP proxies, service composition and service migration are some of the reasons why cross-referencing is necessary.

IP Geo-Location

Mapping IP addresses to a geographic location has become of key importance for the adoption of enterprise cloud computing and the Internet of services. Service locality is key to enforcing restrictions on provider issues regarding resource allocation and service migration for legal requirements of consumers.

There are two methods of IP geo-location; active (based on ping delay and trace routes) and passive (based on databases of IP ranges with country and city assignment). The most common method of IP geo-location used is passive as it is faster and more scalable despite being less accurate. The passive approach used in the auditing architecture sourced IP information from the hostip.info open-source community database, being one of very few mature non-commercial offerings. In Listing 3 an extract of the properties file and java code used by the locality agent of the audit probe to determine the geo-locality of a service is given. Figure 15 shows an example of the output returned from querying the database.

Figure 15. Example HostIP.info query result

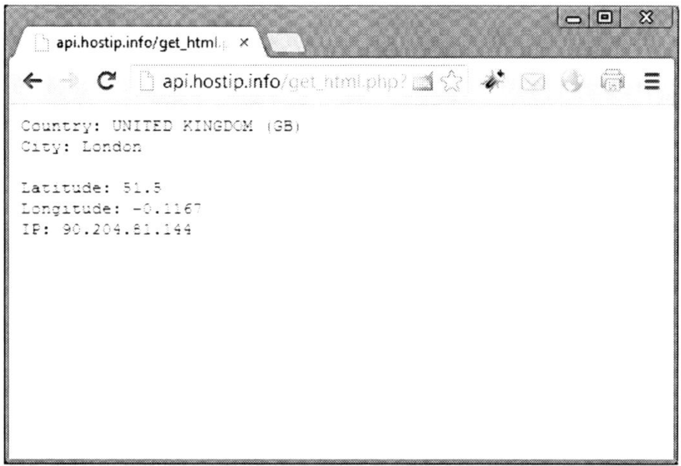

Listing 3.

```
# Probe configuration
geoProbe.id=location
geoProbe.sleep=30
geoProbe.proxy.host=proxy.lon.sap.corp
geoProbe.proxy.port=8080
...
public void init(IProperties properties)
{
        this.properties = properties;
        logger.debug(``GeoProbe.properties \n {}," properties);
        // Initialise XML Parser
        parser = new ParseGeoJSON();
        // Load AMQP Automatic reconnect properties
        {
        reconnect = properties.getBoolean(``amqp.reconnect.enabled," true);
        reconnectSleepBase = properties.getInt(``amqp.reconnect.sleep," 1 * 1000);
        reconnectExponentialBackoff = properties.getBoolean(``amqp.reconnect.exponen-
tial-backoff," true);
        reconnectMaxSleep = properties.getInt(``amqp.reconnect.max-wait," 10 * 60 *
1000);
                if (!run)
                {
                        reconnectSleepActual = reconnectSleepBase;
                }
        }
        // Load probe configuration
```

continued on following page

Listing 3. Continued

```java
            {
                    id = properties.getString(``geoProbe.id");
                    sleepDuration = properties.getInt(``geoProbe.sleep," 30);
            }
            // Connect to AMQP Broker
            {
                    String host = properties.getString(``amqp.broker.host");
                    int port = properties.getInt(``amqp.broker.port," 5672);
                    int timeout = properties.getInt(``amqp.timeout," 10);
                    connection = new Manager(host, port, timeout);
                    key = properties.getString(``amqp.publish.key," ``monitor.update.geo");
                    exchange = properties.getString(``amqp.publish.exchange," "amq.topic");
            }
            // Add manager listener
            {
                    connection.addListener(new ManagerListener()
                    {
                            @Override
                            public void closed()
                            {
                                    logger.warn(``Connection lost");
                                    restart = true;
                                    runThread.interrupt();
                            }
                    });
            }
    }
    private GeoData getData() throws IOException
    {
            return parser.parse();
    }
    private MetricCollection buildProtobuf(String id, GeoData data)
    {
            MetricCollection.Builder metrics = MetricCollection.newBuilder();
            metrics.addMetrics(buildMetric(id, ``location.country," data.country));
            metrics.addMetrics(buildMetric(id, ``location.city," data.city));
            metrics.addMetrics(buildMetric(id, ``location.longitude," data.longitude));
            metrics.addMetrics(buildMetric(id, ``location.latitude," data.latitude));
            return metrics.build();
    }
    private Metric buildMetric(String id, String name, String value)
    {
```

continued on following page

Listing 3. Continued

```
        Metric.Builder metric = Metric.newBuilder();
        metric.setId(id);
        metric.setName(name);
        metric.setValueType(Type.STRING);
        metric.setStringValue(value);
        metric.setTimestamp(now);
        return metric.build();
}
private Metric buildMetric(String id, String name, float value)
{
        Metric.Builder metric = Metric.newBuilder();
        metric.setId(id);
        metric.setName(name);
        metric.setValueType(Type.FLOAT);
        metric.setFloatValue(value);
        metric.setTimestamp(now);
        return metric.build();
}
```

Intel Trusted Execution Technology (Intel TXT)

Intel Trusted Execution Technology (TXT) provides enhanced hardware components enabling the protection of sensitive information from software-based attacks. Features such as micro-processor or I/O subsystem integration enable this technology, allowing the operating system or hypervisors to access these capabilities.

The utilisation of a prototype feature on the trusted platform module (TPM) of the Intel TXT chipset for geo-tagging provides a foundation for future cryptographic hardware methods of attestation.

Geo-Location Migration

Geo-location migration is assessed based on the service location throughout it's lifetime or over a given time period. A service may be singular or be a composite being made up of multiple services. Each deployed entity of a service not only needs to be assessed based upon the location it has been deployed to, but also any location to which an entity of the service resides through the audit period. This is necessary due to virtualisation and the use of migration by the cloud provider for resource utilisation and disaster recovery / backup mitigation. Although a compliance audit can be done as a 'point in time' action (as shown in Figure 14, audits conducted over a given time period (i.e. annually, or bi-annually) may assess compliance through a service lifetime and therefore require all locations in which services reside to be compliant.

EVALUATION OF THE CONTINOUS COMPLIANCE AUDITING SERVICE

An evaluation of the CCAS approach has been determined through a comparative assessment against existing audit processes. These processes were illustrated by simplification of the audit work-flows as defined by ISACA (as implemented

Figure 16. Manual audit plan

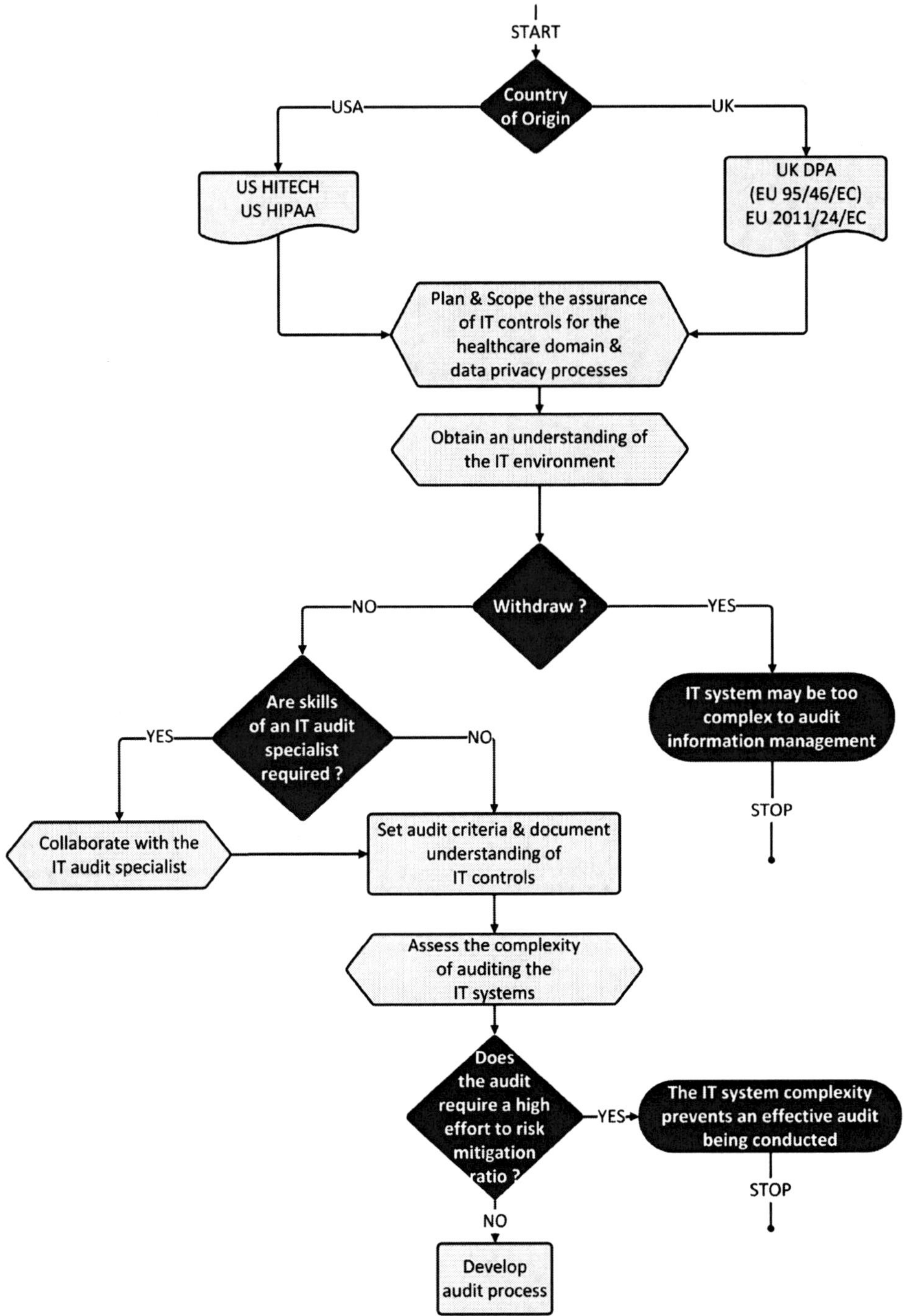

by companies such as PwC). The knowledge for the evaluation was verified by an experienced IT systems auditor.

The existing approach by auditors to assess the compliance of IT controls within a system is divided into two work-flows; planning and testing. The planning work-flow (Figure 16) assesses the effect that IT complexity has on the auditor's ability to study and evaluate the controls implemented within the system. This approach allows the auditors to determine whether or not it is both possible and worthwhile to conduct the required audit tests. The testing work-flow (Figure 17) is only conducted if a positive outcome is produced from the planning work-flow. This work-flow assesses the complexity of the IT environment in order to determine how and what tests to perform on the system, these results are evaluated and compliance breach risk is determined as being of high or low value. If high, tests are re-run, otherwise any deficiencies are documented, identified, remediation attempted and penalties issued.

Figure 17. Manual audit test

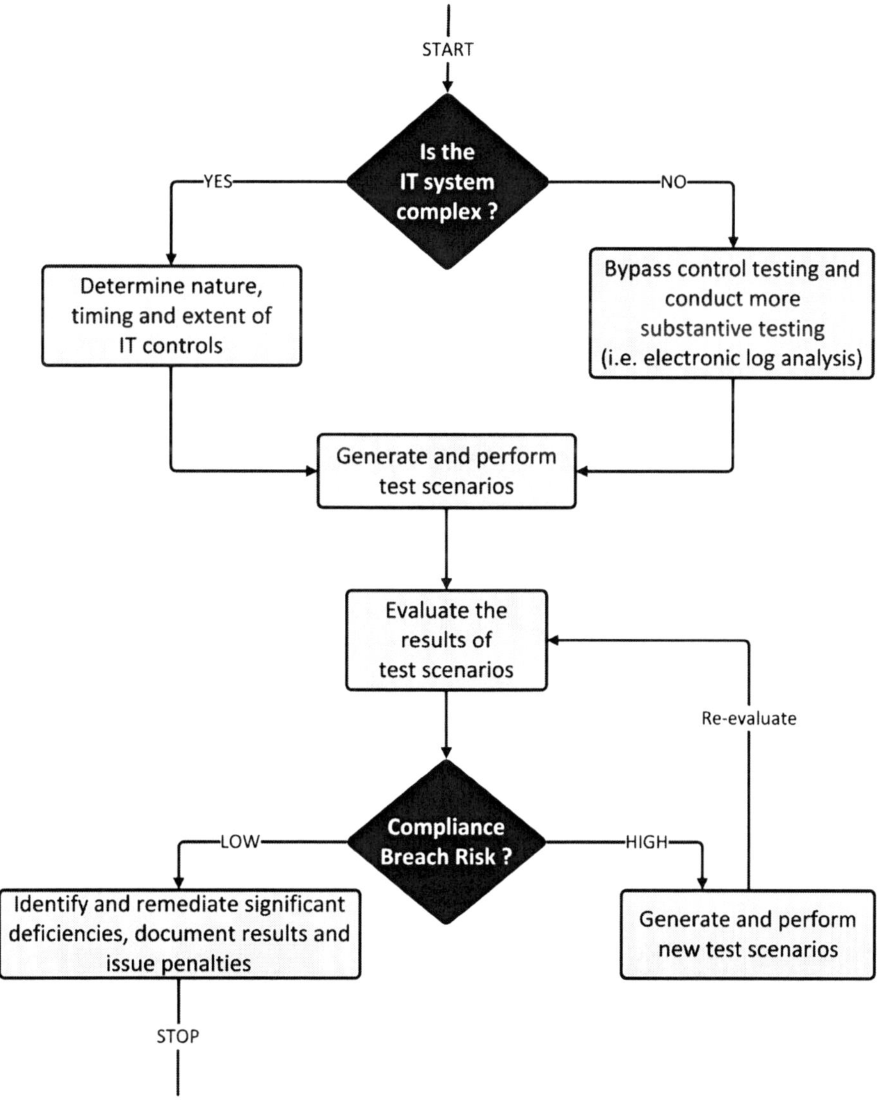

Each step of the existing process requires manual interaction by the auditor. Under most circumstances, distributed cloud-based systems are regarded as being too complex and therefore more audits are unable to be conducted using current auditing methods.

The CCAS Audit approach (Figure 18) provides a more automated approach to auditing in which the auditor is aided in both planning and testing. In CCAS the auditor only needs to assess that the defined SLA requirements match the necessary compliance requirements in order to prepare an audit plan. CCAS then allows the auditor to utilise compliance tests already conducted by the third-party auditing tool, or to conduct substantive testing on historical electronic logs. Evaluation

Figure 18. CCAS audit process

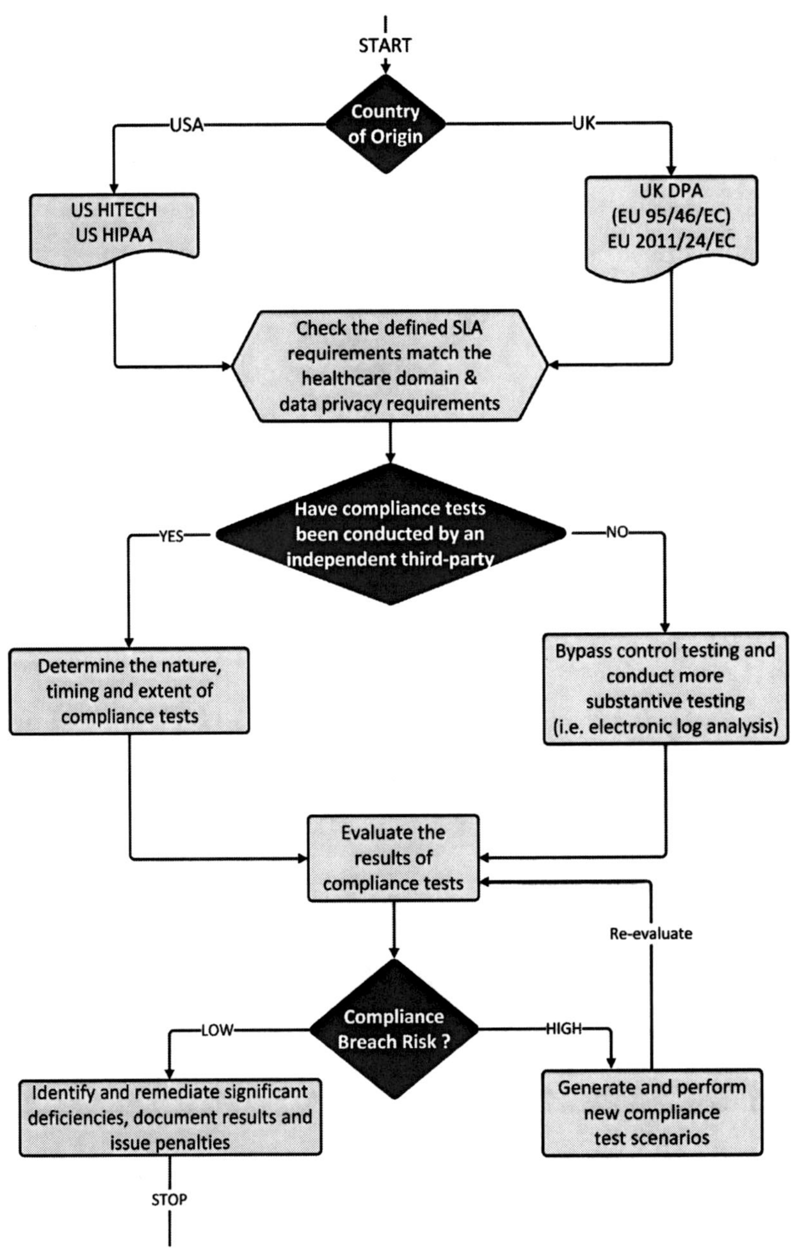

of this existing material enables the auditor to quickly determine the compliance breach risk and any further actions. CCAS has the advantage of enabling the auditor to assess all systems regardless of their complexity.

CONCLUSION

Auditing for e-Health compliance conformance in a cloud context is a topic that tackles relatively new research questions discussing the problems that hinder the adoption of cloud computing for Health Care. As systems become more dynamic, virtualised and distributed it becomes impractical for auditors to undertake a manual approach to assess the compliance of IT systems. In order to provide a tool which bridges the gaps between both the legal and technical domains and provides an auditor with a more automated approach to help achieve compliance conformance a continuous compliance auditing service (CCAS) has been developed.

CCAS demonstrated in this chapter aims to tackle the following three objectives which are fundamental challenges of auditing for compliance conformance in a cloud context: legal specification, scalable architecture and visualising audit results. The CCAS approach for auditing services for compliance was implemented in a real world scenario for EHR systems providing an overview of its function and output in the context of geolocation compliance. An in-depth example of SLA definition, a complex event processing and audit visualisation where provided. To finish an evaluation of the CCAS approach and its output was provided against the existing process and has demonstrated that it can provide audit capabilities to IT environments (such as distributed and cloud-based) which have been previously classified as too complex to be audited for legal compliance.

REFERENCES

Abbadi, I. M., Namiluko, C., & Martin, A. (2011, December). Insiders analysis in cloud computing focusing on home healthcare system. In *Proceedings of Internet Technology and Secured Transactions (ICITST)*, (pp. 350-357). IEEE.

Bouwman, H., & MacInnes, I. (2006). Dynamic business model framework for value webs. []. IEEE.]. *Proceedings of System Sciences, 2*, 43–43.

Edworthy, S. M. (2001). Telemedicine in developing countries: May have more impact than in developed countries. *British Medical Journal, 323*(7312), 524. doi:10.1136/bmj.323.7312.524 PMID:11546681

Gunter, T. D., & Terry, N. P. (2005). The emergence of national electronic health record architectures in the United States and Australia: models, costs, and questions. *Journal of Medical Internet Research, 7*(1). doi:10.2196/jmir.7.1.e3 PMID:15829475

Huffaker, B., Fomenkov, M., & Claffy, K. (2011). Geocompare: a comparison of public and commercial geolocation databases. In *Proceedings of Network Mapping and Measurement Conference (NMMC)*. NMMC.

Kifor, T., Varga, L., Álvarez, S., Vázquez-Salceda, J., & Willmott, S. (2006). Privacy issues of provenance in electronic healthcare record systems. In *Proceedings of the 1st Int. Workshop on Privacy and Security in Agent-Based Collaborative Environments (PSACE 2006)*. PSACE.

Kijl, B., Bouwman, H., Haaker, T., & Faber, E. (2005). *Dynamic Business Models in Mobile Service Value Networks: A Theoretical and Conceptual Framework*. FRUX Deliverable.

Li, M., Yu, S., Ren, K., & Lou, W. (2010). Securing personal health records in cloud computing: Patient-centric and fine-grained data access control in multi-owner settings. In *Proceedings of Security and Privacy in Communication Networks* (pp. 89–106). Springer. doi:10.1007/978-3-642-16161-2_6

Lindner, M., Galán, F., Chapman, C., Clayman, S., Henriksson, D., & Elmroth, E. (2010). The cloud supply chain: A framework for information, monitoring, accounting and billing. In *Proceedings of 2nd International ICST Conference on Cloud Computing (CloudComp 2010)*. ICST.

Lindner, M., McDonald, F., McLarnon, B., & Robinson, P. (2011). Towards automated business-driven indication and mitigation of VM sprawl in Cloud supply chains. In *Proceedings of Integrated Network Management (IM)* (pp. 1062–1065). IEEE. doi:10.1109/INM.2011.5990505

Lindner, M. A., McDonald, F., Conway, G., & Curry, E. (2011). Understanding Cloud Requirements-A Supply Chain Lifecycle Approach. In *Proceedings of Cloud Computing 2011, The Second International Conference on Cloud Computing, GRIDs, and Virtualization* (pp. 20-25). Academic Press.

Milojicic, D., Llorente, I. M., & Montero, R. S. (2011). Opennebula: A cloud management tool. *IEEE Internet Computing, 15*(2), 11–14. doi:10.1109/MIC.2011.44

Peterson, Z. N., Gondree, M., & Beverly, R. (2011). A position paper on data sovereignty: The importance of geolocating data in the cloud. In *Proceedings of the 8th USENIX confErence on Networked Systems Design and Implementation.* USENIX.

Poese, I., Uhlig, S., Kaafar, M. A., Donnet, B., & Gueye, B. (2011). IP geolocation databases: Unreliable? *ACM SIGCOMM Computer Communication Review, 41*(2), 53–56. doi:10.1145/1971162.1971171

Rozsnyai, S., Vecera, R., Schiefer, J., & Schatten, A. (2007). Event cloud-searching for correlated business events. In *Proceedings of E-Commerce Technology and the 4th IEEE International Conference on Enterprise Computing, E-Commerce, and E-Services,* (pp. 409-420). IEEE.

Siwpersad, S. S., Gueye, B., & Uhlig, S. (2008). Assessing the geographic resolution of exhaustive tabulation for geolocating Internet hosts. In *Proceedings of Passive and Active Network Measurement* (pp. 11–20). Springer. doi:10.1007/978-3-540-79232-1_2

Stewart, J. A., Day, M., Print, C., & Favato, G. (2009). Compliance in the supply chain: implications of Sarbanes-Oxley for UK businesses. *ICFAI Journal of Supply Chain Management, 6*(1), 8–19.

IT Union. (2008). *Implementing e-health in developing countries.* ITU Tech Report.

World Health Organisation. (2005). *58th World Health Assembly Report.* WHO Tech Report.

Zhou, L., Zhu, Y., Lin, Y., & Bentley, Y. (2012). Cloud Supply Chain: A Conceptual Model. In *Proceedings of European, International Working Seminar on Production Economics.* Innsbruck, Austria: Academic Press.

KEY TERMS AND DEFINITIONS

Auditing: Collecting and evaluating evidence to determine whether a computer system (information system) safeguards assets, maintains data integrity, achieves organizational goals and consumes resources efficiently.

Cloud Supply Chain (CSC): Two or more parties linked by the provision of Cloud services, related information and funds.

Cloud: A model for enabling ubiquitous, convenient, on-demand network access to a shared pool of configurable computing resources (e.g., networks, servers, storage, applications, and services) that can be rapidly provisioned and released with minimal management effort or service provider interaction.

Compliance: The assurance that processes, defined by both government and regulators, which require that businesses manage data safely, are being adhered to.

Customer Relationship Management (CRM) System: Maintains customer information for the purposes of administration, marketing, sales and support.

Electronic Health Record (EHR) Systems: Special forms of CRM systems customised for the health-care domain used to collect and store patient health information.

Service Lvel Agreement (SLA): Is a contract between a service provider and a consumer that specifies, usually in measurable terms, the conditions upon the service has been provisioned.

This work was previously published in Cloud Computing Applications for Quality Health Care Delivery edited by Anastasius Moumtzoglou and Anastasia N. Kastania, pages 116-139 copyright year 2014 by Medical Information Science Reference (an imprint of IGI Global).

Chapter 75
Critical Success Factors in Health Information Technology Implementation:
The Perspective of Finnish IT Managers

Nguyen Thi Thanh Hai
University of Eastern Finland, Finland

Tommi Tapanainen
Hanyang University School of Business, Korean

Diana Ishmatova
Waseda University, Japan

ABSTRACT

Health Information Technology (HIT) implementation success factors are evolving and proliferating, making it difficult for both researchers as well as practitioners to focus their limited resources on narrowing down those factors that impact success the most. A nationwide survey conducted on Finnish information technology (IT) managers to evaluate the critical success factors (CSFs) for HIT implementation in the order of importance unveils (1) system quality, (2) service and information quality, and (3) the support of leaders to be among the top ranking CSFs. Finnish IT managers generally prioritize system-related success factors higher than collaboration-related success factors. This research is among the first to provide survey-based empirical foundation for success factor prioritization in HIT implementation. It also aims to unravel IT manager decision-making in CSF-ranking process. Further, it enables the identification of success factors, which are rated important but may not have yet been considered sufficiently. One counter-example is "the involvement of physicians as project champions," which has often been seen as crucial to HIT implementation, although project champions were rated at the bottom of the CSF list being surveyed.

DOI: 10.4018/978-1-4666-8756-1.ch075

1. INTRODUCTION

An ongoing debate on how healthcare organizations can achieve greater success in implementing Health Information Technology (HIT) has evolved (Ash et al. 2003a; Brender et al. 2006; Heeks, 2006; Kaplan & Harris-Salamone, 2009). Today, healthcare professionals are still seeking knowledge of and continued to be highly interested in ways to help HIT implementation projects to succeed (Martikainen et al. 2012). Thus, there is a need to examine key factors that will lead to HIT implementation success, more specifically, factors that should be most attended to in the context of competing priorities.

Many studies (e.g. Alexander et al. 2011; Archer & Cocosila, 2011; Ash et al. 2003a; Ash et al. 2003b; Ash et al. 2005; Baron et al. 2005; Gagnon et al., 2009, 2010; Lorenzi et al., 2008, 2009; McGinn et al. 2011) have attempted to identify the success factors for HIT implementation. Ash et al. (2003a), for example, reported on twelve (12) principles towards achieving a successful Computerized Physician Order Entry (CPOE) Implementation. Brender et al. (2006) presented a collection of 110 success factors; unfortunately, such success factor lists are long and unwieldy, and it can be difficult to see which ones should have received more attention than others. Thus, as also pointed out by other researchers (Khandelwal & Ferguson 1999; Remus & Wiener, 2010), prioritization of crucial success factors from the less crucial is necessary.

The current understanding of HIT implementation success factors is based on the gradual accumulation of mainly case and action research results (Nguyen et al. 2014), all of which would need further examination with sound methodological applications. Some prior work obtains the list of success factors from the opinion of expert panels (Ash et al. 2003a; Brender et al. 2006; Kaplan & Harris-Salamone, 2009). However, members of expert panels were mainly from academic institutions and the number of participants was limited.

Other integrative work has relied on literature reviews (e.g. Cresswell & Sheikh 2009; Lau et al. 2012; Lluch, 2011; Van der Meijden et al. 2003), but few attempted to study practicing managerial opinions on success factors. Sudhakar (2012), for example, applied the approach of prioritizing critical success factors from an existing success factor list for software projects. The ranking method in this paper was based on the number of occurrences of a given success factor in the prior literature, rather than first-hand empirical data. No article was found to survey IT manager opinions in ranking HIT implementation success factors by priority.

The role of IT managers is crucial as they are often responsible for the initiation and implementation of information systems (Enns et al. 2003; Leidner et al. 2010; Watts & Henderson, 2006). IT managers, through their experience, can know best which relevant factors have been crucial for successful implementation of the projects; therefore, it is imperative to understand the perceptions of IT managers regarding relative importance of success factors in HIT implementation.

This research aims to reassess and synthesize the critical success factors (CSFs) influencing HIT implementation, focusing on the question: "What are the CSFs in HIT implementation from IT managers' point of view?" A survey conducted on Finnish IT managers results in the priority success factor list. This paper discusses the top ten factors from this list. The study is organized in five sections. Section 2 reviews the prior research to deduce a comprehensive list of HIT implementation success factors from different stakeholders in different contexts (e.g. major hospitals and small clinical practices in rural areas). Section 3 describes the research methodology. Section 4 highlights the study results on the top ten CSFs found while Section 5 delves further into an illustrative discussion on one of these CSFs. Section 6 details the conclusion and limitation of the research.

2. H.I.T. IMPLEMENTATION SUCCESS FACTORS

A review of the extant literature was performed on professional databases (i.e. PubMed, Medline, CINAHL, and Web of Science) with the following keywords: "implementation", "health information technology" or "health information system", or "electronic health" or e-Health, or "medical informatics" and "success." The research team (as explained in the research methodology section) combined factors that had similar definitions. The success factors are explained below and listed in Appendix 1.

2.1. Commitment and Support of Leaders

Having the commitment and support of the leaders helps the project team to overcome the obstacles of implementing HIT successfully (Devine et al. 2008; Gagnon et al. 2010; Amirfar et al. 2011). Klehr et al. (2009), for example, found that the role of the Vice-President, who also served as Chief Nursing Officer, was crucial to project success by providing financial and organizational support to the task force.

2.2. Project Champions

A number of studies (e.g. Box et al. 2010; Gagnon et al. 2010; Klehr et al. 2009; Lowery et al. 2012; Postemaa et al. 2012; Sharkey et al. 2013; Silvester & Carr, 2009; Upton, 2008; Wolf et al. 2006) found that assigning project champions for the HIT implementation could improve its chances of success since project champions can help to coordinate implementation and encourage overall acceptance of the new applications by their peers.

2.3. Project Management

Project management is essential for the control of project resources and the successful completion of project tasks (Ludwick & Doucette, 2009). A project plan should define the scope, schedule and budget of the project and include methods to identify, evaluate and avoid problems (Amirfar et al. 2011; Fullerton et al. 2006; Jacobs et al. 2007; Postemaa et al. 2012). As about 80% of project resources are allocated to process change management including, for example, training hospital staff and integrating new e-Health procedures into clinical practice (Silvester & Carr, 2009), a detailed change management plan is required to ensure that these resource-intensive tasks are understood at the outset.

2.4. Multi-Disciplinary Teamwork

Often, the implementation of any systems has to be managed by a project group, which should include representatives from the IT department, and possible future users from administration and various clinical departments (Fullerton et al. 2006; Jacobs et al. 2007; Lorenzi et al. 2008; Wolf et al. 2006). Having such a team helps in the building of a high quality system that will be accepted by the targeted users. While IT experts know how to implement the systems, they do not know the details of processes actually happening in the organization so that the inclusion of the clinical and other personnel will help to encourage system adoption and use (Devine et al. 2008).

2.5. Cooperation Among Administration, IT, and Clinical Functions

A collaborative relationship between physicians, researchers, hospital administrators, IT specialists, end-users, and external stakeholders (e.g. government officials) is necessary in HIT implementation (Bar-Lev & Harrison, 2006; Klehr et al., 2009; Hernández-Ávila et al., 2013; Dennehy et al. 2011). In particular, Mazzolen (2006) argued that closing the gap among the medical informatics staff, the health professionals, and the hospital management could make the difference between the success and the failure of a good computer-based solution.

2.6. Performance of Project Team

The project team must not only possess basic skills such as IT knowledge, communication skills, and a clear understanding of user needs and business objectives, but effective coordination of the team and stakeholder management are also needed to excel (Fullerton et al. 2006; Devine et al. 2008; Urda et al. 2012). Having the skills is not a guarantee that the project will succeed, for example, a sports team composed of world-class players may still fail to perform up to expectations and can lose to an opponent who "plays well" together even though the isolated players may have far inferior capabilities individually. Therefore, the creation of a team with the know-how to apply best practices and learning "as a team" from prior implementations can make the difference between failure and success in HIT implementations (Lorenzi et al. 2008).

2.7. Co-Development of the System and the Workflow

A matching of the characteristics of the new system to the new envisaged process scheme should be planned. Thus, an understanding of the current work processes and information flows is necessary to design more efficient processes, which can be afforded by the capabilities of the new system (Jeskey et al. 2011; Urda et al. 2013; Vreeman et al. 2006). The efficiencies provided by the redesign can help to promote user acceptance of the new system (Baron et al. 2005; Devine et al. 2008; Urda, et al. 2013; Upton, 2008).

2.8. End-User Participation and Involvement

End-user participation throughout the various system implementation stages has found to be fundamental to success of HIT projects in many studies (e.g. Alexander et al. 2011; Bar-Lev & Harrison, 2006; Batley et al. 2011; Devine et al., 2008; Nykanen & Karimaa, 2006; Silvester & Carr, 2009; Vreeman et al. 2006; Wolf et al. 2006). As end-user adoption of systems is critical to whether systems are considered to be successful (David et al. 1989; DeLone & McLean, 1992), involving and engaging end-users actively in the planning, design, and development phases will not only help to reinforce the multiple changed conditioning by which users are being alerted to and expected to operate with the newly implemented systems, but it will also help facilitate future planning sessions for revisions to be made in updating the adopted system.

2.9. Meeting the Need of End-Users

System designers should strive to understand the needs of users (Upton, 2008). For example, the contribution of a system to a clinical practice is dependent on whether the clinicians' information needs are well understood (Gustafson et al. 2007). User needs can be addressed by work role –focused modeling in the planning phase of HIT implementation. For example, new systems can contribute to work routine intensification to certain work roles, and excessive burden to these work roles may be detected and avoided by such a method (Fisher & Torin, 2008).

2.10. System, Service and Information Quality

Many previous studies (e.g. Batley et al., 2010; Cripps & Standing, 2011; David et al. 1989; De-Lone & McLean, 1992, 2003; Kijsanayotin et al. 2009) found that the implemented system will be used and user satisfaction improves if the quality of the system, information and services are good. All of these will lead to further positive impacts on the individual users and the organization.

2.11. Collaboration with the Vendors

A key factor in HIT implementation success hinges on the relationships developing between the healthcare organization and the vendor (Baron et al. 2005). Such cooperation can help in bringing together the latest IT expertise and practical clinical expertise in the organization, which is crucial in solving problems that arise during HIT implementation (Amirfar et al. 2011). This relationship-building can also help in unraveling the long-term potential of the technology and therefore give knowledge of new IT that can further contribute to the IT strategy of the healthcare organization (Jeskey et al. 2011).

2.12. Infrastructure Quality

Telecommunications capability, rigorous security, interoperability, standardization, and connectivity of clinical information systems are important to keep up with the increment of quick adoption and to make the system useful for the participants by allowing them to access and input events (Baron et al., 2005; Devine et al. 2008; Fullerton et al. 2006; Nesbitt et al. 2006; Silvester & Carr, 2009). Data standardization was described as a central component of system success (Vreeman et al., 2006).

2.13. Provision of Training and Technical Support

In addition to engaging the users, earlier studies (Maust, 2012; Vreeman et al., 2006) reported that adequate staff training was crucial to successful implementation. The intensity of training, the timing and availability of training, and post-implementation training can affect user technology acceptance. For example, training programs stressing the relevance of Electronic Health Record (EHR) to the physicians' jobs, and providing substantial evidence that EHR is easier to use and more effective than what non-adopters

might think will further increase the chances of success for new EHR implementations (Archer & Cocosila, 2011). Having the technical support to the users not only when they are first using the application but also when projects "go live" will allow the implementation team to directly experience what may (may not) be working well (Ash et al. 2003a).

2.14. Sufficient Resources

Sufficient resources (e.g. finance and staff) are important to ensure sustainability of HIT projects (Klehr et al. 2009; Hernández-Ávila et al. 2013; Nesbitt et al. 2006). The source of such finances is often the responsibility of the implementing healthcare organization, but healthcare services are also often supported by government initiatives and alternative sources – such as insurance companies and the patients themselves – all of which needs to be considered as well (Baron et al., 2005).

2.15. Incentives and Regulation

Incentives, whatever their form, are necessary to encourage adoption and lay the concrete foundation for implementation (Baron et al., 2005; Box et al. 2010). As expected, financial incentives were a common issue found in the studies (Ash et al. 2003a; McGinn et al. 2011). However, incentives, even financial incentives, are occasionally insufficient. Then, strong administrative guidance may be necessary to direct HIT implementation (Box et al. 2010).

2.16. Organization Openness and Experience in Change and Innovation

HIT adoption is influenced by the innovative culture of an organization (Gagnon et al. 2010). Rogers (2003) notes that some individuals are more prone to adopt new technology than others.

The presence of these early adopters and opinion leaders who can draw their peers into adopting the new HIT can facilitate the HIT adoption process in the organization (Gagnon et al. 2010; Nesbitt et al. 2006; Sharkey et al. 2013). Similarly, previous HIT experience can help in mastering new technologies (Ludwick & Doucette, 2009). Conversely, lack of such experience can make it very difficult to learn the new technologies (Nesbitt et al. 2006). This principle appears to hold true also for organizational change in general. Gustafson et al. (2007) noted that a history of prior organizational changes creates readiness for future organizational changes.

2.17. Information Communication Technology (ICT) Strategy

The ICT strategy, which defines a long-term ICT vision to be aligned with the organization strategy (Boddy et al. 2009), shapes how ICT can be used within an organization as part of achieving the organization strategic goals and objectives. The ICT strategy covers all facets of organization ICT environment such as hardware and software, vendor management, resource allocation and benefits and cost. To execute an ICT strategy IT managers need to work closely with other departments and user groups within the organization (Deutsch et al. 2010; Wen et al. 2010).

2.18. Organization Strategy

The organization strategy, which consists of planned activities, aims at achieving certain organizational goals including the HIT implementation (Lau et al. 2011). Change management for the implementation project (Callen et al. 2008; Lorenzi & Riley, 2000; Lorenzi et al. 2008) is based on these high-level organizational goals.

2.19. Meeting the Need of Management

The HIT implementation should contribute to key organization objectives (Wen et al. 2010), and the way in which these objectives are achieved should be considered in the planning stage of HIT implementation (Gustafson et al. 2007). As HIT success is influenced by how well it can fulfill these achievement expectations, implementers need to examine the needs of the management and align the goals of the HIT implementation project with organizational objectives before beginning the implementation in order to increase the chance of success.

2.20. Influence of External Environment

The external environment can significantly affect and impact on HIT implementation outcomes through the regulatory and legislative system as well as the general economic conditions and government subsidies (Boddy et al. 2009; Gustafson et al. 2007; Hernández-Ávila et al. 2013; Postemaa et al. 2012; Vitacca et al. 2009). The actions of the national and local government, which may be outside of the organization management controls, will nevertheless have a direct bearing on the success of individual HIT implementations in healthcare organizations (Boddy et al. 2009; Hernández-Ávila et al. 2013).

2.21. Meeting the Need of External Stakeholders

External stakeholders such as governmental organizations may have set requirements for patient safety, quality improvement, patient rights, and prevention of illnesses to the healthcare organizations. As these requirements are aimed at increasing the effectiveness and efficiency of healthcare services, eliminating or reducing redundant examinations and realizing mandated prioritization (Vitacca et al. 2009), healthcare organizations are forced to design their service provision, including HIT, to accommodate the requirements (Gustafson et al. 2007). Thus, HIT implementers should consider how these compulsory external requirements are and/or will be met.

3. RESEARCH METHODOLOGY

3.1. Instrument

The survey questionnaire was based on a literature review (Nguyen et al. 2014), which identified and extracted 15 key success factors for HIT implementation. The questionnaire was pilot-tested with four experts in information management, one IT project manager and one CIO. After considering their comments and suggestions, the questionnaire was revised into a total of 25 CSFs (i.e. 6 new factors were reviewed and added, and 4 factors were broken down into more elementary factors). These factors are measured in 7-point Likert scale where 1 was defined as "extremely important", 2="very important", 3="moderately important", 4="neutral", 5="slightly important", 6="low importance" and 7="not at all important". In the questionnaire, both the term "Chief Information Officer (CIO)" and IT managers were used because usage of the title varies considerably across organizations (Gottschalk, 1999; Lepore, 2000). A licensed translator, who returned from English into Finnish as a graduate student, translated the success factors first from Finnish to English. Finally, the match of these translations with original English equivalents was checked by one of the researchers, who is a native Finnish speaker. A link to the questionnaire was sent to the respondents to rate the importance of these 25 success factors.

3.2. Survey Administration

As no comprehensive source of information was available on IT managers in Finnish healthcare organizations, the list of research subjects was created manually. The Finnish healthcare system consists of municipal central administration, public sector social and healthcare administration, municipally owned IT companies, central hospitals, university hospitals, private hospitals and other healthcare organizations. At least one IT manager was expected to be found in each major hospital. Small healthcare organizations would not necessarily have any IT manager on their payroll; however, at the municipal level, IT services would be sourced from common, municipally owned providers, which were included in this research. The first focus group (54 people) comprises people who were found directly by the researchers. Because not all potential respondents could be found directly, the second focus group (55 people) was composed of people who were named by the contact persons in the target organizations. In this case, the contact persons were asked to forward the questionnaire to "the individual who is responsible for the automated information systems in your hospital". After adjustment for non-working email addresses and additional references from the contact persons, a total of 109 people made it to the final list of potential respondents for the survey. The survey was conducted in April and May 2013 with a total of 34 people responding to it.

4. RESULTS

A total of 34 responses received from 109 people surveyed corresponds to a 31.2% response rate. Responses were obtained from four (4) out of five (5) university hospitals, ten (10) out of a total of sixteen (16) central hospitals, seventeen (17) other public healthcare organizations, two

(2) municipally owned IT companies, and one (1) private IT healthcare. In Finland, the public healthcare sector accounts for 85% of all healthcare services (Winblad et al., 2011), and therefore the surveyed sample represents the population of Finnish healthcare IT managers quite well.

Since the questionnaire was sent via two different channels (i.e. directly to IT managers in some organizations and via contact persons of other organizations), it is necessary to ensure the respondents were, in fact, in the correct target group, that is, IT managers who have clear responsibilities for HIT implementation in their organizations. The criteria for screening the respondents were based on (1) background data from the respondents, and (2) a holistic appraisal based on respondents' titles and their known departmental functions (see Stephens et al. 1992 for similar criteria). The screening was made by two of the researchers working together. Of the 34 responses, two were screened out, because one was an expert doctor, a temporary position; and the other was a security chief, who was being excluded from the IT management function of the organization. Thus, only 32 responses were actually included in the study reported here.

Table 1. Ratings of critical success factors by IT managers

Rank	Success factors	Average rating
1	System quality	1.41
2	Information and service quality	1.69
2	Leaders support and commitment	1.69
4	End-user involvement and participant	1.71
5	Cooperation among administration, IT, and clinical functions	1.75
6	Staff training	1.78
6	Infrastructure quality	1.78
8	Co-development of the system & workflow	1.81
9	Resources	1.84
10	Collaboration with the vendors	1.90

The data analysis has two parts: Part 1: Background information of IT managers; and Part 2: Top ten success factors. In part 2, five missing data items were replaced by the mean of each respective variable.

4.1. Background of IT Managers

The majority (40.54%) of respondents have a technical education background, followed by nursing (24.32%) and commercial (21.62%). Other education backgrounds account for 13.51% including administration and natural science. No IT manager having a medical doctor degree participated in the survey (Figure 1). More than 50% had held management positions either in IT or the nursing field prior to becoming IT managers. Most (67.57%) worked as IT professionals/managers while about 22% worked as nursing staff or a supervisor in nursing before being appointed IT managers. The respondents that were selected in the screening had different titles such as IT management chief, development chief and principal planner, but the IT management chief was the most frequently occurring title. 16 respondents worked in an independent IT unit while others worked in an internal IT department, which was part of the general administration or under the management of the Chief Financial Officer or the Development Director.

4.2. Top Ten CSFs in HIT Implementation

The full rating list of 25 factors is displayed in Appendix 2. Table 1 presents the top ten ranked factors in term of importance from the perception of IT managers in healthcare organizations in Finland.

The IT managers' views generally agreed with the previous studies about the importance of the quality criteria for the system, information, and service, as they were ranked in the first and second positions in the top priority list. They also

Figure 1. Education background

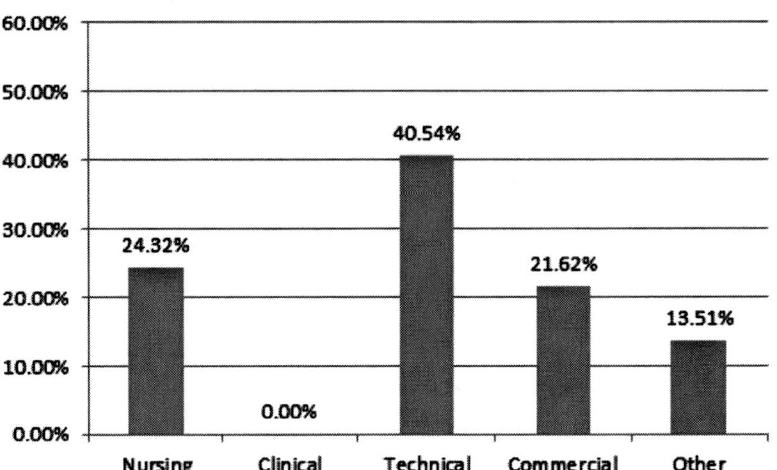

ranked top management team support highly, in third place, and therefore, these managers seem to believe that success would be difficult to achieve without the presence of this support. IT managers also considered end-user participation and adequate staff training to be among the top priorities for HIT success (i.e. in 4th and 6th positions respectively). These factors aim to promote end-user acceptance, which strongly influences whether the implementation is successful or not. Following these factors IT managers listed cooperation among the organizational functions in the 5th position. Similar to end-user participation and staff training, cooperation between organizational functions can foster inter-departmental communication and therefore facilitate the success of HIT implementation.

Furthermore, the quality of the infrastructure is important because the new system must be integrated into the existing infrastructure for it to become operational. IT managers clearly support the importance of this factor, albeit to a lesser degree than the quality of the system to be implemented. IT managers agreed also that the co-development of the system and the workflow is a necessary element for success, and earlier researchers have also recognized this. Despite all of the hype, it is obvious that HIT projects without sufficient resources

cannot obtain success, and this is reflected in the inclusion of resources in the top ten CSFs ranked in Table 1. Finally, IT managers recognized collaboration with the vendors as a key success factor, although it is at the bottom in this list. Many healthcare organizations lack technical know-how and are dependent on vendor relationships to obtain IT expertise, hence the inclusion of this factor.

5. ILLUSTRATIVE CSF DISCUSSION

This research uncovered a list of top ranking CSFs for HIT implementation from the practitioners' perspective. Still, the findings should assist both scholars and healthcare organizations when directing IT managers to use their scarce resources more effectively. By applying the pyramidal study approach (Nguyen et al. 2014), scholars and healthcare organizations can further investigate each CSF listing to isolate the highly relevant solutions for the success of HIT implementations in the different context.

As an illustrative example, based on the findings of this research, IT managers know that they should concentrate on getting end-users involved, engaged and participating actively in the HIT project. Unfortunately, while physicians can be involved in HIT implementation in other ways, the apparent lack of physicians as IT managers (as noted earlier in recruiting respondents for this research) can exacerbate the rift between the physicians as system users and IT staff. In addition, there might be a "chasm" of understanding between IT managers and physicians at the more strategic and tactical management level. While clinicians have been said to be skeptical of, and disinterested in, IT (McAlearney et al. 2007), a significant proportion of physicians have actually been found to want to contribute to IT development (Martikainen et al. 2012) and were enthusiastic about an HIT implementation (Lapointe & Rivard, 2006)). Martikainen (ibid.) pointed out that the lack of physician involvement in HIT implementation is due to their negative experiences with the current methods of eliciting their participation. Hostgaard et al. (2012) also argued that the power among different interest groups involved in HIT projects should be balanced more carefully in order to increase the participation opportunities of physicians. Appointing physicians to positions with a strong voice in HIT implementation, such as IT managers, or the Chief Medical Information Officer (Leviss et al. 2006) could indeed encourage the involvement and support of physicians to HIT implementation efforts.

Another way physicians could get involved in HIT implementation is acting as project champions. For example, if a physician is not an IT manager, appointing a physician to be a project champion can increase the physicians' commitment and involvement in the HIT implementation. This can be beneficial because physicians often serve in senior administrative roles, and therefore securing organizational resources becomes easier for the project. As well, it can help to mitigate change resistance and encourage overall acceptance of the new system among physicians in the organization (Cresswell et al., 2011; Lapointe & Rivard, 2006). Surprisingly, IT managers rated project champions as one of the three least important factors. Therefore, the apparent lack

of physicians as IT managers and the low importance of "physician champion" as judged by the respondents in this research should be examined further in future research in order to find out how best to nurture the relationship between IT managers and physicians and to encourage and facilitate the real participation of physicians in HIT implementation. According to Echoing Boonstra and Broekhuis (2010), more attention should be paid to the role and influence of project leaders/ champions in order to increase the HIT adoption rate. A focus on this success factor and other CSFs as identified by this paper could help to improve the mechanisms of how to facilitate successful HIT implementation.

6. CONCLUSION, LIMITATIONS AND FUTURE RESEARCH

Prior research has extended the list of success factors for HIT implementation. These success factors have, however, been mostly extracted from case and action research–based empirical data with very limited attempts to use surveys to comprehensively examine these factors from a practitioner-based perspective. Moreover, prior literature has so far not provided an empirically grounded priority list of the most important success factors. Such an approach is important in order to understand the success factors, which require most attention when time and resources are limited, and in particular, to do so based on firsthand empirical data. This effort contributes the priority list of success factors for HIT implementation from a nationwide survey of IT managers in healthcare sector organizations in Finland. The outcomes of this study can contribute to an inter-organizational knowledge base of strategies and methods to optimize implementations and to the subsequent achievement of organizational objectives. Understanding the underlying enablers leading to success can also assist different stakeholders to improve future HIT implementation.

While the results of this paper can be useful in general, care should be taken in applying them directly to other contexts as what is truly important for a given project can differ depending on the specific context. For example, in countries where services are provided significantly by private hospitals, IT executives could indicate that the role of incentives to implement HIT successfully may be greater. Small clinical practices might also have a tendency to emphasize the vendor relationship. This is because small practices have less purchasing power, smaller IT workforce, and less administrative resources to plan and design their own solutions. Therefore, they are more dependent on acquiring off-the-shelf products, IT capabilities, and training from these vendors.

The prioritized list of CSFs was generated based on a survey using a Likert-value questionnaire form. The survey approach allowed us to access the opinions of a large group of experts. However, our method of ranking and prioritizing success factors could be usefully complemented with other methods. For example, an avenue of fine-tuning the results could be to use an expert panel to identify the underlying dependencies among the success factors. Then, these experts could be asked to conduct an exercise of analytic hierarchy process to establish the success factor priorities – and whether this result is similar to what was found here.

ACKNOWLEDGMENT

We would like to thank the respondents of the survey and the experts who gave comments on the survey instrument. In addition, we are grateful for the constructive comments of the anonymous reviewers on an earlier version of this paper and the Finnish Culture Foundation and Foundation for Economic Education in Finland for their role in helping to make this research possible.

REFERENCES

Alexander, S., Frith, K. H., O'Keefe, L., & Hennigan, M. A. (2011). Implementation of Customized Health Information Technology in Diabetes Self-Management Programs. *Clinical Nurse Specialist CNS, 25*(2), 63–70. doi:10.1097/NUR.0b013e31820aefd6 PMID:21311246

Amirfar S., Taverna J., Anane S., & Singer J. (2011). Developing public health clinical decision support systems (CDSS) for the outpatient community in New York City: our experience. *BMC Public Health.* 30; 11:753.

Archer, N., & Cocosila, M. (2011). A comparison of physician pre-adoption and adoption views on electronic health records in Canadian medical practices. *Journal of Medical Internet Research, 13*(3), e57. doi:10.2196/jmir.1726 PMID:21840835

Ash, J. S., Chin, H. L., Sittig, D. F., & Dykstra, R. H. (2005). Ambulatory computerized physician order entry implementation. In *AMIA Annual Symposium Proceedings*, 11-5.

Ash, J. S., Fournier, L., Stavri, P. Z., & Dykstra, R. (2003). Principles for a successful computerized physician order entry implementation. In *AMIA Annual Symposium Proceedings*, 36-40.

Ash, J. S., & Stavri, P. Z. (2003). A Consensus Statement on Considerations for a Successful CPOE Implementation. *Journal of the American Medical Informatics Association, 10*(3), 229–234. doi:10.1197/jamia.M1204 PMID:12626376

Bar-Lev, S., & Harrison, M. I. (2006). Negotiating time scripts during implementation of an electronic medical record. *Health Care Management Review, 31*(1), 11–17. doi:10.1097/00004010-200601000-00003 PMID:16493268

Baron, R. J., Fabens, E. L., Schiffman, M., & Wolf, E. (2005). Electronic health records: Just around the corner? Or over the cliff? *Annals of Internal Medicine*, *143*(3), 222–226. doi:10.7326/0003-4819-143-3-200508020-00008 PMID:16061920

Batley, N. J., Osman, H. O., Kazzi, A. A., & Musallam, K. M. (2011). Implementation of an emergency department computer system: Design features that users value. *The Journal of Emergency Medicine*, *41*(6), 693–700. doi:10.1016/j.jemermed.2010.05.014 PMID:20619572

Boddy, D., King, G., Clark, J. S., Heaney, D., & Mair, F. (2009). The influence of context and process when implementing e-Health. *BMC Medical Informatics and Decision Making*, *9*(1), 9. doi:10.1186/1472-6947-9-9 PMID:19183479

Boonstra, A., & Broekhuis, M. (2010). Barriers to the acceptance of electronic medical records by physicians from systematic review to taxonomy and interventions. *BMC Health Services Research*, *10*(1), 231. doi:10.1186/1472-6963-10-231 PMID:20691097

Box, T. L., McDonell, M., Helfrich, C. D., Jesse, R. L., Fihn, S. D., & Rumsfeld, J. S. (2010). Strategies from a nationwide health information technology implementation: The VA CART story. *Journal of General Internal Medicine*, *25*(S1Suppl 1), 72–76. doi:10.1007/s11606-009-1130-6 PMID:20077156

Brender, J., Ammenwerth, E., Nykanen, P., & Talmon, J. (2006). Factors influencing success and failure of health informatics systems: A Pilot Delphi Study. *Methods of Information in Medicine*, *45*, 125–136. PMID:16482383

Callen, J. L., Braithwaite, J., & Westbrook, J. I. (2008). Contextual Implementation Model: A framework for assisting clinical information system implementations. *Journal of the American Medical Informatics Association*, *15*(2), 255–261. doi:10.1197/jamia.M2468 PMID:18096917

Cresswell, Kathrin, & Morrison, Zoe, MPharm, Sarah Crowe, Robertson Ann & Sheikh, Aziz. (2011). Anything but engaged: User involvement in the context of a national electronic health record implementation. *Informatics in Primary Care*, *19*, 191–206. PMID:22828574

Cresswell, K., & Sheikh, A. (2009). The NHS Care Record Service (NHS CRS): Recommendations from the literature on successful implementation and adoption. *Informatics in Primary Care*, *17*, 153–164. PMID:20074427

Cripps, H., & Standing, C. (2011). The implementation of electronic health records: A case study of bush computing the Ngaanyatjarra lands. *International Journal of Medical Informatics*, *80*(12), 841–848. doi:10.1016/j.ijmedinf.2011.09.007 PMID:22001067

Davis, F. D. (1989). Perceived usefulness, perceived ease of use, and user acceptance of information technology. *Management Information Systems Quarterly*, *13*(3), 319–340. doi:10.2307/249008

DeLone, W. H., & McLean, E. R. (1992). Information systems success: The quest for the dependent variable. *Information Systems Research*, *3*(1), 60–95. doi:10.1287/isre.3.1.60

DeLone, W. H., & McLean, E. R. (2003). The DeLone and McLean Model of Information Systems Success: A Ten-Year Update. *Journal of Management Information Systems*, *19*(4), 9–30.

Dennehy, P., White, M. P., Hamilton, A., Pohl, J. M., Tanner, C., Onifade, T. J., & Zheng, K. (2011). A partnership model for implementing electronic health records in resource-limited primary care settings: Experiences from two nurse-managed health centers. *Journal of the American Medical Informatics Association*, *18*(6), 820–826. doi:10.1136/amiajnl-2011-000117 PMID:21828225

Devine, E. B., Wilson-Norton, J. L., Lawless, N. M., Hansen, R. N., Hollingworth, W., Fisk, A. W., & Sullivan, S. D. (2008). Implementing an Ambulatory e-Prescribing System: Strategies Employed and Lessons Learned to Minimize Unintended Consequences. In Henriksen K, Battles JB, Keyes MA, Grady ML, editors. Advances in Patient Safety: New Directions and Alternative Approaches (Vol. 4: Technology and Medication Safety). Rockville (MD): Agency for Healthcare Research and Quality (US).

Enns, H. G., Huff, S. L., & Golden, B. R. (2003). CIO influence behaviors: The impact of technical background. *Information & Management, 40*(5), 467–485. doi:10.1016/S0378-7206(02)00040-X

Fisher, J. A., & Monahan, T. (2008). Tracking the social dimensions of RFID systems in hospitals. *International Journal of Medical Informatics, 77*(3), 176–183. doi:10.1016/j.ijmedinf.2007.04.010 PMID:17544841

Fullerton, C., Aponte, P., Hopkins, R., Bragg, D., & Ballard, D. J. (2006). Lessons learned from pilot site implementation of an ambulatory electronic health record. *Proceedings of Baylor University Medical Center, 19*(4), 303–310. PMID:17106488

Gagnon, M.-P., Desmartis, M., & Labrecque, M. (2010). Implementation of an electronic medical record in family practice: A case study. *Informatics in Primary Care, 18*, 31–40. PMID:20429976

Gagnon, M. P., Duplantie, J., Fortin, J. P., Lamothe, L., Légaré, F., & Labrecque, M. (2009). Integrating scientific evidence to support telehomecare development in a remote region. *Telemedicine Journal and e-Health, 15*(2), 195–198. doi:10.1089/tmj.2008.0070 PMID:19292630

Gustafson, D. H., Brennan, P. F., & Hawkins, R. P. (2007). *Investing in E-Health: What it Takes to Sustain Consumer Health Informatics.* Springer. doi:10.1007/978-0-387-49508-8

Heeks, R. (2006). Health information systems: Failure, success and improvisation. *International Journal of Medical Informatics, 75*(2), 125–137. doi:10.1016/j.ijmedinf.2005.07.024 PMID:16112893

Hernandez-Avila, J. E., Palacio-Mejia, L. S., Lara-Esqueda, A., Silvestre, E., Agudelo-Botero, M., Diana, M. L., & Sanchez Parbul, A. et al. Hernández-Ávila. (2013). Assessing the process of designing and implementing electronic health records in a statewide public health system: The case of Colima, Mexico. *Journal of the American Medical Informatics Association, 20*(2), 238–244. doi:10.1136/amiajnl-2012-000907 PMID:23019239

Hostgaard, A. M., Bertelsen, P., & Nohr, C. (2011). Methods to identify, study and understand End-user participantion in HIT development. *BMC Medical Informatics and Decision Making, 11*(1), 57. doi:10.1186/1472-6947-11-57 PMID:21955493

Jacobs, Brian R., Hallstro, Craig K., Hart, Kim Ward, Mahoney, Daniela & Lykowski, Gayle. (2007). The Clinical Informatics Outcomes Research Group, Lessons from a Successful Implementation of a Computerized Provider Order Entry System, *J Pediatr Pharmacol Ther*, Vol. 12 No. 2

Jeskey, M., Card, E., Nelson, D., Mercaldo, N. D., Sanders, N., Higgins, M. S., & Miller, A. et al. (2011). Nurse adoption of continuous patient monitoring on acute post-surgical units: Managing technology implementation. *Journal of Nursing Management, 19*(7), 863–875. doi:10.1111/j.1365-2834.2011.01295.x PMID:21988434

Kaplan, B., & Harris-Salamone, K. D. (2009). Health IT success and failure: Recommendations from literature and an AMIA workshop. *Journal of the American Medical Informatics Association, 16*(3), 291–299. doi:10.1197/jamia.M2997 PMID:19261935

Khandelwal, V., & Ferguson, J. (1999). Critical success factors and the growth of IT in selected geographic regions. In *Proceedings of the 32nd HICSS*, Hawaii, USA doi:10.1109/HICSS.1999.772760

Kijsanayotin, B., Pannarunothai, S., & Speedie, S. M. (2009). Factors influencing health information technology adoption in Thailand's community health centers: Applying the UTAUT model. *International Journal of Medical Informatics*, *78*(6), 404–416. doi:10.1016/j.ijmedinf.2008.12.005 PMID:19196548

Klehr, J., Hafner, J., Spelz, L. M., Steen, S., & Weaver, K. (2009). Implementation of Standardized Nomenclature in the Electronic Medical Record. *International Journal of Nursing Terminologies and Classifications*, *20*(4), 169–180. doi:10.1111/j.1744-618X.2009.01132.x PMID:19883454

Lapointe, L., & Rivard, S. (2006). Getting physicians to accept new information technology: Insights from case studies. *Canadian Medical Association Journal*, *174*(11), 1573–1578. doi:10.1503/cmaj.050281 PMID:16717265

Lau, F., Price, M., Boyd, J., Partridge, C., Bell, H., & Raworth, R. (2012). Impact of electronic medical record on physician practice in office settings: A systematic review. *BMC Medical Informatics and Decision Making*, *12*(1), 10. doi:10.1186/1472-6947-12-10 PMID:22364529

Lau, F., Price, M., & Keshavjee, K. (2011). From benefits evaluation to clinical adoption: Making sense of Health Information System Success in Canada. *Healthcare Quarterly*, *14*(1), 39–45. doi:10.12927/hcq.2011.22157 PMID:21301238

Leidner, D. E., Preston, D., & Chen, D. (2010). An examination of the antecedents and consequences of organizational IT innovation in hospitals. *The Journal of Strategic Information Systems*, *19*(3), 154–170. doi:10.1016/j.jsis.2010.07.002

Lepore, D. (2000). Are CIOs Obsolete? *Harvard Business Review*.

Leviss, J., Kremsdorf, R., & Mohaideen, M. F. (2006). The CMIO–A New Leader for Health Systems. *Journal of the American Medical Informatics Association*, *13*(5), 573–578. doi:10.1197/jamia.M2097 PMID:16799119

Lluch, M. (2011). Healthcare professionals' organizational barriers to health information technologies – A literature review. *International Journal of Medical Informatics*, *80*(12), 849–862. doi:10.1016/j.ijmedinf.2011.09.005 PMID:22000677

Lorenzi, N. M., Kouroubali, A., Detmer, D. E., & Bloomrosen, M. (2009). How to successfully select and implement electronic health records (EHR) in small ambulatory practice settings. *BMC Medical Informatics and Decision Making*, *9*(1), 15. doi:10.1186/1472-6947-9-15 PMID:19236705

Lorenzi, N. M., Novak, L. L., Weiss, J. B., Gadd, C. S., & Unertl, K. M. (2008). Crossing the implementation chasm: A proposal for bold action. *Journal of the American Medical Informatics Association*, *15*(3), 290–296. doi:10.1197/jamia.M2583 PMID:18308985

Lorenzi, N. M., & Riley, R. T. (2000). Managing change: An overview. *Journal of the American Medical Informatics Association*, *7*(2), 116–124. doi:10.1136/jamia.2000.0070116 PMID:10730594

Lowery, Mandy, Dobbs J & Monkhouse A. (2012). Embedding an electronic health record within a health visiting service. *Community Practitioner*, *85*(9), 20–23. PMID:23029773

Ludwick, D. A., & Doucette, J. (2009). Adopting electronic medical records in primary care: Lessons learned from health information systems implementation experience in seven countries. *International Journal of Medical Informatics*, *78*(1), 22–31. doi:10.1016/j.ijmedinf.2008.06.005 PMID:18644745

Martikainena, S., Viitanenb, J., Korpelaa, M., & Lääveri, T. (2012). Physicians' experiences of participation in healthcare IT development in Finland: Willing but not able. *International Journal of Medical Informatics, 81*(2), 98–113. doi:10.1016/j. ijmedinf.2011.08.014 PMID:21956004

Maust, D.D. (2012). Implementation of an electronic medical record in a health system: lessons learned. *Journal for nurses in staff development: JNSD: official journal of the National Nursing Staff Development Organization,* vol. 28, no. 1, pp. E11-E15.

Mazzoleni, M.C. (2006). Why a system awarded as "MIE '99 Best Paper" failed to be used and hence to affect patient's health? *Methods of Information in Medicine, 45*(1), 90–94. PMID:16482377

McAlearney, A. S., Chisolm, D. J., Schweikhart, S., Medow, M. A., & Kelleher, K. (2007). The story behind the story: Physician skepticism about relying on clinical information technologies to reduce medical errors. *International Journal of Medical Informatics, 76*(11-12), 836–842. doi:10.1016/j. ijmedinf.2006.09.021 PMID:17112779

McGinn, C. A., Grenier, S., Duplantie, J., Shaw, N., Sicotte, C., Mathieu, L., & Gagnon, M. P. et al. (2011). Comparison of user groups' perspectives of barriers and facilitators to implementing electronic health records: A systematic review. *BMC Medicine, 9*–46. PMID:21524315

Nesbitt, T. S., Cole, S. L., Pellegrino, L., & Keast, P. (2006). Rural Outreach in Home Telehealth: Assessing Challenges and Reviewing Successes. *Telemedicine Journal and e-Health, 12*(2), 107–113. doi:10.1089/tmj.2006.12.107 PMID:16620164

Nguyen, H. T. T., Saranto, K., Tapanainen, T., & Ishmatova, D. (2014). A Review of Health Information Technology Implementation Success Factors: Importance of the regulatory and financing environment, *Hawaii International Conference on System Science (HICSS)-47*, Hawaii, USA.

Nykänen, P., & Karimaa, E. (2006). Success and failure factors in the regional health information system design process--results from a constructive evaluation study. *Methods of Information in Medicine, 45*(1), 85–89. PMID:16482376

Postemaa, T. R. F., Peetersb, J. M., & Friele, R. D. (2012). Key factors influencing the implementation success of a home telecare application. *International Journal of Medical Informatics, 81*(6), 415–423. doi:10.1016/j.ijmedinf.2011.12.003 PMID:22226925

Remus, U., & Wiener, M. (2010). A multimethod, holistic strategy for researching critical success factors in IT projects. *Information Systems Journal, 20*(1), 25–52. doi:10.1111/j.1365-2575.2008.00324.x

Rogers, E. M. (2003). *Diffusion of Innovations* (5th ed.). New York, NY: The Free Press.

Sharkey, S., Hudak, S., Horn, S. D., Barrett, R., Spector, W., & Limcangco, R. (2013). Exploratory Study of Nursing Home Factors Associated with Successful Implementation of Clinical Decision Support Tools for Pressure Ulcer Prevention. *Advances in Skin & Wound Care, 26*(2), 83–92. doi:10.1097/01.ASW.0000426718.59326.bb PMID:23337649

Silvester, B. V., & Carr, S. J. (2009). A shared electronic health record: Lessons from the coalface. *The Medical Journal of Australia, 190*(11Suppl), S113–S116. PMID:19485857

Stephens, C. S., Ledbetter, W. N., Mitra, A., & Ford, F. N. (1992). Executive or functional manager? The nature of the CIO's job. *Management Information Systems Quarterly, 16*(4), 449–467. doi:10.2307/249731

Sudhakar, G. P. (2012). A model of critical success factors for software projects. *Journal of Enterprise Information Management, 25*(6), 537–558. doi:10.1108/17410391211272829

Upton, M. (2008). The Royal Hobart Hospital digital medical records success story. *Health Information Management Journal, 37*(1), 46–54. PMID:18245865

Urda, D., Ribelles, N., Subirats, J. L., Franco, L., Alba, E., & Jerez, J. M. (2013). Addressing critical issues in the development of an Oncology Information System. *International Journal of Medical Informatics, 82*(5), 398–407. doi:10.1016/j.ijmedinf.2012.08.001 PMID:22981645

Van der Meijden, M. J., Tange, H. J., Troost, J., & Hasman, A. (2003). Determinants of Success of Inpatient Clinical Information Systems: A Literature Review. *Journal of the American Medical Informatics Association. Review Paper, 10*(3), 235–243.

Vitacca, M., Mazzu, M., & Scalvini, S. (2009). Socio-technical and organizational challenges to wider e-Health implementation. *Chronic Respiratory Disease, 6*(2), 91–97. doi:10.1177/1479972309102805 PMID:19411570

Vreeman, D. J., Taggard, S. L., Rhine, M. D., & Worrell, T. W. (2006). Evidence for electronic health record systems in physical therapy. *Physical Therapy, 86*(3), 434–446, discussion 446–449. PMID:16506879

Watts, S., & Henderson, J. C. (2006). Innovative IT climates: CIO perspectives. *The Journal of Strategic Information Systems, 15*(2), 125–151. doi:10.1016/j.jsis.2005.08.001

Wen, K.-Y., Gustafson, D. H., Hawkins, R. P., Brennan, P. F., Dinauer, S., Johnson, P. R., & Siegler, T. (2010). Developing and validating a model to predict the success of an IHCS implementation: The readiness for implementation model. *Journal of the American Medical Informatics Association, 17*(6), 707–713. doi:10.1136/jamia.2010.005546 PMID:20962135

Winblad, I., Hamalainen, P., & Reponen, J. (2011). What Is Found Positive in Healthcare Information and Communication Technology Implementation? The Results of a Nationwide Survey in Finland. *Telemedicine Journal and e-Health, 17*(2), 118–123. doi:10.1089/tmj.2010.0138 PMID:21385025

Wolf, D. M., Greenhouse, P. K., Diamond, J. N., Ferd, W., & McCormick, D. (2006). Community Hospital Successfully Implements e-Record and CPOE. *CIN: Computers, Informatics. Nursing, 24*(6), 307–316.

This work was previously published in the International Journal of Healthcare Information Systems and Informatics (IJHISI), 10(1); edited by Joseph Tan, pages 1-16 copyright year 2015 by IGI Publishing (an imprint of IGI Global).

APPENDIX

Box 1. Summary of literature review on success factors of HIT implementation

Factors	References
Commitment and support from executives leaders	Amirfar et al. 2011; Gagnon et al. 2010; Devine et al. 2008; Klehr et al. 2009
Project Champion	Alexander et al. 2011; Box et al., 2010; Gagnon et al. 2010; Klehr et al., 2009; Lowery et al. 2012; Ludwick and Doucette 2009; Postemaa et al. 2012; Sharkey et al. 2013; Silvester & Carr, 2009; Upton, 2008; Wolf et al. 2006
Project Management	Amirfar et al. 2011; Baron et al. 2005; Devine at al., 2008; Fullerton et al. 2006; Jacobs et al. 2007; Jeskey et al. 2011; Ludwick & Doucette, 2009; Postemaa et al. 2012; Silvester & Carr, 2009
Multi-disciplinary teamwork and collaboration	Devine at al., 2008; Fullerton et al. 2006; Jacobs et al. 2007; Lorenzi et al. 2008; Urda et al. 2012; Wolf et al. 2006
Cooperation and collaboration among administration, IT, and clinical functions	Bar-Lev & Harrison, 2006; Dennehy et al. 2011; Hernández-Ávila et al., 2013; Klehr et al., 2009; Mazzoleni, 2006
Performance of Project Team	Devine at al., 2008; Fullerton et al. 2006; Lorenzi et al. 2008; Urda et al. 2012; Wolf et al. 2006
Co-development of the system and the workflow	Bar-Lev & Harrison, 2006; Baron et al. 2005; Boddy et al. 2009; Devine et al. 2008; Jeskey et al. 2011; Sharkey et al. 2013; Upton, 2008; Urda et al. 2013; Vreeman et al. 2006
End-user participation and involvement	Alexander et al. 2011; Bar-Lev & Harrison, 2006; Batley et al. 2011; Boddy et al. 2009; Devine et al., 2008; Jeskey et al. 2011; Nykanen & Karimaa, 2006; Silvester & Carr, 2009; Sharkey et al. 2013; Urda et al. 2012; Vreeman et al. 2006; Wolf et al. 2006
Meeting the need of end-users	Boddy et al. 2009; Gustafson et al. 2007; Fisher & Torin, 2008; Upton, 2008
Quality of system, information and service	Batley et al., 2010; Cripps & Standing, 2011; McGinn at al., 2011; Postemaa et al. 2012; Kijsanayotin et al. 2009; Urda et al. 2012
Collaboration with the vendors	Amirfar et al. 2011; Baron et al. 2005; Jeskey et al. 2011
Infrastructure	Baron at al., 2005; Devine et al., 2008; Fullerton et al. 2006; Nesbitt et al. 2006; Silvester and Carr, 2009; Upton, 2008; Vreeman et al., 2006
Provision of Information, Training and Support	Alexander et al., 2011; Archer & Cocosila, 2011; Ash et al. 2003a; Baron et al., 2005; Devine et al., 2008; Fullerton et al. 2006; Gagnon et al. 2009; Jacobs et al. 2007; Maust, 2012; Nesbitt et al. 2006; Sharkey et al. 2013; Vreeman et al., 2006
Sufficient resources	Baron et al., 2005; Klehr et al. 2009; Hernández-Ávila et al. 2013; Nesbitt et al. 2006
Incentives and regulation	Ash et al. 2003a; Baron et al., 2005; Box et al. 2010; Cripps and Standing, 2011; McGinn et al. 2011
ICT Strategy	Boddy et al. 2009; Deutsch et al. 2010; Wen et al. 2010
Organization Strategy	Callen et al. 2008; Lau et al. 2011; Lorenzi & Riley, 2000; Lorenzi et al. 2008
Meeting the need of management	Gustafson et al. 2007; Wen et al. 2010; Wolf et al., 2006
Influence of External environment	Boddy et al. 2009; Gustafson et al. 2007; Hernández-Ávila et al. 2013; Postemaa et al. 2012; Vitacca et al. 2009
Meeting the need of external stakeholders	Boddy et al. 2009; Gustafson et al. 2007; Vitacca et al. 2009
Organization openness and experience in change and innovation	Gagnon et al. 2010; Gustafson et al. 2007; Ludwick and Doucette, 2009; Nesbitt et al. 2006; Sharkey et al. 2013

Box 2. The list of 25 success factors evaluated by IT managers in healthcare organizations

Rank	Success Factors	Average Rating
1	System quality	1.41
2	Information and service quality	1.69
2	Leaders support and commitment	1.69
4	End-user participation and involvement	1.72
5	Cooperation among administration, IT, and clinical functions	1.75
6	Infrastructure quality	1.78
6	Staff training	1.78
8	Co-development of the system and workflow	1.81
9	Resources	1.84
10	Collaboration with the vendors	1.91
11	Technical support	2.22
11	Project management and planning	2.22
13	Project team performance	2.31
14	Multi-disciplinary project teamwork	2.34
15	Meeting the needs of end-users	2.44
16	Meeting the needs of management	2.81
17	Influence of external environment	2.94
18	Openness of the organization to change and innovation	3.03
19	Organization strategy	3.06
20	Information Communication Technology (ICT) strategy	3.16
21	Meeting the needs of external stakeholders	3.22
22	Experiences in change and innovation	3.47
23	Assigning project champions	3.53
24	Regulations	3.91
25	Incentives	4.47

Chapter 76

Business Intelligence for Healthcare:
A Prescription for Better Managing Costs and Medical Outcomes

Jack S. Cook
SUNY Brockport, USA

Pamela A. Neely
SUNY Brockport, USA

ABSTRACT

Using an interpretive case study approach, this chapter describes the data quality problems in two companies: (1) a Multi-Facility Healthcare Medical Group (MHMG), and (2) a Regional Health Insurance Company (RHIS). These two interpretive cases examine two different processes of the healthcare supply chain and their integration with a business intelligence system. Specifically, the issues examined are MHMG's revenue cycle management and RHIS's provider enrollment and credentialing process. A Data and Information Quality (DIQ) assessment of the revenue cycle management process demonstrates how a framework, referred to as PGOT, can identify improvement opportunities within any information-intensive environment. Based on the assessment of the revenue cycle management process, data quality problems associated with the key processes and their implications for the healthcare organization are described. This chapter provides recommendations for DIQ best practices and illustrates these best practices within this real world context of healthcare.

INTRODUCTION

Organizations rely on data for a multitude of applications: customer service and relationship management, decision making, business intelligence (BI), and regulatory compliance. One of these, BI has the potential for improving the quality of information in any industry, although there is currently a push specifically in healthcare to be smarter about its management of key performance outcomes. One contributing factor motivating industry leaders is that healthcare organizations

DOI: 10.4018/978-1-4666-8756-1.ch076

tend to be rich in data, but information poor. Although, healthcare organizations have been slow to embrace BI, these organizations are beginning to search for methods to deliver information to decision makers in more intelligent ways. The two main drivers for developing BI within healthcare are a desire to lower costs and improve patient outcomes. Therefore, one option is for BI to form the heart of any system that delivers organizationally sustaining data to providers and healthcare managers so they can make decisions that positively impact patient and service outcomes, while better managing the revenue cycle.

The challenge is to convince administrators, clerical staff, clinicians and physicians to buy-in to the importance of integrating previously disparate data to create a real-time view of the relationship between a patient, the provider, and the payer or payers. This chapter focuses on business intelligence (BI) systems that support healthcare, and the data and information quality (DIQ) issues that are inherent in any environment that is information intensive. BI has tremendous potential to impact healthcare, from multiple perspectives – patients, providers and payers. From a patient's perspective, BI can provide clinicians treatment and immunization recommendations that are preventative in nature, improving both diagnostic accuracy and better implemented care plans. Billing is critical in today's healthcare environment; providers transmit claims to multiple payers, and payment denials are common. BI dramatically improves data and information quality. Therefore, from the provider's perspective, IT professionals can streamline the complex billing process using BI. From a payer's perspective, a better connection to providers and a more intelligent way to enroll and credential them will reduce claims adjustments and disputes.

This chapter provides a brief literature review of healthcare, business intelligence (BI), as well as data and information quality (DIQ). Then the chapter discusses the healthcare industry as a whole with a particular emphasis on stakeholders and their interrelationships. After the literature and industry review, the chapter examines two cases that make the point that BI is a reasonable approach to manage key healthcare performance outcomes. The first case examines the process of adult immunization, specifically with respect to the Zoster vaccine. This case focuses on four key outcomes: medical outcomes, financial performance, compliance and overall customer satisfaction. The second case details the process that a payer performs to enroll and credential a healthcare provider. This second case looks at the key outcomes of compliance, customer satisfaction and financial performance. Next, we examine background information pertaining to healthcare, business intelligence and data and information quality.

BACKGROUND

Healthcare: As defined by the U.S. Department of Health and Human Services, a healthcare provider is "a provider of services as defined in §1861(u) of the Act (Social Security Act), a provider of medical or health services as defined in §1861(s) of the Act, and any other person or organization who furnishes, bills, or is paid for healthcare services or supplies in the normal course of business." (U.S. Department of Health and Human Services, 2001) Until recently, healthcare providers were paid when sick people sought treatment. Quality and outcomes were not rewarded, but rather providers were paid based on how much was done to treat the patient. In the future, healthcare providers will be given financial incentives to keep people well, and quality, not treatment, will matter a great deal. This shift from volume to value will require a rethinking of treatment plans and a shift towards preventative care.

Ensuring the health of its citizens continues to be at the forefront of politics in the United States, as well as on many corporate and personal agendas. Healthcare systems are judged based on three criteria: access, cost and quality (Shortell, 2004). With respect to access, the United States has been for some time the only industrialized country that does not guarantee health coverage to all of its citizens. Access to healthcare grew to a national crisis. In 2005, 46.6 million Americans were uninsured (ABC News, 2006). With the passage of the Patient Protection and Affordable Care Act (PPACA) in 2010, commonly referred to as Obamacare or the Affordable Care Act, together with the Health Care and Education Reconciliation Act, the U.S. healthcare system received its most significant government expansion and regulatory overhaul since the passage of Medicare and Medicaid in 1965 (Vicini & Stempel, 2012). The goal of Obamacare is to provide affordable health insurance for all U.S. citizens, and to reduce the growth in healthcare spending. Largely due to health reform and other federal policies, the number of uninsured Americans fell for the first time in four years according to the 2011 Census (Broaddus & Park, 2012).

From a cost perspective, the U.S. also has the costliest healthcare system. It is expected that the federal government will foot the bill for approximately 93% ($931 billion) of the Medicaid expansion costs over the period 2014 – 2022, while states will fund the remaining $73 billion (Angeles, 2012). Even for individuals covered by health insurance, the cost of healthcare can be prohibitive. Some predict that Obamacare should reduce the growth in healthcare spending in the long run. The current $2.8 trillion U.S. healthcare system costs almost $9,000 a year for every man, woman, and child in the U.S (ObamaCare Facts, 2013). Websites such as healthcarebluebook. com can give customary and reasonable charges for many procedures, but the actual charges vary widely.

Business Intelligence (BI): BI supports human intelligence with "technologies, applications and processes for gathering, storing, accessing and analyzing data to help users make better decisions" (Wixom & Watson, 2010, p. 14). BI is used in many industries, including healthcare (Olinsky & Schumacher, 2010; Sillup, Klimberg, & McSweeney, 2010). As indicated in the previous section, a number of healthcare systems, such as EHRs, CDS and RCM systems contain elements that qualify them as BI systems.

Wixom and Watson (2010) contend that BI is about getting the data in (via a data warehouse or data mart) and getting the data out (using organizational specific tools to meet decision making purposes). They provide a model of a BI-based organization that includes the traditional data warehouse elements and data integration coupled with analytical tools that have historically been of the online analytical processing (OLAP) and decision support type. These historical tools are now under the umbrella of BI technologies and applications, and are not listed separately. Additionally, and equally as important, the model includes processes related to metadata, data quality and governance. The recognition of these processes as important to the BI environment reinforces the need for practitioners to evaluate BI as a system, not simply a technology.

Two distinct types of BI have evolved: strategic and operational (Imhoff, 2005). Operational business intelligence (OBI) is relevant to both healthcare cases discussed in this chapter. OBI supports more agile decision making at all organizational levels (Marjanovic, 2010). OBI is a flexible, transparent and cost effective way of tightly integrating BI with an organization's constantly evolving business processes (Indart, 2006).

An important aspect of BI is the ability to analyze data and return information that can be used in decision making. Related to BI is the field of big data analytics. As data has become more abundant there is a need for new technologies and techniques to analyze this data effectively (Chen, Chiang, & Storey, 2012). Another challenge in healthcare is the abundance of free text that is not easily analyzed. Doctors' notes, prescription information and notes attached to test results can all be found in the typical healthcare system. New technologies in text analytics are necessary to adequately mine the data to affect decision making (Chen et al., 2012).

New government incentives, specifically the Health Information Technology for Economic and Clinical Health (HITECH) Act, which is part of the American Reinvestment and Recovery Act of 2009 and administered by the Centers for Medicare & Medicaid Services (CMS), stipulates that, beginning in 2011, healthcare providers will be offered financial incentives for demonstrating meaningful use of electronic health records (EHR). Incentives will be offered until 2015, after which time penalties may be levied for failing to demonstrate such use. The Act also establishes grants for training centers for the personnel required to support a health IT infrastructure.

With the HITECH Act providing funding and incentives for new technologies like patient sensors, new methods will be required to analyze data streamed from such mobile devices. Wactler et al (2011) envision that these new technologies must be part of an interoperable, digital infrastructure that is part of a universal system of health data and knowledge. Data in these systems must be diverse and allow for decision support. Furthermore, they contend that patients must be an integral part of the process, taking a major role in their own health and treatment. Data mining approaches, with their associated visualization techniques, could be one way to facilitate the analysis of this enormous amount of data (Hanauer, Zheng, Ramakrishnan, & Keller, 2011). BI systems can include components of scenario-based association mining, allowing healthcare providers new information on leading indicators of specific diseases (Lin, Brown, Yang, Li, & Lu, 2011). Overall BI can lead to greater improvements in patient care and payment flow, but the challenge will be developing new technologies, along with new policies and procedures to ensure that the information in these systems is of the highest quality.

Data Quality Management (DQM): Weber, Otto and Osterle, (2009) define DQM as quality-oriented management of data as an asset, that is, the planning, provisioning, organization, usage, and disposal of data that supports both decision-making and operational business processes, as well as the design of the appropriate context, with the aim to improve data quality on a sustained basis. The management of DIQ is also referred to as data governance.

DQM needs to integrate business and IT functions in order to address both organizational and technical perspectives (Abate, Diegert, & Allen, 1998). Although business and IT departments collaborate to a certain extent, the responsibility of improving data quality (DQ) and managing corporate data is often left to the latter (Friedman, 2008). Holding IT accountable for DIQ, even though data collectors are often outside the scope of control of IT, makes no sense. The analogy would be if management held manufacturing responsible for quality when ninety plus percent of the raw materials and components are supplied by outside vendors and what operators do is assemble components of questionable quality into a product. Obviously, if what is purchased is defective, no amount of proper assembly will make a quality product. The same is true for DIQ. If data collectors input garbage, no amount of work on the part of IT will make system output satisfactory to data consumers. Holding IT responsible for DIQ ignores the critical organizational factors, outside of the control of IT, that are necessary to ensure quality data and information is provided to decision makers. In fact, the quality of data and information is dependent on how it is used, also known as fitness-for-use (Neely & Cook, 2011). And decision makers should specify to data collectors what data is needed and how that data should look; in other words, decision makers need to specify the dimensions of data quality that are important to them.

Data quality is more than accuracy. In fact, Wang & Strong (1996) surveyed end-users and identified fifteen dimensions of quality, grouped into four categories: (1) intrinsic, (2) contextual, (3) representational and (4) accessibility. Intrinsic data quality refers to the dimensions inherent to the data itself, and includes believability, accuracy, reputation, and objectivity. Contextual data quality relates to perceptions of quality: timeliness, appropriate amount of data, value-added, relevancy, and completeness. The dimensions of representational data quality affect how the end user perceives the receipt of the data and includes ease of understanding, representational consistency, concise representation and interpretability. The final category, accessibility, has two dimensions: accessibility and access security.

It is difficult to trust your business intelligence system when DIQ is poor, and processes are ill conceived. Within healthcare, a reduced number of denials for claim payment and increased patient care (Leape et al., 1993) can result from improved DIQ because the system can notify providers of immunization and care plans automatically. This should result in better patient satisfaction. Fewer adjustments to the claims processing system (Romano Mj, 2011), decreased time to enroll providers, and reduced labor with respect to enrolling providers will result in better provider satisfaction and an increase in revenues in general (Rauscher & Wheeler, 2008).

DIQ in healthcare will continue to be of the utmost importance, for patient safety and satisfaction as well as the financial health of the system. Given the unique nature of the payment system in healthcare, it is critical that systems facilitate providers being paid. Getting paid from sometimes multiple payers, when payers have the ability to deny payment for a multitude of reasons, is much more challenging than in almost any other industry.

Interplay between DIQ and BI: Quality can be dramatically improved; for example, medical errors account for the deaths of at least 200,000 people in the U.S. even though the US health-

care system has traditionally been known for high quality (Harmon, 2009). As many as one in seven patients experience an adverse event, at an estimated cost to Medicare of $324 million in just October 2008 (Levinson, 2010) and as many as one in three patients experience a medical error (Classen et al., 2011). Medical errors are of four types: diagnostic, treatment, preventative and other (Leape, Lawthers, Brennan, & Johnson, 1993). Business intelligence (BI) systems could help to alleviate many of these errors. For example, diagnostic errors could be mitigated with BI by utilizing data mining techniques to look for cause and effect of lifestyle factors. These lifestyle factors could guide the diagnostician towards additional testing, ultimately resulting in a correct diagnosis. With respect to treatment errors, BI can be used as a longitudinal resource, ensuring that treatment protocols do not conflict with past history. Preventative errors also utilize the analytical capabilities of BI systems to determine what diseases a patient may be susceptible to and guide caregivers to provide prophylactic treatment.

Each of the previous types of medical errors is person-related. The final category, "Other", is system related. These errors include failure of communication, equipment failure and other system failures. Increasingly, healthcare systems are incorporating aspects of business intelligence, providing analysis of collected patient and financial data, as indicated in the previous paragraph. Intrinsic to systems is the quality of the data held in those systems. The issue of quality is exacerbated as data moves from primary to secondary sources. Thus, if we could improve the data and information quality (DIQ), we may be able to reduce the incidence of patient death and ultimately improve the quality of healthcare in general.

In addressing some of the concerns with quality, the U.S. government has allocated approximately $19 billion a year to be used by healthcare providers to implement electronic health record systems (EHRs) (Keehan et al., 2011). By using decision-support tools or BI, these systems can increase the adherence to protocol-based systems. Additionally, there should be a reduction in adverse drug events and medication errors (Wu et al., 2006). However, these systems can be costly and there is a need to study the return on investment. Bardhan and Thouin (2012) show that the use of EHRs can positively impact the treatment for heart attacks, heart failures and pneumonia. Furthermore, using financial management systems can result in lower operating expenses. On the other hand, Romano (2011) studied clinical decision making systems (CDS) and did not find a correlation between visits with and without a CDS on the quality of care. Linder et al. (2007) had a similar finding. Their study examined EHR use and ambulatory care quality and found no significant association. According to Giannangelo and Fenton (2008), in order for the EHRs to be effective, there must be a standard of codification and it must be used consistently to ensure that data is correct and reliable. This codification, particularly within the financial portion of the system, can lead to more effective revenue cycle management (RCM).

RCM is the collection of methods used to manage claims processing payment and revenue generation. Unlike the standard business-to-business or business-to-consumer model, whereby an invoice or request for payment is generated and the payment is made, a significant proportion of the revenue in healthcare is derived from non-patient payment (e.g., a third party), resulting in multiple streams of payments that must be managed. RCM is a frequent component of BI, allowing managers to increase the speed and amount of patient revenue collection (Rauscher & Wheeler, 2008). A potential consequence of the Patient Protection and Affordable Care Act is that serving publicly insured patients may have a negative impact on revenue cycle management (Rauscher & Wheeler, 2010). However, to the contrary, findings from their research indicate that hospitals with a higher Medicare and Medicaid payer mix actually collect revenues in higher percentages and quicker than hospitals with more privately insured or self-pay patients.

A properly implemented business intelligence system can play a vital role in ensuring quality throughout the data and information lifecycle. Thus, this chapter examines the connections between these two very important and mutually dependent areas of practice, BI and DIQ, in such a data-rich environment as healthcare. The PGOT framework, discussed next, provides an excellent mechanism for evaluating opportunities for improving quality.

Data and Information Quality Framework – PGOT

As evidenced by frameworks such as COBIT (Boritz, 2005), IT governance has been at the forefront of management concerns for a number of years. Increasingly, the challenge is to govern not only the systems, but also the data residing in the systems (Maguire, 2008). As indicated earlier, DIQ is dependent on how the data is used. Thus, acceptable quality in one instance may be unacceptable in another. For example, prescription information may be entered into a system for a patient. The data is accurate, but incomplete. The system has not captured the fact that the patient is seeing a specialist who has prescribed other medications that negatively interact with what the primary care physician has prescribed. Proper data governance, across all care providers, could help to alleviate this problem.

Compared with the extensive research literature on IT governance, academic interest and research on data governance and its relationship to business intelligence is still in its infancy. As introduced in Neely and Cook (2011), the PGOT (**P**eople, **G**overnance, **O**perations, and **T**echnology) framework provides a foundation for evaluating the quality of data and information. Figure 1 presents an enhanced version of the PGOT with an increased emphasis on the people within the system. The governance plans, operational efficiency and technical competency of the systems continue to be a driving force in the overall quality of the data and information. Based on contingency theory of organizational design, the underlying assumption of the PGOT framework is that there is no universal design applicable to all organizations for data and information quality, and healthcare is no exception. It is the contextual factors in healthcare that impact the contribution of data governance in enhancing IT governance and organizational performance. This framework focuses on long-term data and information quality improvement and error prevention, rather than correction. In the two cases discussed later, business intelligence systems are the mechanism by which DIQ is improved. The usefulness of a BI system is directly correlated to the quality of the data that it contains and the information it produces.

It is impossible to ensure "perfect" data quality on all dimensions given that the quality of data and information is dependent on its use; that is, decision making in context. The role of the data governance council, and by extension the chief data steward, business data steward and technical data steward, is to ensure the data and information is of sufficient quality to best meet the demands of most decision makers. The business data steward must define the business requirements and expectations, and trust the technical data steward to work with developers to build a system that meets data and information quality-related business requirements. In addition, the chief data steward must design and implement plans, policies and procedures that comply with legal and ethical requirements and meets the needs of data consumers.

Although perfect data is impossible, there are multiple feedback loops illustrated throughout the framework, many of them resulting from data quality audits, to help in the identification of opportunities to continuously improve DIQ. Therefore, the ability to audit the data and information quality from an operational, technical, and compliance perspective is vital to DQM. As a result, the BI system should have embedded continuous auditing controls, and metrics from such audits should be frequently analyzed for system usability and reliability.

The roles of the people who influence, manage and use the BI system with an emphasis on the data governance system are illustrated in Figure 2. The PGOT framework will be used to focus attention on DIQ within the BI system, specifically in the healthcare industry. The next section describes the healthcare environment and this is followed by a description of two case studies, illustrating how a methodical approach to examining DIQ can help to improve the quality and usefulness of the BI system, and ultimately impact the satisfaction of the patients and providers.

BETTER MANAGING COSTS AND MEDICAL OUTCOMES USING DIQ AND BI

Medicare and Medicaid continue to ratchet down provider payments, and will continue to do so. Fee for service is becoming less prevalent, while value-added and bundled services, referred to within the industry as episodic payments, will increase. Many payers already pay a lump sum for maternity. Physician procedural income will decline while their employment and integration with healthcare facilities will increase. As a result, hospitals, physicians and other healthcare providers will either find a way to deliver healthcare for less money or go out of business. The fundamental challenge of healthcare reform is to simultaneously improve the quality of care while lowering its costs. Although profitability is a dirty word in healthcare, without it, healthcare will not have the funds needed to provide better care for patients, whether it is acquiring the latest technology or hiring adequate staff to treat patients.

To improve quality, many healthcare organizations turn to the National Committee for Quality Assurance (NCQA), an independent 501(c) nonprofit organization in the United States designed to

Figure 1. DIQ in context: PGOT research framework

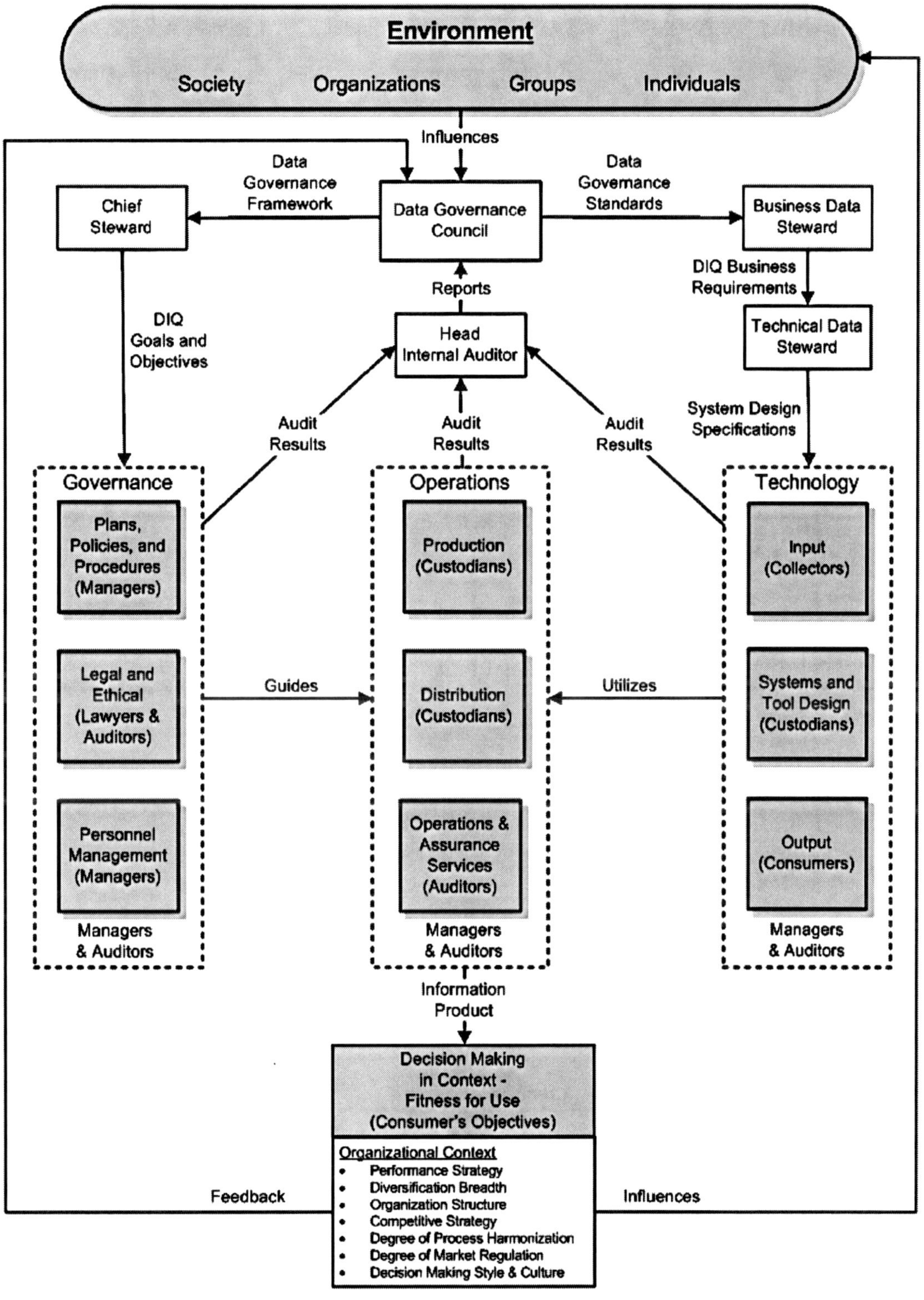

Figure 2. Roles within data governance

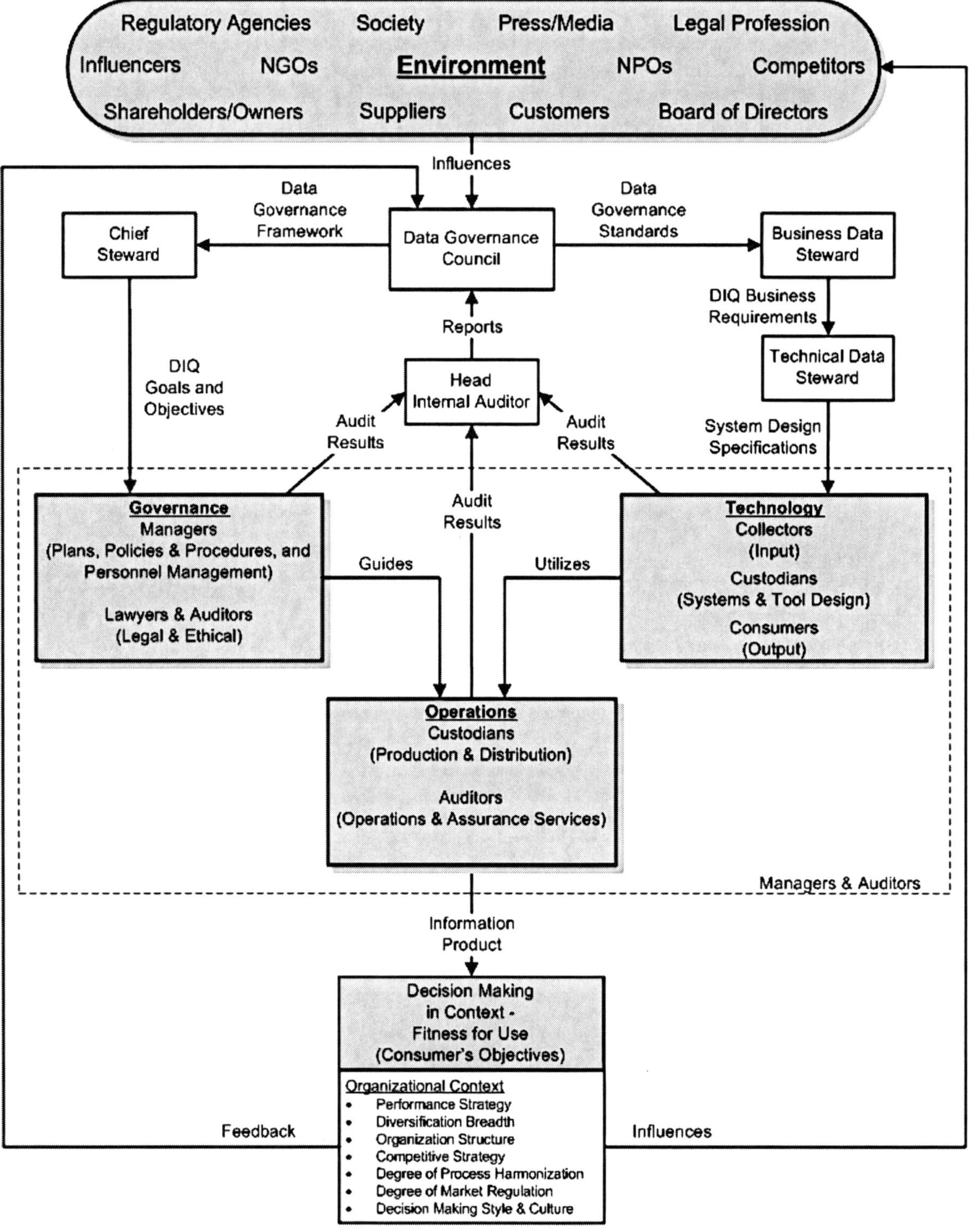

improve healthcare quality. It manages voluntary accreditation programs and certifies physician organizations, and accredits managed care organizations and preferred provider organizations. NCQA's accreditation program represents the most rigorous standards of their kind. The NCQA seal is a widely recognized symbol of quality. Health plans today face a rigorous set of more than 60 standards and must report on their performance in more than 40 areas in order to earn NCQA's seal of approval.

The NCQA's Patient Centered Medical Homes (PCMH) is an innovative program for improving primary care that describes clear and specific criteria for organizing care around patients, working in teams, and coordinating and tracking care over time. The use of the word home in this context does not imply a physical place, rather PCMH is an organization model for providing comprehensive, coordinated high quality primary care that is patient-centered, safe and accessible (Agency for Healthcare Research and Qulaity, 2012). NCQA facilitates a partnership between a patient, and their personal primary care physician, and when appropriate, the patient's family. The primary care clinician leads a team that takes collective responsibility for patient care, providing for the patient's healthcare needs and arranging for appropriate care with other qualified clinicians, when needed. The medical home is intended to result in more personalized, coordinated, effective and efficient care (Agency for Healthcare Research and Qulaity, 2012).

Figure three shows stakeholders of the healthcare supply chain, including NCQA. At the far left, pharmaceutical companies, medical device manufacturers, and biotech companies sell products to distributors and wholesalers for redistribution to the rest of the supply chain. Even though patients are the ultimate consumer of healthcare, they are but one of many groups that pay for healthcare. Payers refer to all those entities that pay the healthcare providers and include employer groups, Medicaid, Medicare, State

Children's Health Insurance Programs (SCHIP), commercial insurers and self-pay. Just as there are a multitude of payers, there are many providers. Home health agencies, long-term care facilities, hospitals, outpatient treatment, specialty care and physicians all provide care for patients. To the far right, of the figure, we see the most fundamental relationship in the healthcare supply chain – physician/patient relationship. It is this relationship that is the focus of the PCMH mentioned in the previous paragraph. As if that was not enough complexity in the supply chain, there are a number of accrediting agencies and regulatory agencies that interact with the healthcare industry. Lastly, the press, legal profession, competitors and board of directors of the healthcare facilities themselves all influence the supply chain. Within this complex environment, we are going to focus on two case studies. The first one involves the processes needed to get paid for vaccinating adults against shingles in a multi-facility medical group. The second case involves the processes required for an insurance company to enroll and credential providers from a large medical provider.

Case 1: Multi-Facility Healthcare Medical Group (MHMG)

This case examines a primary care healthcare group that operates in ten locations. The multi-facility healthcare medical group (MHMG) offers services to patients that include family and internal medicine, pediatrics, pharmacy, eye care, urgent care and other specialties. From this point forward, the organization will be referred to as MHMG. Although MHMG, in general, manages acute illnesses, provides preventive care, and treats chronic conditions, this particular case focuses exclusively on preventive care management and in particular, immunizations. As with most healthcare organizations, MHMG increasingly focuses on two important aspects of healthcare, namely cost and quality. From a quality perspective, the National Committee for Quality Assurance (NCQA) has awarded all ten practices of MHMG with its highest designation – level 3 Patient Centered Medical Home (PCMH).

Before we begin detailing the challenges faced by MHMG, let's examine two out of three processes that are interconnected: provider onboarding, and the revenue management cycle (see Figure 4). Let's begin by examining the provider onboarding cycle. First, MHMG must recruit healthcare providers. Generically a provider is a professional engaged in the delivery of health services and includes physicians, dentists, nurses, pediatricians, optometrists, and psychologists. In the medical field, hospitals and long-term care facilities are also called providers. Once a provider is recruited, an employment offer must be extended and accepted. Then MHMG credentials the provider. Credentialing is the process of reviewing a healthcare provider's qualifications. Academic background, training, and clinical experience are examined to determine if criteria for clinical privileges are met. Privileging defines a provider's scope of practice and the clinical services he or she may provide. Last, the provider must be enrolled with payers so that when claims are submitted, they are paid correctly. Once the provider has completed the onboarding process they will be scheduled to treat patients. This is the touch point between provider onboarding and the revenue management cycle.

Figure 3. Healthcare stakeholders and supply chain

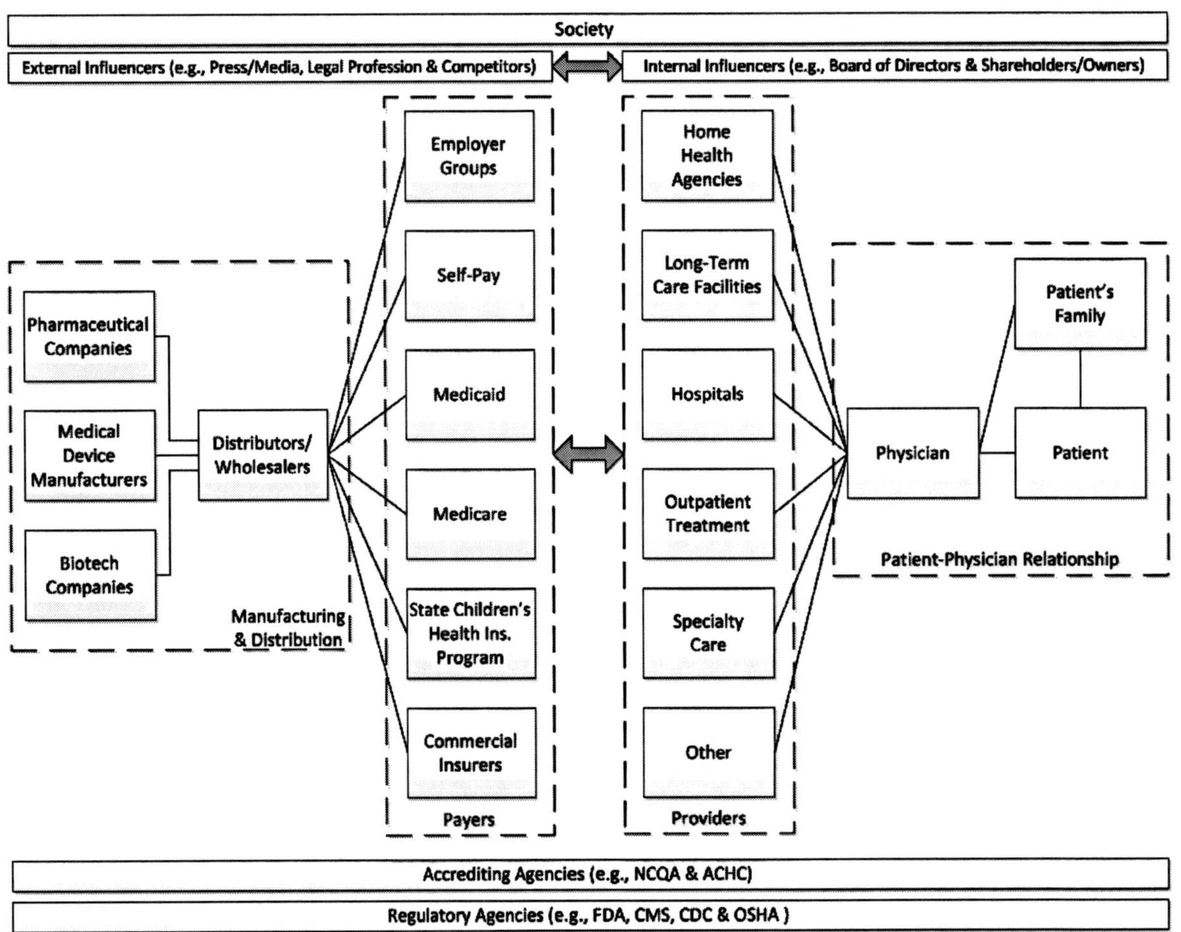

Figure 4. Revenue management and provider enrollment cycles

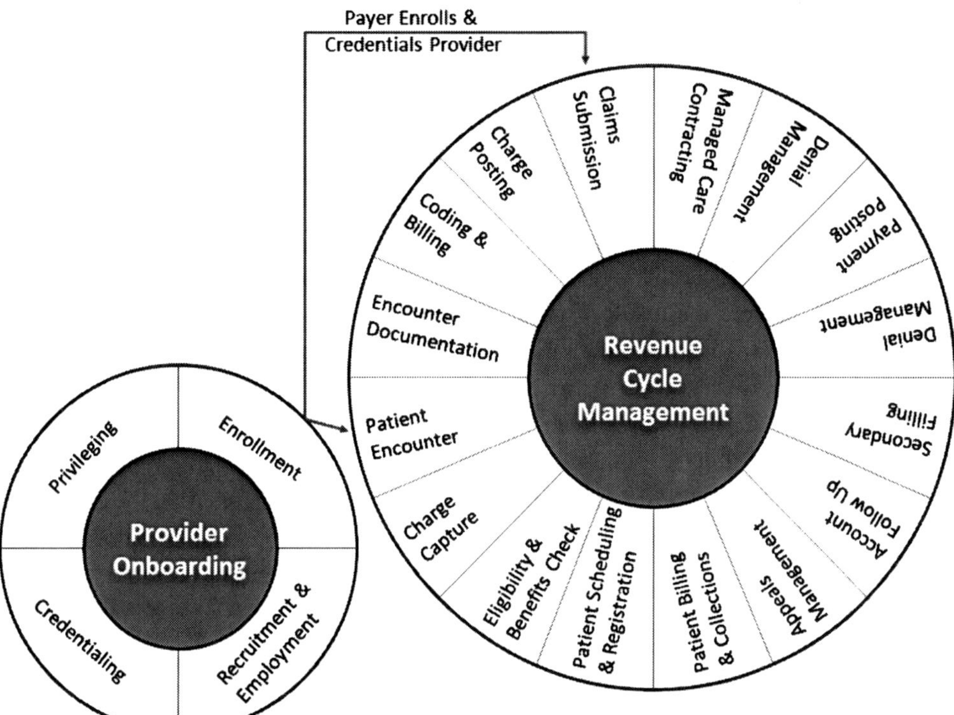

The revenue management cycle has many more steps than the provider onboarding cycle, and requires the participation of numerous individuals such as patients, patient service representatives (PSRs), business service representatives (BSRs), providers, coders, billers and collections. Most patients would be surprised at the large percentage of times healthcare facilities are denied payment from insurance companies, Medicaid, and Medicare.

This particular case examines the revenue management cycle for vaccines. The immune system tends to weaken over time, putting older adults at risk for infectious diseases. The Advisory Committee on Immunization Practices (ACIP) at the Center for Disease Control (CDC) suggests that adults 60 years or older receive the following vaccinations: influenza vaccine, Tdap vaccine, Pneumococcal vaccine and Zoster vaccine. MHMG follows the CDC recommendations.

What precipitated the initiation of this business intelligence project was the large number of denials for the Zoster vaccine. The Zoster vaccine is designed to prevent shingles. Anyone who has had chicken pox is at risk for shingles. Shingles (herpes zoster) is a painful, blistering skin rash that occurs when the virus that caused chicken pox becomes active in the nerves of older adults. Why the virus becomes active in older adults is unclear and typically only one attack occurs.

The challenge from a business perspective is that insurance coverage varies by contract and even patient group; sometimes coverage is under pharmacy benefits, other times medical benefits, or not covered at all. Some payers set the age at 55 rather than 60. To further complicate matters, each of the ten facilities has different processes for verifying coverage, administering the vaccine, and billing. Inconsistent coverage and a nonstandard vaccination process have resulted in many payment denials. The Zoster vaccine is expensive, costing over $200 per shot. However, the total cost was much higher. Patients receive bills that they were not expecting, resulting in vigorous complaints. Clinical and business staff was confused about how to verify insurance coverage and frustrated from all the patient complaints. As a result, some providers stopped giving the immunization and when they did give it, the coders spent an inordinate amount of time verifying every encounter form, calling both pharmacy and medical staff. Something needed to be done.

Most of these denials were the result of poor quality data resulting from an ill-defined vaccination process. The data in the system was incorrect concerning whether the benefits were covered by medical or pharmacy. Often, the amount of the copay was incorrect. When the provider accessed the patient's electronic health record, the data concerning vaccination was often missing or inaccurate.

Even in healthcare, it is not economically or practically feasible to ensure DIQ on all dimensions of quality. Thus, some element of satisficing is necessary. As providers and business managers of healthcare facilities go about the business of managing their operations and reporting financial results, they must be aware of the inherent tradeoffs in DIQ. In healthcare, relevancy is a critical dimension, as well as access security due to the privacy and security rules associated with the Health Insurance Portability and Accountability Act of 1996 (HIPAA). Relevancy occurs when data provides benefit to a decision maker who uses it and finds it helpful for the task at hand. Other important dimensions that should be part of the design of any healthcare BI system include objectivity, completeness and interpretability. Objectivity refers to the extent to which data are unbiased, unprejudiced and impartial. Completeness specifies that data are of sufficient breadth, depth and scope for the task at hand. Interpretability refers to the extent to which data are in an appropriate language and their definitions are clear. Interpretability is always of concern in the medical field, where entire courses exist that focus exclusively on medical terminology.

DIQ impacts all types of transactional systems, and healthcare is heavily transactional in nature. Within the healthcare industry, Kerr, Norris and Stockdale (2008) describe the development and implementation of programs to improve data quality, thus making the strategic management of data quality a part of day-to-day business. Ge and Helfert (2008) examine the four categories of DIQ described earlier and show that improving representational DIQ may intensify the positive effects of contextual DIQ in inventory management. Can this lesson be extrapolated to healthcare systems? Probably so. Authors are in agreement that data quality is a critical success factor (Wixom & Watson, 2001), and that the choice of attributes is a non-trivial decision (Pighin & Ieronutti, 2008).

As can be seen in Figure 5, the PGOT framework can easily be adapted to healthcare. The focus continues to be on people and their interactions with the system. As indicated earlier, IT does not bear the full brunt of responsibility for DIQ in the system. Instead, it is a shared responsibility, with all members along the DIQ information product operations chain (e.g., auditors, data collectors, data custodians, data consumers and managers) accountable for the quality of the data and information. The primary job of many of these stakeholders is not technology (e.g. patient service representatives, nurses, physicians, payers, providers and patients) and it is important that they understand the importance of DIQ.

From a collector's perspective, a busy nurse or physician must appreciate the importance of accurate data entry for downstream use in the billing process. The nurse in the room with the patient will be able to see that he or she is reacting poorly to a drug. This adverse effect must be entered, accurately, into the system so that the physician who uses the BI system two years later will not prescribe a similar drug. Healthcare BI systems in particular must also meet many legal regulations and ethical considerations, and it is vital that policies, plans and procedures be in place for compliance purposes. The focus of

Figure 5. PGOT applied to healthcare: Case 1

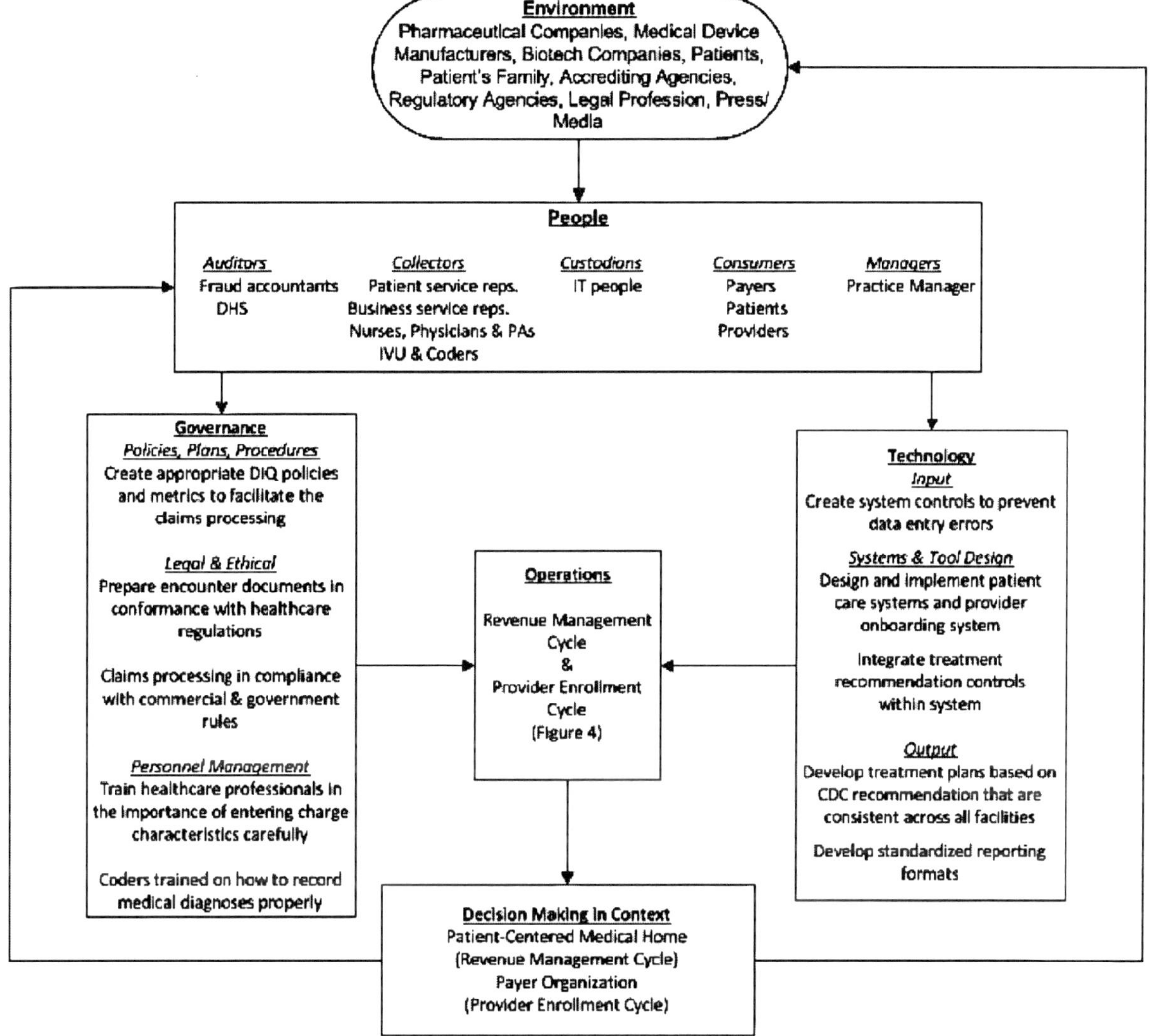

the MHMG case is on the revenue management cycle and the next case on the provider enrollment cycle. Operationally, in another healthcare study, we could also have other cycles such patient-physician, physician-pharmacy, and patient-health insurance provider. The focus of the technology piece will be to ensure that the previous issues can be adequately implemented in the BI system.

The process improvement team first mapped out the current state. The clinical and business staff at each of the 10 facilities were interviewed to determine what the current process was for administering the Zoster vaccine. What resulted was not a single process map but rather 10 distinctly different processes. Figure 6 shows the process maps for three out of the ten sites. At this point, three things became clear. MHMG needed to determine how big the problem was, what was critical for a newly designed process if a new process was warranted and third, create this new standardized process for administering vaccines.

Since every facility was doing things differently, data had to be tracked and trended by site. The metrics vary greatly by site. For example

Figure 6. Immunization flowchart: Before implementing business intelligence

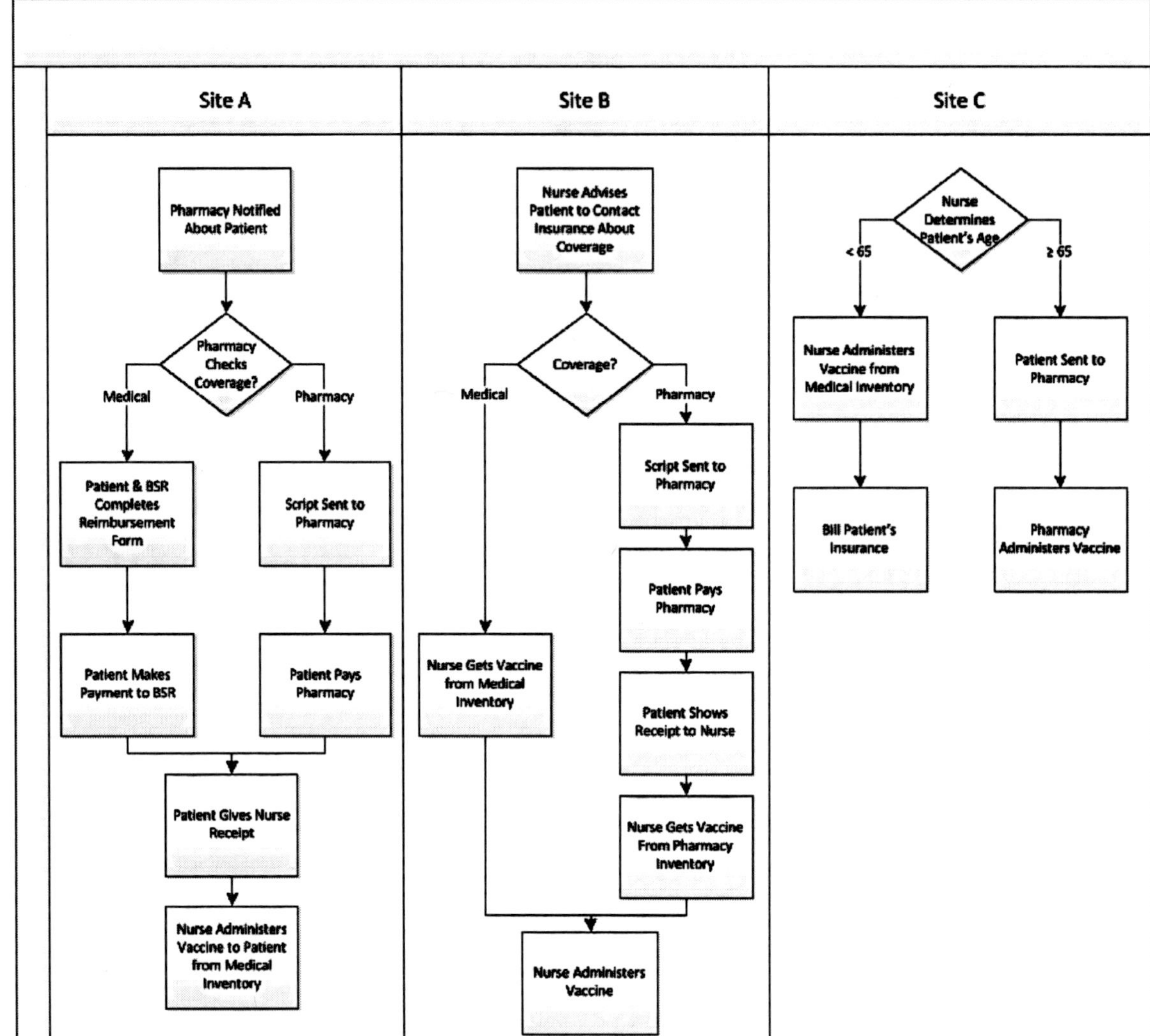

one site administered the vaccine to over 50% of their patients who were 65 and older that visited MHMG in the first nine months of 2012 whereas another site administered the vaccine to less than 1% of those patients who were over 65. Note that MGMH used 65 as the cutoff for their analysis rather than 60. Claims denials ran slightly higher than 54% for the entire organization. That means over half of the vaccines that were administered in the first nine months of 2012 MHMG was not paid for them, resulting in a write-off of approximately $100,000. So clearly the problem impacts patients and MHMG in a significant way. Keep in mind, the numbers cited here are only for the Zoster vaccine. Even though the organization focused on this particular vaccine, the lessons learned were leveraged across all vaccines.

Now that the organization had verified this was a problem worthy of pursuit, the next step was to determine what was critical to stakeholders. For patients, it was critical for them to know up front what their coverage was and if a copay or self-pay was needed, and that it was paid at the time the vaccine was administered. For providers, they also needed to know coverage at the time of the encounter. For coders, they needed a seamless billing system that did not require them to call the pharmacy and medical staff every time they encountered a chart that indicated the vaccine has been administered.

The process improvement team, using their definition of what was critical-to-care (CTC), developed a much more straightforward standardized process with far fewer steps (see Figure 7). The new process consists of three major phases: business intelligence system, patient care, and billing. Now before a patient arrives, the business intelligence system identifies coverage and copay amount for each patient who meets the criteria for the vaccine. In order to test the effectiveness of the new process, two pilot sites were chosen. As often is the case, the two sites that volunteered were sites that had performed much better than the other sites using the old process. In fact, their claims denial percentage was much lower than the organization as a whole (32.6% in the first nine months of 2012 compared to 54%). To proceed with the pilot, standard operating procedures for collecting and posting copays were developed as well as new pharmacy and billing procedures. Furthermore, in order to verify results of the pilot, new reconciliation and control reports were created.

The pilot ran for the last three months of 2012 and the results were significant (see Figure 8). With the new BI system, denials went from 32.59% to 5.65%, providers increased the number of shots they were giving patients, and feedback from staff and providers was positive. The staff commented they could now concentrate on patient care rather than insurance issues concerning this vaccine. The organization rolled out the new process to all 10 facilities starting January of 2013 and expects to have a financial impact on the organization amounting to approximately $600,000 gross revenues and $200,000 in net profit in 2013. This estimated impact is based on a single vaccine and

when the principles learned from this project are rolled out to other vaccines, the impact on the organization will be in the millions.

Prior to the creation of the business intelligence system, there was no easy way for staff to determine which patients that were visiting over the next couple days met the criteria for vaccination. Clinicians often missed opportunities to provide preventive care as recommended by clinical guidelines, forgoing the associated revenue stream. With the creation of a business intelligence component to their electronic health records system, MHMG can identify patients that qualify for vaccines, lab work, and exams covered by their particular insurance company. Alerts in the system can remind clinicians of interventions and screening tests while the patient is in the examination room.

For the Zoster vaccine, the new system generates a list of patients with appointments two business days from now that meet vaccine criteria. For each of these patients, their payment type is examined: commercial insurance, self-pay, or government program such as Medicare or Medicaid. Government programs cover this vaccine under pharmacy benefits and the pharmacy system verifies coverage and copay and notes in the patient's electronic health record whether the vaccine is covered and if so, what the copay amount is. For commercial insurance, the insurance verification unit (IVU) verifies coverage and copay, noting whether the vaccine is covered and if so, what the copay amount is.

As the results show, the implementation of the business intelligence system had a large impact on the medical outcomes, financial performance, compliance (with CDC recommended care), and overall customer satisfaction. The lessons learned from this project are now being replicated with other vaccines. Next, we examine another part of the healthcare supply chain – provider credentialing and enrollment.

Figure 7. Immunization flowchart: After implementing business intelligence

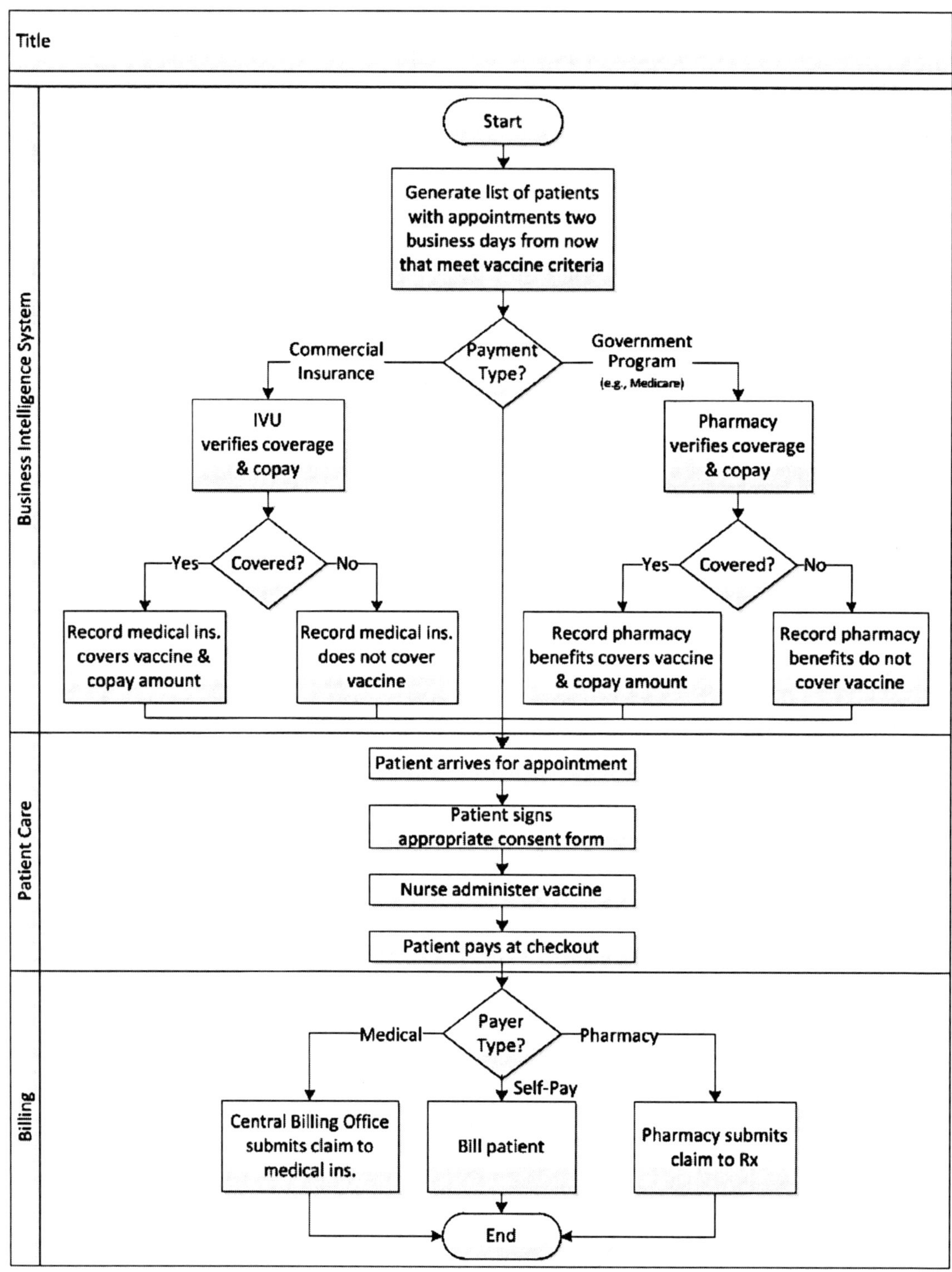

Figure 8. Percentage of denials before and after BI system rollout

2012	Total Claims	Total Denials	% Denials
Jan.	30	10	33.33%
Feb.	22	8	36.36%
Mar	22	8	36.36%
Apr	50	8	16.00%
May	36	10	27.78%
Jun	50	16	32.00%
Jul	34	14	41.18%
Aug	52	14	26.92%
Sep	60	26	43.33%
Averages	39.56	12.67	32.59%

(Before Improvements)

Oct	112	8	7.14%
Nov	164	14	8.54%
Dec	156	2	1.28%
Averages	144.00	8.00	5.65%

(After)

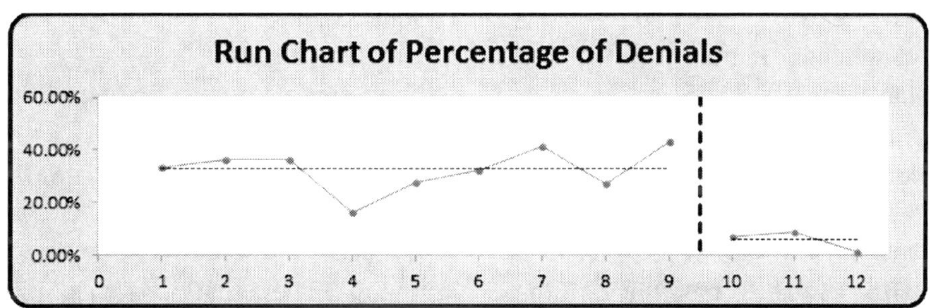

Case 2: Regional Health Insurance Company (RHIS)

This case involves a regional health insurance company and a provider group. This regional health insurance company, referred to here as RHIS, is located in the United States and is a nonprofit health insurer. It has provided health insurance for over 8 decades and currently serves approximately 2 million members. The provider group represents almost 1,000 specialists and primary care providers in negotiating payment rates with third party and credentialing providers. The specialist and primary care provider (SPCP) group will be referred to here as the SPCP group for short. The SPCP group is certified by the National Committee for Quality Assurance (NCQA).

SPCP group has many providers, in many different locations, with differing rates depending on the service(s) rendered. Keeping provider data current in RHIS is challenging. SPCP requests monthly additions and updates to provider information. The SPCP group submits these changes to RHIS in three ways: (1) carve-out list, (2) all employee list and (3) modifications based on a printed copy of the provider database. A carve out list is a list of medical services that are separated from a contract and paid under a different arrangement. Reports have overlaps in information and many people touch these reports before the department ultimately responsible for handling provider file maintenance receives them. For example, sometimes, the duplicate requests found on these three reports are inconsistent. Properly maintaining the provider file is important since the provider record drives the reimbursement the provider will receive.

As a result of a poor process, the following impacts were felt by both RHIS and the SPCP group: (1) system updates lagged well behind requests for updates due to the many "touches", (2) reimbursements to the providers were not timely nor accurate due to lag time mentioned in the first point, (3) inaccurate and untimely reimbursements result in almost 10,000 adjustments per year, (4) credentialing had to perform duplicative tasks in order to complete their new provider process in a timely manner and (5) the SPCP group was very dissatisfied. This dissatisfaction led to the group withholding repayment of over $1 million in overpayments to induce RHIS to reduce the time it took to make updates and to increase the accuracy of the provider file database itself.

The provider file data management (PFDM) department loads and maintains the provider information in all RHIS systems. As mentioned before, the provider record drives provider reimbursement. PFDM processes service requests from SPCP, resulting in three main activities: the creation of new provider recorders, punching through the carve-out list, and making demographic updates. The analysis of the service request process requires all three activities are examined.

The primary objective of this process improvement project was to reduce the time it takes to react to requests for changes from SPCP. Specifically, it addressed reducing the times associated with three activities: the creation of new provider recorders, punching through the carve-out list and making demographic updates. The primary objective of the new provider creation process was to reduce the time it takes to create a new provider record from its current baseline of 55 calendar days to seven calendar days. The primary objective for

punching through the carve-list was to reduce the time it takes from its current baseline of 40 calendar days to seven calendar days. Lastly, the primary objective for updating provider demographics was to reduce the time it takes from its current baseline of 50 calendar days to ten calendar days. Secondary, but important, benefits included reduced time to research the provider record requests and reduce the number of claim payment adjustment and the resulting increase in satisfaction from SPCP as a result.

By implementing a business intelligence system, the data was cleansed, multiple handoffs eliminated, cycle time targets met, and greater customer satisfaction achieved. These two examples illustrate why it is important for healthcare to embrace BI.

Solutions and Recommendations

BI systems have the potential to move the healthcare industry forward. They provide information that will enable better patient care and can help healthcare as a business survive with expedited payments. However, these benefits will only accrue if the data that drives the information is of high quality and is appropriate for the decisions being made.

The PGOT framework, with its focus on the systemic effects of DIQ, can provide structure to the development and use of a BI system in healthcare. Thoughtful consideration of the implications of policies and procedures with respect to DIQ, appointing appropriate people in key roles such as Chief Data Steward and a Governance Council, and ensuring that systems are operationally and technically aligned with the DIQ goals, can help ensure that the BI systems can provide the information needed by providers to make good patient and business decisions.

As seen in the MHMG case, one of the difficulties facing healthcare, is the lack of consistency across multiple locations. Given the size and scope of current healthcare organizations, it is common to find each unit operating independently, particularly with respect to the systems that are in place. Figure 5 illustrates how the PGOT can be applied to healthcare, specifically with respect to revenue cycle management, a key driver of the success of the healthcare business. By examining the BI system with respect to DIQ systemically, we can help ensure that the organization as a whole is running at optimal efficiency. For example, DIQ governance in healthcare can center on claims processing. As indicated earlier, the healthcare industry does not deal with one payer and one payee, but rather multiple payers and payees. As seen in Figure 4, the revenue cycle management can only be enabled if the providers are successfully enrolled in the system with the right credentials and privileges. Without providers, there would be nothing to bill for. Without billing, the healthcare business would not be able to support itself.

Thus, our recommendation is that a multi-step approach be followed:

1. Create a high-level context diagram that shows the system connections to the environment and closely examine the roles of people as they apply to the process (Figures 3 and 4);
2. Create a process flow chart that shows the stakeholders, activities and system data flows in question (Figure 6);
3. Align the PGOT framework (Figure 1) to the process flow chart to identify areas of concern (Figure 5);
4. Implement interventions to close the gap between the "as is" and the "to be" (Figure 7);
5. Track performance and continue to make adjustments as needed (Figure 8).

With this methodical approach to examining the problem and solution, with a careful examination of the DIQ issues along the way, the BI system can be implemented to take full advantage of the power that it holds.

FUTURE RESEARCH DIRECTIONS

DIQ is a critical aspect of any system. The PGOT encompasses DIQ in all types of systems, including BI. It is this area where the two intersect that is interesting to analyze in terms of similarities and differences. There is potential for collaboration between the BI and DIQ research communities. Clearly, DIQ is a critical success factor in BI. As indicated earlier, data quality processes are an explicit part of the BI model. Some elements of the PGOT model exist elsewhere in the BI model, such as people, technologies, governance and metadata. As we begin to develop a roadmap for BI and DIQ integration, there are questions to be answered. Can PGOT simply be embedded in the data quality processes of BI development? How, if at all, are BI systems different with respect to DIQ than TPS or ERP systems? For example as we look at the 15 dimensions of quality raised earlier, how would users of a BI system prioritize the dimensions compared to users of an accounting information system (AIS), which is fundamentally a TPS? Would healthcare BI users value different data quality dimensions than AIS users? Should the people aspects of DIQ be tightly coupled with the people aspects of BI or are they completely different stakeholders? These and other questions should be addressed as we move towards interdisciplinary research between the two fields.

The focus of the preceding paragraph was on the people that interact with the healthcare BI system, and research questions that have not yet been addressed. However, the PGOT also addresses technical considerations and there is a great opportunity for collaborative work between the Computer Science (CS) community and DIQ researchers. For example, data profiling and enrichment are critical factors as we move forward towards more managed care of the healthy individual. In addition, as discussed earlier, there is a great deal of unstructured data in a healthcare BI system. The CS and information science communities are doing research on word mining and automatic classification of terms. Semantic knowledge bases can allow for better coding of physician notes and other free text. In addition, privacy and security issues are critical in a healthcare environment. These are all areas where DIQ researchers can collaborate with their technical colleagues.

Another fruitful collaboration in this arena would be the cross-business disciplinary research. Accountants understand the numbers and MIS researchers understand the technical aspects of metadata. The metadata of a system can be a strong indicator of the potential success of the BI system, as this information flows with the data from primary systems into secondary systems, such as BI. As the accountants determine what metadata is important (data collected, alternative definitions, etc.) the MIS researcher can implement technical controls for capturing this metadata.

CONCLUSION

This paper describes two case studies in the healthcare industry. By weaving the elements of the PGOT framework throughout the narrative, several opportunities for improvement were suggested and discussed. This led to recommendations for best practices. This paper adds to the theoretical literature by operationalizing a theoretical model and showing the interconnections within an overall DIQ system. It adds to the practical literature by offering specific recommendations for practice. DIQ is obviously an important issue in healthcare. It affects the ability of providers and business managers at all levels to make decisions. Within the healthcare industry there are many opportunities for improved decision making, which can directly impact medical outcomes and the bottom line.

There are many organizational systems including transaction processing systems (TPS), management information systems (MIS), enterprise resource planning systems (ERP) and business intelligence (BI) systems. As discussed in the literature review, BI is not just a technology. It is the system which collects, stores, and analyzes business data to support decision making. Key components of this system include source systems, the data warehouse and associated metadata, and the analytical tools such as data mining and general statistical analysis. Moving data from the sources to the data warehouse requires data integration which is both a technology and a process. Metadata, data quality and data governance processes ensure that data moves through the system efficiently and effectively (Wixom & Watson, 2010). Integrating DIQ methodologies into the BI system will help to ensure that the system addresses the end user needs. The descriptions of the cases in this chapter show how this can be accomplished.

REFERENCES

Abate, M. L., Diegert, K. V., & Allen, H. W. (1998). A hierarchical approach to improving data quality. *Data Quality*, *4*(1), 10.

Agency for Healthcare Research and Qulaity. (2012). *Patient centered medical home.* Retrieved 1/16/2013, from http://pcmh.ahrq.gov/portal/server.pt/community/pcmh__home/1483/PCMH_Defining%20the%20PCMH_v2

Angeles. (2012). *How health reform's medicaid expansion will impact state budgets federal government will pick up nearly all costs, even as expansion provides coverage to millions of low-income uninsured Americans.* Retrieved March 5, 2013 http://www.cbpp.org/cms/index.cfm?fa=view&id=3801.

Bardhan, I. R., & Thouin, M. F. (2012). Health information technology and its impact on the quality and cost of healthcare delivery. *Decision Support Systems, 55*(2),438-449. doi: http://dx.doi.org/10.1016/j.dss.2012.10.003

Bitterer, A., Schlegel, K., Hostmann, B., Gassman, B., Beyer, M. A., Herschel, G., & Andrews, W. (2007). *Hype cycle for business intelligence and performance management, 2007*. Stamford, CT: Gartner Research.

Boritz, J. E. (2005). IS practitioners' views on core concepts of information integrity. *International Journal of Accounting Information Systems*, *6*, 20. doi:10.1016/j.accinf.2005.07.001

Broaddus, M., & Park, E. (2012). *Number of uninsured fell in 2011, largely due to health reform and public programs*. Washington, DC: Dept of Health and Human Services.

Byrd, L. W., & Byrd, T. A. (2012). The impact of clinical information technology on information quality in US hospitals. *International Journal of Healthcare Technology and Management*, *13*(1), 71–87. doi:10.1504/IJHTM.2012.048948

Chen, H., Chiang, R. H. L., & Storey, V. C. (2012). Business intelligence and analytics: From big data to big impact. *Management Information Systems Quarterly*, *36*(4), 1165–1188.

Classen, D. C., Resar, R., Griffin, F., Federico, F., Frankel, T., Kimmel, N., & James, B. C. (2011). Global trigger tool shows that adverse events in hospitals may be ten times greater than previously measured. *Health Affairs*, *30*(4), 581–589. doi:10.1377/hlthaff.2011.0190 PMID:21471476

Davenport, T. H. (2010). Business intelligence and organizational decisions. *International Journal of Business Intelligence Research*, *1*(1), 1–12. doi:10.4018/jbir.2010071701

Friedman, T. (2008). *Gartner study on data quality shows that IT still bears the burden*. Stamford, CT: Gartner Group.

Ge, M., & Helfert, M. (2008). Effects of information quality on inventory management. *International Journal of Information Quality*, *2*(2), 15. doi:10.1504/IJIQ.2008.022962

Giannangelo, K., & Fenton, S. (2008). EHR's effect on the revenue cycle management coding function. *Journal of Healthcare Information Management*, *22*(1), 26–29. PMID:19267004

Hanauer, D. A., Zheng, K., Ramakrishnan, N., & Keller, B. J. (2011). Opportunities and challenges in association and episode discovery from electronic health records. *IEEE Intelligent Systems*, *26*(5), 83–87.

Harmon, K. (2009). *Deaths from avoidable medical error more than double in past decade, investigation shows*. Scientific American Blog.

Imhoff, C. (2005). Streaming processes for frontline workers: Adding business intelligence for operations. *Operational Business Intelligence White Paper, Intelligent Solutions Inc.* Retrieved from http://www.tdwi.com

Indart, B. (2006). Operationalizing business intelligence – Turning insight into actions. *Business Intelligence Journal*, *11*(2), 35.

Keehan, S. P., Sisko, A. M., Truffer, C. J., Poisal, J. A., Cuckler, G. A., Madison, A. J., & Smith, S. D. (2011). National health spending projections through 2020: Economic recovery and reform drive faster spending growth. *Health Affairs*, *30*(8), 1594–1605. doi:10.1377/hlthaff.2011.0662 PMID:21798885

Kerr, K. A., Norris, T., & Stockdale, R. (2008). The strategic management of data quality in healthcare. *Health Informatics Journal*, *14*(4), 259–266. doi:10.1177/1460458208096555 PMID:19008276

Leape, L. L., Lawthers, A. G., Brennan, T. A., & Johnson, W. G. (1993). Preventing medical injury. *QRB. Quality Review Bulletin*, *19*(5), 144. PMID:8332330

Levinson, D. R. (2010). *Adverse effects in hospitals: National incidence among medicare beneficiaries*. Washington, DC: Center on Budget and Policy Priorities.

Lin, Y.-K., Brown, R. A., Yang, H. J., Li, S.-H., & Lu, H.-M. (2011). Data mining large-scale electronic health records for clinical support. *IEEE Intelligent Systems*, *26*(5), 87–90.

Linder, J. A., Ma, J., Bates, D. W., Middleton, B., & Stafford, R. S. (2007). Electronic health record use and the quality of ambulatory care in the United States. *Archives of Internal Medicine*, *167*(13), 1400–1405. doi:10.1001/archinte.167.13.1400 PMID:17620534

Maguire, H. (2008). Extending the boundaries of IQ: Can collaboration with information management improve corporate governance? *International Journal of Information Quality*, *2*(1), 23. doi:10.1504/IJIQ.2008.019561

Marjanovic, O. (2010). The importance of process thinking in business intelligence. *International Journal of Business Intelligence Research*, *1*(4), 29–46. doi:10.4018/jbir.2010100102

Neely, M. P., & Cook, J. S. (2011). Fifteen years of data and information quality literature: Developing a research agenda for accounting. *Journal of Information Systems*, *25*(1), 79–108. doi:10.2308/jis.2011.25.1.79

News, A. B. C. (2006). *Fast facts on the U.S. health care crisis*. Retrieved 01/15/2013, from http://abcnews.go.com/WNT/PrescriptionForChange/story?id=2563381

ObamaCare Facts. (2013). *ObamaCare facts: Dispelling the myths*. Retrieved 03/06/2013, from http://obamacarefacts.com/obamacare-facts.php

Olinsky, A., & Schumacher, P. A. (2010). Data mining for health care professionals: MBA course projects resulting in hospital improvements. *International Journal of Business Intelligence Research*, *1*(2), 30–41. doi:10.4018/jbir.2010040104

Pighin, M., & Ieronutti, L. (2008). A methodology supporting the design and evaluating the final quality of data warehouses. *International Journal of Data Warehousing and Mining*, *4*(3), 20. doi:10.4018/jdwm.2008070102

Rauscher, S., & Wheeler, J. R. (2008). Effective hospital revenue cycle management: Is there a trade-off between the amount of patient revenue and the speed of revenue collection? *Journal of Healthcare Management*, *53*(6), 392. PMID:19070334

Rauscher, S., & Wheeler, J. R. C. (2010). Hospital revenue cycle management and payer mix: Do Medicare and medicaid undermine hospitals' ability to generate and collect patient care revenue? *Editorial Board*, *37*(2), 90–104.

Romano, M. J., & Stafford, R. S. (2011). Electronic health records and clinical decision support systems: Impact on national ambulatory care quality. *Archives of Internal Medicine*, *171*(10), 897–903. doi:10.1001/archinternmed.2010.527 PMID:21263077

Shortell, S. M. (2004). Increasing value: a research agenda for addressing the managerial and organizational challenges facing health care delivery in the United States. *Medical Care Research and Review*, *61*(3suppl), 12S–30S. doi:10.1177/1077558704266768 PMID:15375281

Sillup, G. P., Klimberg, R. K., & McSweeney, D. P. (2010). Data-driven decision making for new drugs: A collaborative learning experience. *International Journal of Business Intelligence Research*, *1*(2), 42–59. doi:10.4018/jbir.2010040105

Sunyaev, A., & Chornyi, D. (2012). Supporting chronic disease care quality: Design and implementation of a health service and its integration with electronic health records. *Journal of Data and Information Quality*, *3*(2). doi:10.1145/2184442.2184443

U.S. Department of Health and Human Services. (2001). *Final rules for administrative simplification*. Retrieved 1/15/2013, from http://aspe.hhs.gov/admnsimp/final/PvcPre02.htm

Vicini, J., & Stempel, J. (2012). *US top court upholds healthcare law in Obama triumph*. Retrieved from http://www.reuters.com/article/2012/06/28/usa-healthcare-court-idUSL2E8HS4WG20120628

Wactler, H., Pavel, M., & Barkis, W. (2011). Can computer science save healthcare? *IEEE Intelligent Systems*, *26*(5), 79–83.

Wang, R. Y., & Strong, D. M. (1996). Beyond accuracy: What data quality means to data consumers. *Journal of Management Information Systems*, *12*(4), 5–34.

Weber, K., Otto, B., & Österle, H. (2009). One size does not fit all---A contingency approach to data governance. *Journal of Data and Information Quality*, *1*(1), 4. doi:10.1145/1515693.1515696

Wickramasinghe, N., & Schaffer, J. L. (2006). Creating knowledge-driven healthcare processes with the intelligence continuum. *International Journal of Electronic Healthcare*, *2*(2), 164–174. PMID:18048242

Wixom, B. H., & Watson, H. J. (2010). The BI-based organisation. *International Journal of Business Intelligence Research*, *1*(1), 13–28. doi:10.4018/jbir.2010071702

Wu, S., Chaudhry, B., Wang, J., Maglione, M., Mojica, W., Roth, E., & Shekelle, P. G. (2006). Systematic review: Impact of health information technology on quality, efficiency, and costs of medical care. *Annals of Internal Medicine*, *144*(10), 742–752. doi:10.7326/0003-4819-144-10-200605160-00125 PMID:16702590

KEY TERMS AND DEFINITIONS

Carve Out: Accessing coverage for a specific type of service through a contract separate from that established with the primary providers.

Co-Payment: A cost-sharing arrangement that requires the person insured to pay a specified flat dollar amount, usually on a per-unit-of-service basis, with the third-party payer reimbursing a portion of the remaining charges.

Provider: Generically, a professional engaged in the delivery of health services, including physicians, dentists, nurses, podiatrists, optometrists, and clinical psychologists. Hospitals and long term care facilities are also providers.

Provider Credentialing: The process of reviewing a healthcare provider's qualifications (e.g., academic, training and clinical experience) to determine if criteria for clinical privileges are met.

Medicare: A U.S. federal government-sponsored healthcare insurance program primarily for people over 65, independent of their income; as well as younger disabled people and dialysis patients.

Medicaid: A U.S. health assistance program for certain people and families with low incomes and resources.

PGOT: A framework used to evaluate data and information quality; it partitions an information system into People, Governance, Operations, and Technology.

This work was previously published in Information Quality and Governance for Business Intelligence edited by William Yeoh, John R. Talburt, and Yinle Zhou, pages 88-111 copyright year 2014 by Business Science Reference (an imprint of IGI Global).

Chapter 77

Approaches to Evidence-Based Management and Decision-Making in Healthcare Organizations:
Lessons for Developing Nations

Nouf Al Saleem
King Saud Medical City, Saudi Arabia

Mohamud Sheikh
University of New South Wales, Australia

ABSTRACT

Decision-making is an essential process that everyone takes upon at all times. Healthcare managers make decisions to ensure serving high quality of patient care, reduce costs and allocate resources. Evidence based decision making in healthcare has recently received a lot of attention by all health care stakeholders including clinicians, researchers, managers and policy makers. However, it is more adapted by clinicians and researchers than managers and policy makers. Evidence-Based science began to develop in the early 90s and was later named "Evidence Based Medicine" after its methods have been applied in health-related fields. Yet, Evidence Based Management still showing a slow progress in terms of its application in decision-making in practice worldwide. This chapter seeks to examine the key aspects of decision-making in the health care settings. It further seeks to provide key examples of decision-making and ways to seek evidence, types of evidence, and approaches to making evidence-based decisions.

INTRODUCTION

Decision-making is an essential and continuous process that is taken by everyone all the time. However, for managers and decision makers it is an essential component of their roles. Healthcare managers make decisions to ensure serving high quality of patient care, reduce costs and allocate resources. To take decisions to overcome problems or to choose between two or more choices

DOI: 10.4018/978-1-4666-8756-1.ch077

and to make the needed actions, decision making should be based on scientific information that is collected, analyzed and applied to ensure successful managerial choices and decisions (Akrani, 6/01/2010 10:24:00 PM).

Evidence based decision making in health care is an approach based on relevant and up-to-date valid research (Gray, 2009). It is used to help to standardize the management process and improve the quality of patient care. Evidence based decision making in health care has recently received a lot of attention by all health care stakeholders: Clinicians, researchers, managers and policy makers. However, it is more adapted by clinicians and researchers than managers and policy makers (Walshe & Rundall, 2001). This scientific process is well known, as evidence-based practice (EBP), a science which started to develop in 1992 and was named "Evidence Based Medicine" after its methods have been applied in other health-related fields such as nursing, education sciences, psychology and other fields (Hjørland, 2011). Yet, Evidence Based Management is not commonly used by healthcare managers, and not well followed in developing countries. In addition, this scientific way of applying evidence is still showing a slow progress in term of actual decision making in practice worldwide (Walshe & Rundall, 2001).

In 1996, Sackett defined the Evidence Based Practice (EBP), which is originally concerned with managing individual patients as "The conscientious, explicit and judicious use of current best evidence in making decisions about the care of the individual patient. It means integrating individual clinical expertise with the best available external clinical evidence from systematic research," (Straus & Sackett, 1998) Evidence Based Management is concerned with making managerial decisions in healthcare management based on scientific information instead of experience and educated guessing and focuses on managing systems rather

than individuals (Kovner, Fine, & D'Aquila, 2009). It focuses on organizational issues to manage and influences the delivery of health care with high quality. That can be an important toll in quality management (Shortell, Rundall, & Hsu, 2007).

The increase of medical services costs caused by the growth of the medical fields and medical innovation was one factor leading to scholars, policy makers and managers giving greater attention to applications of evidence based perspective and methods in health care management and policy. Evidence Based Management aims to reach justified decisions and approved effectiveness of health policies by conducting valid research, exactly as the approved medical interventions effectiveness on patients by the EBP (Walshe & Rundall, 2001).

In developing countries, most health care managers are hired without having a relevant educational background and training to be qualified for these roles. They often only have general management skills, and rely on their experience and prior knowledge for decision-making. This hampers efforts to establish a standard and structured form of decisions (Walshe & Rundall, 2001). In order to apply Evidence Based Management in health care organizations, health care managers need to have adequate training in research methods. In addition, the Evidence Based Management approach must be incorporated into gradate programs in health care management (Walshe & Rundall, 2001).

DISCUSSION

Several textbooks and researchers in the field of healthcare management have suggested approaches or steps for a valid decision making process. A commonly used decision making model identifies seven steps in decision-making leading to the best possible managerial outcome.

Steps of the Decision-Making Process

The steps in decision making are as following ("7 Steps in Decision Making," 2007; "Decision Making Process," 2012):

1. **Problem Identification:** Many questions about the problem or situation need to be answered for example; what is the problem? Why it's important to be solved? Who is affected? And when it has to be solved?
2. **Information Gathering:** Relevant, accurate information need to be collected to help in analyzing the problem or the situation for best solution. It is important to know which source of information will be used. Usually three main sources are essential. First is the organizational data. Statistical reports from the relevant issue are important. Second is the scientific information from studies and researches and other organizations experiences. Third is the expert knowledge.
3. **Situation Analysis:** The possible alternative solutions for this problem based on the collected information will be found. It is important to list all possible alternatives in this stage based on the gathered information.
4. **Option Developing:** Perform cause and effect analysis on each of the choices listed. Imagination and experiences it would also be used to imagine the outcome of each choice.
5. **Alternatives Evaluation:** Different alternatives will be compared to each other, the positives and negatives, to make the right choice. The option can be listed in order based on the priority of each option to reach the organization's goals and the desired outcomes.
6. **Best Alternative Selection:** Based on the knowledge gained from previous steps, best alternative (s) can be selected and applied.
7. **Result Evaluation:** This is the last step and involves evaluation and learning from the outcome of the decision reached. It is important to evaluate the outcome of the option or the action was taken. If the issue was solved, the option will be adapted and maintained to be part of the process. Depend on the issue, the choice can be adapted permanently or it can be for a specific period of time. If the issue was not solved as intended to be, it is important to learn from the result. It is also important go back to step one and go through the steps till the desired outcome achieved. Sometimes it's not necessary to start from the first step. It can be started from any other steps as step 2 or step 5 for example as needed.

THEORIES IN DECISION MAKING FOR HEALTH CARE MANAGERS

The literature presents a number of different theories of decision making relevant for health care managers. These theories can be divided into two main categories. First, the *Normative Decision Theory*, which shows how we should act when making decisions. Second, is *the Descriptive Decision Theory,* theories which describe how people actually act when making decisions. These categories may be further subdivided by the focus on groups or individuals(Layman, 2011a). The most prominent decision making theories are summarized in Table 1.

Normative Decision Theory

Classic Economic Theory

It is the simplest way of decision-making, which is chooses between two choices. The choice is informed and rational. This theory divided into two types. First is the "Theory of riskless choice and new economic theory" where the decision taken is certain to maximize the utility, because each one of the choices have a certain outcome. This theory

Table 1. Theories in decision making for health care

	Normative Decision Theory (Prescriptive Theory)	Descriptive Decision Theory
Individual Normative Theory (Economic Theory)	Classic economic Theory: ■ Theory of riskless choice and new economic theory. ■ Theory of risky choice and expected utility theories.	Non expected utility theories
	Game theory	
	Mixed-scanning strategy	
	Statistical decision theory and Bayesian analysis	
Group normative theory	Bounded rationality theory	Bureaucratic politics model of decision making
	Social choice theory	
	Garbage can model	
	Resource dependence theory	

mainly used by managers when making decisions about the budget of their departments. Second is the "Theory of risky choice and expected utility theories" this theory was developed by statisticians where the choice made has some doubt to maximize utilities as it kind of gambling between the choices that have no certainties for the outcome. Each choice has many possible outcomes. Decision making in this theory is based on the manager expectation of satisfaction. This theory is used when managers try to maximize the utilization by the choice they think is the best based on his behavior and convenient. Usually best choice is differ from manager and another. However, the decision in this theory has the potential of loss (Layman, 2011a).

Game Theory

"The theory of games involves the choice of strategies in situations where the outcomes of one's decision are dependent upon one's own choices and those of one or more other persons"(Layman, 2011a). It is similar to risk theory where the decision is taken as gambling but in this theory, is mainly concerned with social activities. In this game the player can be individual or group of persons, or an organization or more. The outcome is the aggregate of gain and loss between the players. The more players in the game the more complicated it is. This theory mainly used in negotiations process, like salaries, contracts, or other employees' agreements. Healthcare mangers benefit from playing the game to better manage the limited resources they have (Layman, 2011a).

Mixed-Scanning Strategy

It is a systematic process of decision-making that needs scanning strategies for the collected, processed and evaluated data. The theory takes decision hierarchal from the top managers to the lower. Decisions are taken step by step; starting from finding the overall decision needed then take smaller decisions that lead to the final overall ones. The higher top managers introduce the strategic planning with the set goals to lead the next managers for their decisions within these goals. Top managers take their decision rational based on the evaluated data collected and they allocate the resources needed for next steps. This theory is used for healthcare managers to be aware of the organization vision and goals and the long term decisions in which it leads the managers for taking decisions that able to meet future changes in one direction (Layman, 2011a).

Statistical Decision Theory and Bayesian Analysis

"It is a method to make optimal decisions under conditions of uncertainty"(Layman, 2011a). This theory bases the decision on statistical facts. These facts provide the expected outcome, the uncertainty of the choice, the expected consequences, and the rules needed to take decisions. This theory is the theory that support Evidence based practice in healthcare organizations. The data is provided form the organization health information system and electronic medical records. Healthcare managers mainly use statistical decisions as organizational evidence to build the needed decisions and improvement based on it. It is used for continuous performance improvement projects in the work process and as a parameter to evaluate the outcome of the health statues or an intervention impact (Layman, 2011a).

Bounded Rationality Theory

It is described as "the most influential hypothesis concerning the way administrative man arrives at a new policy"(Layman, 2011a). It is where the decision makers take the possible decision instead of perfect ones. This is because some decisions are taken under some limitations of the resources, so bonded rationality is used to overcome these limitations. Healthcare managers usually use this theory when they are short of; information, time, and money. They are usually aware that the choice was taken is not the perfect choice but it is the best available choice with the given resources. However, it is important that manager be aware of the compromises of this choice (Layman, 2011a).

Social Choice Theory

It is a theory where decisions are made based on aggregating of many person's decisions and choice as in voting for example. However, the choices are valid only under special conditions. Health care managers when use social choice theory usually they concerns with the public attitude and satisfactions. Example as the public satisfaction of the healthcare service provided. It also can be used as in how the policy makers make decisions for the funding of Medicare and Medicaid (Layman, 2011a).

Garbage Can Model

In this theory decision is not taken in systematic process. As in some organizations, which they do not have clear vision and missions or clear work process and systems. The decision will be study joining of those factors; problems, solutions, opportunities and individuals, independently instead of studying it in sequences and systematic manner. This model of decisions used by healthcare managers who work in academic or public healthcare organizations (Layman, 2011a).

Resource Dependence Theory

This theory is depending on the assumption that, any organization cannot produce and maintain all the resources that organization need. The decision makers have to make decision in which they can provide the needed resources from external source based on good and powerful relations with others. Healthcare managers are required to ensure the constant flow of resources needed inside the organization by choosing the most appropriate and powerful external providers. However, in the resources dependence theory, both external and internal resources are limited. To overcome this issue healthcare managers try to grow the organization to face the limitation of the resources. Managers who apply this theory are able to make organizational growth as a solution to overcome the limitation and shortage in resources needed (Layman, 2011a).

Descriptive Decision Theory

Non-Expected Utility Theories

It called non-expected as the research showed that decision makers do not take decisions as in expected utility theory. This theory explains that decision makers are predictably not following the normative expected utility theory. They seem to be inconsistencies in rationality. The theory describes that decision makers try to predicate the undesirable outcome to try to avoid it. They only follow the clear and certain information. So, managers reject the other alternative if the information about it is not clear even if it is not the right choice. That's why it is considered to not be rational decisions. Usually managers adapt this theory are more likely to be dissatisfied about losing more than being satisfied about winning. This theory has a huge benefit as managers are always tend to take the positive choice (Layman, 2011a).

Bureaucratic Politics Model of Decision-Making

This decision-making theory is mainly used for national policy making level and for big organizations as well. This theory describes the US experience. It is a combined concept from bounded rationality and from US foreign policy analysis. The policy and decisions must satisfy the public. The problem with this theory, goals and interest are differing as it comes from different entities in the government. Moreover implementation in organizations is depending on how faithful the organization's members are to implement these decisions. Managers work in publically healthcare organizations as in federal or state health system usually adopt this theory and make goals competing to the goals of the court system (Layman, 2011a).

Evidence Based Management in Health Care Organizations

Health care managers are required continually to make decisions regarding many healthcare matters. In order to make effective decisions, managers need information as a basis for their decisions. Managers can find many sources of information, including; from one's own work experiences, work experience of others, experts' opinions and from research studies. The assumption at the foundation of evidence-based management is that health care managers should base their decisions on relevant evidence from well-conducted studies. Such evidence should be accurate, accessible, applicable and actionable(Kovner, et al., 2009).

Evidence based management, as an approach, is concerned with translating the best evidence into practice in an organization to help in the decision-making. EBMgt is based on models and methods developed to improve medical care and reduce variability in outcomes based on best scientific evidence available. However, translating the evidence needs special skills in research and research methods and to recognize the relevant valid evidence that can be used. It is necessary to understand that, EBMgt cannot be one mold that can be applicable to all different situations and circumstances within different contexts(Rousseau, 2006). It needs to efficiently identify the available evidence most relevant to a management problem or decision situation, assess it and apply it in the appropriate way within the context (De Groot, 2005). In order to translate the scientific evidence into a practice, four factors are needed. Those are; best scientific evidence available, organizational evidence, stakeholders' values and practitioners' expertise and judgment.

EBMgt was defined by Briner, Denyer and Rousseau in 2009 as

Evidence-based management is about making decisions through the conscientious, explicit, and judicious use of four sources of information: practitioner expertise and judgment, evidence from the local context, a critical evaluation of the best available research evidence, and the perspectives of those people who might be affected by the decision (R. B. Briner, Denyer, & Rousseau, 2009).

EBMgt is similar to EBM in many aspects but are different in others. Both are concerned with making decisions based on scientific evidence but are different in the relevant research base, the professional culture and in the nature of decision-making processes. However, the research evidence related to health care management is limited due to many factors including a management culture in the developed nations that has historically placed great emphasis on the manager's independent judgment within the constraints of organizational policies and practices. This and other factors have led to the slow progress in applying EBMgt in health care organizations and especially in comparison with the wide application of EBM (Walshe & Rundall, 2001). EBMgt can be applied across managerial departments throughout any organization. It is well suited to Human Resource Management (HRM) where a number of research studies have been conducted in this field and applied in HRM practice(Rousseau & Barends, 2011). However, applying and implementing EBMgt in any organization as a decision making approach will lead to changing the whole organizational culture(Kovner, et al., 2009). In order to achieve this change, an effective leadership is needed. Leadership in any organization is the key concept of leading the organization's staff to assist in achieving the ultimate organizational mission and goals. Closely linked to EBMgt, is the concept of evidence-based leadership (EBL). The latter is defined as " the conscientious, explicit, and judicious use of theory-derived, research-based information in making decisions about care de-livery system"(De Groot, 2005). EBL helps the organization to incorporate the leaders' vision with the best available evidence. Such leadership should ensure that all the organization's executives, managers and employees are working toward one vision and mission and are committed to the same goals which are being furthered by managerial practice based on best evidence(De Groot, 2005).

The Need for Evidence Based Management

The rapidly changing health care environment throughout the world, and especially in developing nations, has increased the difficulty in providing timely, reliable and accessible health care services. In addition, costs of the medical and non-medical resources for health care services have increased as well. Managers admit that old practices and self-experience are not enough to insure that the organization is aligned with the global developments and demands. However, managers are required to use their critical thinking acumen and react fast with any situations that may arise(Walshe & Rundall, 2001),(Rousseau & Barends, 2011). Executives lead healthcare organizations, and line managers manage resources with the assistance of HRM and other staff specialists. Technically oriented health care providers provide the core health care services. It is therefore vital to ap-ply evidence-based standards and criteria to all organizational managerial, clinical and technical support. In other words we must develop, maintain and use both EBM and EBMgt knowledge and processes to support effective decision-making. It is also necessarily that a change in organizational culture be effected to create and sustain ongoing partnerships between the management, clinicians and patients to achieve the highest quality patient care, ensure patient safety and use resources ef-ficiently to achieve the organization's integrated vision, mission and goals(Trinder, 2008). This link between EBM and EBMgt will ensure the contestant provision of health care service to the patients which will improve the quality of service and patient safety (Shortell, et al., 2007).

EBMgt, as an approach, can provide a model to close the gap between the research and the practice. It can provide the scientific principles together with the organization facts to make decision that can solve problems. Managers who can systematically collect data about the organization facts can accumulate enough information about certain issue and will be able to join it with relevant scientific studies and will be capable to make a decision that hit the problem and solve it (Rousseau, 2006). It is important that, managers rely on scientific bases and learn more from literature to improve their managerial and decision making skills. It is not enough anymore that a manager solely depends on his/her own experiences and practice personal believes and understanding. It was found that, some managers apply wrong practice, for example using disinvites (i.e. threatening and punishing). This is not advisable and can be considered as a misuse of authority, which can ultimately lead to adverse effects on the entire organization. This misinterpretation for the experiences needs to be corrected by learning more about management, leadership and behaviors to be able to make the right decision to reach the organization's goals. EBMgt will help in providing this learning culture and continues improvement (Rousseau, 2006). In addition, EBMgt, managers do benefit from applying EBMgt when making decision to make a justification and strong reference of their actions. This will give them the power and authority to make their point and get the support from all stakeholders, as well as organizational legitimacy. (Rousseau, 2006).

Evidence Based Human Resource (EBHR)

EBMgt is introduced in many management departments in health care organizations. HRM is the first department that has applied this type of management as an approach for managerial decision-making. Managers are encouraged to use research and best evidence in their managerial decisions to manage employees and bring the best outcome for the organization. In HRM, EBMgt helps in making the best decision through all the HR functions and the organization environment (Rousseau & Barends, 2011). It helps direct and lead leadership ensure the organization's employees job analysis, job description, recruitment and selection, compensations, career and development, training and motivation, employees' benefits and rights, organizational strategic planning and budgeting system based on scientific information (Niles, 2012).

HRM has benefited from the different studies that were conducted in this field; from scientific information, which is informative for different HR domains, especially in staff motivation, innovation, change management, organizational learning and development, individual education, culture and organizational behavior. Applying EBHR in an organization means that four main features have to be applied in the decision making process in HRM. These are; the use of the best scientific evidence, systematic gathering of the organizational facts, practitioners' judgment to assess and evaluate to enhance learning and improve the quality of the decision making, and finally the ethical considerations for the decision impact (Rousseau & Barends, 2011).

The best scientific evidence means to find the relevant and valid research from scientific sources. It has to be from a well-designed study that is free from any bias. In organizational practice, managers have to use the situation analysis and the real facts present within the organization to find the relevant research and apply it in the right context. Applying the research will need the practitioners' judgment to extract and make best use of the evidence that will limit the normal human bias in making decisions. Expert judgment will ensure the use of the right research in the right context based on the critical thinking is made beside the situational analysis. Any decision made will have effects on the stakeholders and / or the society. Ethical consideration has to be in mind when making the decisions, as the impact can be either direct or indirect. Managers will be responsible for any outcome that result from their decisions.(Rousseau & Barends, 2011)

There are many studies that have aimed at explaining techniques in managing peoples, such as job applicants, employee selection, employees training and development. In HRM, many factors are involved when applying EBMgt. These include human factors and ergonomics, which can have an effect on the psychological and physical tasks of employees. This can make EBMgt applicable in some of HRM domains while it may be difficult to apply in others (R. Briner, 2008).

Using Global Evidence for Local Decision

Healthcare systems vary from one organization to another, and from one country to another. As technology innovation assists globally, to share same information and knowledge, healthcare organizations are easily able to learn from each other's knowledge and experience. Unlike EBM, EBMgt depend on local facts of the organization. Studies and research in medical field might be the same for most of the cases, but in management cases are differ in different organizations or in different situations. EBMgt encourages the managerial decisions to be based on scientific research and studies, however it encourages the healthcare organization to tailor the policy and guidelines that suits the organization achieve the goals which can improve the quality of service and better resources allocation. Same policy may not necessarily suit all healthcare organizations, but may increase the burden on the organization both financially and logistically. Shared scientific knowledge helps create a base for the information and infrastructure in the organization. This helps healthcare managers in each organization tailor

the appropriate decision for the current situation from the materials they have along with the organizational experiences (Clancy & Cronin, 2005).

How to Practice Evidence Based Management in the Organization

Applying EBMgt as a practice is a challenging initiation for any manager in the beginning. However, practicing it becomes easier with time as managers become more skilled in finding the best evidence for certain situations. Literature provides steps to guide managers in how to find and apply scientific information for informed decision making instead of relying on the only information available on hand. Usually practitioners follow the five steps model which is: *ask the question, search, appraise, apply and finally evaluate* (Trinder, 2008). Finding the best evidence to be applied can be found by performing systematic review and meta-analysis. Systematic review is a comprehensive summary of literature review for a specific question after identifying and appraising the validity of each individual study (Jones & Evans, 2000)while Meta-analysis concentrates in the review of the statistical analysis and the mathematical part in each study (Borenstein, Hedges, Higgins, & Rothstein, 2011). Guidance for applying EBMgt within the organization was introduced by Denis M. Rousseau in 2011 through the following guided format;(Rousseau & Barends, 2011)

First Step: The manager should start by creating questions that can generate answers that can lead to the better-informed decisions. Such questions should be fitting with the context and the setting of the organization, for example, whether the organization is for profit, governmental or nongovernmental. It should also consider the organization's goals, desired outcomes, and the values of those most affected by the decision, including the staff.

Second Step: Search for publications with citations for scientific evidences relevant to that decision. The managers can seek assistance from professionals such as researchers, information specialists or librarians to help them find the best source for scientific evidence. Those researches should be then shared with colleagues to encourage team thinking about the issue. This will create a base for management study in that certain topic, and to be cited in the memos for communicating and supporting any decisions the evidence is based and well justified.

To find the publication, it should start by searching using keywords from the question that was created. Usually numerous number of articles can be found. To narrow that down, more specific new words should be added during searching. Adding the word "studies" helps in finding the quality of information's needed.

Third Step: Critically appraise the evidence that was found. It is helpful to review the summary of the evidence in systematic reviews studies and meta-analysis studies to have a comprehensive understanding of the issues as informed by the available studies relevant to the question or topic. However, original studies have to be apprised in three main aspects: *Relevance, validity, and impact.* To check relevance, managers should go through and read the abstract of the study to see how closely it applies to the situation. Next is to check the validity by reviewing the design of the study. Proper study design will show significant relationship between variables and suggest likely cause and effect relationships and minimizing possible bias or confounders. In addition, by checking the methodology of the study we can find the impact of that study and the size of the affected group. Good methodology should cover two main points: *the use of control* or

at least comparison groups, and the other is the different points of time used in data collection. Moreover, many other points should be checked when critically appraising the study, such as the validity of the measurement instruments used, for example questionnaire or other method used for data collection.

It is important to note that the manager should be aware of the different study designs, and the best study design that can answer the target questions and reach the desired outcome. For example, if looking for cause and effect relation, intervention with controlled study such as randomized control trial (RCT) should be used as this is considered the strongest study design. Others such as cross-sectional, case and case-control studies might be weaker compared to RCT. However, unlike clinical studies, case study and cross-sectional designs can be affective and useful for management and policy research situation where control are not feasible and when analyzing processes and events retrospectively. However, to be useful, all studies in evidence base must be well designed and must have used proper analytical methods. In addition PDSA (Plan- Do-Study-Act) cycles are types of studies frequently used in management particularly in quality improvement models (Shortell, et al., 2007).

Fourth Step: Managers have to integrate the evidence with their experience, cultural work-related norms and stakeholders' concerns. The gathered evidence needs to be applicable to the specific problem or decision situation, and this necessitates some experience, particularly when quality and/or reduction of costs are concerned. Understanding how to apply and communicate evidence, with the stakeholders and colleagues is important so that a desired outcome can be reached.

Last Step: It is very important that managers monitor and evaluate the result of their decisions. Managers need to compare the actual outcome of their decisions with the assumptions they made prior to decision and the initial goals or targets. They can then learn what needs to be corrected or adapted to improve decision-making. An ongoing cycle of performance improvement will be required and reported.

Strengthening Health Systems through Evidence

Knowledge driven from scientific evidence has important positive impact on the health system globally. Evidence is the basic foundation for best practice in health policy that drives the six building blocks of health system to the desired outcome. Healthcare managers and leaders are required to use evidence in all the health systems areas that includes; medical, technology, finance, recruitment and development, information and research, service delivery and in leadership and governance. By ensuring successful management of those areas, health system goals to ensure high quality of service and patient safety with better coverage and access to health services will be accomplished.

Strengthening the health system by using evidence through research to introduce health policy is now the main aim of most of the countries to achieve the 2015 Millennium Development Goals (MDGs). However, all stockholders who are responsible for creating policies that strengthen the health system should work together as there are always misunderstanding between researchers and decision makers(WHO, 2012). The World Health Organisation (WHO) has established an international collaboration with many countries that introduced the Alliances for Health Policy and System Research (HPSR) that is aimed to improve the health system in developing countries by using research. Evidence from research is intended to close the gap and the challenges those countries are facing in the health system. WHO has submitted many reports that encourage using

research as a source of knowledge to have better informed decision making process to strength the health system around the world(De Savigny & Adam, 2009).

EXAMPLE OF SUCCESSFUL APPLICATION OF EVIDENCE BASED MANAGEMENT IN HEALTHCARE ORGANIZATIONS

There are some successful experiences in the literature of applying EBMgt in healthcare organizations.

Case Example 1: Acme Medical Center

Acme Medical Center has applied EBMgt to realign the inpatient beds to better meet current and future need. Managers and practitioners have gathered national and organizational data about the bed utilization to come with a prediction for the future need. The process started by formulating a research question. It was formulated by a steering committee led by the CEO to address the problem they are facing. The question in this case was: " *over the next three to five years, how many beds will Acme need, by service and level of care), and what bed stack assignments will best accommodate current and future requirements with as little reassignment as possible?*" The next step was to search for data that is relevant from current organizational reports of inpatient data with an assessment report compared to benchmarks and projections. The committee assessed the quality and validity of the data and if it is relevant to the case. The committee used the evaluated data to calculate the estimated bed capacity needed for future. Based on the results, the committee set up a planning guideline to bring up solutions for the problem. The committee has set both short and long-term recommendations that provide alternative solution to meet the target of bed capacity to answer the question. By applying the recommended solutions, result showed a better practice and clever way to accommodation the expected growth of patient volume instead of transfer patients and squeeze them in another place (Kovner, et al., 2009).

Case Example 2: Memorial Hospital

Memorial Hospital employed EBMgt to improve the Operating Room (OR) scheduling. The hospital used to do what is called "Block Scheduling" which is a block of OR time – either time or room-to be allocated for individual or group of surgeons in order to overcome the pressure that hospital face to efficiently allocate the OR time. As in the previous case, OR executive committee followed the EBMgt approach and started by formulating a research question. The question in Memorial Hospital was mainly to understand the current level of deficiency in order to find the appropriate start point for improvement. The questions were as follows: *"What is the current level of block utilization?, what is the variation across departments, and what opportunities exist for improving overall utilization and minimizing interdepartmental variation?"* The committee gathered data from the literature, peer hospitals and the organization's data. Data were evaluated to ensure validity, relevancy and free of bias. Based on the evaluated data, the committee introduced short-term solutions as a quick improvement for the current situation, as well as a long-term solution as a base for a permanent system and work process. Two quick actions were taken to solve the current issue. First one was by extending OR schedules one extra room for 4 hours in each department in the OR. By this action the OR could manage the extra load in operation with better resource allocation with minimize staff overtime. Second action was, to encourage intradepartmental efficiency in the work process. By following these steps, monitoring and evaluating results,

the hospital has succeeded to improve the OR scheduling efficiency and brought a system to maintain it (Kovner, et al., 2009).

Case Example 3: Mental Health Medical Facility

In a similar case as the previous two, EBMgt was implemented as intervention to manage chronic diseases. As depression is the second most common disease in the world, and depressed people usually do not admit their problem to see specialist, instead they asked for treatment in primary care, it was important to set up newer strategies to improve depression treatment in primary care settings. As in the previous cases, the medical center started the process by formulating a question. The question was: *" How can we integrate the best approach to depression treatment within primary care?"* The center started searching for evidence for the effectiveness of the treatment, the latest treatment, collaborative strategies for integration of primary care services with mental health services. Although evidence was limited there was good quality of some evidence in the literature. Based on the evidence, the decision was taken. Main action was to improve communication of critical information among patients, providers and payers. By applying the evidence in management, clinical decisions and to patients, an improvement was noticed in the care provided but not in the illness itself(Kovner, et al., 2009). The literature mentioned the role of EBMgt along with EBM in improving the acute coronary syndromes.

In other settings, one hospital could reduce the time from door to balloon time for acute myocardial infarctions (AMI) patients by applying EBMgt. Managers reviewed the literature on management of the workflow to faster the initiation of electrocardiograms on patient who need it. By providing guidelines that recommend the use of certain medications in patients with AMI as β-blockers, we can improve the patient conditions.

EBMgt helps sustain the patient care that physicians provide by; providing insight into shared goals for improvement, providing substantial administrative support, having strong physician leadership, and using credible data feedback (Shortell, et al., 2007).

EDUCATION AND EVIDENCE BASED MANAGEMENT

Evidence based management should be a part of management schools, and this should include developing an acceptable level of statistical and research skills for future healthcare managers. Generally, in business schools the focus is mainly on general management skills and functions but not research methods. Although in rare circumstances, some professors tend to teach what they have learned and are not updating their curriculum with evidence-based materials. In addition, some business schools do not offer evidence-based management courses assuming that is not related to management although such courses should be an integral component of any degree in management (11). In order to close the gap between research and practice, there is a need to have models for EBMgt to be taught in schools for managers. Changing curriculums and teaching norms is important. Building collaborations with international universities and accrediting degrees from reputable educational institutes might be very helpful to ensure the highest standard of managerial education in developing countries. Educators need to be updated on various educational techniques that incorporate evidence within management, and this can only be achieved by continuous professional development courses for professors. Professors need to guide students on how to use different research methods, how to read the articles and on how to implement evidence in their future practice (Rousseau, 2006). On the other hand, students must be aware that relevant scientific evidence is available and they need to learn how to translate the relevant findings into practice. It helps more when students can experience a real advantage of applying the evidence with certain issues. In addition, it brings the maximum benefit of learning when students can extract principles from cases by themselves and translate it into solutions. This is more practical than to find a suggested solution in an article which often targets a particular circumstance and context (Rousseau, 2006). However, it can be argued that education itself is not evidence based. The literature suggests that in education, it is much harder to apply evidence-based approaches than in medicine. The ability to generalize knowledge gained from the research seems to be more limited in education than in medicine. Knowledge itself is not enough to ensure good practice in the work settings (Hammersley, 2001).

Challenges in Applying Evidence Based Management

Evidence based management has some challenges and limitations to be applied. The main factor that prevents managers from applying EBMgt is simply their little or no knowledge about the area. Even if managers want to be evidence-based practitioners they don't know how. Most managers have busy schedules, which do not accord them the opportunity to explore scholarly journals and get up to date with the latest developments in the field. Some managers lack the skills needed to retrieve, interpret, and translate evidence into practice. In addition, and as mentioned earlier, the undergraduate managerial education itself is not yet evidence-based, therefore graduated managers do not have the basic skills in using scientific evidence. Another challenge, in this respect, is that many managers perceive EBMgt approach would be limiting their freedom in taking the actions and decisions they are convinced with based on their experience and norms within the working environment they are serving. So their fear of losing autonomy and control over their decisions might be also of importance to note (Rousseau, 2006).

Management, unlike medicine and other medical specialties, it is not considered to be a profession to the same degree. Managers may have different backgrounds, qualifications and degrees. In addition, management situations are complicated and changeable. Stakeholders' influence on decision making is an additional challenge. Adding more to its complexity, feedback of any managerial decision takes long time and hence, the impact of managerial decision cannot be estimated immediately, and might need years to be evaluated(Rousseau, 2006). Research study designs for management as HRM are not identical to those for medicine and other medical specialties (Trinder, 2008) and hence need to be developed and updated. Until this happens, it is necessary to combine the critical thinking with the best available evidence (Rousseau & Barends, 2011). On the other hand of that challenge, EBMgt as with EBP, is not only difficult to be implemented or translated into practice, it was also argued that EBP is not a cumulative approach to practice, as it relies on some specific facts unique to the problem situation which was studied. In addition, sometimes there is not enough evidence to know which type of evidence is more applicable and likely to be more effective. Meta-analysis might be one of the most comprehensive designs in addressing specific managerial problems and offer evidence-based solution. However similar to other studies, this analytical approach, which makes use of data provided by prior original studies, can lead to misleading results if not well planned and executed (Trinder, 2008), (Hammersley, 2001), especially if the particular settings in question is not the same or similar to those where the research was conducted. Finding relevant studies of high quality in management is not an easy task. As an example, there are only few studies that have explored how employees can make a balance between their experience and scientific evidence when

they are in a situation of taking decisions(Trinder, 2008). The major challenge is how to get evidence from studies of high quality and ignore those of weak methodological quality(Rousseau, 2006).

There are several barriers for the use of EBMgt in healthcare organizations. Firstly, insufficient access to research and getting full text of the articles due to financial or technical problems is an obvious barrier. Secondly, insufficient skills among managers related to the use of research electronic databases and the application of critical appraisal to evaluate the quality of articles is an obstacle for proper decision-making. Thirdly, political issues within the organization may play a role in interfering with the hierarchies that governs the work of staff members. Lastly, inadequate relevant evidence and hectic schedules of managers can contribute to the limited use of evidence in healthcare managerial decisions (Trinder, 2008).

Introducing changes to any organization by applying EBMgt as part of the EBP will need to consider many aspects. These aspects include organizational strategic planning, the organizational economic and financial situation, and the organizational environment such as the learning and knowledge components. Lastly, organizational culture and people's attitude and beliefs also need to be considered. Creating evidence-based infrastructure within an organization needs a major change in the organizational structure, which might be costly. This is a substantial challenge for organizations with limited resources (Trinder, 2008).

Critical Appraisal of Evidence Based Management

Evaluation of EBMgt as in EBP, is not an easy task. Lots of healthcare managerial outcomes are not easily measured. It is hard to measure the effectiveness of applying evidence based as an approach. Moreover, EBP is not constant. Same evidence-based information can be interpreted differently according to the context of the study and whether or not it was applied to individual or population. Additionally, the critical appraisal of EBMgt is that there is no clear and consistent definition and therefore, it is not clear what theories can be applied in practice and how they differ if their application varies (Trinder, 2008).

Despite the above mentioned difficulties in critical appraisal of EBMgt, there are some aspects that are in favor for its use. EBMgt has the advantage of a continuously updated process which can provide a systematic approach for knowledge for a specific issue(Trinder, 2008). Similar to EBP, EBMgt is affected by the availability of technology in order to access it. Obviously modern healthcare organization needs to have an adequate IT system in order to disseminate information and provide access for practitioners to the information they need. Organizations can provide training to the practitioners on how to use available technology, how to access the evidence and how to implement it. It is important to create a learning organization culture and provide enough budget and resources to make sure that EBMgt can play a role in decision making among managers(Trinder, 2008).

Another factor critical to EBP is its linear approach in decision-making, based on scientific information, which can override experiences and norms within the managerial systems, and other knowledge. Moreover, EBP cannot sometimes welcome consumers in the decision-making. However, several studies have shown effectiveness when consumer opinion is involved after empowering them to play part of the decision making (Trinder, 2008).

FURTHER READING AND FUTURE DIRECTIONS

Some Relevant Studies from the Literature

"Evidence Based Management from theory to practice" is an important article by Kieran Walshe and Rhomas G. Rundall that discussed the importance of evidence in decision-making at both clinical and managerial settings. Authors of this article, which was published in 2001, indicated that there is an uneven application of EBP in the different healthcare areas. Despite the fact that managers encourage clinicians to apply EBM, managers themselves do not use evidence in their decisions making process(Walshe & Rundall, 2001).

In 2002, Ranjit Bose from the University of New Mexico published an article that explored how knowledge management can enhance health care management systems and support decision-making. It discussed the importance of integration of clinical and administrative/financial management in order to create a successful health care organization. The study showed that Information Technology (IT) is an important tool in the health care organizations for gathering information utilized by managers to take decisions. (Bose, 2003).

An article by Elizabith J. Layman, introduced theories for decision making in health care organization for managers and supervisors. Those theories can help managers in practice the right decisions needed in all management functions. The author has also given some examples to help managers find the right theory that would be applicable depending on the situation they have (Layman, 2011b).

A systematic review study was conducted in 2005 in McMaster University, Canada, and provided evidence to support the importance of the interaction between the researchers and policy makers. Systematic reviews are seen as effective tool to inform health care management and policy makers with information needed in their fields (Lavis et al., 2005).

In 2008, a semi-structured qualitative interview study, conducted by MacDonald and colleagues, showed that decision making within the study group has no structured form for decisions. Although the study mentioned that the decisions making was used for both solving problems and for improvement opportunities, the study did not indicate how successful this was to achieve the desired out come by unstructured decision making form (MacDonald, Bath, & Booth, 2008).

An article by Aktas et al. published in 2005, discussed the "management-oriented decision support model". It concluded that, health care managers are required to make effective decisions to provide high quality of patient care service with less cost, which will be accomplished only with available relevant and accurate information. The article proposed a health information system, which will provide the required information and results for health care managers, who can analyze it and interpret it without research skills needed (Aktaş, Ülengin, & Önsel Şahin, 2007).

A paper by Bob Hamlin, University of Wolverhampton, UK arguing the empirical research that was conducted on NHS trust hospital in UK discussing the support of evidence based health care management the managerial effectiveness within the NHS trust hospital. The research supported other studies finding which is the judgment and perception of managerial behaviour it is different from the managers than superior and subordinates. The study showed some positive points of managerial behaviours that show effectiveness of the management while there was some negative points which should be avoided. The writer has indicated the limitation of this study, as it was conducted in only one hospital and hence its results cannot be generalized to all health care organizations. However, despite that limitation, the research supports the development of evidence based management in all healthcare organizations (Hamlin, 2001).

1n 2005 an article by Denise M. Rousseau discussed evidence based management and the gap between research and practice. The only way to overcome the gap between science and practice is by applying the evidence based management model. The writer has stressed the importance of introducing the evidence-based management in management schools. Main reason of why managers are not applying evidence management was simply because they don't know about it. The article suggests the collaboration among managers, researches, and educator to build the supported culture to make the right decision based on the latest and best evidence (Rousseau, 2006).

Another article by Denis M. Rousseau issued in 2011 discussed the role of using best evidence in decision making in Human Resource (HR). This approach was called Evidence Based Human Resources (EBHR). The article introduced a guide for EBHR to be part of the organization practice. It was mentioned that, the first department has applied the evidence based management as an decision making approach was the HR. Common misunderstanding was to compare evidence based management with EBM, the writer cleared that, ecannot be a randomized control trial (RCT) for managers. Instead in EBHR model, managers have to use the critical thinking, with situational analysis beside the best available scientific evidence. (Rousseau & Barends, 2011)

An article by Kanak Guatam, Saint Louis, University school of Public Health issued in 2008, addressed the Research-Practice Gap in Healthcare Management. The writer has mentioned the most common barriers in many stages to translate research in to a practice in health care organization. Some suggest solutions was mentioned as the necessary of educating managers about research and research methods, the collaboration researchers with education process in management schools, enhance change in health care organizations to adapt evidence based management in its daily practice (Gautam, 2008).

In 2006, a paper by Jeffrey Pfefferand Robert I. Suttonin in Evidence Based Management discussed the importance for managers to practice EBMgtin order to treat the organization illness as physician treat patients ill. It suggested that managers have to move to the best evidence insisted of the six substitutes that is always used. Those were mentioned are personal experience, specialist skills, hype, dogma, and mindless mimicry of top performers (Pfeffer & Sutton, 2006)

An article by Stephen M. Shortell and his colleagues issued in 2007 discussed the need to link between EBM and EBMgt to improve patient safety and the health care service. The article indicated that, EBM alone it is not enough bring the needed patient care. It needs health care organization to be consistent in providing its service. Managers has to be involved to identify the organizational strategy and structure to enable the physicians to provide consistent health care service (Shortell, et al., 2007)

A case of evidence based policy issued in 2003 by Urban institute and was revised in 2008, has indicated the importance and the urgency of evidence based policy in public programs to provide an acceptable return for paid taxes by the public. The evidence based policy which was defined as "it is a rigorous approach that draws on carful data collection, extermination, and both qualitative and quantitative analysis" will benefit to answer the main questions which are, first, what is the problem exactly? Second, what is the possible way to address the problem? Third, what are the probable and impact of each? And fourth, what political and social values do the proposed options reflect? The case has discussed the benefit of the evidence based policy in many public sectors as, health insurance coverage, criminal justice, education, and housing discrimination (Press & Decoder, 2003).

A paper by Martyn Hammersley issued in 2001, answering some questions about evidence-based practice in education. The writer argued that in evidence-based practice the practitioners have to be able to access a valid relevant research is necessary to improve their practice. However, she argued that, evidence based practice not necessary lead to improvement of the service. Practitioners need to learn about research and how to ask the right question that is relevant to the situation in order to get the right answer from the right research (Hammersley, 2001).

An article by De Groot, discussed the evidence based leadership and its role in providing the patient safety in health care organization. It reported that patient safety can be provided as part of the leader role in the organization and as part of the vision and mission and the change which can be introduced to the organization. The writer discussed that, leadership should be evidence based in order to lead the health care practitioners to provide service to the community that ensure patient safety (De Groot, 2005).

A book review by Y Connie J. Evashwick was issued in 2010 evaluating the book titled (Evidence Based Management In Healthcare) by Anthony R. Kovner and colleagues which was issued in 2009. The book discussed Appling evidence based management as a decision making approach in health care organization. It introduced a study that was conducted on senior managers and showed that managers are rarely using evidence in their decision-making. The book discussed the role of managers in health care organization and how it is important to evidence rather than other factors. It introduced a guide with six steps in how to apply evidence based management as decision making approach (Kovner, et al., 2009).

Evidence based Practice: a critical appraisal is a book with ten chapters that discussed many aspects of evidence based practice and management(Trinder & Reynolds, 2000).Chapter 9 of this book was about Evidence Based Human Resource and concentrated on EBP in a management wise. It discussed the HRM role in managing people, and how proceed HRM techniques based on scientific evidence to manage for individuals, group or as organizational behavior. The chapter has mentioned some relevant examples. (R. Briner, 2008)

Chapter 10 of (Evidence based Practice: a critical appraisal by Trinder L.) book, is critically apprise evidence based practice in general. It was mentioned how it is difficult to critical apprise EBP for many reason. However, the chapter mentioned the strength and the weakness of using EBP into practice. It mentioned some practical problems and suggests some solutions. Moreover, many challenges of applying EBP was mentioned as a conclusion (Trinder, 2008).

WAY FORWARD AND RECOMMENDATIONS

Evidence Based Management in Health Care organizations is minimal and at times non-existent. Our literature review found no studies that aimed at shedding light on how decision-making is processed by health care managers in developing countries. It is also not clear whether or not new methods of evidence based management are applied as a decision making approach. In order to improve the health care system in all its essential areas; delivery of service, workforce, information, medical products, financing, governance and leadership (WHO, 2007), we need to understand the factors that affect decision making, and investigate strategies that health care managers in developing nations follow. Such research will help us find the strengths and weaknesses in health care decision making in developing nations, and suggestions for actions needed for improvement. This would possibly help in achieving the main goal of the health care systems, which is to improve the public health status of the population by providing high quality and accessible health care services at reasonable costs across all levels of the population.

It is time for healthcare managers to be aware of the importance of EBMgt that is equally as important as EBM in providing the required medical services to patients. In fact, healthcare managers are more powerful and authorized in healthcare organizations. They provide policy and guidelines for healthcare providers and need to allocate resources for the best outcomes. As managers are the responsible members in the healthcare organization, to face the quick advance in technology and science with limited resources with increasing demands, they are required to base their decision-making on four important sources of information. These are: *best scientific evidence available, organizational evidence, stakeholders' values, and practitioners' expertise and judgment.* Important to note is that education plays an important role in how healthcare managers approach their decisions. Health care managers need more education and training in EBMgt to support patient care by applying EBM as the foundation for continuous improvement of health care services, and to insure quality patient care and safety with more efficient allocations of resources.

Healthy population cannot be achieved by applying scientific evidence in managing single cases; it requires the entire health system to be managed according to latest and relevant scientific evidence.

REFERENCES

7 Steps in Decision Making. (2007). *The Happy Manager.*

Aktaş, E., Ülengin, F., & Önsel Şahin, Ş. (2007). A decision support system to improve the efficiency of resource allocation in healthcare management. *Socio-Economic Planning Sciences, 41*(2), 130–146. doi:10.1016/j.seps.2005.10.008

Borenstein, M., Hedges, L. V., Higgins, J. P., & Rothstein, H. R. (2011). *Introduction to meta-analysis.* Wiley.

Bose, R. (2003). Knowledge management-enabled health care management systems: Capabilities, infrastructure, and decision-support. *Expert Systems with Applications, 24*(1), 59–71. doi:10.1016/S0957-4174(02)00083-0

Briner, R. (2008). Evidence-based human resource management. *Evidence-based practice: A critical appraisal,* 184-211.

Briner, R. B., Denyer, D., & Rousseau, D. M. (2009). Evidence-based management: Concept cleanup time? *The Academy of Management Perspectives*, *23*(4), 19–32. doi:10.5465/AMP.2009.45590138

Clancy, C. M., & Cronin, K. (2005). Evidence-based decision making: Global evidence, local decisions. *Health Affairs*, *24*(1), 151–162. doi:10.1377/hlthaff.24.1.151 PMID:15647226

De Groot, H. A. (2005). Evidence-based leadership: Nursing's new mandate. *Nurse Leader*, *3*(2), 37–41. doi:10.1016/j.mnl.2005.01.004

De Savigny, D., & Adam, T. (2009). *Systems thinking for health systems strengthening*. World Health Organization.

Gautam, K. (2008). Addressing the research-practice gap in healthcare management. *Journal of Public Health Management and Practice*, *14*(2), 155–159. doi:10.1097/01.PHH.0000311894.57831.4b PMID:18287922

Gray, J. A. M. (2009). *Evidence-based healthcare and public health: how to make decisions about health services and public health*. Churchill Livingstone.

Hamlin, B. (2001). *Support of Evidence-Based Healthcare Management: an empirical study of managerial effectiveness within an NHS trust hospital*. University of Wolverhampton.

Hammersley, M. (2001). *Some questions about evidence-based practice in education*. Paper presented at the symposium on" Evidence-based practice in education" at the Annual Conference of the British Educational Research Association, University of Leeds.

Hjørland, B. (2011). Evaluation of an information source illustrated by a case study: Effect of screening for breast cancer. *Journal of the American Society for Information Science and Technology*, *62*(10), 1892–1898. doi:10.1002/asi.21606

Jones, T., & Evans, D. (2000). Conducting a systematic review. *Australian Critical Care*, *13*(2), 66–71. doi:10.1016/S1036-7314(00)70624-2 PMID:11235454

Kovner, A. R., Fine, D. J., & D'Aquila, R. (2009). *Evidence-based management in healthcare*. Health Administration Press.

Lavis, J., Davies, H., Oxman, A., Denis, J. L., Golden-Biddle, K., & Ferlie, E. (2005). Towards systematic reviews that inform health care management and policy-making. *Journal of Health Services Research & Policy*, *10*(suppl 1), 35–48. doi:10.1258/1355819054308549 PMID:16053582

Layman, E. J. (2011a). Decision making for health care managers and supervisors: Theory into practice. *The Health Care Manager*, *30*(4), 287–300. doi:10.1097/HCM.0b013e3182350e7b PMID:22042136

Layman, E. J. (2011b). Decision Making for Health Care Managers and Supervisors: Theory Into Practice. *The Health Care Manager*, *30*(4), 287–300. doi:10.1097/HCM.0b013e3182350e7b PMID:22042136

MacDonald, J., Bath, P. A., & Booth, A. (2008). Healthcare managers' decision making: Findings of a small scale exploratory study. *Health Informatics Journal*, *14*(4), 247–258. doi:10.1177/1460458208096554 PMID:19008275

Niles, N. J. (2012). *Basic Concepts of Health Care Human Resource Management*. Jones & Bartlett Publishers.

Pfeffer, J., & Sutton, R. I. (2006). Evidence-based management. *Harvard Business Review*, *84*(1), 62. PMID:16447370

Press, U., & Decoder, J. (2003). *The Case for Evidence-Based Policy*.

Rousseau, D. M. (2006). Is there such a thing as" evidence-based management"? *Academy of Management Review*, *31*(2), 256–269. doi:10.5465/AMR.2006.20208679

Rousseau, D. M., & Barends, E. G. R. (2011). Becoming an evidence-based HR practitioner. *Human Resource Management Journal*, *21*(3), 221–235. doi:10.1111/j.1748-8583.2011.00173.x

Shortell, S. M., Rundall, T. G., & Hsu, J. (2007). Improving patient care by linking evidence-based medicine and evidence-based management. *Journal of the American Medical Association*, *298*(6), 673–676. doi:10.1001/jama.298.6.673 PMID:17684190

Straus, S. E., & Sackett, D. L. (1998). Getting research findings into practice: Using research findings in clinical practice. *BMJ: British Medical Journal*, *317*(7154), 339–342. doi:10.1136/bmj.317.7154.339

Trinder, L. (2008). A critical appraisal of evidence-based practice. *Evidence-based practice: A critical appraisal*, 212-241.

Trinder, L., & Reynolds, S. (2000). *Evidence-based practice: A critical appraisal*. Blackwell Science Oxford. doi:10.1002/9780470699003

Walshe, K., & Rundall, T. G. (2001). Evidence-based Management: From Theory to Practice in Health Care. *The Milbank Quarterly*, *79*(3), 429–457. doi:10.1111/1468-0009.00214 PMID:11565163

WHO. (2007). *Everybody's business, Strengthening Health Systems To Improve Health Outcomes WHO's framework for action*. WHO.

WHO. (2012). *Changing Mindset Strategy on Health Policy and Systems Research*. Retrieved from http://www.who.int/alliance-hpsr/alliancehpsr_changingmindsets_strategyhpsr.pdf

KEY TERMS AND DEFINITIONS

Decision-Making: The process of making a choice between given options or taking a required action.

Evidence Based Human Resource: Make Human Resource policy and procedures based on scientific relevant and valid data.

Evidence Based Practice: Perform and practice based on a scientific relevant and valid data.

Evidence-Based Management: Making managerial decisions based on scientific relevant and valid data.

Healthcare: The care delivered by professional practitioners including diagnosis, treatment and prevention of any kind of illness or injuries for patients.

Healthcare-Managers: The person who are responsible to manage the process of care giving toward a set of goals and objectives.

Management: The process of organizing and coordinating tasks and people's effort to achieve the desired outcome effectively and efficiently.

This work was previously published in Transforming Public Health in Developing Nations edited by Mohamud Sheikh, Aziza Mahamoud, and Mowafa Househ, pages 69-89 copyright year 2015 by Information Science Reference (an imprint of IGI Global).

Section 6
Emerging Trends

This section highlights research potential within the field of E-Health and Telemedicine while exploring uncharted areas of study for the advancement of the discipline. Introducing this section are chapters that set the stage for future research directions and topical suggestions for continued debate, centering on the new venues and forums for discussion. A pair of chapters on space-time makes up the middle of the section of the final 11 chapters, and the book concludes with a look ahead into the future of the E-Health and Telemedicine field. In all, this text will serve as a vital resource to practitioners and academics interested in the best practices and applications of the burgeoning field of E-Health and Telemedicine.

Chapter 78
Mobile Health Services:
A New Paradigm for Health Care Systems

Nabila Nisha
North South University, Bangladesh

Afrin Rifat
North South University, Bangladesh

Mehree Iqbal
North South University, Bangladesh

Sherina Idrish
North South University, Bangladesh

ABSTRACT

Today, information and communication technology (ICTs) are influencing health system development across many developing countries, particularly through the application of mobile communications. As such, there has been an initiation of a new paradigm of mobile health services which has made health-care delivery more accessible, affordable and effective. However, such service delivery platform has been mainly targeted towards the rural population, so there is growing concerns about its acceptance and future use intentions in the urban areas. The aim of this paper is to examine and critically assess the underlying factors that can influence future use intentions of mHealth services in the context of Bangladesh. The conceptual model of the study identifies that information quality, facilitating conditions, trust and effort expectancy plays an important role in capturing users' overall perceptions of mobile health services. Finally, the study highlights the managerial implications, future research directions and limitations from the perspective of Bangladesh.

1. INTRODUCTION

Information and communication technology (ICTs) has radically transformed healthcare delivery across many developing countries. The introduction of ICT in healthcare, particularly the application of mobile technology based health care services (mHealth), has made healthcare delivery more accessible and affordable in recent times. This new form of healthcare delivery serves as a tool with a huge potential for health care organizations to deliver quality and cost-effective care to geographically dispersed populations in low and middle-income countries [Powell et al., 2003; Ganesh, 2004; Jung, 2008]. As a result, there is a growing enthusiasm among the analysts of global health for the possibilities that has opened up through this new paradigm of mobile health services.

DOI: 10.4018/978-1-4666-8756-1.ch078

Mobile health (mHealth), has been broadly defined by the Global Observatory for e-Health (GOe) of the World Health Organization (WHO) as the medical and public health practice supported by mobile devices, such as mobile phones, patient monitoring devices, personal digital assistants (PDAs) and other wireless devices [WHO, 2011]. The mHealth application generally provides patient monitoring, sends text messages reminding patients to take needed medications and offers suggestions for maintaining health while pregnant, even in war-ravaged places [Harvard School of Public Health, 2012].

Within Bangladesh, there has been considerable exploration of the ways in which mobile phones can be used as a means to provide relevant health information to people. The simplest example has been the use of SMS messages as part of a government health education programme, wherein the country's leading mobile phone operators broadcast the government's SMS messages at no additional cost to the mobile phone users [WHO, 2011]. Over time, Bangladesh experienced significant advances and development in the health care sector as the government initiated a number of mHealth programmes that are currently operational through telemedicine services by means of specialized 24/7 call centers [DGHS, 2014].

Although mHealth services alleviate some of the access and timeliness related challenges in the provision of healthcare services in the rural areas of Bangladesh [Rashidee, 2013], there is growing concerns about the acceptance and future use intentions of such services in the urban areas of the country. It is noteworthy that perceptions of poor quality of healthcare information may dissuade users from availing mHealth services because health concerns are among the most salient of human concerns [Kaplan and Litwka, 2008]. Also, if the system of mHealth services cannot be trusted to guarantee a threshold level of quality, it will remain underutilized, be bypassed or used mostly as a measure of last resort [Dagger et al., 2007; Akter et al., 2010]. This importance of information quality and trust for mHealth services has been evidenced in numerous studies, but there is a paucity of research regarding the effects of these factors on the acceptance and use of mHealth services in Bangladesh.

This study fills into the void by aiming to conceptualize the proposed constructs of information quality and trust to examine the factors that can influence future use intentions for mHealth services in the context of Bangladesh. To pursue this purpose, the unified theory of acceptance and use of technology (UTAUT) model has been used. Findings of this research will provide further insights into understanding and managing potential mHealth users, particularly hailing from the urban areas of Bangladesh. This study can also assist various public and private hospitals of the urban areas, along with various telecommunication networks to consider the idea of providing suitable mHealth services to the urban people of Bangladesh.

2. LITERATURE REVIEW

This study argues that it is necessary to determine the factors that can influence future use intentions for mHealth services in the context of Bangladesh. As such, the current practice of mHealth services and its implications in Bangladesh, followed by the research platform of the study and finally, the theoretical background of the proposed constructs has been discussed to determine the gaps for the study.

2.1. Mobile Health Initiatives in Bangladesh

As part of their initiative to develop an ICT-informed health system, the government of Bangladesh has developed a Health Management Information System (MIS) department under the Directorate General of Health Services (DGHS). One major function of this department is to ensure a mobile phone health service, which involves government-run health complexes and district hospitals using mobile phones as a local 24-hour call centre [DGHS, 2014]. People residing in the rural areas can contact with the health professionals through this network. They can make calls, free of charge, and the doctor on duty will provide free medical advice. Moreover, web-camera has been given in each sub-district, district, medical college and post-graduate institute hospitals in Bangladesh. These hospitals, therefore, can give telemedicine services using Skype or any other video conferencing platforms. The International Telecommunication Union (ITU) and WHO also launched a new partnership called the 'mHealth' initiative to use mobile technology, in particular text messaging and applications, to help combat non-communicable diseases (NCDs) such as diabetes, cancer, cardiovascular diseases and chronic respiratory diseases in Bangladesh [WHO, 2011]. In addition, some mHealth services in Bangladesh like the Mobile Alliance for Maternal Action (MAMA) offers guidance on safe pregnancy, along with information and advice to pregnant mothers regarding health and nutrition related matters [Reza, 2012; Sultana, 2014].

2.2. Necessity of Mobile Health Services in Bangladesh

The current healthcare system of Bangladesh consists of various government health facilities and a number of private providers of health services [Koehlmoos et al., 2011; Ahmed et al., 2013]. The private healthcare providers include large and small non-governmental organizations (NGOs), private hospitals and clinics, as well as a substantial number of informal providers of health services and drugs, known as village doctors. These informal providers typically work outside a proper health regulatory framework and provide diverse treatment pathways, which often results in drugs being issued without prescriptions in varying dosages. In general, residents of the rural areas or urban slums of Bangladesh tend to approach such informal providers since they have limited access to trained healthcare providers. This significant shortage of trained healthcare providers and provision of healthcare services in an inappropriate manner has led to a growing interest in the possible ways that ICTs, in particular the use of mobile phones, can improve access to safe, effective and affordable health services and advice in Bangladesh. Within this context, mHealth has emerged as a viable solution to serve the pressing healthcare needs through its high reach and low cost mechanism [UNF, 2009]. Today, mHealth is seen as an enabler of change in the healthcare sector for the residents of both the rural and urban areas of Bangladesh.

2.3. Research Setting of the Study

Given that a substantial section of the rural population has little or no access to proper healthcare services, it is quite possible that mHealth applications can bring quality health services to rural areas. However, whether such access to advice from an unknown hospital doctor will be utilized by the urban people still remains a question. As such, it is imperative to examine the factors that can influence the acceptance and use of mHealth services among the urban areas of Bangladesh.

Literature reveals that understanding individual acceptance and use of information technology is one of the most important branches of information systems research. The model that has been most widely used for this purpose tends to be the Technology Acceptance Model (TAM) [Davis, 1989; Davis et al., 1989], which was adapted from the Theory of Reasoned Action (TRA) [Ajzen and Fishbein, 1980; Fishbein and Ajzen, 1975]. Based on this review and synthesis of prior technology acceptance research, Venkatesh et al. [2003] developed the unified theory of acceptance and use of technology (UTAUT) model. UTAUT has served as a baseline model to study a variety of technologies in both organizational and non-organizational settings. However, given the number of technology devices, applications, and services that are targeted at consumers in recent times, it became necessary to identify the factors that can influence consumer adoption and use of technologies [Stofega and Llamas, 2009]. This led to the introduction of the UTAUT2 model by Venkatesh et al. [2012].

Venkatesh et al. [2012] adapted the four key constructs (i.e. performance expectancy, effort expectancy, social influence and facilitating conditions) that influence behavioral intention to use a technology and/or technology use from the original UTAUT model and tailored it to fit the consumer context. Thus, *performance expectancy* is defined as the degree to which using a technology will provide benefits to consumers in performing certain activities; *effort expectancy* is the degree of ease associated with consumers' use of technology; *social influence* is the extent to which consumers perceive that important others (e.g. family and friends) believe they should use a particular technology; and *facilitating conditions* refers to consumers' perceptions of the resources and support available to perform a behavior [Venkatesh et al., 2012]. Past studies like Venkatesh et al. [2003] claimed that the constructs of performance expectancy, effort expectancy and social influence determines the behavioral intention to use a technology, while behavioral intention and facilitating conditions influence the technology use in a particular context. Venkatesh et al. [2012] further claimed that the addition of new constructs in a consumer context can contribute to the expansion of the theoretical horizons of UTAUT. Against this backdrop, this study has selected the original UTAUT and UTAUT2 model as a theoretical foundation to develop a proposed research model for this study.

2.4. Proposed Constructs of Information Quality and Trust

An impressive body of academic research [e.g. Jiang et al., 2001; DeLone and McLean, 2003; Nelson et al., 2005; Lallmahamood, 2007; Jung, 2008; Lee and Chung, 2009; Lin, 2011; Lau et al., 2013] adapted various forms of quality dimensions in order to investigate users' quality perception regarding a technology. Although there is no study that directly measured quality perception of health services over the mobile platform, some studies like Chae and Kim [2001], Varshney [2005] and Ivatury et al. [2009] examined mobile information services and mobile telemedicine services in developing countries and found the dimension of information quality to be predominant.

Information quality (IQ) plays a critical role in building user satisfaction and customer loyalty for mobile internet services [Chae et al., 2002; Jung, 2008]. In their researches, DeLone and McLean [2003] and Lee and Chung [2009] suggested that information quality can significantly predict users' perception regarding the use of mobile based technology in sensitive areas like mobile banking or mobile health services. Generally, the three most important indicators of information quality are completeness, accuracy and currency [Masrek et al., 2012]. Accuracy has been defined as the extent to which the information is correct, unambiguous, objective and meaningful or believable [Wand and Wang, 1996]. On the other hand, completeness refers to the extent to which all possible states relevant to the user population are available in the stored information [Nelson et al., 2005]. However, the assessment of completeness is more of a subjective issue, since the system can be complete as far as one user is concerned but incomplete in the eyes of another [Nelson et al., 2005]. In order to overcome this ambiguity of completeness, researcher has identified currency of information as another dimension of information quality. According to Nelson et al. [2005], currency can be defined as the degree to which information is up to date, or the degree to which the information precisely reflects the current state of the world. Together all these three attributes capture the key elements of information quality and direct users' perception regarding any mobile technology related services.

On the other hand, trust has been found to have a direct, positive effect on usage intentions in various e-commerce research [e.g. Gefen and Straub, 1997; Pavlou, 2003; Jung, 2008]. Findings often claim the lack of trust in the service or service provider to be one of the main reasons why consumers hesitate to engage in any technology related services [Lanseng and Andreassen, 2007; Klein, 2007].

According to Rousseau et al. [1998], trust can be defined as a psychological state comprising the intentions to accept vulnerability based on positive expectations of the behaviour of another. It is a social and personal factor that has been investigated by Lin [2011] and El-Wajeeh et al. [2014] in various dimensions such as personality-based trust, knowledge-based trust, etc. In the healthcare sector, trust is best described as the individuals' perceptions of the credibility of the healthcare service provider as the source of the health information that is obtained [Jung, 2008]. Korp [2006] and Jung [2008] further claim that high perceived credibility can generate trust for technology-based health services. Perceiving the provider as credible means that the individual can express trust so that the uncertainty involved in using the mobile technology based health service and the possible risks involved can be overcome.

Overall, the existing theories have clearly identified that information quality and trust play a significant role in influencing future usage intentions for mHealth services. As such, there is a research call to capture user's perception in mobile health services by employing these two constructs. Moreover, very few studies have focused on these two dimensions in particular in the context of Bangladesh. This study thus taps into this opportunity and attempts to significantly contribute to the literature by conceptualizing a proposed research model for mobile health services.

3. RESEARCH MODEL AND HYPOTHESES

In conceptualizing the proposed model for mHealth services, the four key constructs of the original UTAUT model (i.e. performance expectancy, effort expectancy, social influence and facilitating conditions) and the two proposed constructs of information quality and trust, drawn from previous literature of mHealth services, has been incorporated. Figure 1 shows the proposed research model. In addition, all the variables hypothesized in this study and their likely relationships towards consumer acceptance and use of mHealth services in Bangladesh has been discussed next.

3.1. Performance Expectancy

Performance expectancy generally depicts a users' view of the usefulness of adopting a technology. According to Venkatesh et al. [2003], performance expectancy has been derived from perceived usefulness (TAM/TAM2), relative advantage (IDT), extrinsic motivates (MM), job-fit (MPCU) and outcome expectations (SCT) in the UTAUT model. According to several empirical evidences, performance expectancy is particularly identical to perceived usefulness factor of the original TAM model, which claim that when a user perceives a technology useful, the likelihood of adopting that technology increases [Venkatesh, et. al., 2003; Jimison and Sher, 2008; Holden and Karsh, 2010]. Moreover, Sun et al. [2013] claim that in the context of mHealth services, the usefulness can only be captured by the extent to which it can help users to solve their health related issues. If users believe that using mHealth services can help them to solve their problems, they are more likely to adopt this technology. Hence, the hypothesis is:

Figure 1. The proposed research structure

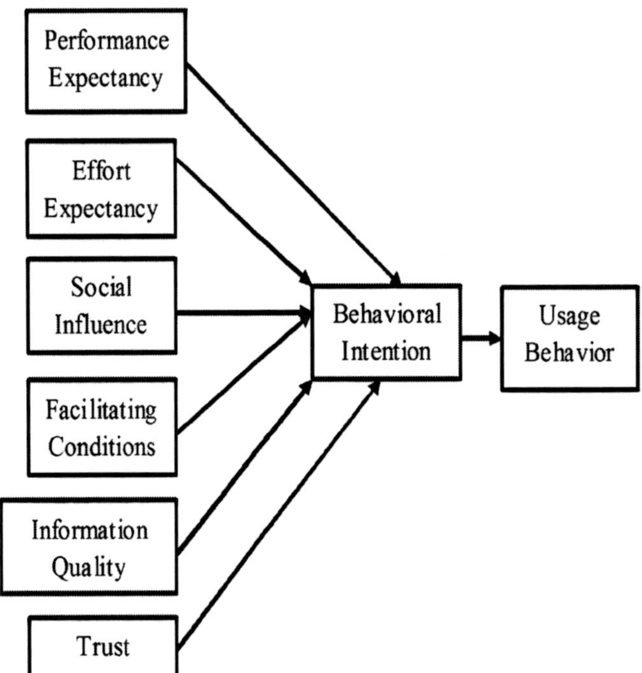

H1: Performance expectancy significantly affects individual intention to use mHealth services.

3.2. Effort Expectancy

Effort expectancy is considered to be directly related with the ease of using a particular technology [Phichitchaisopa and Naenna, 2013]. It is a construct of UTAUT model that can be represented as perceived ease of use in TAM or TAM2 model, complexity in MPCU and ease of use in IDT model. According to Davis et al. [1989], Szajna [1996] and Venkatesh [1999], all of these effort-oriented constructs act as more significant factors during the early stages of adopting a new technology. Several studies like Park et al. [2007], Wu et al. [2007], Wills et al. [2008], Moores [2012] and Sun et al. [2013] claim that perceived ease of use or effort expectancy has considerable impact on attitude towards the adoption of mHealth or any other healthcare related technology. As a result, the following hypothesis has been proposed:

H2: Effort expectancy significantly affects individual intention to use mHealth services.

3.3. Social Influence

Social influence refers to the degree to which an individual perceives that important others believe he or she should use the new system or technology [Venkatesh et al., 2003]. It can be represented by the constructs of subjective norm (TRA, TAM2, TPB/DTPB and C-TAM-TPB), social factors (MPCU) and image (IDT) [Kohnke et al., 2014]. The idea behind social influence is that even though an individual may not be in favour of adopting a new technology, they intend to use it as he/she believes it will enhance his/her image among his/her family and peers [Venkatesh and Davis, 2000]. Many studies indicate a positive relationship between social influence and behavioural intention towards a particular technology. In fact, researchers like Jung [2008] and Sun et al. [2013] empirically show that there is a significant positive relationship between social influence and adoption of mHealth technology. Thus, the proposed hypothesis is:

H3: Social influence significantly affects individual intention to use mHealth services.

3.4. Facilitating Conditions

According to Venkatesh et al. [2003], facilitating conditions refer to the resources and technical infrastructure that a user believes exists to support the adoption of a particular technology. In other words, facilitating conditions indicate the prospective conditions that may restrain or facilitate adopting a technology [Sun et al., 2013]. Past studies by Venkatesh et al. [2003], Venkatesh and Zhang [2010] and Venkatesh et al. [2012] argue that a consumer with a lower level of facilitating conditions may have a lower intention to use a particular technology. Moreover, researchers like Boontarig et al. [2012], Phichitchaisopa and Naenna [2013] and Sun et al. [2013] show that there is a positive significant relationship between facilitating conditions and health care technologies. Based on these findings, this study hypothesizes that:

H4: Facilitating conditions significantly affects individual intention to use mHealth services.

3.5. Information Quality

Lin and Lu [2000] and Venkatesh and Davis [2000] introduced information quality, namely output quality, as an antecedent of perceived usefulness in TAM2 model. In the consumer service context, this construct captures an individual's perception of the quality of the healthcare response given to the request, that is, the health information obtained. Also, Song et al. [2006], Jung [2008] and Lee and Chung [2009] claim that the quality of the information is the single most important attribute for users of health information. As such,

information quality can have a significant positive effect on the behavioral intention of consumers towards mHealth services. Thus, the study hypothesizes that:

H5: Information quality significantly affects individual intention to use mHealth services.

3.6. Trust

As mentioned above, perceived credibility plays an important role in creating trust and some researchers like Watzdorf et al. [2010] further claim that past experiences with a technology can have the biggest impact on trust. Prior empirical studies like Jung [2008], Mohamed et al. [2011] and El-Wajeeh et al. [2014] particularly employed the construct of trust in the context of internet-based health services and found that trust has a direct significant influence on behavioural intention to use any health related technology like mHealth services. Thus, the following hypothesis has been conceived:

H6: Trust significantly affects individual intention to use mHealth services.

3.7. Behavioral Intention

Behavioral intention, which refers to the intention to use a system, is the major determinant of the actual behaviour. Researchers like Davis et al. [1989], Venkatesh et al. [2003], Venkatesh and Zhang [2010] and Yu [2012] repeatedly emphasized the strength of the construct of behavioral intention on usage behaviour. These past studies claim that individual behavior is predictable and can be influenced by individual intention that, in turn, can have a significant influence on technology usage. Moreover, Venkatesh and Davis [2000] found significant positive correlation of behavioral intention and actual use. In the context of mHealth services, Jung [2008] and Sun et al. [2013] investigated and empirically proved that behavioral intention of the technology positively affects its usage. Following the lead, this study hypothesizes that:

H7: Behavioral intention significantly affects individual behavior of using mHealth services.

4. RESEARCH METHOD

4.1. Data Collection

The predominant existence of mobile health services in the rural areas has inadvertently deprived urban people of the use of such services. In addition, the absence of city hospitals as the provider of mHealth services has made it imperative to examine the acceptance and use of mHealth services among the urban areas of Bangladesh. As such, the population selected for this study only represented urban people who are currently exposed to the use of mobile phones and can thereby avail mobile health services in the future.

Data for this study has been collected by conducting a survey through paper-based questionnaires on a sample of 1000 respondents. By using probability sampling and a stratified random sampling method, respondents were then selected for the sample. The use of this particular sampling method helped in avoiding biasness in data and provided equal opportunity for all urban people who can be the potential users of mobile health services in Bangladesh.

Three research assistants were trained and dispatched to collect data from the respondents, following the suggestion of past studies like Yang [2004] and Yu [2011]. Each research assistant carried two versions of the questionnaire. One set was developed by the researchers in English and the other set was translated by the research assistants into Bengali – the primary language used by the local residents of Bangladesh. Since all the researchers were bilingual and familiar with business terminologies, they back-translated the Bengali version in order to confirm translation equivalence of the questionnaire.

Respondents were mostly educated and had English proficiency and so they were asked to self-administer the English version of the questionnaire. In other cases, the participants self-administered the Bengali version of the questionnaire or the research assistants themselves filled in the questionnaire based on the respondents' verbal responses.

4.2. Measurement

All the items used to measure the research variables of the survey has been adapted from previous studies on information and technological advancements, eHealth services and mHealth services - with minor changes in wording to tailor them to the context of Bangladesh. This ensured the content validity of the questionnaire used to assess each constructs depicted in the model. The quantitative survey contained 24 statements in order to evaluate the four constructs of the UTAUT model and the two new constructs proposed for the model, as listed in Table 1. The scales for the UTAUT constructs (performance expectancy, effort expectancy, social influence, facilitating conditions and behavioral intention) were adapted from Venkatesh et al. [2003], Luarn and Lin [2005], Jung [2008], Venkatesh and Zhang [2010], Yu [2012] and Sun et al. [2013]. The scales for information quality were drawn from Nelson et al. [2005], Jung [2008] and Lee and Chung [2009]. On the other hand, the items used to assess trust were based on Jung [2008], Mohamed et al. [2011] and El-Wajeeh et al. [2014]. All these items were measured using a five-point Likert scale, ranging from "strongly disagree" to "strongly agree". The questionnaire included two demographic questions of gender and age as well.

After a four-week survey, 927 completed and usable responses were obtained from the structured questionnaires. Table 2 represents the demographic information of respondents in terms of gender and age.

Table 1. Constructs and corresponding items

Constructs	Corresponding Items	Items Sources
Performance Expectancy	[PE1] Using mHealth services will improve my life quality [PE2] Using mHealth services will make my life more convenient [PE3] Using mHealth services will make me more effective in my life [PE4] Overall, I find mHealth services to be useful in my life	Sun et al. [2013]
Effort Expectancy	[EE1] Learning to use mHealth services is easy for me [EE2] Becoming skillful at using mHealth services is easy for me [EE3] Interaction with mHealth services is easy for me [EE4] Overall, I think mHealth services are easy to use	Sun et al. [2013]
Social Influence	[SI1] People who are important to me think that I should use mHealth services [SI2] People who are familiar with me think that I should use mHealth services [SI3] People who influence me think that I should use mHealth services [SI4] Most people surrounding me use mHealth services	Venkatesh et al. [2003], Jung [2008], Sun et al. [2013],
Facilitating Conditions	[FC1] Using mHealth services suits my living environment [FC2] Using mHealth services fits into my working style [FC3] Using mHealth services is compatible with my life [FC4] Help is available if I have problems in using mHealth services	Venkatesh et al. [2003], Venkatesh & Zhang [2010]
Information Quality	[IQ1] I believe mHealth services provide complete information [IQ2] I believe mHealth services provide up-to-date information [IQ3] I believe mHealth services provide relevant information	Jung [2008], Lee & Chung [2009]
Trust	[T1] I believe mHealth services to be trustworthy [T2] I believe mHealth services to be credible	Jung [2008]
Behavioral Intention	[BI1] I prefer to use mHealth services [BI2] I intend to use mHealth services [BI3] I plan to use mHealth services	Sun et al. [2013]

5. DATA ANALYSIS AND RESULTS

The research model was tested using the structural equation modeling (SEM) facilitates of SmartPLS (version 2.0). The method of partial least squares (PLS) was mainly chosen to conduct this analysis since a number of interaction terms have been included in the research model and PLS is capable of testing these effects [Chin et al., 2003]. As such, the measurement model was examined first to assess the reliability and validity of the constructs and then, the structural model was analyzed to examine the relationships hypothesized in the research model.

5.1. Measurement Model

Results from the measurement model are presented in Table 3 and Table 4 and it includes information about the reliability, validity, correlations and factor loadings. The composite reliabilities of the constructs ranged between 0.815 and 0.895, which exceeds the 0.7 cut-off value as recommended by Nunnally and Bernstein [1994]. The average variance extracted (AVE) was greater than 0.5 in all cases and greater than each square

Table 2. Demographic profile of respondents

Demographics	Frequency	Percentage (%)
Gender		
Male	546	58.9
Female	381	41.1
Age		
20 or below	158	17.0
21 – 30	476	51.3
31 – 40	145	15.6
41 – 50	94	10.1
Above 50	54	5.8

correlations, which indicates that the model has both convergent validity and discriminant validity [Fornell and Larcker, 1981]. Moreover, the internal consistency reliabilities (ICRs) of multi-item scales modeled with reflective indicators was 0.75 or greater, suggesting adequate reliability. The pattern of loadings and cross-loadings also supported internal consistency and discriminant validity, with some exceptions: one item from each construct of social influence, facilitating conditions and information quality were deleted due to their low loadings and high cross-loadings.

5.2. Structural Model

The path coefficients and significance levels in the structural model are presented in Figure 2. The factors of information quality (0.247, p<0.05), facilitating conditions (0.235, p<0.05), trust (0.199, p<0.05) and effort expectancy (0.169, p<0.05) displayed a significant and positive path towards the behavioral intention of using mobile health services, in their order of influencing strength. However, the construct of performance expectancy (0.155, p>0.05) and social influence (0.134, p>0.05) reported an insignificant path towards the individual behavior of using mobile health services.

Therefore, all hypotheses (except H1 and H3) dealing with behavioral intention to use mobile health services are supported. Subsequently, the hypothesized relationship between behavioral intention and usage (0.251, p<0.05) is found to be statistically significant, thereby supporting hypothesis H7.

5.3. Findings and Implications

This study has revealed quite a few understandings on the back stage possibilities of the potential usage of mobile health services among the urban population of Bangladesh. Constructs such as information quality, facilitating conditions, trust and effort expectancy has been found to have a

Table 3. Factor loadings, composite reliability and AVEs

Constructs	Items	Factor Loadings	Composite Reliability	AVE
Performance Expectancy	PE1	0.807	0.889	0.668
	PE2	0.847		
	PE3	0.850		
	PE4	0.761		
Effort Expectancy	EE1	0.822	0.895	0.680
	EE2	0.834		
	EE3	0.840		
	EE4	0.802		
Social Influence	SI1	0.867	0.891	0.732
	SI2	0.876		
	SI3	0.823		
Facilitating Conditions	FC1	0.776	0.864	0.680
	FC2	0.877		
	FC3	0.818		
Information Quality	IQ1	0.908	0.887	0.797
	IQ2	0.876		
Trust	T1	0.915	0.815	0.691
	T2	0.737		
Behavioral Intention	BI1	0.868	0.891	0.731
	BI2	0.873		
	BI3	0.823		

Table 4. Measurement model estimations

	ICRs	BI	EE	FC	IQ	PE	SI	T
BI	0.8	**0.9**						
EE	0.8	0.5	**0.8**					
FC	0.8	0.5	0.4	**0.8**				
IQ	0.8	0.5	0.4	0.8	**0.9**			
PE	0.8	0.4	0.6	0.4	0.4	**0.8**		
SI	0.8	0.4	0.4	0.3	0.3	0.3	**0.9**	
T	0.8	0.3	0.3	0.3	0.3	0.2	0.8	**0.8**

Notes:

1. BI (Behavioral Intention); EE (Effort Expectancy); FC (Facilitating Conditions); IQ (Information Quality); PE (Performance Expectancy); SI (Social Influence); T (Trust).

2. Diagonal elements represent the AVEs, while off-diagonal elements represent the square correlations.

Figure 2. Results of structural equation modeling

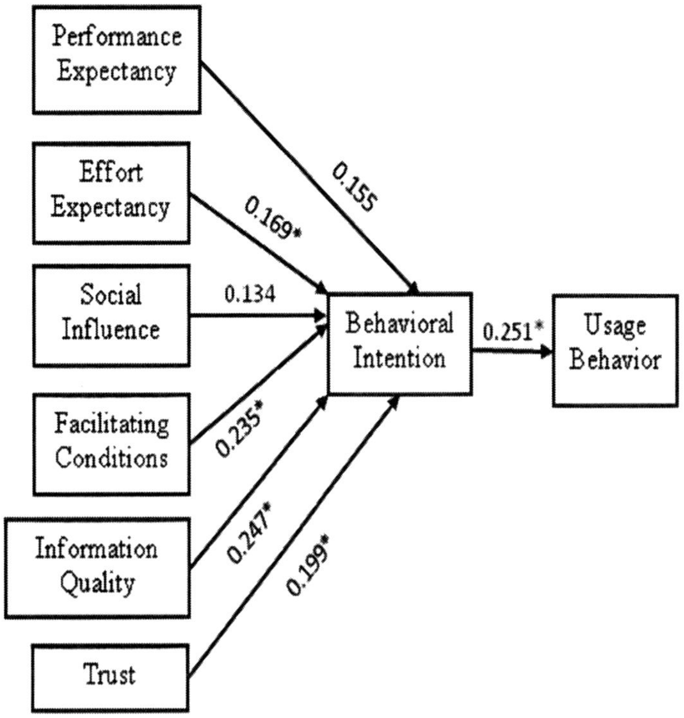

salient influence on behavioral intention, which directly stimulates the usage of mHealth services. On the other hand, performance expectancy and social influence has been identified as insignificant factors of behavioral intention in the context of Bangladesh. The inclined reasons behind such findings are quite obvious and most of such are shaped by the local culture and infrastructure of the country.

Information quality is found to be the strongest direct determinant in influencing respondents' behavioral intention of mHealth services. Sustainable relative advantages of mHealth service, particularly receiving immediate and accurate healthcare advices, play an important role in shaping behavior in terms of adopting such new technologies. Jimison and Sher [2008], Holden and Karsh [2010] and Sun et al. [2013] also reported similar results in their studies. The underlying cause behind such result is the novelty of such technology in the culture of Bangladesh, where most of the information regarding a service is distributed in a traditional manner from physical locations. So, when the information is disseminated over a mobile platform, the quality for sure matters to a large extent. Take away for healthcare service providers from this finding is to ensure the provision of accurate information through the call center personnel to the users. They must also keep in mind that one negative case in terms of accurate response may lead to decreasing brand equity and hence, hospitals and clinics should train the front liners accordingly. Developing a sustainable system which ensures complete and accurate dissemination of healthcare information can thus encourage the consumption of such services among the urban people of Bangladesh.

Facilitating conditions is the second most important construct according to the research findings of this study. This finding is consistent to Boontarig et al. [2012], Phichitchaisopa and Naenna [2013] and Sun et al. [2013]. The penetration of mobile phones is a comparatively new concept in Bangladesh and particularly, when such devices are being used as a platform of commuting other errands such as receiving instant healthcare advices, ensuring facilitating conditions has a prime role to play. Strong and correct comprehension on available facilitating conditions is important to build the right perception in the mind of the target market by showing repeatedly that all they need is a mobile phone of any type and a mobile connection mainly to take the benefits of mobile healthcare services. Both the government and private sector hospitals and clinics of Bangladesh are already displaying a lot of interests and concerns in this regard, as they have set their foot targeting the rural segments and working on developing the infrastructure challenges. However, city hospitals need to work more towards the development of such conditions for the city dwellers of Bangladesh.

Trust is another important construct that can influence behavioral intention of mHealth services as per the findings of this study and this is similar to Jung [2008], Mohamed et al. [2011] and El-Wajeeh et al. [2014]. A crucial link to trust is the perceived credibility of such services, which is why potential users are more likely to trust the service if they are convinced with the credibility of the services and of the providers. This matches with the findings of Korp [2006], Jung [2008], Wang et al. [2003], Luarn and Lin [2005], Koenig-Lewis et al. [2010], Dasgupta et al. [2011] and Yu [2012]. Marketers can use this insight and focus on developing positive experiences among the early adopters. Once the early adopters are convinced and trust is built and spread in the market, early majority and late majority will be netted accordingly. To build credibility and trust, successful cases may be communicated in the form of testimonials to reach both the external and internal information search sources. Experts and celebrity endorsements with assurance in different communications may also be used. NGOs, who already have built a trust

through their sustainable credibility, may play an important role to communicate the assurance of such services to the urban markets as well.

The study further drills that most of the current and potential users of mHealth services tend to judge the importance of the service based on the required effort expectancy for it. Respondents who expect less effort input in the service consuming process, especially at the adoption stage like that of mHealth services in Bangladesh, are more likely to show positive attitude in embracing the service. This finding is consistent with the evidence provided by Davis et al. [1989], Szajna [1996], Park et al. [2007], Wu et al. [2007], Wills et al. [2008], Moores [2012] and Sun et al. [2013]. By making sure that the target market perceives the efforts needed to avail these services as an ease, healthcare service providers can net a positive attitude towards these services. Communications of the providers, particularly of the city hospitals, should focus more on the actual handiness of such services.

Insights from this study can assist various public and private hospitals of the urban areas of Bangladesh in designing the service that can be offered through the mHealth technology. For instance, city hospitals must ensure that patients do not have a long waiting line before they are connected to the mHealth technology and once they are connected, the focus of the hospitals must be more on the accurate dissemination of healthcare advice. Since the quality of healthcare information matters a lot for the people, such immediate service can help them relate to the mHealth technology more easily. Also, city hospitals must design a simple and user-friendly interface for providing mHealth technologies so that anybody can avail it and use it with ease. This can include the use of mobile applications on Smartphone or easily accessible call centers that will readily connect people to the mHealth technology. Once this is done, the factors of facilitating conditions, trust and effort expectancy – all will be taken into account and various hospitals of the urban areas will be in a position to provide suitable mHealth services to the urban people of Bangladesh.

5.4. Limitations and Future Research Directions

Despite the theoretical and practical implications of the study, the findings of this research should be interpreted in the light of the limitations. First, the conclusions drawn from this study are based solely on the urban population of Bangladesh. A similar research can be done to examine the antecedents and consequences of the acceptance and use of mHealth services for other developing countries across the world. Second, a longitudinal study can be adopted in future works to examine and compare the research model in different time periods, thereby providing a better insight into the adoption of mHealth services in Bangladesh. Finally, other than the constructs used in this study, there can be various other factors that can influence the acceptance and use of mHealth services. Further research considering different constructs can enhance the understanding of precise determinants for mHealth services in Bangladesh.

REFERENCES

Ahmed, S. M., Evans, T., Standing, H. and Mahmud, S. (2013), "Harnessing pluralism for better health in Bangladesh", *The Lancet*, viewed 21 November 2014, <>10.1016/ S0140-6736(13)62147-9

Ajzen, I., & Fishbein, M. (1980). *Understanding Attitudes and Predicting Social Behavior*. Englewood Cliffs, NJ: Prentice-Hall.

Akter, S., D'Ambra, J., & Ray, P. (2010), *18th European Conference on Information Systems: conference proceedings*, University of Pretoria, pp.1-12, viewed 04 August 2014, < http://ro.uow.edu.au/cgi/viewcontent.cgi?article=4188&context=commpapers>

Boontarig, W., Chutimaskul, W., Chongsuphajaisiddhi, W., & Papasratorn, B. (2012), "Factors influencing the Thai elderly intention to use smartphone for e-Health services", *IEEE Symposium on Humanities, Science and Engineering Research*, pp.242-246. doi:10.1109/ SHUSER.2012.6268881

Chae, M., & Kim, J. (2001), *Information quality for mobile internet services: A theoretical model with empirical validation*, Twenty second international conference on information systems. doi:10.1080/101967802753433254

Chae, M., Kim, J., Kim, H., & Ryu, H. (2002). Information quality for mobile Internet services: A theoretical model with empirical validation. *Special Selection: M-Commerce, 12*(1), 38–46.

Chin, W. W., Marcolin, B. L., & Newsted, P. R. (2003). A partial least squares latent variable modeling approach for measuring interaction effects: Results from a Monte Carlo Simulation study and an Electronic-Mail Emotion/Adoption study. *Information Systems Research, 14*(2), 189–217. doi:10.1287/isre.14.2.189.16018

Dagger, T. S., Sweeney, J. C., & Johnson, L. W. (2007). A hierarchical model of health service quality: Scale development and investigation of an integrated model. *Journal of Service Research, 10*(2), 123–142. doi:10.1177/1094670507309594

Dasgupta, S., Paul, R., & Fuloria, S. (2011). Factors affecting behavioural intentions towards mobile banking usage: Empirical evidence from India. *Romanian Journal of Marketing, 3*(1), 6–28.

Davis, F. D. (1989). Perceived usefulness, perceived ease of use, and user acceptance of information technology. *Management Information Systems Quarterly, 13*(3), 319–340. doi:10.2307/249008

Davis, F. D., Bagozzi, R. P., & Warshaw, P. R. (1989). User acceptance of computer technology: A comparison of two theoretical models. *Management Science, 35*(8), 982–1003. doi:10.1287/ mnsc.35.8.982

DeLone, W. H., & McLean, E. R. (2003). Information systems success: The quest for the dependent variable. *Information Systems Research, 3*(1), 60–95. doi:10.1287/isre.3.1.60

Directorate General of Health Services (DGHS). (2014), *Health information system & e-Health,* viewed 23 August 2014, <http://www.dghs.gov.bd/index.php/en/ehealth/our-ehealth-eservices/84-english root/ehealth-eservice/97-telimedicine-services-in-comunity-clinics>

El-Wajeeh, M., Galal-Edeen, G., & Mokhtar, H. (2014). Technology acceptance model for mobile health systems. *IOSR Journal of Mobile Computing and Acceptance, 1*(1), 21–33.

Fishbein, M., & Ajzen, I. (1975). *Belief, Attitude, Intention and Behavior: An Introduction to Theory and Research.* Reading, MA: Addison-Wesley.

Fornell, C., & Larcker, D. F. (1981). Evaluating structural equation models with unobservable variables and measurement error. *JMR, Journal of Marketing Research, 18*(1), 39–50. doi:10.2307/3151312

Ganesh, J. (2004). E-health-drivers, applications, challenges ahead, and strategies: A conceptual framework. *Indian Journal of Medical Informatics, 1,* 39–47.

Gefen, D., & Straub, D. W. (1997). Gender differences in the perception and use of e-mail: An extension to the technology acceptance model. *Management Information Systems Quarterly, 21*(4), 389–400. doi:10.2307/249720

Harvard School of Public Health. (2012), *Mobilizing a revolution: How cell phones are transforming public health,* viewed 18 November 2014, <http://www.hsph.harvard.edu/news/magazine/mobilizing-a-revolution/>

Holden, R. J., & Karsh, B. T. (2010). The technology acceptance model: Its past and its future in health care. *Journal of Biomedical Informatics, 43*(1), 159–172. doi:10.1016/j.jbi.2009.07.002 PMID:19615467

Ivatury, G., Moore, J., & Bloch, A. (2009). "A doctor in your pocket: Health hotlines in developing countries", *Innovations: Technology, Governance & Globalization* [online]. *MIT Press Journal, 4*(1), 119–153.

Jiang, J. J., Klein, G., Roan, J., & Lin, T. M. (2001). IS service performance: Self-perceptions and user perceptions. *Information & Management, 38*(8), 499–506. doi:10.1016/S0378-7206(01)00072-6

Jimison, H. B., & Sher, P. P. (2008). Consumer health informatics: Health information technology for consumers. *Journal of the American Society for Information Science, 46*(10), 783–790. doi:10.1002/(SICI)1097-4571(199512)46:10<783::AID-ASI11>3.0.CO;2-L

Jung, M. (2008), From health to e-Health: Understanding citizens' acceptance of online health care, doctoral thesis, Luleå University of Technology, Sweden, viewed 08 August 2014, <http://epubl.ltu.se/1402-1544/2008/68/LTU-DT-0868-SE.pdf>

Kaplan, B., & Litewka, S. (2008). Ethical challenges of telemedicine and tele-health. *Cambridge Quarterly of Healthcare Ethics, 17*(04), 401–416. doi:10.1017/S0963180108080535 PMID:18724880

Klein, R. (2007). Internet-based patient-physician electronic communication applications: Patient acceptance and trust. *e-Service Journal, 5*(2), 27–51. doi:10.2979/ESJ.2007.5.2.27

Koehlmoos, T. P., Islam, Z., Anwar, S., Hossain, S. A. S., Gazi, R., Streatfield, P. K., & Bhuiya, A. U. (2011), "Health Transcends Poverty: The Bangladesh Experience", in D. Balabanova, M. McKee and A. Mills, (eds.) 'Good Health at Low Cost' 25 Years on: What Makes an Effective Health System, London: London School of Hygiene and Tropical Medicine: 47.

Koenig-Lewis, N., Palmer, A., & Moll, A. (2010). Predicting young consumers' take up of mobile banking services. *International Journal of Bank Marketing*, *28*(5), 410–432. doi:10.1108/02652321011064917

Kohnke, A., Cole, M. L., & Bush, R. (2014). Incorporating UTAUT predictors for understanding home care patients' and clinician's acceptance of healthcare telemedicine equipment. *Journal of Technology Management and Innovation*, *9*(2), 29–42. doi:10.4067/S0718-27242014000200003

Korp, P. (2006). Health on the Internet: Implications for health promotion. *Health Education Research*, *21*(1), 78–86. doi:10.1093/her/cyh043 PMID:15994845

Lallmahamood, M. (2007). An examination of individual's perceived security and privacy of the Internet in Malaysia and the influence of this on their intention to use e-Commerce: Using an extension of the Technology Acceptance Model. *Journal of Internet Banking and Commerce*, *12*(3), 1–26.

Lanseng, E. J., & Andreassen, T. W. (2007). Electronic healthcare: A study of people's readiness and attitude toward performing self-diagnosis. *International Journal of Service Industry Management*, *18*(4), 394–417. doi:10.1108/09564230710778155

Lau, M. M., Cheung, R., Lam, A. Y. C., & Chu, Y. T. (2013). Measuring service quality in the banking industry: A Hong Kong based study. *Contemporary Management Research*, *9*(3), 263–282. doi:10.7903/cmr.11060

Lee, K. C., & Chung, N. (2009). Understanding factors affecting trust in and satisfaction with mobile banking in Korea: A modified DeLone and McLean's model perspective. *Interacting with Computers*, *21*(5), 385–392. doi:10.1016/j.intcom.2009.06.004

Lin, H. (2011). An empirical investigation of mobile banking adoption: The effect of innovation attributes and knowledge-based trust. *International Journal of Information Management*, *31*(3), 252–260. doi:10.1016/j.ijinfomgt.2010.07.006

Lin, H. (2011). The effect of multi-channel service quality on mobile customer loyalty in an online-and-mobile retail context. *Service Industries Journal*, *32*(11), 1865–1882. doi:10.1080/0264 2069.2011.559541

Lin, J. C. C., & Lu, H. (2000). Towards an understanding of the behavioral intention to use a web site. *International Journal of Information Management*, *20*(3), 197–208. doi:10.1016/S0268-4012(00)00005-0

Luarn, P., & Lin, H. H. (2005). Toward an understanding of the behavioral intention to use mobile banking. *Computers in Human Behavior*, *21*(6), 873–891. doi:10.1016/j.chb.2004.03.003

Masrek, M. N., Uzir, N. A. and Khairuddin, I. I. (2012), "Trust in mobile banking adoption in Malaysia: A conceptual framework", *Journal of Mobile Technologies, Knowledge & Society*, Vol.2012, No.2012, pp.1-12.

Mohamed, A. H. H. M., Tawfik, H., Al-Jumeily, D., & Norton, L. (2011), "MoHTAM: A technology acceptance model for mobile health applications", Developments in E-systems Engineering (DeSE), pp.13-18.

Moores, T. T. (2012). Towards an integrated model of IT acceptance in healthcare. *Decision Support Systems*, *53*(3), 507–516. doi:10.1016/j.dss.2012.04.014

Nelson, R. R., Todd, P. A., & Wixom, B. H. (2005). Antecedents of information and system quality: An empirical examination within the context of data warehousing. *Journal of Management Information Systems*, *21*(4), 199–235.

Nunnally, J. C., & Bernstein, I. H. (1994). *Psychometric Theory*. New York: McGraw-Hill.

Park, J. K., Yang, S. J., & Lehto, X. (2007). Adoption of mobile technologies for Chinese consumers. *Journal of Electronic Commerce Research*, *8*(3), 196–206.

Pavlou, P. A. (2003). Consumer acceptance of electronic commerce: Integrating trust and risk with the technology acceptance model. *International Journal of Electronic Commerce*, *7*(3), 101–134.

Phichitchaisopa, N., & Naenna, T. (2013). Factors affecting the adoption of healthcare information technology. *EXCLI Journal*, *12*, 413–436.

Powell, J. A., Darvell, M., & Gray, J. A. M. (2003). The doctor, the patient and the world-wide-web: How the Internet is changing healthcare. *Journal of the Royal Society of Medicine*, *96*(2), 74–76. doi:10.1258/jrsm.96.2.74 PMID:12562977

Rashidee, A. H. (2013), "Emerging mobile health in Bangladesh", *The Daily Star*, 30 June, viewed 12 July 2014, <http://archive.thedailystar.net/beta2/news/emerging-mobile-Health-in-bangladesh/>

Reza, P. R. (2012), "Bangladesh: Mobile health service for expecting and new mothers", *Global Voice*, 26 December, viewed 12 August 2014, <http://globalvoicesonline.org/2012/12/26/bangladesh-mobile-Health-service-for-expecting-and-new-mothers/>

Rousseau, D. M., Sitkin, S. B., Burt, R. S., & Camerer, C. (1998). Not so different after all: A cross-discipline view of trust. *Academy of Management Review*, *23*(3), 393–404. doi:10.5465/AMR.1998.926617

Song, J., & Zahedi, F. (2006). Trust in health infomediaries. *Decision Support Systems*, *3*, 390–407.

Stofega, W., & Llamas, R. T. (2009). *Worldwide Mobile Phone 2009-2013 Forecast Update, IDC Document Number 217209*. Framingham, MA: IDC.

Sultana, S. (2014), "Taking care of health through mobile phones", *The Financial Express*, 15 February, viewed 12 August 2014, <http://www.thefinancialexpress-bd.com/2014/02/15/18873>

Sun, Y., Wang, N., Guo, X., & Peng, Z. (2013). Understanding the acceptance of mobile health services: A comparison and integration of alternative models. *Journal of Electronic Commerce Research*, *14*(2), 183–200.

Szajna, B. (1996). Empirical evaluation of the revised technology acceptance model. *Management Science*, *42*(1), 85–92. doi:10.1287/mnsc.42.1.85

United Nations Foundation. (2009), *mHealth for Development: The opportunity of mobile technology for healthcare in developing world*, viewed 13 November 2014, <http://www.vitalwaveconsulting.com/insights/mHealth.htm>

Varshney, U. (2005). Pervasive healthcare: Applications, challenges and wireless solutions. *Communications of the Association for Information Systems*, *16*(3), 57–72.

Venkatesh, V. (1999). Creating favourable user perceptions: Exploring the role of intrinsic motivation. *Management Information Systems Quarterly*, *23*(2), 239–260. doi:10.2307/249753

Venkatesh, V., & Davis, F. D. (2000). A theoretical extension of the technology acceptance model: Four longitudinal field studies. *Management Science*, *46*(2), 186–204. doi:10.1287/mnsc.46.2.186.11926

Venkatesh, V., Morris, M. G., Davis, G. B., & Davis, F. D. (2003). User acceptance of information technology: Toward a unified view. *Management Information Systems Quarterly*, *27*(3), 425–478.

Venkatesh, V., Thong, J. Y. L., & Xin, X. (2012). Consumer acceptance and use of information technology: Extending the Unified Theory of Acceptance and Use of Technology. *Management Information Systems Quarterly*, *36*(1), 157–178.

Venkatesh, V., & Zhang, X. (2010). Unified theory of acceptance and use of technology: U.S. vs. China. *Journal of Global Information Technology Management*, *13*(1), 5–27. doi:10.1080/1097198X.2010.10856507

Wand, Y., & Wang, R. Y. (1996). Anchoring data quality in ontological dimensions. *Communications of the ACM*, *39*(11), 86–96. doi:10.1145/240455.240479

Wang, Y. S., Wang, Y. M., Lin, H. H., & Tang, T. I. (2003). Determinants of user acceptance of Internet banking: An empirical study. *International Journal of Service Industry Management*, *14*(5), 501–519. doi:10.1108/09564230310500192

Watzdorf, S. V., Ippisch, T., Skorna, A., & Thiesse, F. (2010), *Ninth International Conference on Mobile Business 2010: conference proceedings*, Ninth Global Mobility Roundtable (ICMB-GMR), pp.329-336, viewed 29 July 2014.

WHO. (2011). *M-Health: New Horizons for Health through Mobile Technologies, Global Observatory for eHealth Series* (Vol. 3). Geneva: World Health Organization.

Wills, M. J., El-Gayar, O. F., & Bennett, D. (2008). Examining healthcare professionals' acceptance of electronic medical records using UTAUT. *Issues in Information Systems*, *9*(2), 396–401.

Wu, J., Wang, S., & Lin, L. (2007). Mobile computing acceptance factors in the healthcare industry: A structural equation model. *International Journal of Medical Informatics*, *76*(1), 66–77. doi:10.1016/j.ijmedinf.2006.06.006 PMID:16901749

Yang, K. C. C. (2004). A comparison of attitudes towards Internet advertising among lifestyle segments in Taiwan. *Journal of Marketing Communications*, *10*(1), 195–212. doi:10.1080/1352726042000181657

Yu, C. (2012). Factors affecting individuals to adopt mobile banking: Empirical evidence from the UTAUT model. *Journal of Electronic Commerce Research*, *13*(2), 104–121.

Yu, C. S. (2011). Construction and validation of an e-lifestyle instrument. *Internet Research*, *21*(3), 214–235. doi:10.1108/10662241111139282

This work was previously published in the International Journal of Asian Business and Information Management (IJABIM), 6(1); edited by Patricia Ordóñez de Pablos, pages 1-17 copyright year 2015 by IGI Publishing (an imprint of IGI Global).

Chapter 79
The Internet of Things and Opportunities for Pervasive Safety Monitored Health Environments

Vaughan A. Michell
University of Reading, UK

ABSTRACT

This chapter discusses the opportunities for new ubiquitous computing technologies, with concentration on the Internet of Things (IoT), to improve patient safety and quality. The authors focus on elective or planned surgical interventions, although the technology is applicable to primary and trauma care. The chapter is divided into three main sections with section 1 covering medical error issues and mechanisms, section 2 introducing Internet of Things, and section 3 discussing how IoT capabilities may address and reduce medical errors. The authors explore the existing theory of errors expounded by Reason (Reason, 2000, 1998; Leape, 1994) to identify perception-, decision-, and knowledge-based medical errors and related processes, environments, and cultural drivers causing error. The authors then introduce the technology of the Internet of Things and identify a range of capabilities from sensing, tracking, control, cooperative, and semantic reasoning. They then show how these new capabilities might be applied to reduce the errors expounded by the discussed error theories. They identify that: IoT enables augmentation of objects, which provides a massive increase in information transfer, thus improving clinician perception and support for decision-making and problem solving; IoT provides a host of additional observers and opportunities, which can shift the focus of overworked clinicians from constant monitoring to undertaking complex actions, such as decision making and care; IoT networks of sensors and actuators, through the addition of semantic and contextual rules, support decision making and facilitate automated monitoring and control of pervasive safety-monitored health environments, thus reducing clinician workload.

DOI: 10.4018/978-1-4666-8756-1.ch079

1. INTRODUCTION

1.1 Patient Safety

The safety of patients and the avoidance of iatrogenic or unintentional harm to patients has grown in importance as medical procedures and technology complexity accentuates traditional human factor failings (Nolan, 2000; Lin *et al*, 2001). These and other publications such as Hoff et al (Hoff et al, 2004) have highlighted the risk of unintended impacts of mistakes and medical errors. Whilst most studies have focused on the cause of error and human factors (Caryon et al, 2010; Patterson *et al*, 2002; Benning et al, 2011; Holden, 2009), less work has been undertaken on technology to reduce error (Ball et al, 2003). One of the key problems in medical situations is that the human agent is often both the executor and monitor of actions. In many medical interventions we still rely on 'the human in the loop' and depend alone on the reliability of their perception, cognition and decision-making. The fallibility of an often-overworked brain, trying to make sense of complexity (Nolan, 2000), or the distracted social animal, lacking in independent and reliable action information and facts, is often the cause of many of the errors. Whilst information systems, decision support systems, robots and medical information have reduced the errors in mundane tasks (Ball et al, 2003), their sensors and ability to offer corroborating or alternative facts has been limited to points and focused solutions until now. With the introduction of the Internet of Things, the promise of small, cheap and ubiquitous sensors allied to actuators and smart logic offers opportunities to provide appropriate facts, and historical information, to support independent decision making and care-control at the point of need. This capability, as an augmentation of the human agent, has the potential to improve patient safety despite the increased cost and scarcity of clinical skills that health institutions are now facing.

1.2 Medical Processes, Activities and Actions

This section defines basic terms for medical processes, activities and actions that are used widely throughout the chapter. Humans can be defined as actors in an environment. A medical actor has a set of formal goals and actions to achieve as part of their clinical work activities. Any medical process can therefore be depicted as being a sequence of work activities to achieve a goal with each work activity involving a number of actions or movements by one or more actors to support the activity (e.g. selecting an anaesthetic, or injecting a patient as part of the anaesthetic process). Actors may be human (e.g. a scrub nurse) or intelligent machines. A process (and constituent activities and actions) involves the transformation of a set of resources to achieve a goal (see Figure 1).

Figure 1. State change actions on resources

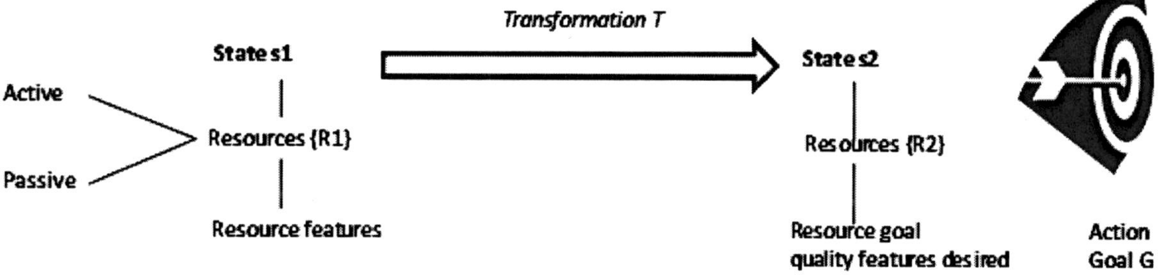

We differentiate between active resources that can transform the environment (which is a resource that drives the transformation) and passive resources (which are themselves transformed) (Michell, 2011). Resources, apart from human agents, can be categorised into: machines that are non-consumable (e.g. tools that leverage human resources, machines that can act independently (e.g. a pump), and general equipment and consumable resources (e.g. drugs, swabs etc.) that are converted as a part of the action. Each activity involves the interaction of specific resources in a specific pattern to transform those resources from a starting state s1 to a new state s2. State s2 has a set of quality measures on the properties of the transformed resources. Outside the organised resources there is an environment comprising structured and unstructured objects (e.g. chairs, doors etc.), which may or may not interact in the process.

Jalote-Parmar et al. (Jalote-Parmar et al, 2008) identified medical intervention processes as an integration of four workflows that are integrated to form a surgical intervention process. The anaesthetic sub process involves and anaesthetist

and an operating department practitioner working together; to both anaesthetise the patient and keep them alive. The surgical sub-process involves the active intervention activities of the surgeon and surgical assistant to execute a plan of action using and consuming resources to improve the patient's condition. The instrumentation subprocess relates to a scrub nurse preparing and managing tools/surgical instruments (e.g. endoscope, diathermy tools), ensuring these are provided and managed at the appropriate stage in the actions and activities. We adapt this approach and use three sub-processes as examples of resources in a medical process (see Figure 2).

At the lowest level of a process is an individual action, which is seen as an atomic constituent of work activities. It is at this level that resources interact, are consumed and transformed; for example, a syringe injecting an anaesthetic. The syringe is a used resource, the anaesthetic is consumed and its state transformed as it enters the blood stream. This also alters the state of the patient. An individual medical action level of intervention is often clinically prescribed and may include evidence-based research on the biology,

Figure 2. Example clinical processes and sub-processes

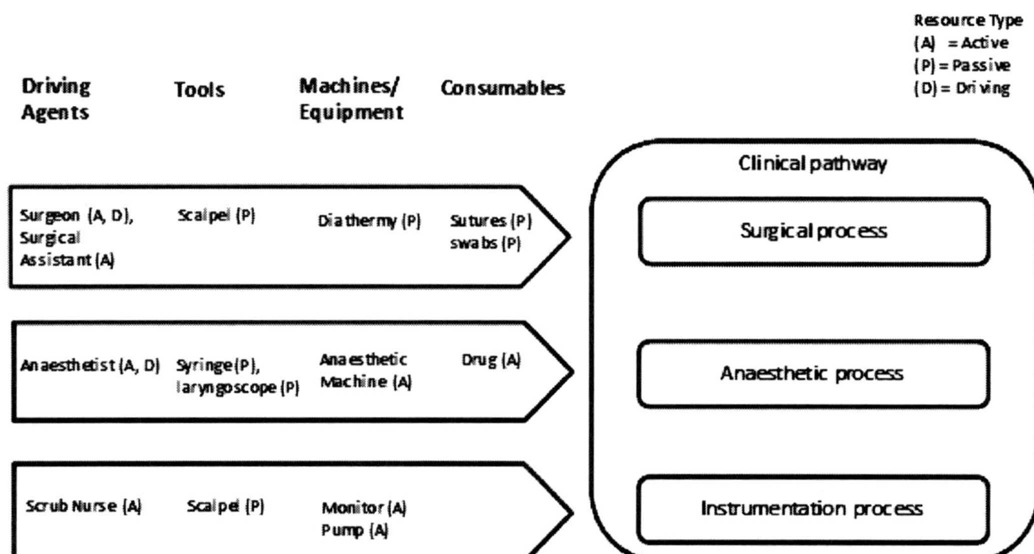

biomechanics, and physiology of the action on the patient. The lowest level focuses on how to execute the action to achieve a specific result, e.g. how to inject a patient.

At the activity level the focus is on how multiple resources should interact together. As in human-human, human- machine, etc. in a specific sequence of actions and states. For example, the interactions between the anaesthetist and the operating department practitioner in intubating a patient; thus the activity is a set of sequenced actions.

Finally at the process or workflow level of interaction, the focus is on the control and sequence and scheduling of resources; (Preece et al, 2008) agent roles (who/what executes what activity), and interactions at the high level (e.g. the setting up of a theatre-operating list).

At all levels the actions, the right resources and right sequence of actions must be known to the driving agents to ensure efficient and effective transformation of the resources to meet the medical goals. In addition the outcomes and end states must be checked at some point against goals to ensure control. In medical practice, unlike industry, this is achieved by part planning for elective and standard events, and part clinician cognitive adaptation to the changing situation (e.g. a deteriorating patient) (Figure 3).

An elective medical process can also be defined as a set of related states. Planning for action involves identifying goals and the correct planned procedures and processes to meet the goal. For example, a surgeon would complete his diagnosis and select the procedures, complete the patient consent process with patient/carer in the planning stage.

Then a resourcing stage involves identification and allocation of resources to each activity in the plan. Resources need to be i) eligible for the transformation, ii) available at the planned time, iii) in the required state, and iv) of the right quality for the transformation. This stage also includes any set up and preparation of equipment. This includes; assembly of devices, groups of tools, drug preparation, and machine set up to achieve specific mechanical and/or biochemical interactions for the intervention. Also any adverse reaction in the resources, e.g. drug interactions, need to be identified and resolved.

An example might be a scrub nurse identifying the procedure to be used from the theatre list. The

Figure 3. Process, activity and action composition

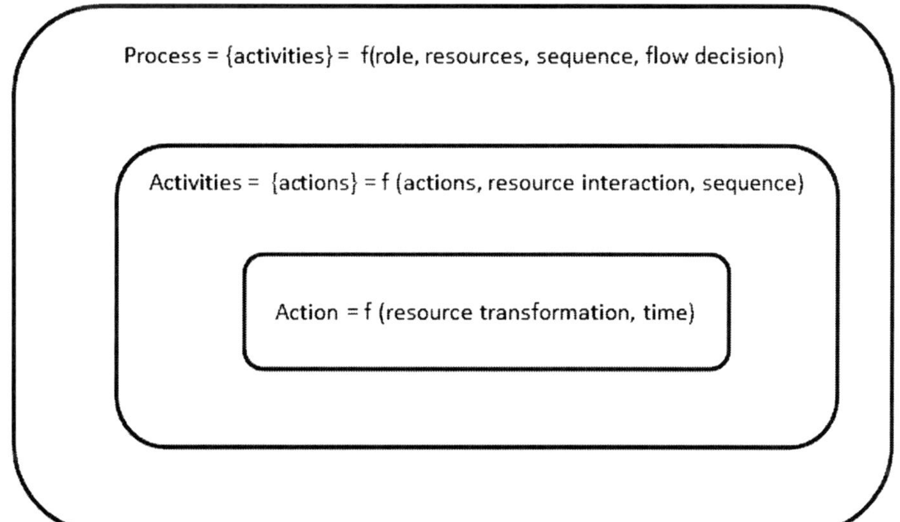

nurse gathers the complete set of instruments (i), ensures they are in the right state iii) (sterilised) and ready to use (ii/iv) and hands them to the surgeon at the right point in time. The action/interaction stage is the point of execution of the plan with the prepared resources. Critical at this point is ensuring the right resource action/interaction, and the correct sequence and timings required to meet the intervention goal. This requires the right resources in the right location and state. For example, a surgical assistant may perceive the surgeon's actions and pre-empt them by preparing a needle ready for the next task. Integral with the execution of each action/ activity is performance monitoring and control. This is where the resource transformation results are checked as they happen against the desire objectives and can be adjusted as needed.

Finally post action monitoring is needed to ensure progress towards the clinical goal or to identify further interventions. Here the checking of goals vs. actions can enable behaviours and their outcomes to be better understood and lessons and improvements in the stages identified. The key steps described are detailed in Figure 4.

1.3 Medical Error: The Individual Human Dimension

Reason defined an error as 'a failure of a planned action' (Reason, 1995). He distinguished between conscious deviations as 'violations', which we can identify as motivation errors and slips and mistakes where the intention was to follow a formal planned action. This chapter focuses on slips and mistakes and not violations, which is addressed in a separate chapter.

Reason distinguished between slips, i.e. failure to execute an action and failure to execute the 'correct' action or mistakes (Reason, 2000; Leape, 1994). He suggested slips were due to attention issues or intention failures. Based on Wiegmann & Shappell's work we can identify errors of perception and reading of cues (Shappel and Wiegmann, 2000) that are part of unconscious thought. Other mistakes relate mainly to the human mind's perception, judgement and decision points concerning actors application of rules and knowledge, which is part of conscious cognitive reasoning (Michell, 2013).

1.3.1 Perception Errors

Leape classified slips into: a) involving the use of a more familiar approach ('capture errors'), b) where the focus of the action is on the wrong object - i.e. description errors, c) the mental association is incorrect 'association activation errors', or d) simply forgetting due to distraction ('loss of activation errors'). These errors concern unconscious skills based behaviours where the actor is looking for cues that link to sensory- motor actions

Figure 4. The 5 phases of the planned medical intervention process

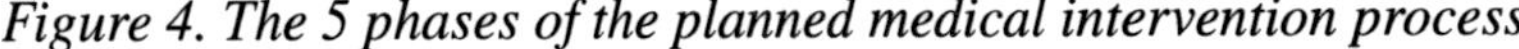

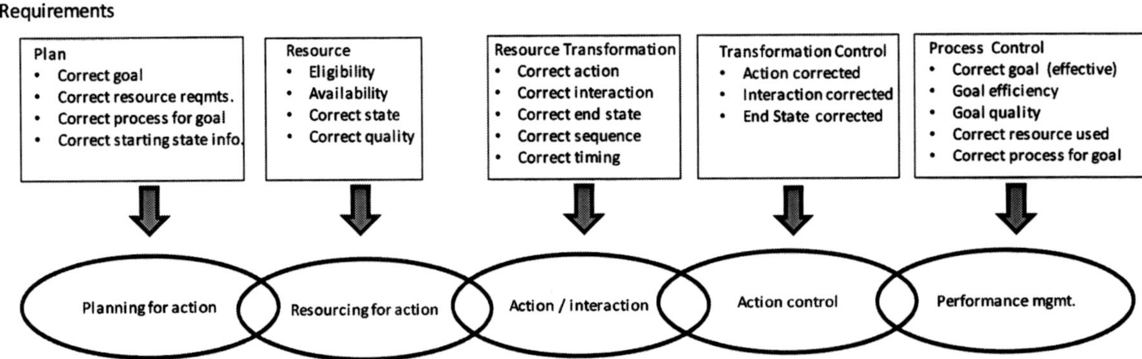

to meet a specific goal G, which is not achieved due to the error behaviours a)-d) (Michell, 2013) as illustrated in Figure 5.

Whilst formal clinical pathways, with documented tasks and protocols and specified goals, can reduce slips (Panella et al, 2003) by specification of actions and sequences, they still occur. An example of a), an incorrect plan/deviation is described in Panella et al.'s research, which concerns the significant variation in use (mainly) of a recommended 'total hip replacement' pathway (Panella et al, 2003). Forgetfulness, i.e. d), or wilful avoidance of documentation, such as clinical pathways, still occurs frequently enough to cause variations and safety issues in clinical processes. For example missing an obvious elbow injury (Smits et al, 2009; Panella et al, 2003). Even the most basic recording of the key patient vital signs of temperature, respiratory rate, blood pressure, oxygen saturation and mental state are often recorded on entry to a hospital, but several signs may be missed after a few hours in a hospital (Benning et al, 2011). Other common examples

of forgotten routine patient care actions include failure to give patients prescribed medicines and failure to maintain patient hydration levels (Benning et al, 2011).

1.3.2 Recording and Disseminating Errors

One aspect of medical processes, which differs from many industrial processes, is the lack of full control over the inputs. Medicine involves a response to human events, and often involves unpredictable and complex biochemistry. Successful medical intervention is dependent on the accurate recording and dissemination of perceptions and observations. These are typically in the form of medical notes and patient records. Although electronic patient records will improve access and readability, issues still arise. Donabedian noted the high incidence of errors in diagnostic reports and the need for completeness and checking/ observation of practice (Donabedian, 2005). He also raises the point that once a diagnosis has been

Figure 5. Perception errors

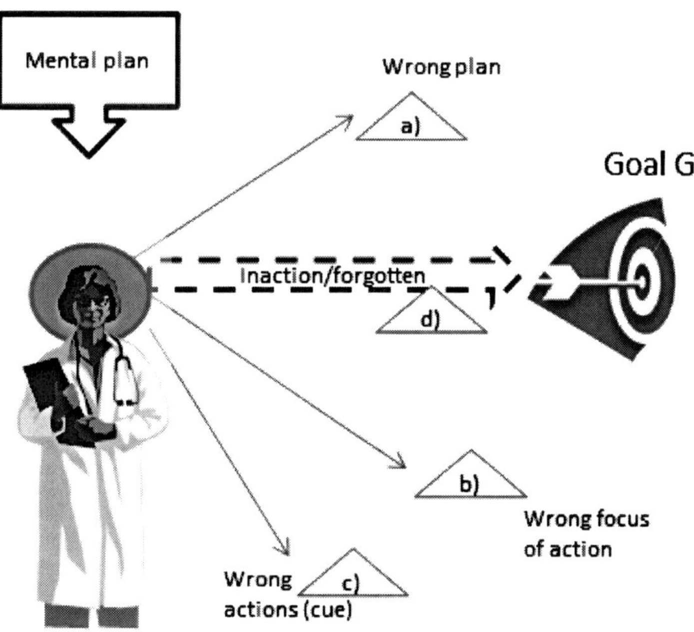

made, further perception and analysis to question the diagnosis is rarely made. The initial diagnosis is assumed to be correct and not correlated with later evidence and perceptions.

1.3.3 Rule Based Errors

A key human behaviour is the capturing, developing and application of rules. As Rasmussen suggests (Rasmussen, 1983) familiar work actions, such as clinical activities, are often driven by human stored rules or norms based on experience and training/education. Shappel et al (Shappel and Wiegmann, 2000) separate errors in decisions into rule based, knowledge based choice decisions and problem solving decisions'. Rule based errors (Leape, 1994) involve either e), i.e. applying the correct rule to the wrong context due to incorrect situation perception (e.g. mis-assigning a clinician with an inappropriate skill to a specific patient problem (Smits et al, 2009) or f), i.e. applying a rule that has been recorded incorrectly, to the right situation, for example calculating doses incorrectly (Smits et al, 2009). Rule error might be due to incorrect guidelines or perception and experience of taught and observed rules. Formal checking and specification of clinical guidelines, to detect rule based and related errors in clinical guideline and pathway documents, has been recommended to reduce obvious errors, however resourcing such checks is costly (Peleg and Tu, 2009).

1.3.4 Knowledge Based Errors

Knowledge based errors are errors in the mental plan of action. Knowledge based choice decisions can result in errors from cognitive processing decision failures related to the use of g) an incorrect mental model, or h) an incomplete mental model that does not represent the actual situation due to lack of experience (information and facts for decision making) or knowledge of the clinical area (Smits et al, 2009).

Other knowledge error contributors are the human factor compulsion to revert to a (see i)) familiar mental model and decision, rather than a realistic one produced by cognitively assessing all the facts to select a superior decision (Reason, 2000). An accurate mental model of the situation is critical to avoid problem solving and choice errors (Michell, 2013). Jalote-Parmar et al highlight the problem of the lack of a shared platform to provide a common understanding or integration and sharing of mental models in the surgical team (Jalote-Parmar et al, 2008). They advocate careful pre-planning and design using a workflow integration matrix to enable shared understanding or 'distributed cognition' (Ladema, 2009). Such cognitive errors also arise due to poor logic and cognitive processing, which limits the range of facts used, assembles facts incorrectly (rule errors), and/or makes faulty inferences based on the available facts (problem based decisions). This relates to the clinicians clinical reasoning ability based on their training, experience and cognitive capability.

1.3.5 Problem Solving Errors

Failure of clinical reasoning in problem solving is often cited as a cause of error (Benning et al, 2011) (see Figure 6). Clinical reasoning, based on established medical concepts and experience, is particularly important as part of problem solving where limited knowledge or processes exist due to the new nature of the event (Rasmussen, 1983). The clinician therefore relies on making cognitive sense of the problem in terms of knowledge regarding facts and perceptions and his mental model of the problem. He uses schemas and strategies and past cases to analyse the problem and identify potential solutions (Sawyer et al, 1996). Individual knowledge based errors often relate to human factors issues, such as biased memory.

Figure 6. Cognitive causes of errors: Mental model

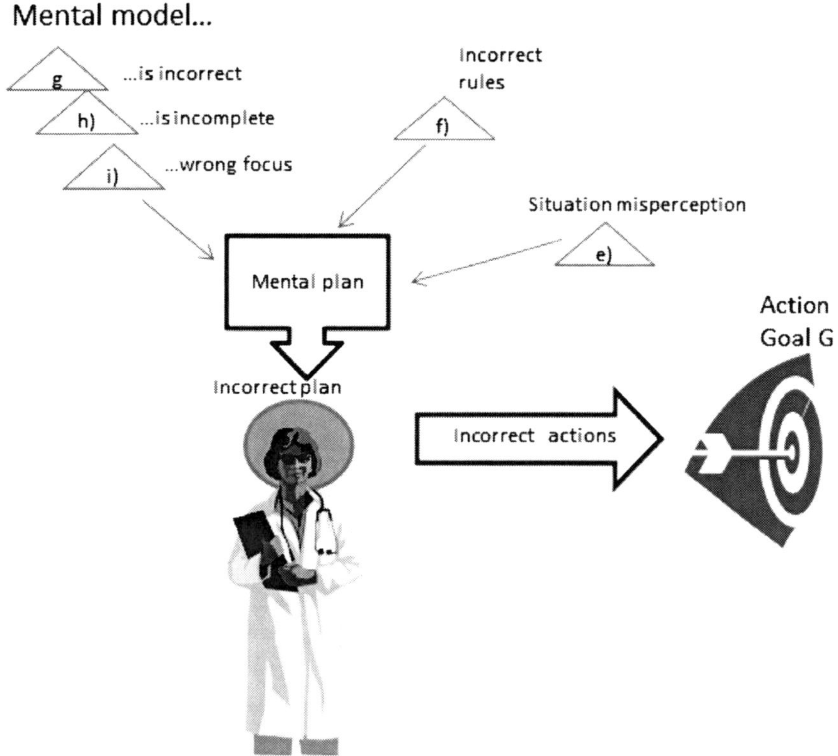

Individual knowledge based error can occur where a course of action or schema becomes a reflex; i.e. the 'available', easy to apply, i.e. 'standard', solution (Leape, 1994). Alternatively over-confidence forces clinicians to jump to conclusions or 'confirmation bias' where the initial idea that makes sense becomes the focus of the solution without evaluation of alternatives (Leape, 1994). A key issue is a lack of information used within choice decision making; for example, Caryon et al. quote one ICU study where most of the errors were due to lack of patient information (Caryon et al, 2010). Humans have a tendency to prefer simple cognitive actions, possibly due to our limited spans of attention and the fact that complex actions can seriously limit cognitive resource to support alternative problem identification or solution generation (Rasmussen, 1983).

1.4 Medical Error: The Equipment Resource Dimension

In even the simplest medical intervention processes, often complex technical resources are widely used; ranging from scalpels, stethoscopes, to equipment such as an infusion pump, MRI scanners. etc. We define resources under three types. Firstly passive resources, which are not capable of motion or sense, e.g. scalpels, dressings. etc (Michell, 2011). Secondly active resources, which are capable of motion, e.g. pumps, machines, etc. Finally intelligent agents, which can process information and act independently, and may be able to sense their own environment (Figure 7).

Faults in the human interaction with resources might also cause patient harm. Firstly the equipment needs to be available at the right time, i.e.

Figure 7. Individual errors

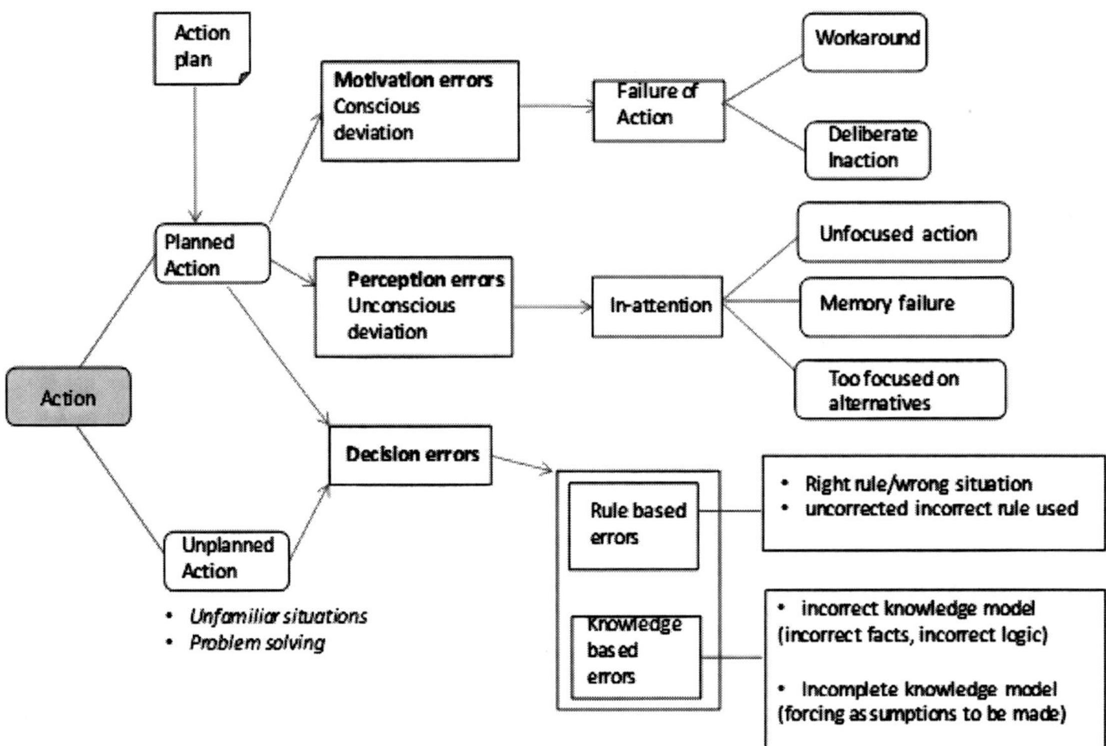

not lost/stolen or faulty, or in an incorrect state (Smits et al, 2009). Even if the equipment is present it needs to be correctly set up to avoid failure of safety risking results. A typical example of equipment related error relates to the removing of safety interlocks and guards to speed up work (Holden, 2009). The complexity and ease of understanding of the human computer interface (HCI), e.g. visibility and interface use issues, can often cause set up errors (Borycki and Kushniruk, 2010).

User error, through a lack of knowledge concerning how to correctly apply the equipment, can be a major source of error (Weigmann et al, 2010). Often this may be due to either the equipment design itself, poor human-computer interface design and/or poorly written or trained procedures (Shappel and Wiegmann, 2000). For example, mixing up discrete and continuous scales (Sawyer et al, 1996), or inadvertently programming a pump for 10 times the ideal dose (Zhang et al 2003). Finally, even if the equipment is set up and used as designed (i.e. as per procedure), we still have the potential for an operational technical failure. For example, a button pressed on a specific make of infusion pump can register the reading twice, thus potentially doubling the drug dose given to a patient (Holden, 2009). Whilst enormous advances have taken place in terms of equipment reliability to reduce technical failure, there are often failures in basic consumable resources (Smits et al, 2009). Also the complexity of much medical equipment still results in set up and use errors due to wilful misuse, workarounds or unintended consequences of use beyond expected parameters. For example, an airway heater melting a breathing tube due to careless positioning (Helmreich, 2000). This range of errors is reflected in Figure 8.

Figure 8. Equipment related errors: Example types

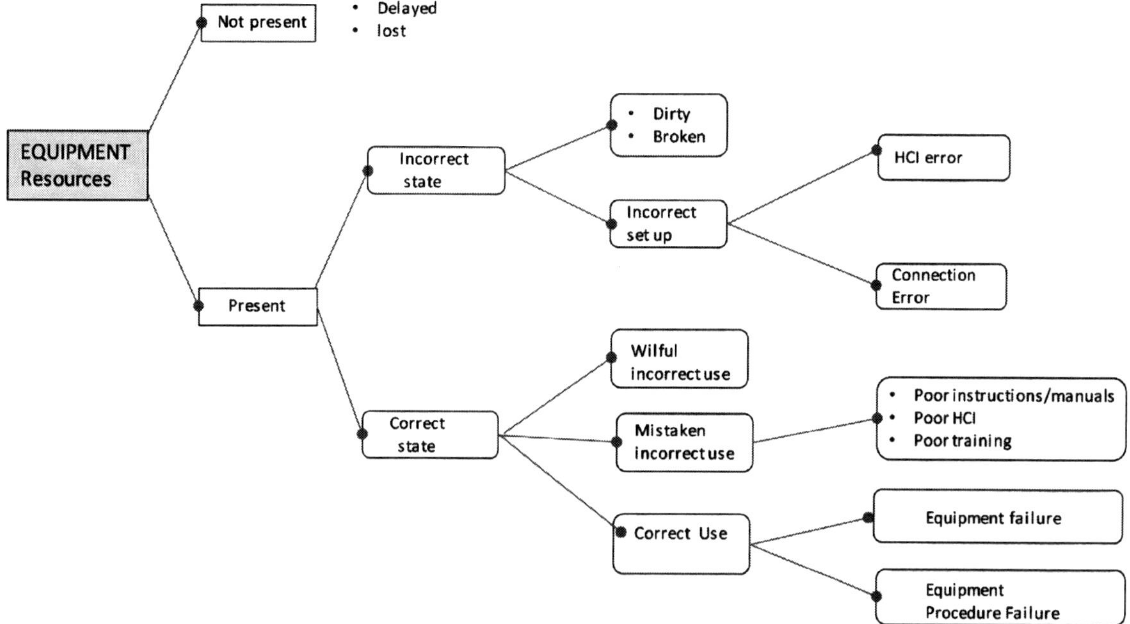

1.5 Medical Error: The Process Planning Dimension

Most medical interventions are based on a planned process interaction of a correct and complete set of agents and resources to achieve an improved medical state for the patient. This involves planning at three levels: process, activity, individual action. In the planning stage many forms of process and procedure plans and cues are available. These range from clinical pathways, which identify the sequence of actions (but rarely the resources) to achieve a specific outcome, to care bundles of advice regarding clinical actions or algorithm/ protocol treatments and specific clinician-resource interaction on a patient (Michell, 2012b). However, as Smits et al's survey recalls, the process planning and guiding artefacts can often be 'too complicated, inaccurate, unrealistic or poorly presented' (Smits et al, 2009). As we have seen earlier the plan and procedures followed, must be accurate with 'correct rules' and the conditions for their application. But often the issue is too many rules and procedures to take in with little correlation and update to enable understanding of implications for changed and additional procedures (Michell, 2012b). Also as Caryon et al (Caryon et al, 2010 suggests the procedure may have not been updated or may have been written by a person lacking the operational experience. This advocates the need to gather information about the actual practices and processes used. The right resource availability at the right time is critical. The knowledge of alternative courses of action also needs to be available / accessible. This often depends, as we have seen, on unreliable human memory. In executing the process any lack of coordination and control of a process is often seen as a key source of error (Kamalanathan et al, 2013).

1.6 Teams and Communication Error

Smits investigation, of unintended medical events, identified up to 25% were as result of human interaction (Smits et al, 2009). Teamwork is vital to good medical outcomes. Teamwork depends on a perception of actual actions and expectation of planned actions of others. Communication is important in planned processes and even more so in unplanned event driven processes. Reason identifies miscommunication as a key source of error with examples of use of similar words, mistaken common association between words (Reason 1998). Lack of communication and miscommunication, is a problem particularly with large surgical teams, such as in paediatric cardiac operations (Benning et al, 2011). Communication errors are highly prevalent when transferring responsibility between clinicians and teams (Caryon et al, 2010). There may also be over-communication to the patient, but not enough communication of what actions have been taken among clinicians e.g. where blood tests have been duplicated (Smits et al, 2009).

Verbal and written communication errors, for example lack of information, poor quality / clarity of information and untimely information, frequently occur in clinical activities, and lead to uncertainty and incomplete information for correct decision-making (Arora et al, 2005). Whilst improvements have been made in training in verbal handovers in terms of inclusion of pertinent, thorough and anticipatory information, the communication of vital information is still at risk because: a) it may be isolated in one person; b) forgetfulness or poor decisions can still render transfer void (Helmreich, 2000).Checklists have been widely used, but are subject to the fallibility of human culture and memory; with many unused or poorly used with much data collection missed or not updated (Berg and Goorman, 1999). Communication is not just between agents, but also what information a resource communicates. A good example includes poorly inscribed figures on a medical tool that could result in dangerous and incorrect use of equipment; e.g. a seven can look like a 1 on a scale measurement (Sawyer et al, 1996).

1.7 Medical Error and the Environment

We separate the environment into two parts, the physical environment of things and objects and the conceptual environment of rules, laws, policies, culture and human behaviours.

1.7.1 Physical Environment

Reason coined the term 'local traps' to identify working environment conditions, which in conjunction with violations of procedures and human error can create unsafe and risky patient situations (Reason 1998). Physical environmental issues such as noise, lighting, heating and vibration may act as interrupts and distractions to clinical actions, which result in slips and mistakes (Caryon, 2006). Also the layout of the environment such as chairs, tables and obstructions can reduce timeliness of actions and result in potential accident harm to clinicians and patients alike.

1.7.2 Conceptual Environment and Safety Culture

The abstract concepts used within any work environment are also an important contributor to medical error. The conceptual environment for safety concerns both formal concept, i.e. controlled by management policies, and informal concepts, i.e. cultural norms and human behaviours. The culture of an organisation, therefore, provides a set of standards of behaviour to which its members follow and aspire. Safety culture ideally involves everyone focusing on the 'value and priority of the patient' (Weigmann et al, 2010). However, the workload and attention demanded of clinicians, often the only resource monitoring and controlling clinical actions, can threaten rather than enhance patient wellbeing. This is particularly true when standards and controls are relaxed through lack of staff / observers and controllers. A culture in which procedures and standards are flouted, and there is little concern, management or control of slack practices, can provide a fertile environment for a 'multitude of errors'. A good example of poor safety culture in the UK is given in the recent Francis report (Francis, 2013). The required safety culture to resolve these issues must be self-analysing and open (Reason 1998).

1.7.3 Management and Control

Managing and controlling clinical behaviour and activity at present relies on human observation and interaction, and hence is open to human factor failings. The focus here is on: a) allocating work efficiently and effectively, i.e. 'planning, scheduling and forecasting' and b) observing and controlling violations of process and appropriate behaviour to avoid error and patient risk situations. Task workload and the cognitive complexity of the task are both error-inducing factors (Weigmann et al, 2010). Also mis-scheduling of the right staff can also be an issue (Helmreich, 2000). Good management and control requires accurate, timely and appropriate situational information in the right context. All too often this relies on human monitoring of both other human agents and machines. Inability to be aware of everything can lead to knock on errors (Smits et al, 2009). All seeing, monitoring, and control, is a 'tall order' in the increasing complex event driven medical environments, such as ICUs (Caryon et al, 2010). Even with analysis tools, such as root cause analysis, many failures have no clear set of facts to support thorough analysis.

1.8 Summary of Key Safety Issues

The review of current error theory above highlights the key human source of error in terms of perception, decision-making and knowledge errors in human actions and interactions with resources to deliver clinical goals in execution of work processes. Many clinical or related goals may be pre-planned, e.g. elective neck of femur surgery or unplanned in response to trauma events, etc., which can be a source of rule or policy error. Event based workflows can also be a source of knowledge error. A human action will also depend on the human mental and physiological state and the presence of environmental interruptions and specific cultures. Errors also occur in human to machine, or human to passive resource interactions, or in the use of technology, equipment, tool and machine resources.

A key issue is that despite automated alarms any human in the process is ultimately responsible for both monitoring the state of the patient, their colleague's actions and technology, amid a sea of potential human fallibility. This is an ever increasing challenge with the increase in technology and the lack of sufficient time and staff available due to cost pressures. Sadly these human factor errors will always be present and therefore require appropriate design, automation and control to manage or circumvent them. Ladema et al. make clear that safety depends on Hutchen and Klausen's clinical team's 'distributed cognition' i.e. the sharing and updating of knowledge (Ladema, 2009); but overworked clinicians are hard-pressed to improve their own cognition. Accordingly we need to harness device awareness, to not only support the communication of agent cognition, but to add to it without increasing the cognitive burden or creating cognitive overload (Kirsch 2001). Caryon et al. in their study of human factors and patient safety, suggest that a solution relates to the building of systems that 'ensure mindfulness in clinical process owners and stakeholders' (Caryon et al, 2010). However the increasing demand for, and lack of availability and high cost of, clinicians means that relying on clinicians alone is not enough. We need to identify how new technologies can support and share the clinicians burden and help to reduce human failings.

Until recently technology that enabled action, needed to be monitored and controlled by the same overworked and fallible human sensors and sensibilities. Information systems, advice guidance and information were the main deliverables to support the harassed clinician. But these have often added to the burden of information overload. However, newer technologies, such as the Internet of Things, promises cheap and massively capable communicating sensors. This heralds a new ability to self-check, reason and provide hard facts and evidence about what is happening in the real environment, not just information provision. Additionally, smart actuators enable technology to make an impact on, and take more control of the physical world. The Internet of Things, promises to add extensive additional capability to the sensing, management and control and avoidance of medical errors. Section 2 explores the capabilities of IOT, and Section 3 identifies examples of how these capabilities may enable improved safety and reduced error.

2. CAPABILITIES OF IOT

2.1 What is the Internet of Things?

2.1.1 What is a Sensor?

A sensor is 'an intelligent resource that is able to detect physical states and changes in the environment'. A sensor, through a specific sensing mechanism can 'observe phenomena' and produce data about the phenomenon (Patel et al, 2011). Phenomena are 'an observable property of a physical entity' e.g. temperature, pressure, tag identity of an object (Patel et al, 2011) Sensing involves a measurement of the signal representing the phenomena or state of a physical/real object or environment in the real world and its changes over time.

Sensing = f (signal from the real world)

This signal must be interpreted and measured against a datum, in order to provide data about the phenomena. The mechanism of measurement (or measurand) will vary with the phenomena that are being captured, e.g. measurement of the presence of a human / animal can be detected by heat via a thermal sensor. Where state is a property of the sensed phenomenon that belongs to an entity or a unique item identity (id) at a specific point in time. For example, temperature is a state property of a room, a person, etc.

State = f (phenomenon, id)

States may be binary, e.g. present/not present, of a specific value, e.g. clean/dirty, or a continuously variable physical property. Sensing the variable state of physical entities involves gathering a data signal vs. a datum or fixed level in order to identify a measure of the state, i.e. or can observed value that indexes the state.

Sensors enable the accurate measurement of a wide variety of object or agent states. Russomanno et al. developed an ontology of sensors based on general sensor mechanisms e.g. chemical, electromagnetic and the specific attribute measured (the measurand) e.g. thermal expansion (Russomanno et al, 2005). Combing Russomanno and Patel et al. (Patel et al, 2011) and Michell's (Michell, 2011) taxonomies to relate to sensing of phenomena of medical resources mentioned earlier gives the reference structure in Figure 9.

2.1.2 Understanding 'Things'

The Internet of Things (IoT) has developed from the ability to add sensor capability to objects and pervasive use of cheap robust sensors. The 'thing' refers to both 'real and virtual entities that are capable of being identified' (de Saint-Exupery, 2009) and used in the human environment. These 'things' or 'entities' can be converted from passive physical objects that cannot sense or move in their environment with sensors and actuators to sense,

Figure 9. Sensor taxonomy: adapted from Russomanno et al., 2005

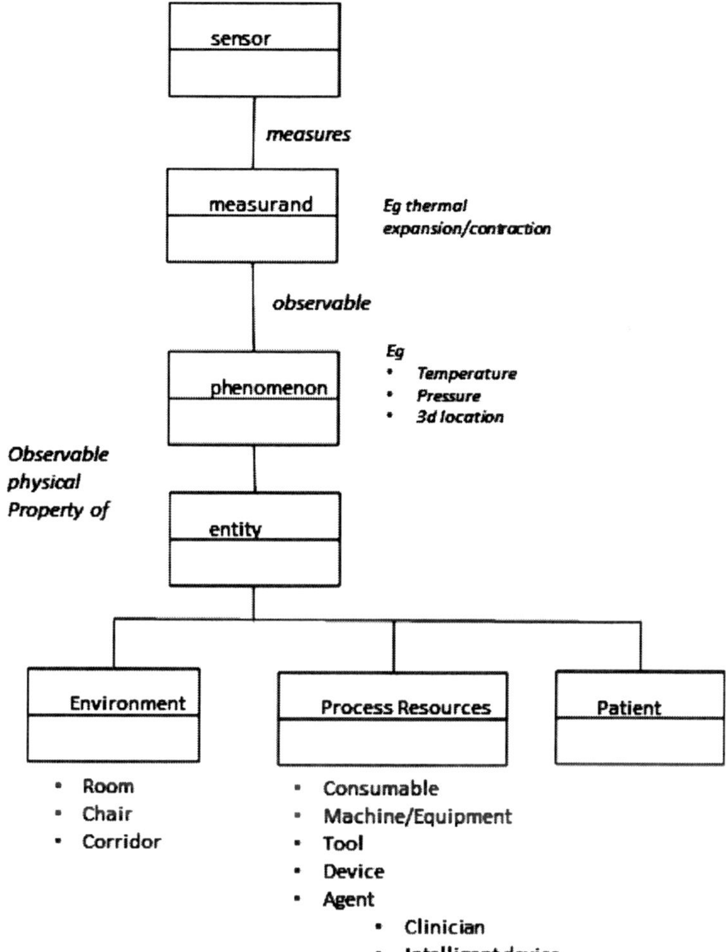

communicate and act on the environment using the web as the communications hub (Korteum et al, 2010). However the IoT is not simply a network of sensors but of 'objects with processors, identities and intelligent interfaces' (de Saint-Exupery, 2009), which enables interrogation concerning the impact of actions on the physical environment. The following sections examine the key components necessary for the Internet of Things.

2.1.3 Processor/Tags

IoT development has grown largely from the ubiquitous use of cheap radio communications and radio frequency electronic identity tags and 'smart labels' (Bohn et al, 2004).The smart label or tag includes a memory chip, containing identity and other relevant information about the object the tag is attached to (Atzori et al, 2010).The tag is read by a sensor that can identify / read the memory. Fitting an object with a tag effectively gives a passive object a unique identity and a memory that can be interrogated at a distance. Tags can be a few millimetres in size, and are either passive, which stores and transmit existing data, or active, which can capture information from their environment via sensors (Cooper and James, 2009). Wireless technology enables local or near field communication and reading/ interrogation of the tag at up to a few metres or more range. This is the basis of operation of passive pervasive security access cards, credit card and other tags that are widely used today in sales and security situations (Mattern, 2003). A standard object identity tag enables automatic scanning and identification of an object and recovery of any information held in its memory. This enables tags to be used as either manual or automatic proximity triggers to recognise objects and when linked to actuators open doors or gate to enable access to areas (Fleisch, 2010). IoT development of the tag includes adding a sensor so the tag can receive signals from the environment and a processor so that the signals can be processed and communication with other tags or the web can be enabled. IoT relies on this radio frequency and solid state processor technology, which is widely used in logistics and tracking to drive down the cost of sensors. This has dramatically increased the number of devices connected to and addressable/controllable through the web. This is estimated by Swan to be 50Bn connected devices in 2020 (Swan, 2012). Figure 10 summarises these key components.

2.1.4 Communications

A key aspect of the Internet of Things is the ability to retrofit passive objects with cheap and reliable wireless communication tags, sensors and actuators to identify their location and to sense the object state and/or the environment state. This technology provides the ability to communicate directly with machines and devices to enable the command and control of physical actuators that enable motion and full robotics; independent of human interaction. The Internet of Things is intended to be an integrated WSAN - wireless sensor and actuator network with machine to machine, and machine to agent, interaction, enable sensing communication and control of the physical human world (Patel et al, 2011). This will also enable a revolution in small or nano objects and include nano size sensors and actuators deployed inside human patients to sense and physically act on the body via the internet of nano things (Jain et al). This will make what has been a semi linked digital world a more human three-dimensional world, by linking to analogue devices and analogue states typical of human decision making (Privat, 2012).

2.1.5 Network Connectivity

Many of the definitions of the internet-of-things emphasise the web capability providing a 'connectivity to smart objects ' and being uniquely addressable, based on standard communication protocols" (Atzori et al, 2010). Unique tag addresses, which are able to communicate to relevant devices (i.e. something performing a particular function or purpose) via the internet, underpins

Figure 10. Basic IoT Components

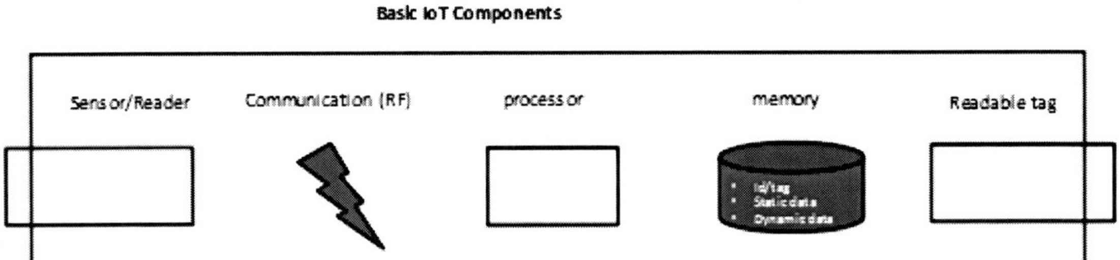

Basic IoT Components

Sensor/Reader   Communication (RF)   processor   memory   Readable tag

Id/tag
Static data
Dynamic data

the development of a 'web of things'; i.e. using an 'Internet of tags' with addresses to identify objects of interest in the environment. In addition an 'internet of devices', with addresses and communication between devices should exist (Privat, 2012). With the traditional web, the focus is on human to application, or human to machine. communication; as a network for connecting people to people, or people to automated information processes. Humans are the driving resource (Michell, 2011) i.e. are largely responsible for initiating and controlling the work process. The main web linkages have been from humans via human computer interfaces to other computers, and human computer interfaces (HCIs) back to humans. The focus of the current web has been on information transfer and processing, with little independent computer sensing of the environment, or ability of the computer to act on the environment. In contrast the Internet of Things enables direct machine to machine, i.e. device to device, connection, communication and processing independent of humans by using the web as a communication channel and a rich source of further data and knowledge.

2.1.6 Types of Sensors

To provide an overview of the example types and capabilities of sensors we identify sensor classes by the phenomenon measured, e.g. temperature, location, etc., and by the environment they are used in. As we have seen tags and tag-readers enable sensing of another tagged object via their identity, a feature widely used for access control. Location sensors that measure absolute GPS position are widely available, alternatively abstract locations can be sensed via the id tag (Hung et al, 2004). Similarly process and abstract states can be sensed by update from a reader that triggers a signal on the completion of a process or event. Sensors have long been available to measure absolute values of physical properties such as temperature, pressure, etc. Dynamic physical properties of an object

such as force, velocity, acceleration can also be sensed and accurately measured. For example for measuring body joint forces (Raskovic et al, 2004) or blood flow volume, or shocks / falls (Hung et al, 2004). An increasing range of specific chemical and biochemical sensors are also available to detect, both the presence of, and the magnitude of, the phenomena for specific diseases. For example, epilepsy (Swan, 2012), Kidney disease (Hepp et al 2005), diabetes (Raskovic et al, 2004). The miniaturisation of physiological sensors for blood pressure (BP), ECG/heart rate, oxygen saturation, etc. is beginning to enable IoT sensing individual patient phenomena (Hung et al, 2004). We can see the relationships in the various type of phenomena, detailed in Figure 11 and 12, for an object resource and a patient / agent.

2.1.7 Tracking Capabilities
F (Measure, Time)

Bohn defines two key capabilities of smart objects: the ability to track the objects in real time and the ability to interrogate them as to their status (Bohn et al, 2004). The term tracking is often used to relate only to the movement of an object or person (Atzori et al, 2010). We use a wider definition of tracking as the *'ability to know the properties of an object (its state) at appropriate points of time so that it can be utilised optimally in an organisation'*.

Tracking = f (state, time) Where state = f(phenomenon, id))

In the set of properties, we include both the physical states (temperature, pressure) and conceptual states for example clean or dirty. Measuring state changes with time enables object location, behaviour and physical property changes to be monitored / tracked. This enables facts about the states of objects, and or the environment, to be recorded as facts allowing appropriate actions to be taken.

Figure 11. Sensor phenomena: Resource properties

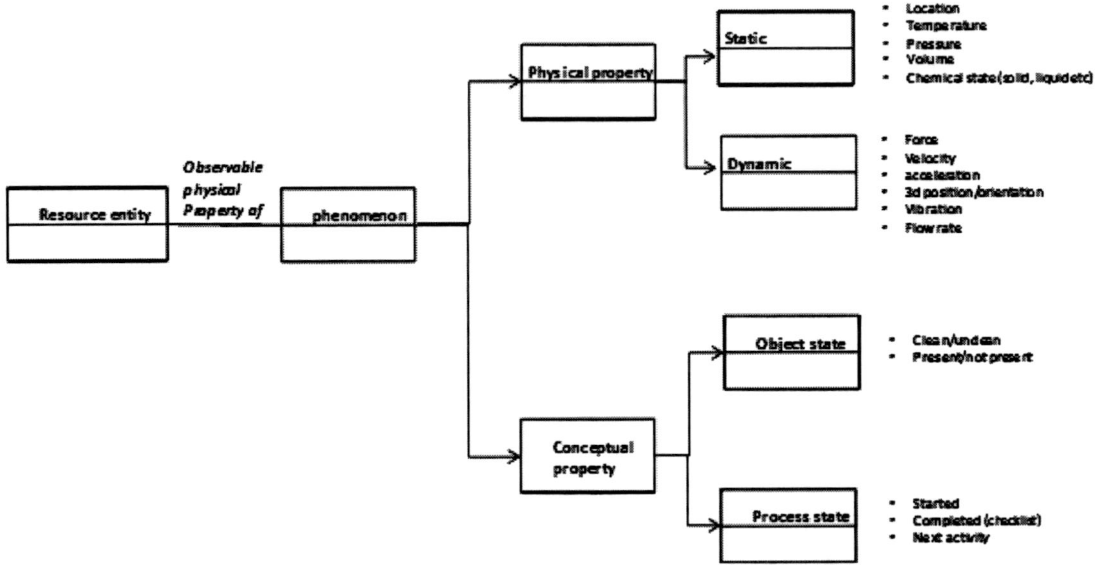

Figure 12. Sensor phenomena: Patient properties

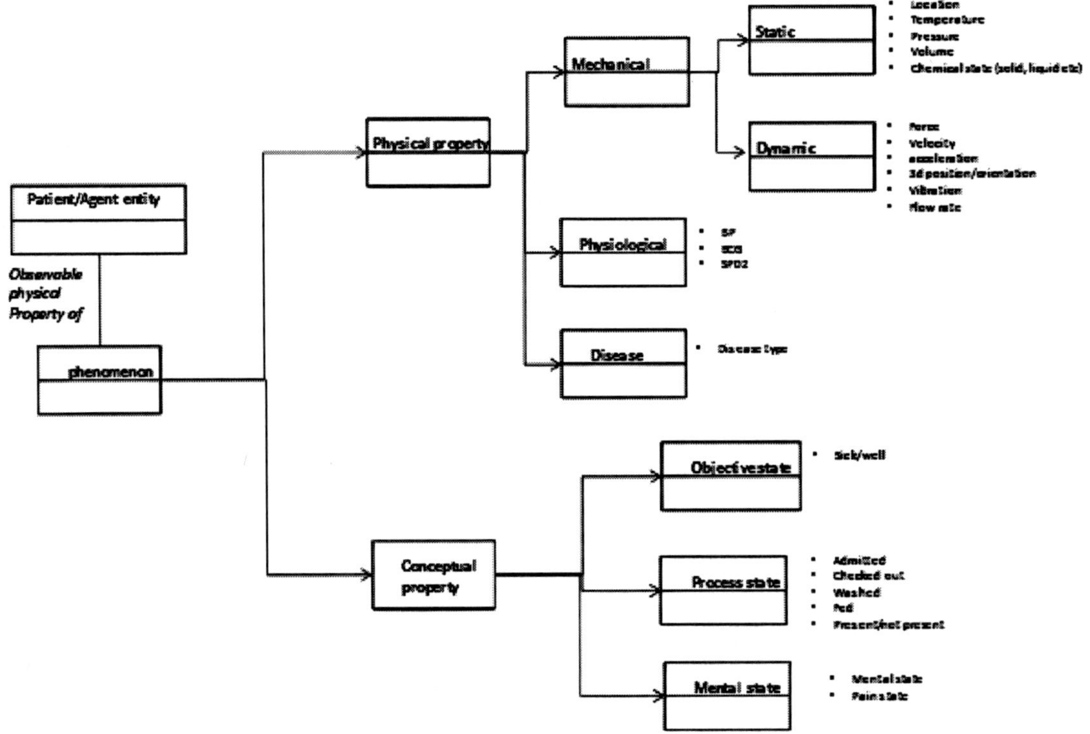

2.1.8 Tracking Types

Retrofitting objects with IoT components enables the recording of a wide variety of states of the object. Location tracking has been widely used as a tracking variable for identifying the location or stage in process of objects on the move. Medical applications of location tracking include tracking of clinicians, medical tools and equipment (Tsiatsis et al, 2010).This enables the correct identification of patients and equipment for scheduling purposes. Tracking of usable resources, tools and equipment such as wheelchairs, aspirators, monitors (Carmichael, 2013), etc. enables both their location and allocation to a process to be identified. In addition tracking of consumable resources (e.g. blood bags), enables use of stock control technologies for re-ordering, as blood and other medical consumables are used. Patient records, pathways and other clinical documents can also be tagged and tracked, to enable infor-

mation to be found and allocated to the correct resource and process (Russomanno et al, 2005). The ability to tag and track resources applied to a medical action or activity can reduce stress and errors in selecting ineligible resources, or lack of availability of the correct resource (Sheehan et al, 2003). These devices have also been actively used to track the location of dementia patients and babies via wrist tags (Carmichael, 2013). RFID sensors have also been used to monitor and control states. For example, the temperature of volatile drugs should be controlled to maximise their use. Abstract states, such as the state of a resource or patient in a process, can also be tracked by transferring state values based on triggering or transfer of information from agents or other sensors. The ability to detect, check and track a resource id also enables us to check eligibility, or exclusion rules, for example whether a resource can be moved out of a secure location. The range of information related to object states is summarised in Figure 13.

Figure 13. Object tracking: Concept type examples

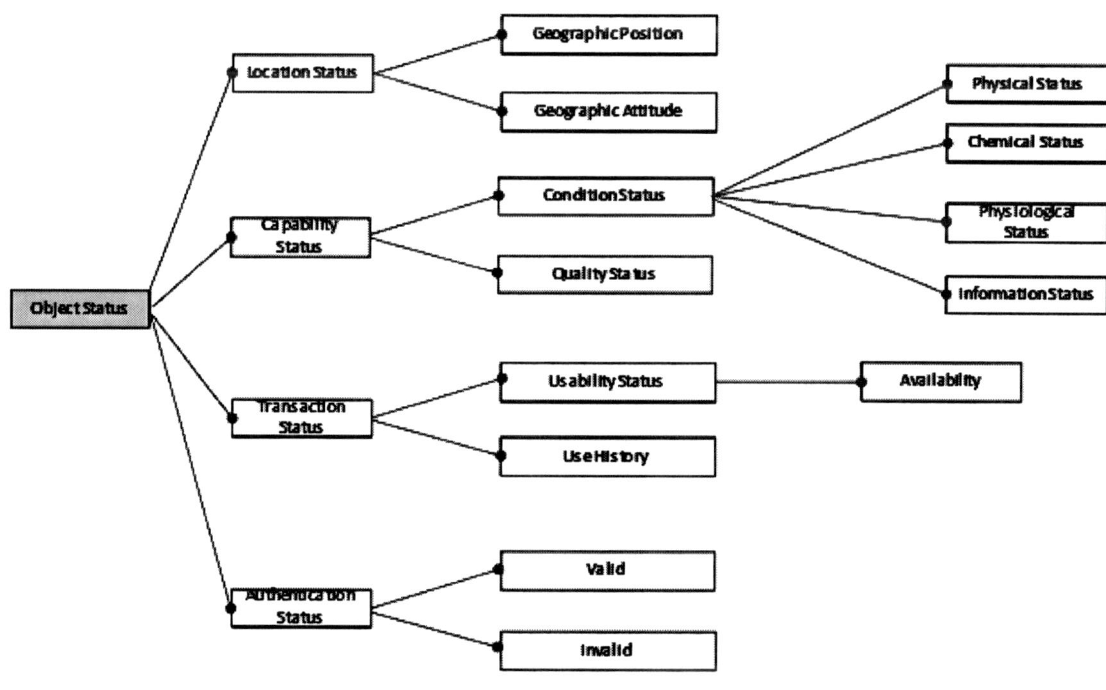

2.1.9 Sensors and Control

Sensors are vital to control of actions and states. Even a simple process will involve decision points as a choice between options, typically a set of options that requires assessment or evaluation of some value attributed to the decision options (Michell, 2012b). Typically decisions have an implicit or explicit goal or objective that the optimum decision should meet. Control involves a decision that evaluates a state achieved by an action vs. a specific goal state.

There are two types of control. Firstly control of the logic of decisions to guide an event – known as sequential or logical control as one may control a series of actions such as a process or workflow. Secondly feedback or linear controls that correct an action to ensure it meets its desired objective Either type requires a decision about a state of an object that is to be controlled.

The control state may be a qualitative conceptual value (e.g. state = clean) or a measured value (e.g. temperature = < 30C). Typically the measured value must be related to a target acceptable range or specific value (Michell, 2012b). Examples of states might include: absolute value, where the state matches a specific measure, or with a task being undertaken i.e. state is true/not true (Binary) or Range.

Although a workflow process is generally non-linear due to complex multiple human and device inputs, for illustration we adopt a general analogy to an engineering control approach to provide an intuitive model of control (Astrom and Murray). Linear controls are often defined as part of a feedback control loop to identify the tracking error between the expected reference goal r and system output y (Astrom and Murray). Control processes typically can be seen as s two-step process of a) detecting the tracking error r-t and are coupled with an action b), to adjust the output y to meet the goal reference r and remove the tracking error.

Feedback Control = f (if(control metric (r-y)), then (control action reducing r-y))

2.1.10 Embedding Objects with Smart Sensors

The capability of IoT based sensors to identify and track phenomena over time can be added to active objects/devices and connected to the device processor, or be added to passive objects. One application is to use IoT sensors to monitor activity of an otherwise passive object to understand problems in its use. For example, smart sensors have been embedded in orthopaedic implants to enable remote monitoring, which can reduce the need for hospital visits (Carmichael, 2013). Embedding enables what may have been a standalone machine, such as a pump or tool, to be monitored. Thus 'augmentation' of what may have been a passive object, can facilitate sentient capabilities, i.e. allowing objects to sense and even reason or make decisions about the health and activity of patients, as a result of sensor measurements (Marin-Perianu et al, 2008).

2.1.11 Wearable Computing and Body Area Networks

The miniaturisation of processors and sensors, and the ubiquitous use of mobile technology, is enabling the development of sensors that can be worn or placed inside the human body to detect blood pressure, pulse and cardiac events (Staccini et al, 2005). Swan mentions the use of smart wristbands, watches and glasses which enable monitoring of heart rate, walking motions and monitoring of specialised diseases such as epilepsy seizures based on skin activity and movement via accelerometers (Swan, 2012). Wearable sensors in the form of skin applied patches enables continuous monitoring of patient blood chemistry (Swan, 2012). Raskivic et al. defined four levels of body sensor capability: i) simple recording/transmission of patient signals; ii) processing of signals and feedback to patient for control/behaviour change; iii) sensors to feedback signals to actively correct malfunctioning organs; and iv) where sensors and devices replace an existing organ (Raskovic et al, 2004).

2.1.12 'Smart' Sensor/ Object Capabilities

The ability to sense the environment and environmental conditions independent of humans, combined with low cost sensors and device communications, offer an opportunity to make hitherto passive objects 'smart'. Lopez et al suggest that a smart object is an object that can sense and measure its environment, and can communicate to other smart objects/devices, has a unique identity, and can make decisions about its own situation and its interactions (Lopez et al, 2012). Smart sensing suggests the ability to independently perceive (subject to the type of sensor) and to act on the environment via sensors, processors and communications to other devices and the web (Korteum et al, 2010). IoT sensors can be triggered by the proximity of another tag manually or automatically as in card readers, or triggered via rules regarding what is sensed, for example triggered on sounds, or even haptics (Fleisch, 2010).

Korteum et al perceive smart objects as IoT sensors applied to tools and devices used as resources in a work process. They divide them broadly into three types: a) 'activity/function aware' that sense human actions on the device and its use; b) 'policy or rule based aware objects' that can relate how the smart object has been used to policies regarding how it should be used and can 'provide alerts to use violations'; c) process or workflow aware objects that sense activities / events and relate these activities to the planned events expected in the workflow (Korteum et al, 2010).

2.1.13 Rule Based Reasoning

Firstly, using our earlier notation concerning safety issues, smart objects should be able to perceive changes of states in the environment. Where a state change is a function of a measure or metric vs. a datum. Secondly, If production rules (Korteum et al's 'policy') are added to a smart sensor of the form; if condition x then perform action y (if, then)), actions to be triggered are dependent on specific sensor conditions (Fleisch, 2010). This enables simple rule based 'reasoning' in smart sensors. Such 'reasoning' provides smart objects with a level of control over the environment, and when linked to actuators, an ability to change the environment. Control can be extended to monitoring, and control of processes by adding a schema of the sequence and timing of process actions, where Process = f(rules, time). However, to fully 'sense' processes at higher levels there is a need to communicate and share state facts between other smart objects embedded in the process.

2.1.14 Cooperative Processing and Sensing

Communication between objects can enable the sharing of information regarding states, sensor observations, actuator positions, etc. It enables the triangulation of information from multiple sources, and, with appropriate reasoning, logic can be used to make sensible inferences about the sensor 'facts' recorded by the peer-to-peer network of objects. For example Strohbach et al. investigated how safety could be improved by fitting chemical drums as smart objects that were able to sense the proximity of two chemicals that might adversely interact. This augmentation enabled both the location of the drums in authorised areas to be checked and also the interaction of drums. Ferscha et al. identified the need for middleware for autonomous computing peer to peer framework to control the network of sensors and or actuators such that they can configure themselves, distributes sensing tasks and dynamically adapt to changes and manage sensor faults (Fercha et al, 2008). Such a network, that enables new sensors to be plugged in, can act as a valuable independent array of eyes and ears in a clinical environment, thus supporting clinician perception with more factual and potentially more reliable inputs, if interpreted properly.

2.1.15 Activity Recognition

Strobach et al's work suggests how smart objects might combine their sensing/perception and ability to communicate/ interact with reasoning to obtain knowledge about their environment (Strohbach et al, 2004). The smart sensors in this case include a-priori information and rules they are designed with, together with sensor information that is used to make inferences about the environment via inference rules. Force, position, and motion sensors were added to jugs and glasses on a table, which were able to sense ('perceive') their movement and interaction by humans and identify the sequence of actions. The comparison and recognition of patterns of movements and force changes over time on the objects enables the objects to infer the set of actions that has taken place. This reflects Korteum et al.'s (Korteum et al, 2010) process aware objects.

2.1.16 Context Awareness

Most existing sensor work has focused on identity, position and visual sensors, but the IoT will enable diverse sensors modalities and relationships between them. The relationship between sensor information of the same or different type can provide context to the information. Gellerson et al. identify a number of contexts including location, visual scene, auditory that includes the real world states, specific aspects (Gellersen et al, 2002).

Marin-Perianu et al. defined different levels of context from individual sensor: a) physical context – position, temperature, velocity; b) agent situation or activity; or c) network sensor interaction with a common known context (Marin-Perianu et al, 2008). The integration of different smart sensors, for example, vision, smell, state, physiology would enable rich contexts to be developed and used to enable more complex decision-making. Whilst detailed analysing and integration of the relative contextual sensor facts are needed, the ability to sense context from sensor integration enables IOT sensors to be used to identify for example unsafe patient behaviours or reactions. Such capabilities could be used to identify context and provide process control. This could be applied to a medical process or pathway to enable sensing and control of a process down to activity and action level. With context awareness comes the ability to identify what, when and where and create facts and knowledge about an environment. In addition the ability to record facts over time enables the recording of behaviour of objects and resources in the environment, i.e. the ability to:

- Share data and facts.
- Share information (data in context).
- Create new knowledge (information in context).

2.1.17 Cooperative Reasoning

Additional opportunities of IoT include the cooperation between artefacts using their sensors, e.g. what Korteum et al term peer to peer reasoning. This enables smart objects to compare their data and reasoning about their states and dispositions; e.g. Strohbach et al.'s smart chemical drums that check that highly reactive chemicals are not stored together by using of smart proximity sensors (Strohbach et al, 2004). Smart objects can exchange information and questions, e.g. about their physical sensing information (Korteum et al, 2010). If passive objects are embedded as smart sensors and designed to cooperate in this way (Strohbach et al, 2004), then this provision of 'facts' about the world can be checked and validated by a multitude of other sensors, such that the facts become 'objective' and can be relied on, or at least included in the human decision process. This additional information about physical actions, and physical conditions, can be made available to check human actor views about a situation. For example Jara et al. (Jara et al, 2010) describe a drugs Interaction Checker based on IoT. The drug interaction checker uses IOT type devices to sense specific drug identities. The existence of various drugs in proximity can be checked for adverse interaction both in terms of patient allergy and drug combination rules.

2.1.18 Reasoning and Inference: Relative and Relational Sensor Values and Rules

Readings from combinations of sensors, e.g. vital signs, can be combined to provide a set of facts about the state and the state changes over time. Machine reasoning, i.e. inferences depend on logical linkages between causes and effects. By adding rules to the sensors, or a controller of many sensors, then inferences are possible from the sum of information. A conditional Boolean rule can be used to deduce or decide an appropriate action based on the sensor state time data, or numerical rules used to make a decision based on a numerical expression (Wang, 2011).

Process flows can also be controlled via event/ state or time driven rules to select appropriate actions. Connecting up clinical pathway checklists to such a controller combined with sensor readings would enable the actual action and state at the end of the action to be checked vs. the clinician's sign off that the state had been achieved. This would act as an electronic checklist to which the sensed state could be included to provide both an action and a state / measure audit trail. The quantity of

time series data collected from sensors in different contexts can also be interrogated and data mined to identify new knowledge and patterns resulting from specific behaviours and patient reactions to interventions. One example of this approach uses a semantic web rule language (SWRL) reasoning engine to identify and manage the states of residents in a nursing home for example monitoring dangerous behaviours that could result in a patient falling (Tiberghien et al, 2012).

2.1.19 Smart Actuators

The development of IoT will not just be a sensor revolution. For the first time actuators, i.e. technology to enable physical motion such as stepper motors, hydraulic and pneumatic systems and and prime movers of all types can communicate with and be controlled by the IoT network (Fercha et al, 2008). The addition of smart technology to actuators enables the transformation of the state of objects in the environment by applying a force and moving an object.

Actuator status and force and position information will enable automated and sensitive control and manipulation of physical objects at macro and micro scale to aid human manipulation and action. Hence IoT web based actuators can act as driving resources enabling change, unlike the traditional web that was limited to passive information provision and reporting. The development of sensor and actuator networks (SANs) will enable a massive increase in information and facts about events and states of resources and their interactions in the real world or 'real world internet' (Gluhak et al, 2009). The development of communication and decision making endowed actuators is predicted to herald a 'fourth' industrial revolution in manufacturing, where 'machines organise and communicate among themselves and supply chains automatically communicate with manufacturing plants' that will further reduce smart object costs and also spread to medical uses.

2.1.20 Resource Oriented Architecture

The proliferation of smart objects enables an architecture of smart resources to be created, for example a network of intelligent power sockets for monitoring and controlling energy consumption (Sheehan et al, 2003). Indeed work by Gluhak, Tsiatis and others suggest the development of a general real world resource based architecture (SENSEI) to control more advanced sensor-actuator resources in a network that enables action on the environment (Gluhak et al, 2009). This would lay the foundations for cooperation between actuators and machines that would provide a potential massive capability increase in terms of real world action and control in a medical environment. A proposed example aims to link sensors and actuators personalised to patient needs to recognise typical patterns of patient behaviour and accordingly identify unusual or dangerous behaviour (Miori and Russo, 2012). This approach is based on context rules and statistical analysis of multiple and varied sensor data.

The basic behaviours of smart objects discussed above can be summarised by extending Lopez et al' model (Lopez et al, 2102) as:

P1. **IDENTITY:** Possess unique identity.

P2. **COMMUNICATE:** Can communicate and transmit information.

P3. **SENSE ENVIRONMENT:** Can sense ambient properties.

P4. **MAKE DECISIONS:** Can decide between options.

P5: **COOPERATE:** Can act as part of a network system.

P6. **SENSE EVENTS AND CONTEXTS:** Possess logic for action.

P7. **MANIPULATE ENVIRONMENT:** Can change the physical environment.

2.1.21 Summary IoT Capabilities

The above discussion identifies levels of capability that underpin the Internet of Things that we can illustrate using the smart object properties P1-P7. Firstly augmenting a passive resource or object in the environment with a processor, database and communication facility to provide an identity and ability to communicate identify and pass passive historical information, i.e. in tagged objects (ie P1/2). A second level of capability is added with the introduction of a sensor (P3), converting the object to an active resource (Michell, 2011) with a capability to a) sense a state (a signal from a change of state/phenomena in the real world) and b) track a state vs. time. A third level of capability is provided by addition of rules (P4) to identify how far the sensed state is from the control state. At this level any control action may be via humans acting on the sensed information; and the control state is often information provided for human control.

However, capabilities of a smart object are only realised, with a fourth level of capability, the ability to cooperate (P5) with other objects as a network based object sharing and disseminating state information. The addition of further rules and middleware enable dissemination of resource state information and coordination and control of states based on information from a range of sensors. Here the relationship between many sensed states of different phenomena enables cooperation to decide a human or machine action.

A fifth level of capability is provided by the addition of reasoning rules to make sense (P6) of multiple sensor state information and to identify complex and rich contexts that provides knowledge and facts about the state of the objects and environment. The use of control rules enable information, from sensor states in different locations and at different times, to be combined to enable actions to be planned, given the sensor reasoning information and knowledge.

Finally a sixth capability to act on and control the space time layout of an environment is provided by linking the smart sensors to actuators to create a smart actuator. The actuator can apply force to an environment and via sensor feedback enable controlled force location change and transformation of the physical environment to various degrees. A further step (not shown) of integrating networked sensors and actuators enables the networked coordination of intelligent manipulators to autonomously transform the environment, i.e. linking the sensors to networked robotics and the potential for robotic hospitals. A summary of the key capability descriptions of smart objects is given in Figure 14.

2.1.22 Smart Cooperative Medical Machines

The ability to finely control actuators together with robotics and miniaturisation offers the opportunity for the development of smart dedicated medical machines to act on the patient in conjunction with a surgeon or anaesthetist. The ability for such machines to cooperate with the clinician enables support for control and automation of routine actions. Provided these were reliably safe then this would ideally reduce the necessary perception and control load in interventions.

Figure 14. Key capabilities of smart objects

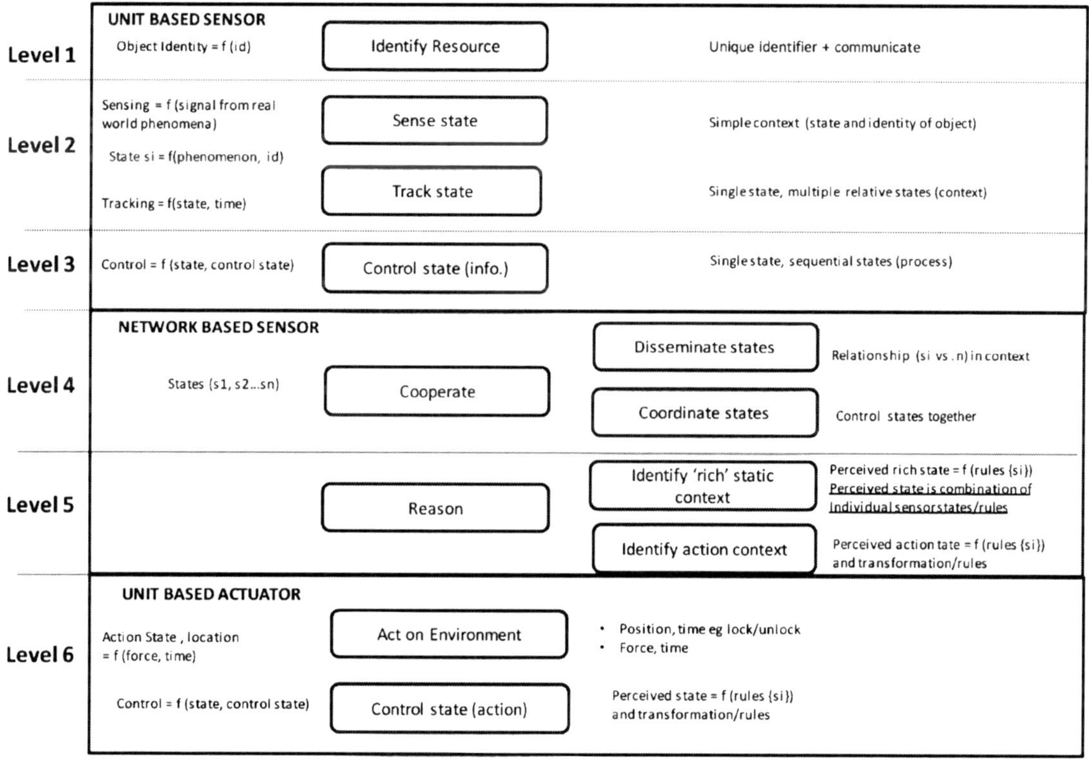

2.1.23 Towards IESME: IoT Enabled Safety Monitored Environments

The capability of IoT can be summarised in Figure 14. IoT operates at four levels.

- Firstly the individual sensor and tracking capability enables state monitoring of resources and the environment
- Secondly the addition of rule based logic enables sensory information control of resources and the environment
- Thirdly the networking of sensors enables contextual reasoning about resource and environmental object relationships. Processes and behaviour can be monitored
- Finally the linking of sensors with actuators provides the capability to act on and physically control resources and the environment

3. IMPLICATIONS FOR SAFETY

This section explores examples of potential applications of IoT to augment human perception, decision-making and knowledge; i.e. to reduce error types.

3.1 IoT and Perception Errors

Perception errors involve misperceptions, incomplete perceptions, and wrong focus of perception. Often these errors are reduced by comparing views of other actors, and more sensor information, to establish the correct cues and highlight missed or unconsidered perception. However, the augmentation of passive objects, with IoT capabilities as smart sensors, offers an opportunity to provide independent machine perceptions, regarding the state of patients and the clinical environment.

3.1.1 Routine Status Monitoring and Tracking

Capture errors (a) focus on the more familiar and can be reduced by enabling sensors to trigger reminders about alternative checks and courses of action to be considered. Description errors, (b), ie, correct plan / wrong subject, due to poor focus of attention, can be reduced by smart cooperative sensors, which are able to remind clinicians of the next process step, or to tag the clinical pathway and all the related equipment directly to the unique patient id. Human activation errors due to incorrect association of action, i.e. c), might still pose a problem. However increased use of sensor facts can reduce the number or actions, thus reducing the chance of clinician cognition overload.

3.1.2 Not Forgetting the Patient!

The error of simply forgetting to check the state of actions should be vastly reduced as a result of IoT technology, as patient and clinical environment sensors can share the burden. Disasters, such as patients dying because of human monitoring negligence (Francis, 2013), should also become a thing of the past. For example, the availability of wireless vital sign sensors (Lorincz et al, 2004) and wearable computing technology allows patient vital signs to be live monitored and recorded at all times whilst in the care environment. The Internet of Things would enable the main vital signs information to be continually highlighted thus avoiding errors due to simple forgetfulness, such as leading to a patient dying from dehydration (Francis, 2013).

3.1.3 Equipment and Resource Error Reductions

The use of RFID to track objects is already helping in identifying patient, clinician and equipment i) location, and ii) medical information (Fuhrer and Guinard, 2006). RFID technology is now actively used for identification of the right resource for the activity, e.g. blood bags, medical inventory, equipment tracking and expiration of drugs (Wamba and Ngai, 2013). Tracking of health process resources can reduce delay and associated patient safety risk of lateness in processes and pathways. Smart object RFID based tracking can also be used to check the process state of medical equipment, e.g. clean/unclean etc and ensure corrective maintenance to reduce technology failure risk.

3.1.4 Increased Validation of Perceptions.

More importantly the ability of peer-to-peer object communication enables cross checking and validation of object 'facts', which can support and validate clinician's perceptions especially if working alone to be checked. The main advantages of RFID technology as a basic wireless sensor technology relates primarily to improved traceability, efficiency (in terms of location and availability) to reduce process delays and increased resource information (Wamba and Ngai, 2013). Use of RFID technology in IoT will also have these advantages, and the ability to ensure the correct action on the correct resource objective as most resources (patient, agent, machine, tool, etc.) will be tagged. In addition the perceived result of the action should be clear by augmenting the agent's sensor with IoT.

3.1.5 Slips and Action Perception Control

Forgetting an action, or step (see section 2d), is a frequent occurrence. Forgotten actions are traditionally reduced via use of checklists, which are often formalised as a key part of clinical pathways. The use of additional documents or pictures reminds clinicians of the process steps and a checklist reminds clinicians of the need to confirm

the execution of key actions (Nolan, 2000). These documents, however, are passive reminders and may be ignored, especially if not a point of focus and/or if verbose or poorly designed (Weigmann et al, 2010). What is needed is a proxy, to save the clinician from missing something. IoT facilitates such a proxy capability. The capability of objects, and resources used in the clinical environment to sense process steps (Korteum et al, 2010), enables an active checklist, with actuator active constraints if necessary, to stop further actions to be available to remind the clinician of the process step - even if distracted. It also serves to avoid lapses into more familiar but incorrect approaches (see section 2a).

3.1.6 IoT Actuators and Active Constraints

Nolan mentions the use of constraints on actions - e.g. polarised plugs etc., which are traditionally used to avoid technology misperception and physical connection errors such as using the wrong plug, assembling equipment incorrectly or not making necessary technical device connections (Nolan, 2000). IoT enables the use of active constraints by using sensors, which sense inappropriate actions and could exert via actuators, i.e. locks or physical controls on actions. For example object embedded sensors scan track the dynamic use of an object and compare it with appropriate models of use and provide passive warnings, e.g. messages, lights or voice and sound warnings or stop the device. In addition the ability to communicate to actuators enables the opening and closing of doors, and the use of automated guided vehicles to ensure equipment is moved at the correct time. They also ensure its current location is known and secured.

3.2 IoT and Decision Errors

Decision errors involve making wrong decisions (rule based errors) or deciding with reduced information or too focused information. These errors can be reduced by ensuring a complete set of options are considered, e.g. by checklist reminders.

3.2.1 Rule Based (e) Misapplication of a Correct Rule to the Wrong Situation

An example of how IoT can reduce rule-based errors is a drug interaction checker. Jara et al (Jara et al, 2010) described how a knowledge based system containing drug information can be used to identify interaction and adverse events resulting from interactions between drugs or a drug on a specific patient (e.g. allergies, dose issues, etc.). The system requires the use of drug containers and RFID tags to identify drugs as smart objects, which communicates with a pharmaceutical drug information system and the patient history to make decisions regarding safety risks. The IoT tag almost removes perception error, as rule based error (i.e. correct rule / wrong context and applying an incorrect rule (see Figure 6) are minimised in this case by extensive machine based pharmaceutical rules. The result is expected to greatly reduce the current 6.7% adverse drug reaction rate with a manual clinician based decision approach (Jara et al, 2010).

As we have seen, a complete pre-planned process can be modelled as a series of decision-action points. Use of an appropriate network of IoT sensors would enable actions and behaviours to be sensed and cross-correlated against process expectations. However, the highly intrusive nature of such support means it would have to be applied sensitively.

3.2.2 Decision Support and Activity Flow

IoT can provide additional cues and rules information, e.g. a reminder of a protocol if triggered actively. This may be sufficient to remind clinicians of the specific rules and / or the conditions in which treatment is best used. In addition process aware cooperating objects and instruments with a model of the expected process could be used in medical interventions to remind or alert clinicians to differences of use.

3.2.3 Information for Knowledge Errors

Knowledge errors driven by incomplete knowledge (see Figure 6) should be reduced significantly by incorporating additional sensors that are now commercially able to sense both continuous patient physiology, and the process state and resource states. The problem of incorrect knowledge should also be potentially reduced in terms of the status facts provided and cross-correlated from multiple sensors. The addition of context and reasoning rules for IoT sensor data should also enable rules and reasoning to be checked and standardised. The issue of lack of questioning of initial diagnosis can also be highlighted as more sensor data history develops during the treatment of the patient and more reliable facts arise to confirm the original diagnosis or support alternative diagnoses. Reasoning algorithms and rules linked to particular disease paths, and reconciled against the actual sensor readings, should enable differences to be identified and alarms triggered for human intervention. However, the quantity of data and the form of interaction with clinicians needs to be managed to avoid overwhelming the clinician and making the situation worse.

3.2.4 Smart Sensors for Choice Decisions Errors

Lorincz et al. (2004) envisioned smart networks of RF based sensors to improve the safety and reliability of patient trauma triage. The development of this vision, via IoT smart sensors, can provide a much larger range of reliable facts through ambient on body and in body sensors. This will surely reduce the errors in trying to: a) identify the extent of trauma; and b) what patient to treat first. Indeed the ability to monitor patient's vital signs and conditions dynamically, and over time, means that dynamic adjustments in clinician attention should be possible as different patients respond to care, or lack of care. In addition, the perennially 'difficult' problem of identifying the medical cause of the newly arrived, yet deteriorating, patient should become less complex due to the correlated information being captured from the multimodal range of sensors available through IoT.

3.3 Resource Interaction Risk

We have seen that medical adverse events and incorrect resources, e.g. drugs administered to patients are a frequent source of human factors error due to the wrong resources interacting. IoT can enable a reduction in these errors by identity and location sensing. An example, which reduces reliance on drug knowledge and information, is Floerkemeier et al's use of embedded technology to perform content management tasks, using IoT like sensors to detect the content and change in content of a box, e.g. a 'magic medicine cabinet' and smart surgical kit (Floerkemeier et al, 2003). This approach could readily be extended to identify what drugs were taken/used by specific clinicians with each patient. It could also be extended to drug preparation, i.e. by sensing a drug in proximity to active phials and syringes and a specific patient's notes or pathway.

3.4 Reasoning and Inference Support

As we have seen, IoT sensor technology can be used to facilitate the input of AI type reasoning, and decision support systems, such as clinical experts to provide additional problem solving strategies and schemas to apply.

3.4.1 Communication Errors

The ability to provide a pervasive network of sensors can provide fact based evidence and accurate state-time history, which previously relied on fallible human memory. This increases certainty of information and, by implication, better decision-making. But IoT also enables improved agent-machine and tool communication. The ability to cheaply sense action sequences in processes enables equipment to sense how it should be used and provide alerts for misuse (Korteum et al, 2010) or violations. Similarly processes configured with smart IoT sensors would enable detection of different from expected activities and also trigger other devices to provide visual / aural guidance as to what should be done.

3.4.2 Cooperative Reasoning and Triangulation of Control

Helmreich (Helmreich, 2000) reported that a combination of equipment malfunctions and human errors could be avoided by using smart IoT objects. Networked pressure, temperature, and location sensors placed within equipment would enable alarms if problems arise; such as intubation blockages, equipment overheating, or performing outside its physical and design range. In addition, communication and coordination between sensors (equipped with reasoning) would enable automatic solution suggestions to be raised to the driving clinicians or other resources able to act on the information. Typically many human process controls rely on a second checker that is divorced from the process For example the ODP nurse or surgical assistant. With the use of smart objects, subject to their operational characteristics, they offer an opportunity to provide an independent check of the effectiveness and quality of a human action, and also the opportunity to logically reason the care action given.

3.5 Connecting the Patient to Reduce Error

The augmentation of intelligent agents (devices and machines) with IoT technology has already started. Smart infusion pumps now include medication error prevention software (Leung, 2011).

Smart devices, such as these, will, however, become even smarter when device data is cross correlated to other physiological sensors (both internal and external, i.e. worn), to provide further facts. This provides data to support better clinician decision making concerning patient state and medication regime. The Internet of Things offers the potential for a massive increase in perception and decision-making information, as well as error detection and control capabilities. It also enables the harnessing of intelligent patient input to add another layer of error detection.

3.6 Smart Facts: Modifying and Learning from the Process

Smart sensor information can provide information about how a process is actually used (smart facts). This is often different to the original design specification (Caryon et al, 2010). Sensor data can collect this information non-intrusively. This enables evidence driven updates and modification concerning the process that are often slower and more error prone with human based feedback.

3.7 Culture Errors: IoT Micro-Communications for Behaviour Change

IoT can enable behaviour change by facilitating personal messages to be sent to clinicians based on intelligent monitoring of data and contextual sensor information. Repeated messages and warnings can ensure gradual changes in action and behaviour in response to them. For example Swan mentions how sensors may identify that a diabetic patient has not tested their glucose and trigger a message, which is sent to the patient to remind them to take their test reducing diabetes risk (Swan, 2012). Such 'micro-communications' can be developed to enable a culture changes, whether by machines or teams sending personal text messages and warnings, to encourage specific safety conscious behaviour.

3.8 Could the Eileen Bromiley Case be Addressed with IoT?

A well-documented example of human factor error is the Eileen Bromiley case detailed by Carthey (Carthey, 2009). The key error issue here is the distraction of the surgeons in the relatively simple process of intubating a patient. The key contributing factors were loss of situational awareness and focusing not on the patient being starved of oxygen whilst ignoring obvious system alarms. This begs the question could this case be avoided in an IoT regime? Clearly more and wider types of sensors would mean more alarms that could also be ignored. However IoT offers a) a massive increase in contextual sensing b) the ability to physically act. Firstly if the patient was well instrumented such that all vital signs were correlated into a single display this would concentrate the mind. Secondly, the use of haptic technology (explored in a later chapter) and BANs may enable feeling for the patient to be transferred to the surgeon. If the surgeons were able to briefly feel what their patient felt via appropriate force and tactile feedback it might have focused the mind on what really was the problem. Thirdly it should be possible in the future to provide actuator interlocks to ensure an airway was maintained. A final thought is that increased real time sensors monitoring real world responses and behaviours will inevitably lead to a massive increase in data to better model both interventions and human and patient responses, which should ultimately lead to more efficient, effective and far safer interventions.

3.8.1 IoT Monitoring and Control of the Planned Medical Intervention Process

Returning to our Figure 4, the 5 phases of the planned medical intervention process, we can identify potential improvements in each of the five stages of medical planning, intervention and reporting.

Errors in the planning for action stage can be reduced by tagging action plan / pathway documents and information sets and relating these to the information from the tagged patient. The ability to identify, correlate and check the information in information systems, with actual real time physical data form sensors, should increase accuracy and timeliness of facts and rules and reduce planning errors.

Tagging of all key resources in the resourcing for action stage enables opportunities to schedule agents and machines in a more reliable and comprehensive manner and ensure their correct state. Also the relationship between tagged resources can be checked to minimise adverse allergic reactions with the patient or between active resources such as drugs. Missing resources should be avoided and any substituted resources should at least be based on more accurate and reliable information.

At the action and interaction level of executing the intervention process, the correct identity / location of resources in the appropriate time sequence can be better ensured. It should be possible to provide more complete and accurate information to support each activity and to both prompt progress of each activity and produce sensor records of the action and result. Rule based and Knowledge support can be improved by making sensor information available and coded knowledge and alternative protocols etc to reduce knowledge completeness and accuracy errors.

Intervention actions can also be better controlled with a greater range of sensor information; i.e. feedback control of the quality of the action vs. the desired state. Support for changes in actions resulting from events and ensuring the correct alternative resources. Control of process steps and violation and improvements should be possible.

Finally performance management should be simplified by the abundance of sensor data. Sensor data can be mined and analysed to create new intervention knowledge. Actual resource behaviours may be checked vs. the plan and lessons drawn about the type and state of resources and their use in future interventions, through the IoT evidence based state results. Additionally the introduction of the new best practices, as rules or warnings / advice in the IoT sensors, can help embed the new behaviour culturally. This enables us to update the model to identify the IoT contribution to monitoring and control of the five phases in Figure 15.

3.8.2 Process, Activity and Action Safety Control

Based on our earlier discussion of controls and the opportunities offered by IoT we can superimpose three levels of control on those described in Figure 2 (Process, Activity and Action Composition). At the process level IoT smart sensors can be used to identify agents and their roles, and match these to resources based on planned processes and activities. IoT sensors also enable pragmatic workflow activity control; providing both i) an information perspective of logic and flow control guidance, and ii) as well as the potential for control actuators to prevent unwanted activities and coerce required actions and behaviours. At the activity level smart sensors enable facts to be gathered to enable feedback and linear control of the outcome of activities. Action checklists no longer require fallible deontic humans to tick a list. Instead, a multiplicity of sensors will identify what has been done and how well, in terms of quality. Resources to be used in activities can be checked and their interactions and results can be confirmed. Further potentially adverse or prohibited interactions, such as a drug, chemical and device risks, can be alerted, or even physically prevented via a link to actuators. Rule based decisions can be advised and checked, and many may be carried out by devices and machines; freeing up human agents to cognitively observe and focus on patient needs and outcomes. Finally at the action level, prompts and guidance can be given concerning actions and reactions to new information. This can be facilitated by an increased number and range of sensors, preventing reliance on the fallibility of human sensors and perception. The IoT augmented version is shown in Figure 16.

Figure 15. IoT monitoring and control of planned medical intervention processes

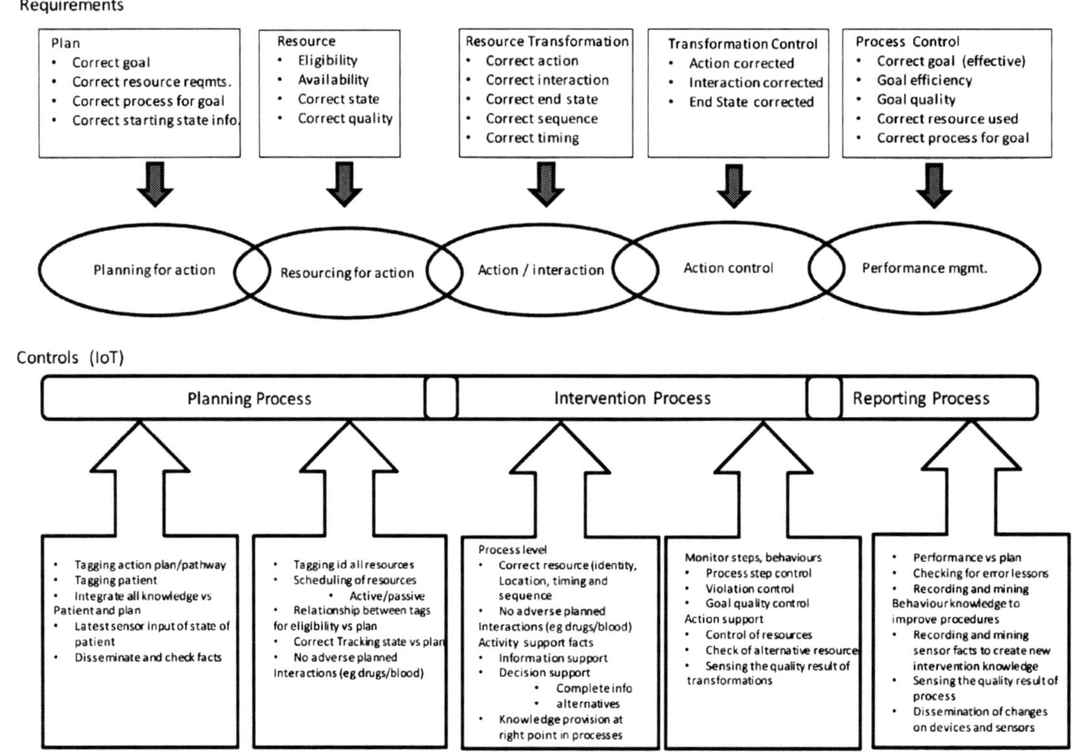

Figure 16. The three levels of augmented IoT process control

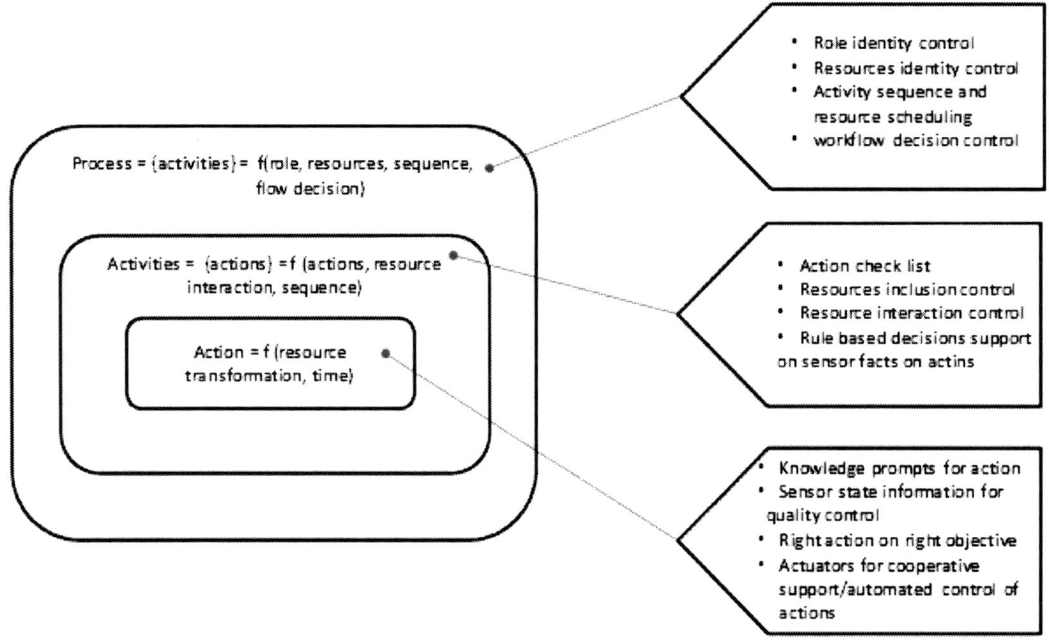

4. LIMITATIONS

Technology advancements are rarely straightforward, and increased information and knowledge creates its own problems. IoT is still a very immature technology with many barriers to overcome, including a standard communications protocol, appropriate middleware to control and coordinate sensor networks, etc. This section briefly discusses some of the limitations of IoT enabled pervasive safety monitored health environments.

4.1 Automation and Creation of Additional Errors

Although IoT can provide valuable additional observation and intelligence to reduce error, as Nolan (Nolan, 2000) points out, automation can also add additional errors and complexity. The increased reliance on machine facts and reasoning will also lead to the creation of many new machine-machine and machine-agent error paths. Hence the introduction and application of IoT needs to be executed carefully to maximise the most benefit, with the least additional complexity, and /or introduction of new error channels.

4.2 Danger of Tight Coupling

Cook and Rasmussen point out the dangers of introducing systems that are tightly coupled where an error in one part of the system has a knock on effect on another (Cook and Rasmussen, 2005). IoT provides a good basis for looser coupling as the low cost and cheap replication of many IoT objects enables duplication and redundancy and hence reduced reliance on any one key device or system. High workload, a source of tight coupling, should also be reduced by delegation of some activities to smart IoT objects and systems and also better automatic triage and monitoring of criticality of patients. However, this is at the cost of increased complexity.

4.3 Risk of Increase in Complexity

Increased complexity, through the technical use of IoT, can add to distraction errors and hence IoT use needs to be considered carefully so IoT smart objects become a part of the team. The ability to connect sensors, devices, etc. will generate many more orders of magnitude of data (requiring cross-coloration and comparison). This leads to an explosion in the number of connected nodes, data collected from those nodes, and processing to extract valuable information from this data.

4.4 Design for Smart Object Interaction

Successful design of the IoT based requires careful linkage and integration between active agents and newly active objects and resources. Rasmussen advocated the importance of matching system functions to human functions (Rasmussen, 1983), to enable better interaction and Zhang et al's 14 medical device usability heuristics (Zhang et al 2003) should be observed. We should perhaps consider smart objects as extensions of our own physical sensors, and analyse how we can optimise the affordances of the devices used in conjunction with natural human affordances.

4.5 When and If?

The IoT depends on a number of developments: a) a standard protocol for linking the devices and sensors; b) a reliable technology to enable the web to be linked to the actual device, i.e. web to device interface; and finally c) motivation and willingness to use the solutions. This final element is one of the biggest barriers to change. The surgical pride and professionalism developed over centuries that has a tendency to rely more on fallible human decisions and sense making may act to reduce the acceptance and development rate of this hugely promising safety-centric domain of technology.

5. CONCLUSION

We have identified key error models and a range of medical error types and shown how these error types might be addressed by the diverse capabilities of Internet of Things technology. The reduction of patient risk and improved patient safety requires improved information, performance feedback and transparency (Seagull et al). We have seen that cheap ubiquitous smart IoT sensors offers the potential of reliable facts and information about real world activities. If managed carefully and with awareness of unintended consequences, IoT can enable a step change in patient safety improvement. The ability to augment and retrofit passive resources with smart sensors down to the nano scale means the number of passive resources in a surgical process of medical environment is vastly reduced. Instead a relative passive human focused sensing environment is replaced by objects able to provide facts and context as well as reasoning to reduce the human sensing load. In addition, the number of driving agents is likely to increase as intelligent machines and objects can sense and act on / transform the environment with or without human intervention; i.e. via IoT actuators. This frees humans to act and drive on the most complex of activities requiring specialist human skills.

In summary IoT technology has the potential to revolutionise patient safety, by making large numbers of passive objects active. Resources will increasingly be able to sense their environment, and the presence of other resources. Entities will be enabled to transmit information and will a) support decision-making, b) make decisions themselves in certain circumstances independent of humans and c) in specific cases independently act on and transform the environment. For the first time in healthcare capabilities will exist for information technology to independently reason and physically apply care without relying on the human in the loop. This critical connection of sensing and actuation offers enormous scope for improvements in patient safety, and will certainly help augmentation the limited supply of human capability and focus that health services are now facing.

REFERENCES

Arora, V., Johnson, J., Lovinger, D., Humphrey, H. J., & Meltzer, D. O. (2005). Communication failures in patient sign-out and suggestions for improvement: A critical incident analysis. *Quality & Safety in Health Care, 14*(6), 401–407. doi:10.1136/qshc.2005.015107 PMID:16326783

Aström, K. J., & Murray, R. M. (2010). *Feedback systems: An introduction for scientists and engineers.* Princeton, NJ: Princeton University Press.

Atzori, L., Iera, A., & Morabito, G. (2010). The Internet of Things: A survey. *Computer Networks, 54*(15), 2787–2805. doi:10.1016/j.comnet.2010.05.010

Ball, M. J., Garets, D. E., & Handler, T. J. (2003). Leveraging information technology towards enhancing patient care and a culture of safety in the US. *Methods of Information in Medicine, 42*(5), 503–508. PMID:14654884

Benning, A., Dixon-Woods, M., Nwulu, U., Ghaleb, M., Dawson, J., Barber, N., & Lilford, R. (2011). Multiple component patient safety intervention in English hospitals: Controlled evaluation of second phase. *British Medical Journal, 342.* PMID:21292720

Berg, M., & Goorman, E. (1999). The contextual nature of medical information. *International Journal of Medical Informatics, 56*(1), 51–60. doi:10.1016/S1386-5056(99)00041-6 PMID:10659934

Bohn, J., Coroamă, V., Langheinrich, M., Mattern, F., & Rohs, M. (2004). Living in a world of smart everyday objects–Social, economic, and ethical implications. *Human and Ecological Risk Assessment, 10*(5), 763–785. doi:10.1080/10807030490513793

Borycki, E. M., & Kushniruk, A. W. (2010). Towards an integrative cognitive-socio-technical approach in health informatics: Analyzing technology-induced error involving health information systems to improve patient safety. *The Open Medical Informatics Journal, 4*, 181. PMID:21594010

Carayon, P., Hundt, A. S., Karsh, B. T., Gurses, A. P., Alvarado, C. J., Smith, M., & Brennan, P. F. (2006). Work system design for patient safety: The SEIPS model. *Quality & Safety in Health Care, 15*(suppl 1), i50–i58. doi:10.1136/qshc.2005.015842 PMID:17142610

Carmicheal, A. (2013). *How to power the Internet of Things*. Professional Engineer.

Carthey, J., & Clarke, J. (2009). *NHS institute for innovation and improvement, version 2009: The how to guide for implementing human factors in healthcare version 1.2 2009.03.28*.

Caryon, P., & Wood, K. E. (2010). Patient safety - The role of human factors and systems engineering. *Studies in Health Technology and Informatics, 153*, 23–46. PMID:20543237

Cook, R., & Rasmussen, J. (2005). Going solid: A model of system dynamics and consequences for patient safety. *Quality & Safety in Health Care, 14*(2), 130–134. doi:10.1136/qshc.2003.009530 PMID:15805459

Cook, R. I., & Render, M. L. (2002). Improving patient safety by identifying side effects from introducing bar coding in medication administration. *Journal of the American Medical Informatics Association, 9*(5), 540–553. doi:10.1197/jamia. M1061 PMID:12223506

Cooper, J., & James, A. (2009). Challenges for database management in the Internet of Things. *IETE Technical Review, 26*(5), 320. doi:10.4103/0256-4602.55275

de Saint-Exupery, A. (2009). *Internet of Things*. Retrieved from http://www.sintef.no/upload/IKT/9022/CERP-IoT%20SRA_IoT_v11_pdf.pdf

Donabedian, A. (2005). Evaluating the quality of medical care. *The Milbank Quarterly, 83*(4), 691–729. doi:10.1111/j.1468-0009.2005.00397.x PMID:16279964

Ferscha, A., Hechinger, M., Riener, A., dos Santos Rocha, M., Zeidler, A., Franz, M., & Mayrhofer, R. (2008). Peer-it: Stick-on solutions for networks of things. *Pervasive and Mobile Computing, 4*(3), 448–479. doi:10.1016/j.pmcj.2008.01.003

Fleisch, E. (2010). What is the Internet of Things? An economic perspective. *Economics, Management, and Financial Markets*, (2), 125-157.

Floerkemeier, C., Lampe, M., & Schoch, T. (2003). *The smart box concept for ubiquitous computing environments*. Paper presented at the Smart Objects Conference. Grenoble, France.

Francis, R. (2010). *Independent inquiry into care provided by mid Staffordshire NHS foundation trust January 2005-March 2009* (Vol. 375). London: The Stationery Office.

Fuhrer, P., & Guinard, D. (2006). Building a smart hospital using RFID technologies. *ECEH, 91*, 131–142.

Gellersen, H. W., Schmidt, A., & Beigl, M. (2002). Multi-sensor context-awareness in mobile devices and smart artifacts. *Mobile Networks and Applications, 7*(5), 341–351. doi:10.1023/A:1016587515822

Gluhak, A., Bauer, M., Montagut, F., Stirbu, V., Johansson, M., Vercher, J. B., & Presser, M. (2009). Towards an architecture for a real world internet. In *Future internet assembly* (pp. 313–324). Academic Press.

Helmreich, R. L. (2000). On error management: Lessons from aviation. *British Medical Journal*, *320*(7237), 781. doi:10.1136/bmj.320.7237.781 PMID:10720367

Hepp, M., Leymann, F., Domingue, J., Wahler, A., & Fensel, D. (2005). Semantic business process management: A vision towards using semantic web services for business process management. In *Proceedings of the e-Business Engineering*. IEEE.

Hoff, T., Jameson, L., Hannan, E., & Flink, E. (2004). A review of the literature examining linkages between organizational factors, medical errors, and patient safety. *Medical Care Research and Review*, *61*(1), 3–37. doi:10.1177/1077558703257171 PMID:15035855

Holden, R. J. (2009). People or systems? To blame is human: The fix is to engineer. *Professional Safety*, *54*(12), 34. PMID:21694753

Hung, K., Zhang, Y. T., & Tai, B. (2004). Wearable medical devices for tele-home healthcare. *Social Science & Medicine*, *69*, 1701–170.

Jain, P. C., Noor, A., & Sharma, V. K. (n.d.). *Internet of Things -An introduction*. Retrieved from www.cdacnoida.in/ascnt2011/Ubiquitous Computing/Paper/1.IOT.pdf

Jalote-Parmar, A., & Badke-Schaub, P. (2008). Workflow integration matrix - A framework to support the development of surgical information systems. *Design Studies*, *29*(4). doi:10.1016/j.destud.2008.03.002

Jara, A. J., Alcolea, A. F., Zamora, M. A., Skarmeta, A. F. G., & Alsaedy, M. (2010). *Drugs interaction checker based on IoT*. Paper presented at the Internet of Things (IOT). New York, NY.

Kamalanathan, N. A., Eardley, A., Chibelushi, C., & Collins, T. (2013). Improving the patient discharge planning process through knowledge management by using the Internet of Things. *Advances in Internet of Things*, 16-26.

Kirsh, D. (2001). A few thoughts on cognitive overload. *Human-Computer Interaction*, *16*(2-4), 305–322. doi:10.1207/S15327051HCI16234_12

Kortuem, G., Kawsar, F., Fitton, D., & Sundramoorthy, V. (2010). Smart objects as building blocks for the Internet of Things. *IEEE Internet Computing*, *14*(1), 44–51. doi:10.1109/MIC.2009.143

Leape, L. L. (1994). Error in medicine. *Journal of the American Medical Association*, *272*(23), 1851–1856. doi:10.1001/jama.1994.03520230061039 PMID:7503827

Leung, B. K. (2011). *Smart infusion pumps reduce intravenous medication administration errors at an Australian teaching hospital*. Retrieved from jppr.shpa.org.au

Lin, L., Vicente, K. J., & Doyle, D. J. (2001). Patient safety, potential adverse drug events, and medical device design: A human factors engineering approach. *Journal of Biomedical Informatics*, *34*(4), 274–284. doi:10.1006/jbin.2001.1028 PMID:11977809

López, T. S., Ranasinghe, D. C., Harrison, M., & McFarlane, D. (2012). Adding sense to the Internet of Things. *Personal and Ubiquitous Computing*, *16*(3), 291–308. doi:10.1007/s00779-011-0399-8

Lorincz, K., Malan, D. J., Fulford-Jones, T. R., Nawoj, A., Clavel, A., Shnayder, V., & Moulton, S. (2004). Sensor networks for emergency response: Challenges and opportunities. *IEEE Pervasive Computing / IEEE Computer Society [and] IEEE Communications Society*, *3*(4), 16–23. doi:10.1109/MPRV.2004.18

Marin-Perianu, R., Lombriser, C., Havinga, P., Scholten, H., & Tröster, G. (2008). Tandem: A context-aware method for spontaneous clustering of dynamic wireless sensor nodes. In *The Internet of Things* (pp. 341–359). Berlin: Springer. doi:10.1007/978-3-540-78731-0_22

Mattern, F. (2003). From smart devices to smart everyday objects. In *Proceedings of Smart Objects Conference*. Retrieved from http://scholar.google.co.uk/scholar?q=Mattern%2C+F.+2003.+From+Smart+Devices+to+Smart+Everyday+Objects&btnG=&hl=en&as_sdt=0%2C5

Michell, V. (2011). A focussed approach to business capability. In *Proceedings of the First International Symposium on Business Modelling and Design* (pp. 105-113). SciTePress.

Michell, V. (2013). Cognition capabilities and the capability-affordance model. In *Business modelling and software design*. Noordwijkerhout, Netherlands: BMSD. doi:10.1007/978-3-642-37478-4_6

Michell, V., Tehrani, G., & Liu, K. (2012). Are clinical documents optimised for patient safety? A critical analysis of patient safety outcomes using the EDA error model. *Journal of Health Policy and Technology*, *1*(4), 214–227. doi:10.1016/j.hlpt.2012.10.003

Miori, V., & Russo, D. (2012). Anticipating health hazards through an ontology-based, IoT domotic environment. *British Medical Journal*, *320*(7237), 771.

Nolan, T. W. (2000). System changes to improve patient safety. *British Medical Journal*, *320*(7237), 771. doi:10.1136/bmj.320.7237.771 PMID:10720364

Panella, M., Marchisio, S., & Di Stanislao, F. (2003). Reducing clinical variations with clinical pathways: Do pathways work? *International Journal for Quality in Health Care*, *15*(6), 509–521. doi:10.1093/intqhc/mzg057 PMID:14660534

Patel, P., Pathak, A., Teixeira, T., & Issarny, V. (2011). Towards application development for the Internet of Things. In *Proceedings of the 8th Middleware Doctoral Symposium*. ACM.

Peleg, M., & Tu, S. W. (2009). Design patterns for clinical guidelines. *Artificial Intelligence in Medicine*, *47*(1), 1–24. doi:10.1016/j.artmed.2009.05.004 PMID:19500956

Preece, A., Gomez, M., de Mel, G., Vasconcelos, W., Sleeman, D., Colley, S., & La Porta, T. (2008). Matching sensors to missions using a knowledge-based approach. In *Proceedings of SPIE Defense and Security Symposium* (pp. 698109-698109). International Society for Optics and Photonics.

Privat, G. (2012). Extending the Internet of Things. *Communications and Strategies*, (87), 101.

Raskovic, D., Martin, T., & Jovanov, E. (2004). Medical monitoring applications for wearable computing. *The Computer Journal*, *47*(4), 495–504. doi:10.1093/comjnl/47.4.495

Rasmussen, J. (1983). Skills, rules, and knowledge, signals, signs, and symbols, and other distinctions in human performance models. *IEEE Transactions on Systems, Man, and Cybernetics*, (3): 257–266. doi:10.1109/TSMC.1983.6313160

Reason, J. (1995). Safety in the operating theatre - Part 2 - Human error and organisational failure. *Current Anaesthesia and Critical Care*, *6*, 121–126. doi:10.1016/S0953-7112(05)80010-9

Reason, J. (1998). Achieving a safe culture: Theory and practice. *Work and Stress*, *12*(3), 293–306. doi:10.1080/02678379808256868

Reason, J. (2000). Human error: models and management. *British Medical Journal*, *320*(7237), 768. doi:10.1136/bmj.320.7237.768 PMID:10720363

Russomanno, D. J., Kothari, C., & Thomas, O. (2005). Sensor ontologies: From shallow to deep models. In *Proceedings of the System Theory*. SSST.

Sawyer, D., Aziz, K. J., Backinger, C. L., Beers, E. T., Lowery, A., & Sykes, S. M. (1996). *An introduction to human factors in medical devices.* Washington, DC: US Department of Health and Human Services, Public Health Service, Food and Drug Administration, Center for Devices and Radiological Health.

Seagull, F. J., Moses, G. R., & Park, A. E. (2011). Pillars of a smart, safe operating room: Performance and tools. *Advances in Patient Safety: New Directions and Alternative Approaches, 3.*

Shappel, S. A., & Wiegmann, D. A. (2000). *The human factors analysis and classification system-HFACS (No. DOT/FAA/AM-00/7).* Washington, DC: US Federal Aviation Administration, Office of Aviation Medicine.

Sheehan, M. J. H., Deitz, D. P. H., Bray, M. B. E., Harris, M. B. A., & Wong, M. A. B. (2003, January). The military missions and means framework. In The interservice/industry training, simulation & education conference (I/ITSEC) (Vol. 2003, No. 1). National Training Systems Association.

Smits, M., Groenewegen, P., Timmermans, D., van der Wal, G., & Wagner, C. (2009). The nature and causes of unintended events reported at ten emergency departments. *BMC Emergency Medicine, 9*(1), 16. doi:10.1186/1471-227X-9-16 PMID:19765275

Staccini, P., Joubert, M., Quaranta, J., & Fieschi, M. (2005). Mapping care processes within a hospital - From theory to a web-based proposal merging enterprise modelling and ISO normative principles. *International Journal of Medical Informatics, 74,* 335–344. doi:10.1016/j.ijmedinf.2004.07.003 PMID:15694640

Strohbach, M., Gellersen, H. W., Kortuem, G., & Kray, C. (2004). Cooperative artefacts: Assessing real world situations with embedded technology. In *Proceedings of UbiComp 2004: Ubiquitous Computing* (pp. 250–267). Berlin: Springer. doi:10.1007/978-3-540-30119-6_15

Strohbach, M., Kortuem, G., Gellersen, H. W., & Kray, C. (2004). Using cooperative artefacts as basis for activity recognition. In *Ambient intelligence* (pp. 49–60). Berlin: Springer. doi:10.1007/978-3-540-30473-9_5

Swan, M. (2012). Sensor mania! The Internet of Things, wearable computing, objective metrics, and the quantified self 2.0. *Journal of Sensor and Actuator Networks, 1*(3), 217–253. doi:10.3390/jsan1030217

Tiberghien, T., Mokhtari, M., Aloulou, H., & Biswas, J. (2012). Semantic reasoning in context-aware assistive environments to support ageing with dementia. In *The semantic web* (ISWC 2012) (pp. 212-227). Berlin: Springer.

Tsiatsis, V., Gluhak, A., Bauge, T., Montagut, F., Bernat, J., Bauer, M., & Krco, S. (2010). *The SENSEI real world internet architecture.* Paper presented at the Future Internet Assembly. New York, NY.

Wamba, S. F., & Ngai, E. W. (2013). Internet of Things in healthcare: The case of RFID–enabled asset management. *International Journal of Biomedical Engineering and Technology, 11*(3), 318–335. doi:10.1504/IJBET.2013.055379

Wang, Y. (2011). Inference algebra (IA), a denotational mathematics for cognitive computing and machine reasoning (I). *International Journal of Cognitive Informatics and Natural Intelligence, 5*(4), 61–82. doi:10.4018/jcini.2011100105

Wiegmann, D. A., Eggman, A. A., El Bardissi, A. W., Parker, S. H., & Sundt, T. M. III. (2010). Improving cardiac surgical care: A work systems approach. *Applied Ergonomics*, *41*(5), 701–712. doi:10.1016/j.apergo.2009.12.008 PMID:20202623

Zhang, J., Johnson, T. R., Patel, V. L., Paige, D. L., & Kubose, T. (2003). Using usability heuristics to evaluate patient safety of medical devices. *Journal of Biomedical Informatics*, *36*(1), 23–30. doi:10.1016/S1532-0464(03)00060-1 PMID:14552844

This work was previously published in the Handbook of Research on Patient Safety and Quality Care through Health Informatics edited by Vaughan Michell, Deborah J. Rosenorn-Lanng, Stephen R. Gulliver, and Wendy Currie, pages 382-420 copyright year 2014 by Medical Information Science Reference (an imprint of IGI Global).

Chapter 80
Service Evolution in Clouds for Dementia Patient Monitoring System Usability Enhancement

Zhe Wang
Edinburgh Napier University, UK

Guojian Cheng
Xi'an Shiyou University, China

ABSTRACT

The authors present an analysis which concludes that most e-health system are packaged for large-scale access through cloud-based services shared in a real-time service deployment environment. The service, which has already been deployed in the clouds for e-health construction, needs to instantly change itself in order to enhance the usability for the patients, especially for the dementia patient monitoring system. The evolution for the service in cloud-based systems can be driven fundamentally based on the service function improvement, quality of service improvement, and service collaboration improvement, which can greatly enhance the usability of the dementia patient monitoring system and dynamically enlarge the life-cycle of the current service system in clouds without replacing the reusable service components. The quality of service evolution of the dementia patient monitoring system is essential because the system reliability and instant messaging sending ability is needed in the dementia patient monitoring system. The system should be as reliable as possible for its undertaken the people's life and healthy ensure for all those who use the system.

INTRODUCTION AND MOTIVATION

Evolution Patterns mainly focus on service inventory re-organization and re-composition, service security enhancement and service accessing database bottleneck re-balance as the contribution of our approach. In this chapter we will provide the detailed design of these patters by using use case diagrams, activity diagrams and class diagrams in different angle of view as the adequate description for each pattern. The detailed design for each pattern can be further refined based on particular case study background and each pattern can also have different edition for its problem-oriented

DOI: 10.4018/978-1-4666-8756-1.ch080

feature. The evolution pattern also obeys the critical rules defined by software engineering which we proposed in this approach, which is feature oriented model driven product line approach. The approach started from evolution feature modeling and finished at aspect weaving. During the whole process the evolution pattern is always the core element that bridges the gap between evolution analyses to evolution realization. As we proposed in the first place that all the evolution patterns can be extended, reused, re-created for its problem-oriented feature and resulted as the problem solution, so that the process of evolution pattern must also obey the critical software engineering approach from use case design to detailed design before code generation by MDA model. The evolution for service collaboration ability in the dementia patient monitoring system is needed because different people need to working together to achieve the patient care in the e-health background. People using or accessing the service in clouds can be achieved using a variety of devices, such as pc, laptop, phone or server. Different people in different locations holding different equipment need

to work together through accessing the service in clouds, the service in clouds should be evolved to enhance the collaboration ability for people's collaboration activity through the service. In the dementia patient monitoring system, people's collaboration activity is quite adequate to verify the value the service collaboration evolution. [Wang, Kevin & Liu 2012, 2013, 2014]

The service pool construction has been observed to be achieved by a general process as the aspect weaving activity. If the operations exactly answer to the process, we can have the increased number of services to expand the function of the service pool. It is the process of how SaaS is in a position to tender non-limited function and ability for the consumer when the service is constructed corresponds to SaaS construction. The construction and deployment of web service has been successfully performed in three ways, one of which is to utilize the current open source code or already deployed service and invoke it through its published URL, the other is to construct the code from original by ourselves, and the last one is that we can combine the two methods together.

Figure 1. The general evolution pattern UML model

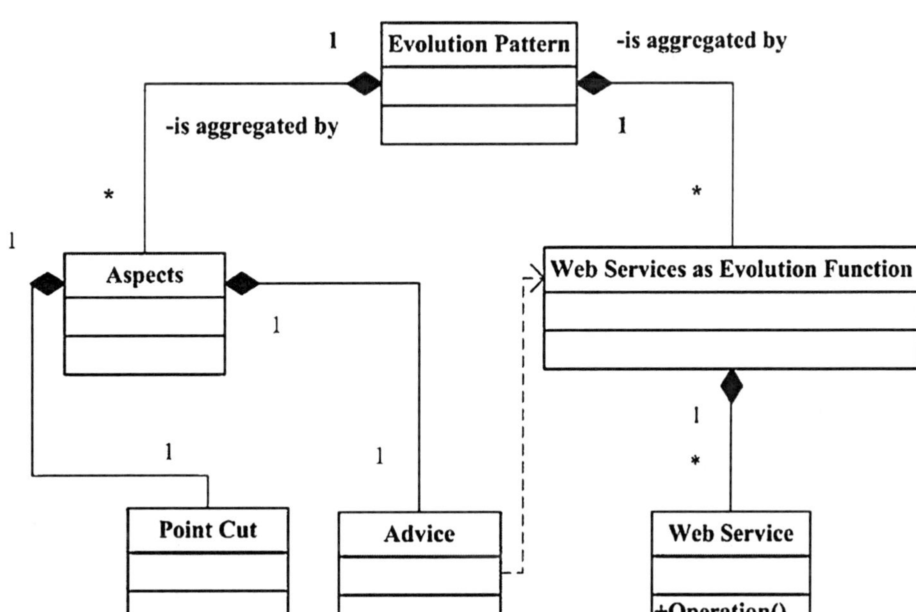

Figure 2. Service pool deployment architecture

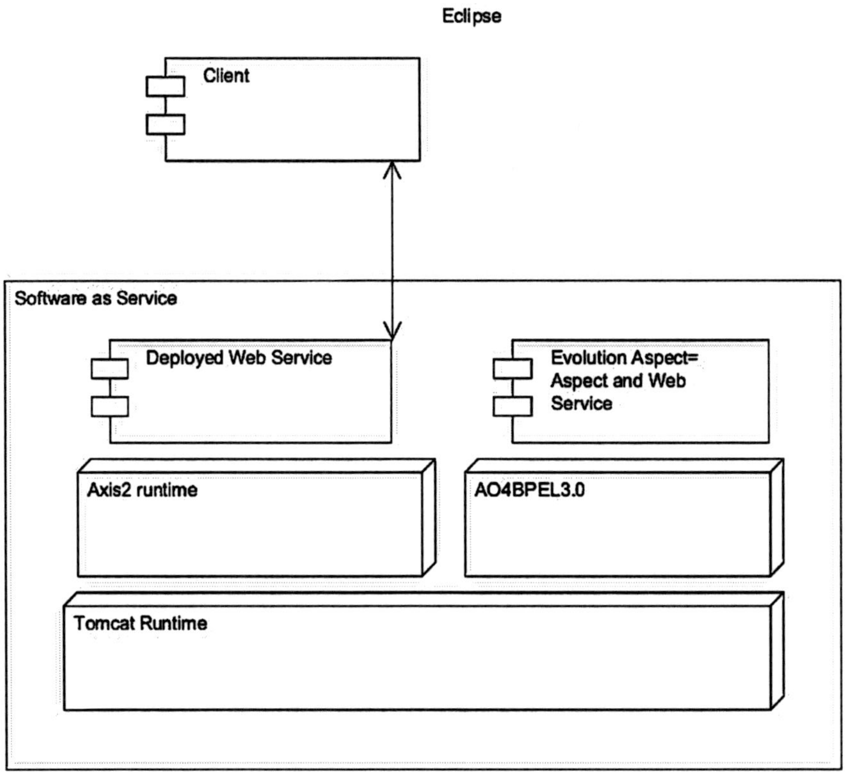

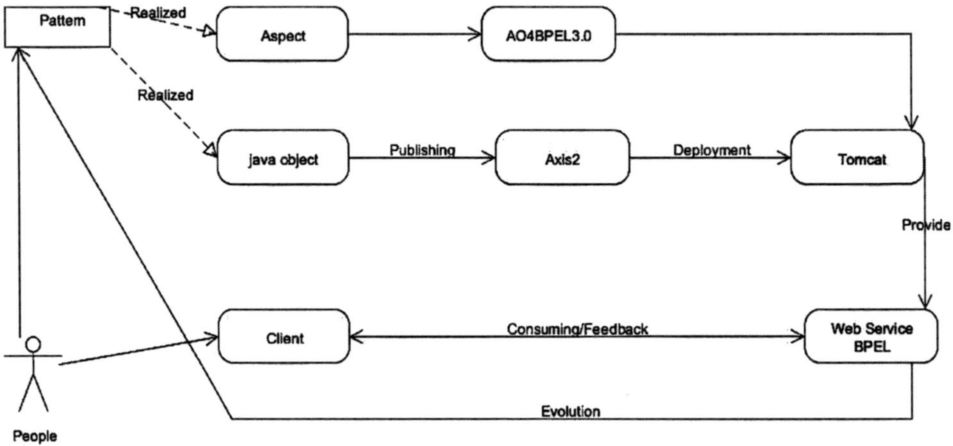

Figure 3. General service pool constructions and aspect weaving interaction diagram

This chapter stands clearly in the mode of the secondary system with the assistance of JDK, tomcat, axis2 and Eclipse. As far as you may see, the general iterative progress for service pool construction has been described in the preced-ing passage. We choose the java web service in our experiment because it is totally constructed form java object and can use axis2 to package it as.AAR file before deployment to tomcat server. Axis2 refers to software from Apache Open

Source project which converts the Java message into SOAP and goes backward movement to re-converts the SAOP message into Java message. The usefulness of Tomcat service is considered to translate the SOAP message into HTTP message and vice-versa. The rule base consists of all possible combinations of the tomcat associated with axis2 to carry out the SOA messaging transferring over the heterogeneous platform. In the Case Study background we are coding the java object for system stimulation. The rationale behind this is that java class can be instantly packaged into. AAR file for being deployed to Tomcat server aim at making it running as a Web Service. Another important step will be engaging in creating the SaaS through generating and deploying the BPEL file to Tomcat Server for the sake of orchestrating all these services. It is not until aspect weaving is followed close upon earlier step that we can finish the SaaS evolution at last.

PROBLEM STATEMENT

This approach proposes a general way of how to support service evolution in dementia patient monitoring system by using service evolution pattern. Although the service evolution pattern and its repository in essence is a large collection of problems solving method towards service evolution typically in clouds, we prefer to just concern the dementia patient monitoring system evolution in this case study.The evolution pattern comes into operation built upon the composition of all these reusable components which are engaged in function achievement and weaving activity achievement. As for the function achievement, their components continue to follow the attention on realizing the functionality that the evolution pattern is designed as the solution to the problems which it aims at.

Let us now consider the weaving activity achievements, these components centralized treat how to weave these function components into the running system in that the evolution pattern is applicable to deal with the problems. It has become apparent that there are two kinds of components like the function component and the weaving activity components are useful to the evolution pattern in detailed designing and implementation. All these components should be reusable enough for different evolution patterns or only one of these evolution patterns to meet with the reusability of the evolution pattern. Take the re-organization evolution pattern and the re-composition evolution pattern for example. The detailed realization for those evolution patterns are relied on the function components and the weaving activity components that constitute the evolution pattern as what has been mentioned earlier. One of the most commonly used reusable components for evolution pattern are the function components inclusive of connector, pipe, wrapper, proxy and another are the interceptor weaving components containing timer, selector and detector. In other words, the above reusable components combine the evolution pattern in general; however, some evolution patterns needs specific components for its function achievement and weaving activity achievement in construction. Because those changeful combinations are being implemented in generating different evolution patterns and results in the repository of those reusable components enlarging. Besides, if accomplished, the above components also can be further enlarged as the main innovation source we can have in the evolution pattern innovation task, reckon they have the advantage that we can use evolution feature to select these components to further refine the evolution pattern until the pattern is suitable for solving different evolution problems. This implies that there is a basically process where these components are manipulated to obtain the desired target as possible. With the case of greedy search approaches, it is found that the design and realization for these components can also be fulfilled by the software engineering method.

In dementia patient monitoring system, the problems domain description for service evolution provides insights on defining the evolution feature that is capable of constantly recognition with the requirement from people. These evolution features in turn provide a useful and direct indication of which corresponding evolution pattern should be selected to resolve the evolution problems.. Evolution pattern for service evolution can be deem as a general method that entails consistently updates to manage particular service evolution challenges encountered in dementia patient monitoring system evolution. [Wang, Kevin & Liu 2012, 2013, 2014].

STATE OF THE ART

Service-Oriented Architecture is a component-based model. It connects different services by the well-organized interface. The interface is defined in the manner which is independent from the hardware, operating systems and programming languages. This make the system service be able to interact with each other in a common way [David, 2009]. In the real situation of IT enterprises, different kinds of operating systems, application software, and system software and application infrastructure interact with each other. Some existing application software will be used to support the business processes, and developing a new system from beginning to end is not possible, the enterprise should have a quick reaction. SOA uses the existing application and application infrastructure to solve the customer requirements and to provide a greener business framework for the enterprise [Charfi, 2004].

Service-Oriented architecture is now generally recognized as a significant development, particularly for business application systems. Services may be implemented in any programming language [Ardagna, 2007].By wrapping legacy systems as services; companies can preserve their investment in valuable software and make this available to wider range of applications. SOA allows different platforms and implementation technologies that may be used in different parts of a company to inter-operate. Most importantly, perhaps, building applications based on services allows companies and other organizations to co-operate and to make use of each other's business functions. Thus, systems that involve extensive information exchange across company boundaries, such as supply chain systems, where one company orders goods from another, can easily be automated [Ankolekar, 2002].

The development of software with services is based on the idea of composing and configuring services to create new and composited services. This may be integrated with a web user interface to create a web application or may be used as components in some other services composition [David, 2009]. The services involved in the composition may be specially developed for the application, or from some external providers.

Web Service

Web services technology is becoming increasingly popular because of its potential in many years. It is a new type of components that can be invoked over the internet. This presents a promising solution for addressing platform interoperability problems faced by system integrators. The flexibility of this new component type also facilitates service composition using existing web services. Promoting component re-use has been a dream for the software engineering industry. Because of this potential for service composition, the agent research community has also explored it for composing agent's behaviors [Buhler, 2003]. Web service integration aims to compose different web service components to achieve a more advanced service unit. This area has now become a very popular research area. This sub section is to give a critical literature analysis in this area for what other people mainly study on this area and what their contribution is, Recently, web service as the main technique for supporting Service Oriented Computing and Service Oriented Architecture, has been widely used in all these areas. The industry and academic have provided research on web service at different angles [Dey, 1999]. With the mature of web service standards and the enterprise platform which support the web service become more and more advanced, lots of enterprise and commercial organization come to join the area we called Software as a service, SAAS. They release their products and service by using the web service standard in order to attract good partners, and find out the potential customers. Such actions can make them earn big profits in the software market. But, today's software service which provided by these software enterprises on the web mainly cannot meet the demand from the customers because the services are simple in their structure and function. Some of them even have bugs. How to integrate these web services and provide an integrated service as an advanced enterprise service to meet the commercial need has become a very important question. This is also a key point for how to optimize service integration [McIlwraith, 2001] [Pillai, 2003] [Rajan, 2009] [Lucchi, 2007] [White, 2005].

Web Service Integration Description

Currently, there is no clearly definition on web services integration, lots of research defined the web service integration in different angles and focused on different areas. Based on the definition by Piers on the service integration [Pirse, 2002], the web service integration is providing more advanced service ability by basic integration on web service. The definitions above are abstractive, even haven't provided a discussion on how to integrate and it also haven't given the basic definition on web service integration. But this definition gives three key points of information. Firstly, the service integration needs other services. Secondly, after the integration the outcome is another new service.

Thirdly, the services used to integrate can come from any part of the web resource [Schilit, 1994].

The comments on the web service integration are from two points of views, which considerate that the integration can be divided into two types Based on the processing model from the viewpoint of web service integration process, the integration process can be defined as a particular control flow and data flow, a set of services that can accomplish a particular task Based on the component unit viewpoint, the web service integration is defined as a self-control and cooperating unit action that can generate a new system Based on all different kinds of definitions, the web service integration can be defined as: according to the requirement of the customer, automatically to choose appropriate (maybe distributed) sub-services and to make these sub-services integrated and cooperated to accomplish the tasks needed by the customer; the integration process will be done under a kind of service integration framework. The web service integration can use the advantage of these small, simple and easy-to-execute sub-services to construct more functional and complex services to meet the demand of customers. This kind of reconstruction integrates the sub-services distributed on the web and Internet to build a more advanced and useful new system to support enterprise and commercial tasks [Charfi, 2004].

Web Service Integration Problem

With the mature and quick development for the web service technique, more and more steadily and reliable services are published on the web. But, in another way, the functions provided by a single web service are limited. In order to make use of the advantage fully provided by the shared web services resources, it is quite necessary to integrate these web services together to form a more advanced service. This can speed up the software development and quickly meet the customer's demand. In another aspect, the sub-services run on different platforms may be constructed by different methods and languages, and provided by different software corporations, the developers should integrate the subservices based on the particular application background and demands [Gibbins, 2003][Emmerich, 2006].

The Framework of the Web Service Integration

For the reason that there are lots of integration techniques and frameworks, it is hard to provide a general integration framework. The chapter abstracts an integration framework which can show the basic idea of the integration method. The framework is a good specification on the integration methodology. The framework contains two roles, namely service demander and service provider, five components, namely translator, integration manager, execute engine, service adapter and service provider, all to cooperate with each other to carry out the integration [Preuveneers, 2005].

Web Service Integration Framework

The generic web service integration execution flow is as follows:

First the service provider provides the service, registers it at the registration centre. If the service demander needs the service, a natural language should be used to describe the demand. After the description is translated by the translator to a computer recognizable language such as OWL, it will be delivered to the service integration management component [Wang, 2007].

The service integration management component drives the integration process based on the description provided by the demander and then submits the integration plan to the execution engine. The execution engine will then submit the plan to the service adaptation component. The adaptation component registration center has the records of all services registered in the center. The service adapter compares the services and chooses the most appropriate one, and then

return the decisions to the execute engine. The execute engine selects the web service based on the sequence determined by the service integration component and then returns the outcome to the customer [Decker, 2007]. There are six key stages in the process of service construction by composition [Emmerich, 2006]:

Stage 1: Outline work flow. In this stage the developer uses the requirements and the selected services as a basis for creating an ideal composite service.

Stage 2: Discover service. During this stage, the developer searches in the service registries to discover the appropriate services, and discovers who provides these services and the details of the services.

Stage 3: Select services. From the set of service candidates that have been discovered, the developer uses these services to implement work flow. Selection criteria will obviously include the functionality of the services, the cost of the services and the quality of service (e.g., responsiveness, availability, etc). The developer needs to decide the choice of a number of services, which can be bound into a work flow.

Stage 4: Refine the work flow. The developer will refine the work flow based on the services that have been selected. This will involve adding details to the abstract description, or changing the work flow by repeating the service discovery and selection activity until the final work flow is established.

Stage 5: Create work flow program. During this stage, the abstract work flow design should be transformed to an executable program. The developer may use a conventional programming language such as Java, C# to adapt a candidate service, and to use a more specialized work flow language such as WS-BPEL to implement the service as discussed in the previous section. The service interface specification should be written in WSDL.

This stage will involve the development of user interfaces [Decker, 2007] [Walkerdine, 2008] [Baresi, 2005] [Paolucci, 2002] [Gibbins, 2003].

Web Service Integration Method

So far, the industry and research institutes have studied the web service integration from different angles, and proposed several kinds of integration methods. Generally speaking, the industry methods focus on proposing integration description languages, editing tools and execution engines. The research groups focus on semantic web, intelligent programming and automatic integration in order to prove the integration systems by using formal methods [Baresi, 2005].

Web Service Integration Based on BPEL

The BPEL method is the typical representation of the work flow method. BPEL4WS (Business Process Execution Language for Web Services), is a web service integration description language based on work flow proposed by IBM, MICROSOFT and BEA in 2002. It integrates the WSFL and XLANG together, form a high level commercial language to describe the business action [Qu, 2006]. The function of BPEL is to integrate the service to form a new web service; structured action will be used to define the work flow. However, BPEL4WS does not support work flow evolution in the run-time [Leitner, 2009].

Web Service Integration Based on Semantic-Web

The basic question is how to represent the web service data, function and information by using a unified method that can make the computer understand the description in order to choose and find web service in the web resources automatically and precisely. Before the emerging of semantic web, the web service description cannot meet the demand above. The semantic web integration

enables the computer to automatically understand and operate to form the new web service by adding semantic information into web services. Semantic web represents the web service data and function at semantic level.

Currently, the main achievement of the semantic web service integration is OWL-S (Web service Ontology Language). It enables the service to be found, invoked, integrated, self-operated and supervised automatically. The OWL-S has three parts. Service Profile provides service and the high level description, including service description, function and service property. Service Model represents the service working logic. The sub-component Process Model describes the service component behavior and process. The sub-component Process Control Model used to support the service execution and supervision. Services Grounding represents how to use the web service. It is the mapping of the abstractive service description to the specific service description [Lucchi, 2007].

Web Service Integration Based on Component Method

The web component method considers the service as a component in order to use the principle of the software development, e.g. reuse, deletion or expansion. The main idea is to encapsulate the information in a definition, which can represent the web component. The web component interface can be published, in order to be used in service finding and reuse. Web service component method supports some basic integration structure: sequence, parallel.etc. The expansion is based on condition and while - do structure [Zeng, 2004].

Web Service Integration Based on Model Driven Architecture (MDA)

A number of Web services are now available and therefore it seems natural to reuse existing Web Services to create composite Web Services. Specially, it is a hot topic to study the problem of Web

Service Composition using MDA. Proposed as a Web Service composition method based on model driven architecture, the model driven software development methodology applied to Web Service composition is a good solution in this area. Nowadays, software enterprises publish their software by using web services. But, the ability of a single web service is limited; therefore the industry and academic organizations hope to generate new web services by using composition method. Composition means to select simple, reusable and appropriate web services from service repositories, and then to composite these services. The services generated by composition method are called composite services. It is possible to take the advantage of MDA by introducing the MDA's feature and technique to the web service composition area. This will simplify the composition progress. For example, if we can build the platform independent web service integration model and transform the model to platform dependent code, the service integration model can then adapt to the dynamic changes from the platform and the integration technique.

Specification of MDA

MDA was proposed by OMG as a new software development method, it uses models to analyses and solve operation problem in software development stage in order to enhance the development efficiency. MDA divides the software model into two parts, which are PIM (platform independent model) and PSM (platform specific model). These two models can be linked by model transformation, which can help software designers ignore the restriction of a specific platform. MDA frameworks use the platform independent language to build PIM model, then transform the PIM model to PSM model based on the mapping rules between the specific platform and the programming language. Therefore, the system code can be generated automatically.

The Development Process of MDA

Firstly, software developers use PIM to build the system model. Secondly, PIM model will be transformed to PSM model based on specific platform and programming technique. The PSM model can be organized as a PSM model set. Thirdly, the software developers will modify the PSM model based on platform feature. The change on PSM will be reflected to PIM, which is the advanced feature of MDA. Fourthly, to propagate the evolution to the PSM model in order to generate more qualified code. Fifthly, to transform the PSM to source code because PSM is close to the system realization technique, so the transform process can be realized directly.

Model Driven Architecture for Web Service Integration

The most valuable benefit for using MDA in web service integration is the separation of integration logic and the integration rules. Firstly, using UML to describe the web service composition model, i.e., to represent the composition model in a high abstractive level. Secondly, mapping the model with specific composition rules that realize the integration. The web service composition based on MDA model can be categorized into two types, namely the static model and the dynamic model. How to realize the web service composition by using MDA? The OMG's MDA uses Meta Object Facility to category the model into M3, M2, M1 and M0 four layers. Model transformation can be triggered between different layers. Based on the different layers, the model can be categorized as different types. The System Objects are in the M0 layer, the model used to describe M0 is M1, e.g. the UML model. The model used to specify the formal rule and grammar of M1 is M2, which is called Meta Model, e.g. the UML's Meta model and SQL's Meta model. The M3 is Meta Object

Facility's model, which is the highest Meta model. M2 is the realization of M3, M1 is the realization of M2, and M0 is the realization of M1 [Liu, 2009].

THE PROPOSED APPROACH

Pattern One: Patient SaaS Inventory Evolution

Use case diagram shown in Figure 4.

Here user means doctors, nurses, carers, stakeholders in SaaS.

The activity diagram is shown in Figure 5.

The class diagram is shown in Figure 6.

Pattern Two: Service Security Enhancement

Use Case Diagram shown in Figure 7.

Here user means doctors, nurses, carers, stakeholders in SaaS.

The activity diagram is shown in Figure 8.

The class diagram is shown in Figure 9.

Pattern Three: Service Accessing Database Bottleneck Re-Balance

Use Case Diagram shown in Figure 10.

Here user means doctors, nurses, carers, stakeholders in SaaS.

The activity diagram is shown in Figure 11.

The class diagram is shown in Figure 12.

A strong effort is underway for implementing the above evolution patterns' detailed design which should be provided as general accessing method for invocation which this can be refined during the specific case study requirement. All these evolution functions should be encapsulated inside the web service component and then further detailed code generation can be driven by MDA models, particularly for each evolution function implemented by web service logic. Here user means doctors, nurses, carers, stakeholders in SaaS.

Figure 4. User case models for patient SaaS inventory evolution

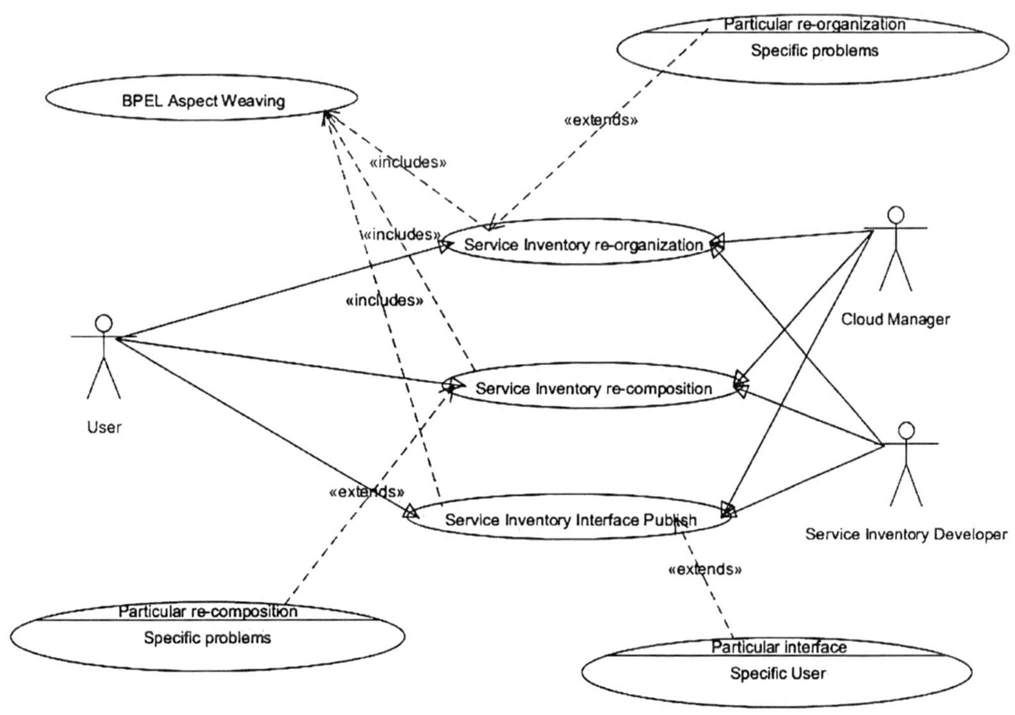

Figure 5. Activity diagram for patient SaaS inventory evolution

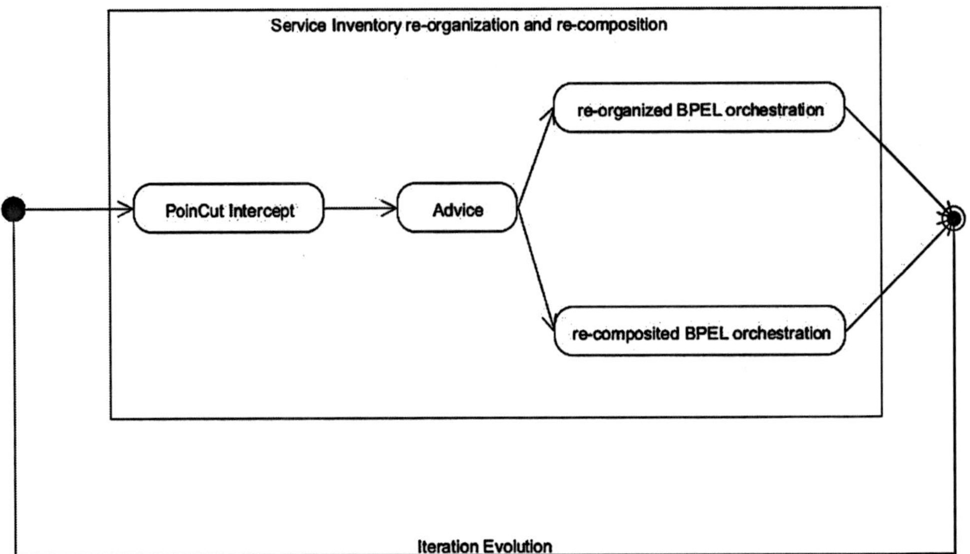

Figure 6. Class diagram for patient SaaS inventory evolution

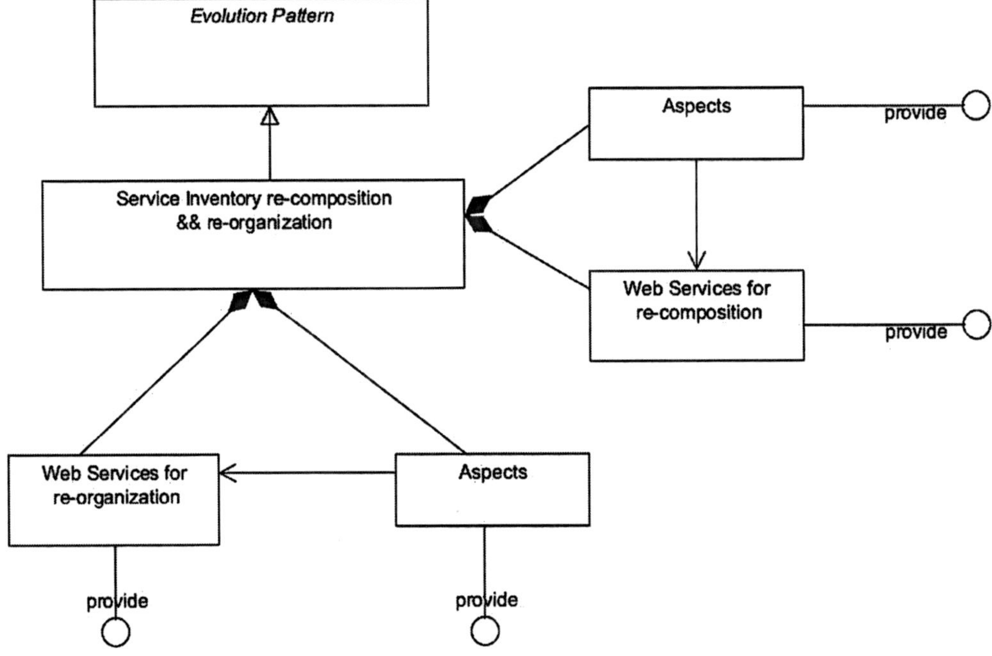

The definition of aspects consists of two parts, point cuts definition and advice definition. These definitions are fully relying on the services that require to be evolved in the case study. Perspective view on SaaS Inventory and Load balancing virtualization Evolution Pattern

The service in the clouds and service inventory are largely distributed in clouds since they

Figure 7. Use case diagram for service security enhancement in patient case SaaS inventory

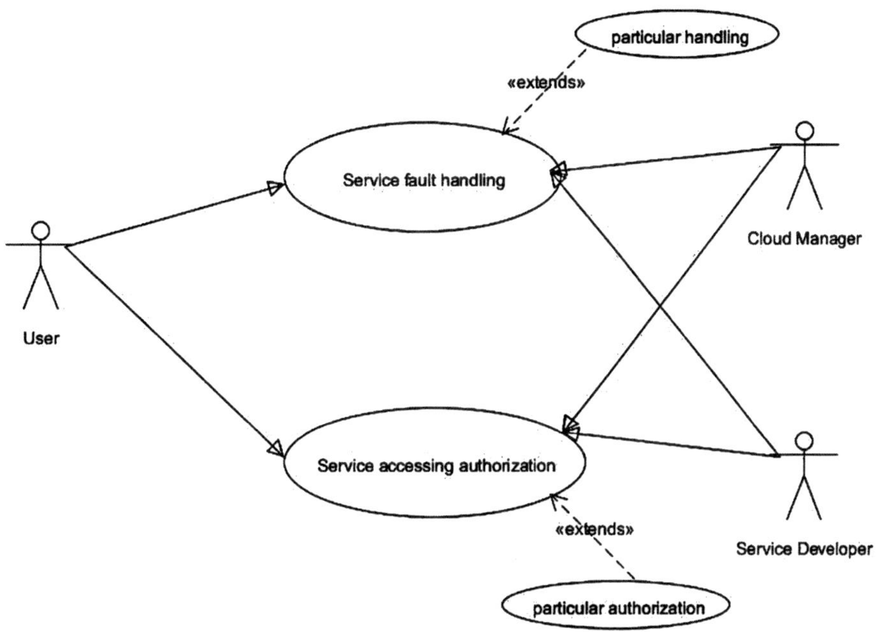

Figure 8. Activity diagram for service security enhancement in patient case SaaS inventory

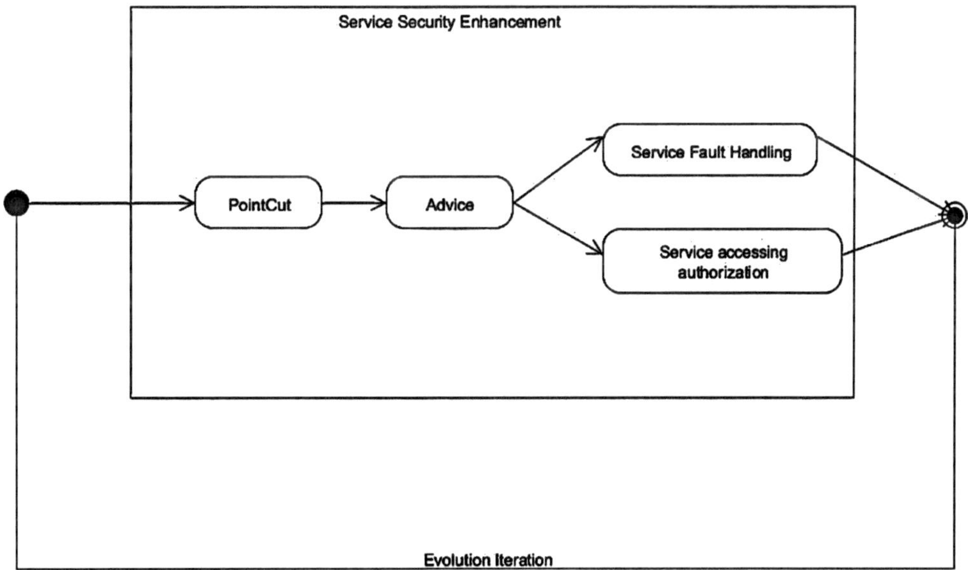

are composited together based on the consumers' requirement and working autonomously. However, a composited service component can be further characterized as required forming a larger web service with enhanced functionality and transpar-ently existing in a wide scale. SaaS (Software as a service) is emerging from institute and industry at the peak moment. It has become apparently that some types of service have more load balancing burden undertaken ability than the others, such as

Figure 9. Class diagram for service security enhancement in patient case SaaS inventory

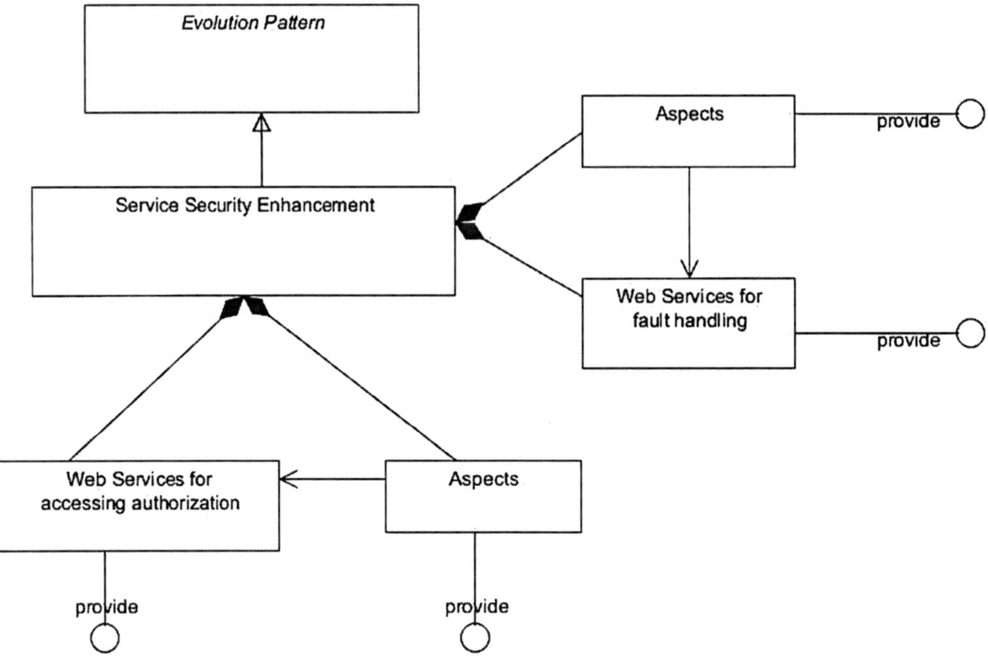

Figure 10. Use case diagram for service accessing database bottleneck re-balance in patience care SaaS inventory

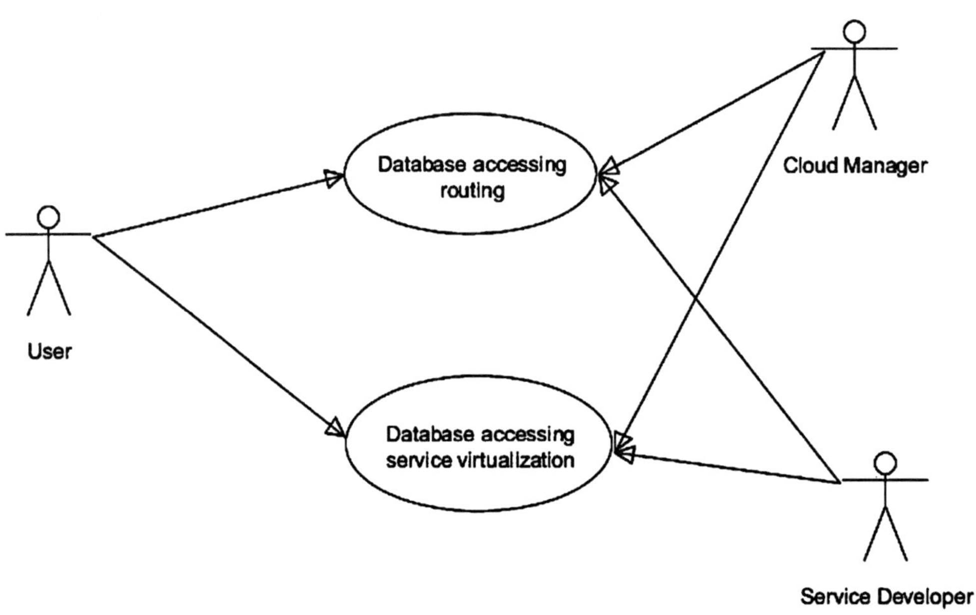

Figure 11. Activity diagram for service accessing database bottleneck re-balance in patience care SaaS inventory

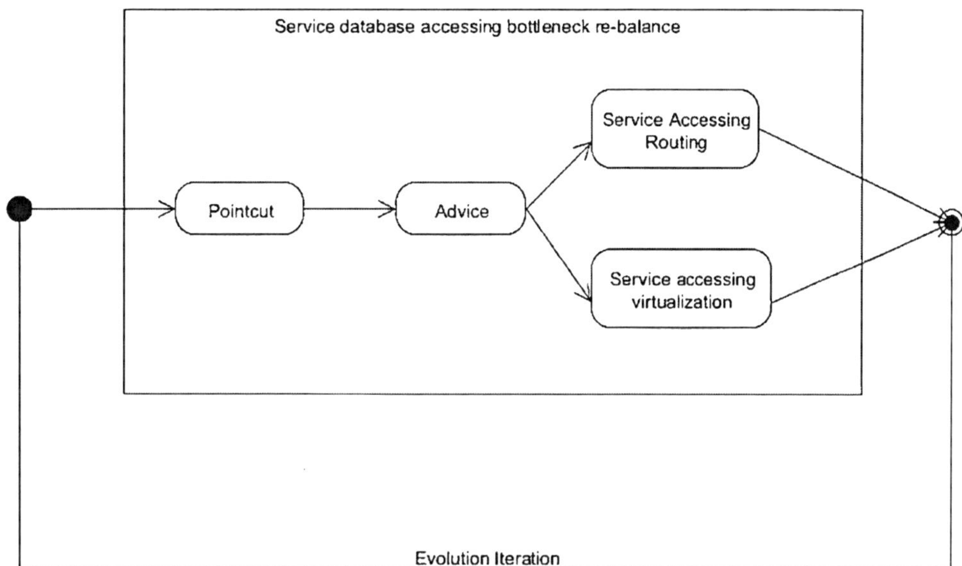

Figure 12. Class diagram for service accessing database bottleneck re-balance in patience care SaaS inventory

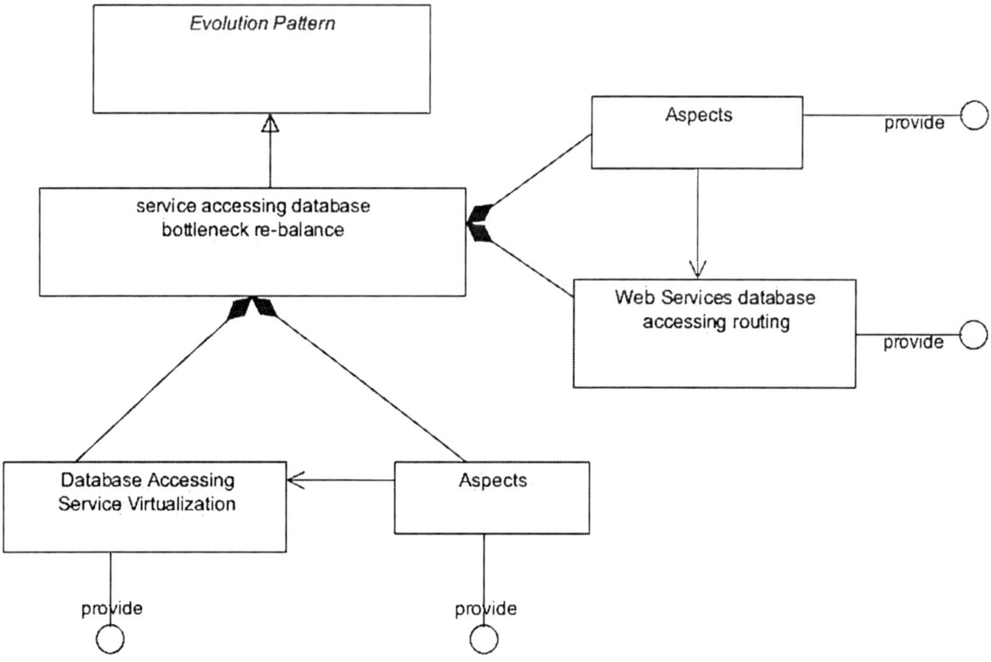

the routing service, security service and specific reusable service function for specific tasks, each of those are likely to be shown as high rating of invocation. Obviously, evolution pattern has to confront such serious problems during the evolution process.

Weaving the instance of a virtualized service to the current BPEL based composited service is for the purpose of increasing computing ability for one or several notes of the service so that it can increase more load balance ability on the service. It is when the service virtualization evolution pattern working on the elastic clouds to provide such ability of virtualizing a service instance the service consumers will be guided by the evolution aspect driven mechanism to customize particular edition service instance from the same virtualized service instance recognized by its session ID.

Reflection routing is performed for reducing the burden of each virtualized service instances and therefore enhances the service performance. The services in the clouds inventory can be modeled through two perspective viewing there are Horizontal branch and Vertical branch which represent a single service and composite services respectively. Service in the horizontal branch can be composited into one vertical branch service or several vertical branches. Obviously, the higher composite rating the service has the more reusable the service is. As show in this manner, it is noteworthy that such kind of services are the most valuable object service for evolution activity, because it make an important contribution to further composited services which are frequently been taken for compositing SaaS.

Patient Care Service Inventory as SaaS

1. A SaaS component in clouds (Figure 12) is a service inventory unit which contains a large number of related services. It provides functions through multi-service interface and it can enhance and extend the function through the plug-in interface. Indeed, the service inventory as SaaS component is substantially used in clouds because of its flexibility, collaborative, reusability and efficiency on-demand.

2. The inner modeling of the SaaS component (Figure 13) is described with the perspective view of SaaS inventory and load balancing virtualization. The services in SaaS components providing multi-interface for invocation through orchestration respectively results in the changing of the SaaS component interface being vibrantly evolved base on applying SaaS inventory re-organization and re-composition evolution pattern.

3. Correspondingly, the SaaS component interface is exposed as the vertical view of the service inventory which means the services are orchestrated together. However, other services which are used to composite SaaS components are in the horizontal view of the service inventory. Service evolution in clouds is based on evolving each SaaS component through evolution pattern.

4. It is indicated that the deep level evolution can change the underlying web services logic inside the SaaS component which is used to composite SaaS. What's more, the large scale evolution can alter the whole SaaS component in the clouds thoroughly. In addition, the load balancing evolution pattern can solve the problem of bottleneck if the SaaS component needs to be highly dynamic. After all, these two kinds of evolution pattern are cooperative to settle one particular evolution problem by using different evolution pattern which is mainly comprised by different aspects.

5. E.g. the evolution for load balancing virtualization needs the changing of the SaaS component interface and the changing of the underlying web services logic that composite the SaaS components.

Figure 13. SaaS inventory perspective view and load balancing virtualization evolution pattern in patient case SaaS inventory

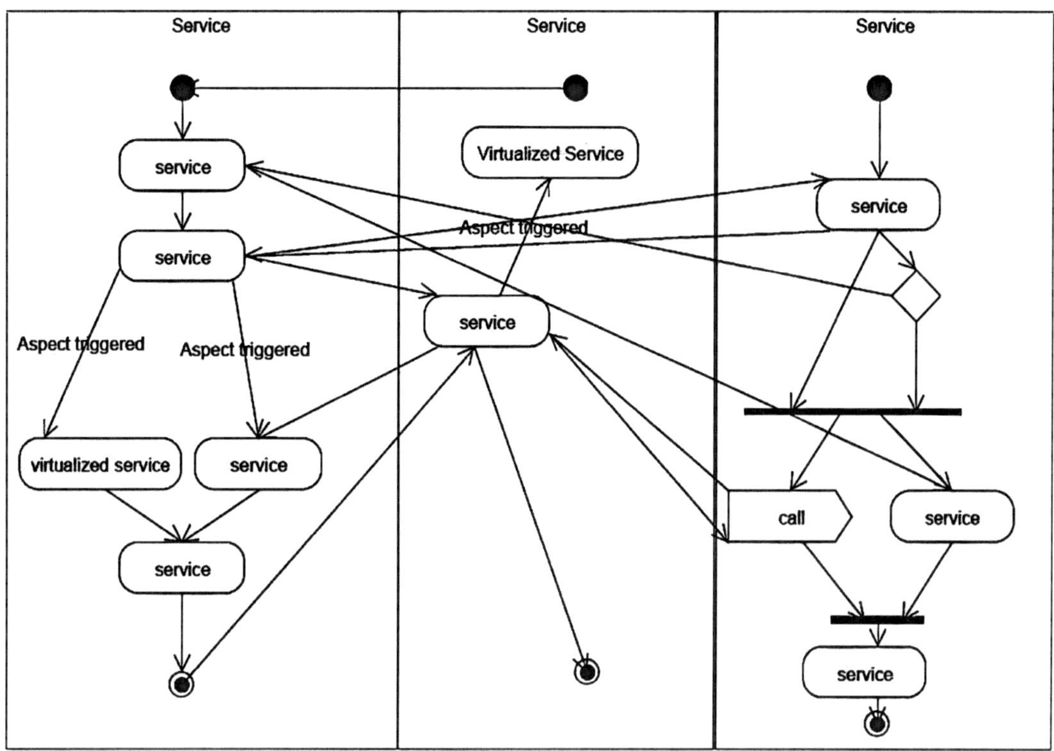

Figure 14. Patient care SaaS inventory model in cloud

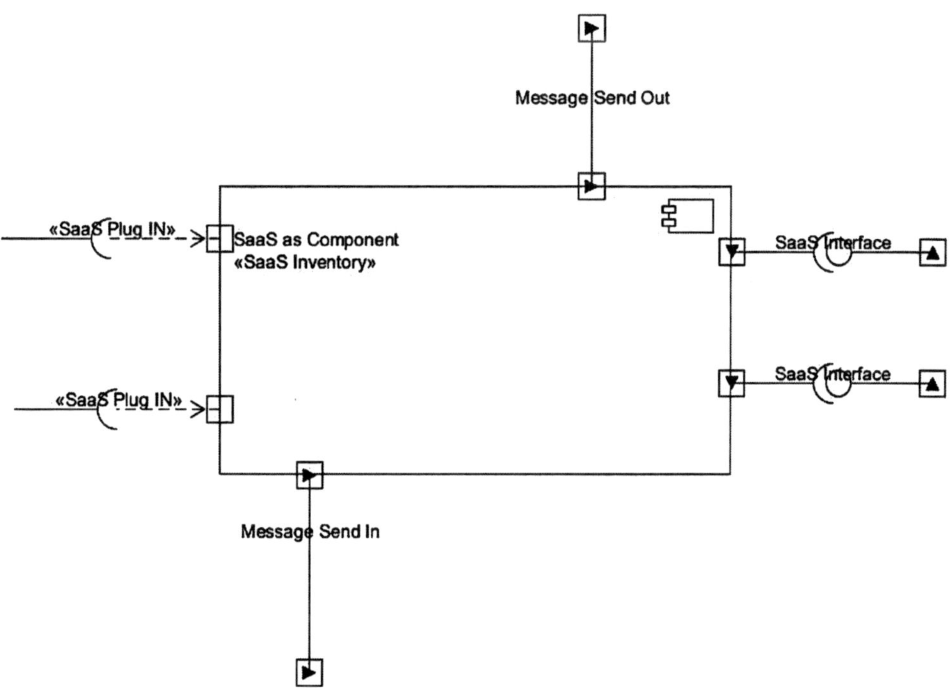

Figure 15. Inner view of the patient care SaaS inventory

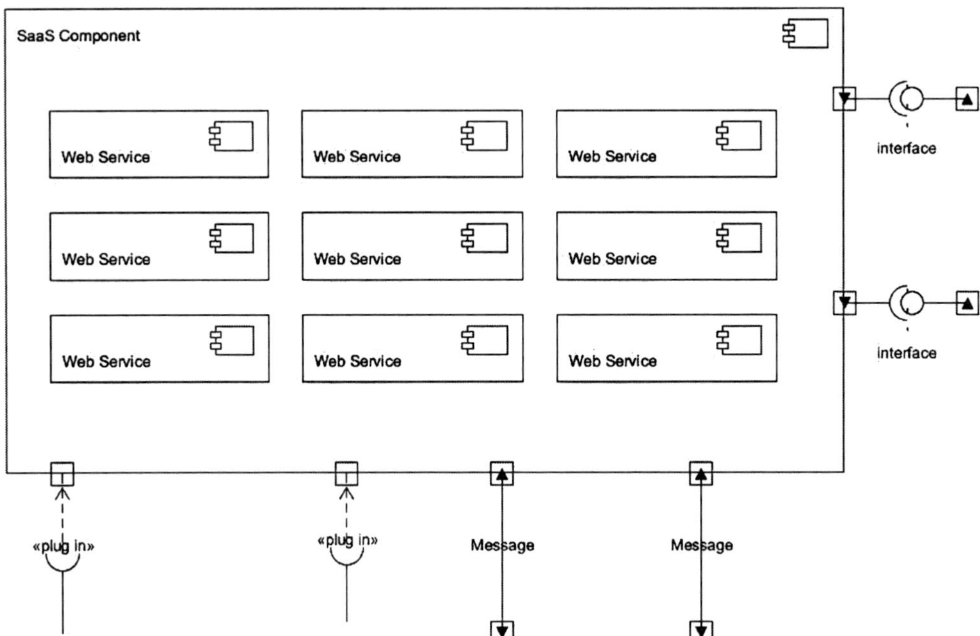

Figure 16. Outlook view of the patient care SaaS inventory

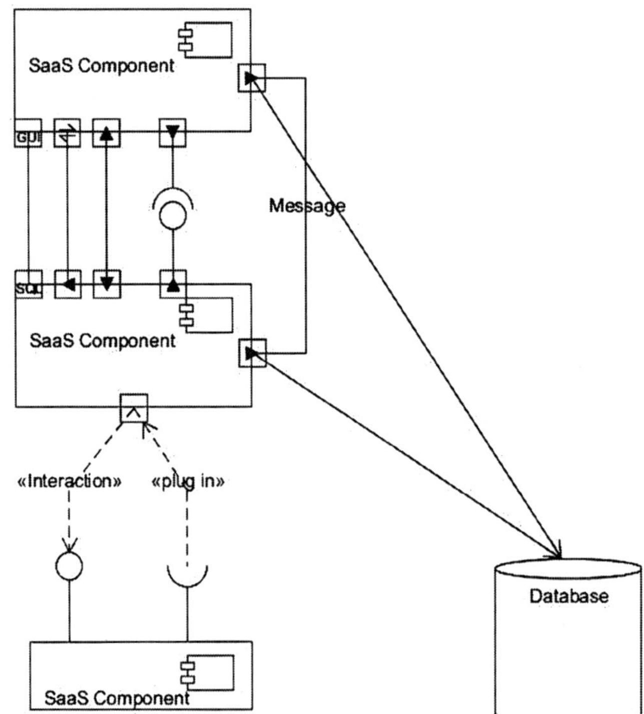

Collaboration between each SaaS component is also needed in the clouds environment. These SaaS components are distributed in different clouds like public cloud, private cloud and hybrid cloud which appear to be particularly reliant on coordination in the clouds environment. It is expected that such evolution is happened in large scale. As well, security and load balancing should be taken into consideration under such context. The collaboration evolution process means the evolution of the service are happened synergistically based on people involving to define what kind of evolution they need, in order to solve that problem we introduce evolution feature to solve such problem and that can make the approach can specifically define the evolution pattern based on people involving.[Wang, Kevin & Liu 2012,2013,2014]. The design of the web service as function is the static part of the evolution pattern while weaving the aspect by sequence is a dynamic process of the evolution pattern. Such dynamic process has its corresponding relation with the solving plan that provided by the evolution pattern description. [Wang, Kevin & Liu 2012, 2013, 2014]

IMPLEMENTATION OUTLOOK

The service evolution occurs in BPEL by using aspect oriented weaving, and the aspect can change the current BPEL behavior both in process level and java class level. Obviously, service deployed on the BPEL engine are all compiled and encapsulated class.(specifically for java based service) In order to evolve such service, we can change the BPEL process and its related service based on the knowledge of its WSDL file. The WSDL file describes which service has been invoked by the BPEL process and which function is used for parameter input and response so as to offers the detail information about the service needed to be evolved. It is showed that the upper BPEL may contain lower services process. That means the evolution can happened in large scale and deep level. [Wang, Z.Chalmers.K, 2014][Wang, Z.Chalmers.K, Liu, X2013]

This is a practical example to show the service evolution based on evolution pattern.

Figure 17. Evolution pattern for broker

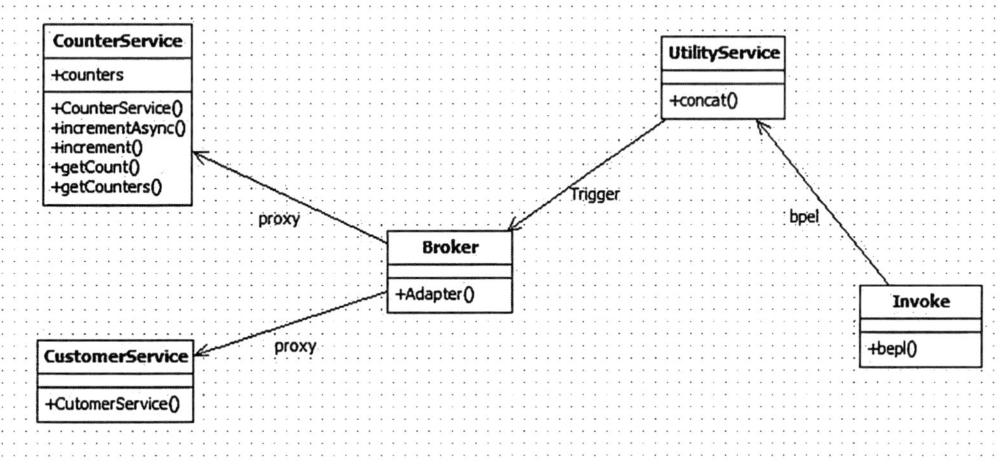

Figure 18. Result of the SaaS evolution

```
<soapenv:Envelope xmlns:soapenv="http://www.w3.org/2003/05/soap-envelope">
  <soapenv:Body>
    <odens:helloResponse xmlns:odens="http://stg.tu-darmstadt.de/ao4bpel">
      <response>Hello AO4BPEL World!
This is an AO4BPEL Around-Advice whos pointcut(xpath("process[@name="HelloWorld"]/sequence[1]/invoke[@name="invokeConcat"])).matched the activity "invokeConcat".
Response of original request (proceed): "? ?
Counter increased to: "The Broker Service has been Invoked!"
ThisJPInVariable.parameters.string1: "?"
ThisJPInVariable.parameters.string2: "?"
ThisJPActivity.process: "HelloWorld"
ThisJPActivity.type: "OInvoke"
ThisJPActivity.partnerlink: "utilityServiceLink"
ThisJPActivity.porttype: "{http://stg.tu-darmstadt.de/utilityService}UtilityServicePortType"
ThisJPActivity.operation: "concat"</response>
    </odens:helloResponse>
  </soapenv:Body>
</soapenv:Envelope>
```

EMPIRICAL EVALUATION

This approach propose a generic approach to support service evolution in dementia patient monitoring system by using service evolution pattern, the service evolution pattern and its repository is a collection of problems' solving method that specifically for service evolution in clouds, in this case we focus on the dementia patient monitoring system evolution. The evolution pattern will be realized based on the composition of all these reusable components, these components are working for both function achievement and weaving activity achievement. For function achievement, these components are mainly focus on realizing the functionality that t is designed as the solution for the problems which the evolution pattern aims at. For weaving activity achievements, these components are mainly focus on how to weave these function components into the running system as the evolution pattern designed for solving the problems. So the evolution pattern detailed design and realization will be based on two kinds of components, the function component and the weaving activity components. All these components are reusable for different evolution patterns or particularly for one of these evolution patterns, the reusability of the evolution pattern is mainly rely on the reusability of these components, for example, the re-organization evolution pattern and the re-composition evolution pattern. The detailed realization for this evolution pattern is relied on the function components and the weaving activity components that constitute the evolution pattern. Most commonly used reusable components for evolution pattern are: Function components: connector, pipe, wrapper, proxy and interceptor Weaving components: timer, selector and detector. We can used the above reusable components to constitute the evolution pattern, however some evolution patterns needs specific components for its function achievement for weaving activity achievement which are also feasible. Different combination of this reusable component can be used to generate different evolution patterns and the repository for this reusable component is also enlargeable. While, however, the above components can be further enlarged as the main innovation source we can have in the evolution pattern innovation task. One of the advantage that these components has is we can use evolution feature to select these components to further refine the evolution pattern until the pattern is suitable for solving different evolution problems. There are a process for selecting these components and refine the evolution pattern. The design and realization for these components can also be realized by the software engineering approach. [Wang, Kevin & Liu 2012, 2013, 2014]

The Evolution Life-Cycle Evaluation for Doctors, Nurses, Carers, Stakeholders in SaaS

- **Evolved Systematic Testing:** The evolved systematic testing is based on overall system testing, such as the whole SaaS inventory testing after part of the SaaS logic has been evolved. This process is to guarantee the overall service logic is working properly include the evolved service logic especially after the whole SaaS inventory logic has been evolved in its service interface, core service working flow, core service logic, etc. This testing rang is based on the overall system which means it is the last testing step before handing in the evolved system to the people, this overall testing can be separated into several testing rang based on how large the SaaS inventory it is because it is not necessary for all the service logic to be combined together to work in one service working flow in a large SaaS inventory. This kind of separated rang service testing methodology is quite useful in the clouds SaaS environments.

- **Critical Service Logic Analysis:** The critical service logic analysis is to identity which part of the SaaS inventory is under risk after evolution, or which service logic is not working properly shows by the systematic testing. This step is quite rely on the testing result report from the last step, the systematic SaaS testing, which provide the working status of the SaaS inventory. Moreover, this step also takes the currently SaaS inventory architecture into consideration which provides the architecture risk of the SaaS inventory such as load balancing burden of particular part of the SaaS inventory, security risk, service facade and core logic coupling, service facade and service contract strong coupling, service core logic and service contract strong coupling. Etc.

- **Possible Service Evolution Suggestions:** The possible service evolution suggestions is based on the previous critical service logic analysis to provide the suggestion and advice for further service evolution in order to eliminate these risks that could be happened in the future. In this step, it is

Figure 19. The patient care SaaS inventory evolution verification

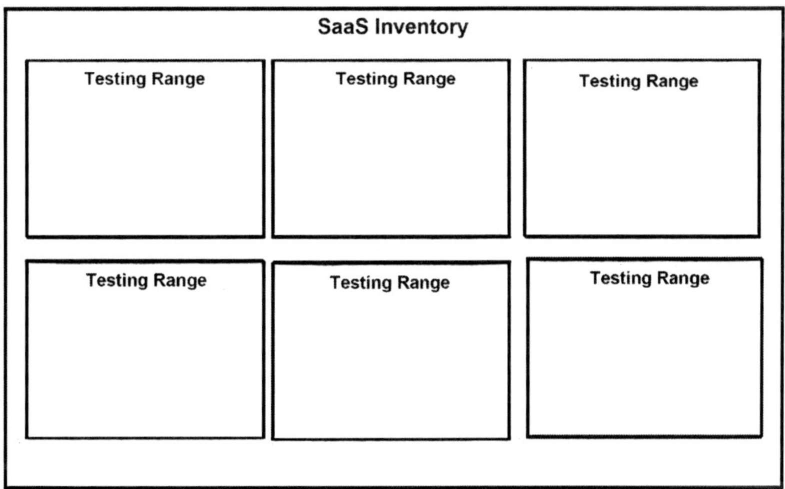

quite familiar with design a new evolution plan for the service logic system and takes the existing risks into consideration.

- **Further Service Evolution Requirement:** The further service evolution requirement is proposed by people who are continuously needs the system to be maintained. The evolution requirements are also needed to be combined with the previous analysis together in order to provide the most appropriate service evolution plan.

The whole SaaS inventory evolution life-cycle is show as the above diagram. It has the Service Evolution Requirement analysis, Service evolution plan, Systematic testing result analysis and Service evolution suggestions and risk analysis. The life-cycle is going to run in a cycle way to make the SaaS logic can continuously evolve to the maximum maintenance that people can provided.

The evolution is continuously evolving without stopping in the whole SaaS logic life-cycle.

LESSONS LEARNED

The problems domain description for service evolution in dementia patient monitoring system is needed in order to define the evolution feature that can capture the evolution requirement from people. We use these evolution features to tackle the evolution problems and choose the corresponding evolution pattern that specifically for solving this problem. So, evolution pattern for service evolution is a general method that can be further refined to solve particular service evolution problems in dementia patient monitoring system evolution.

FUTURE WORKS AND CHALLENGES

Based on the literature review so far, the proposed evolution approach will achieve effective service evolution in clouds by supporting three major features: I) Synergistic. All the stakeholders of

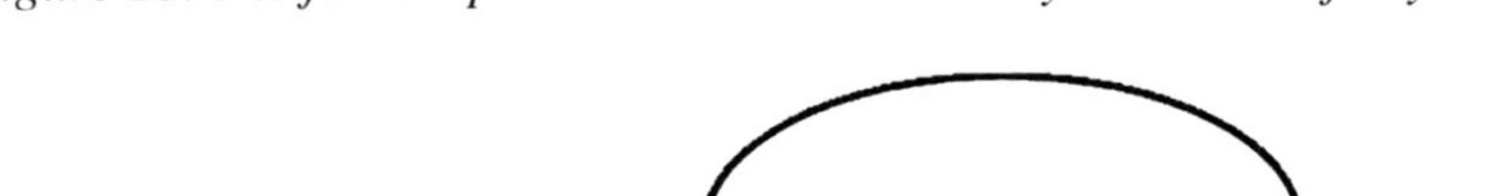

Figure 20. The further patient care SaaS inventory evolution life-cycle

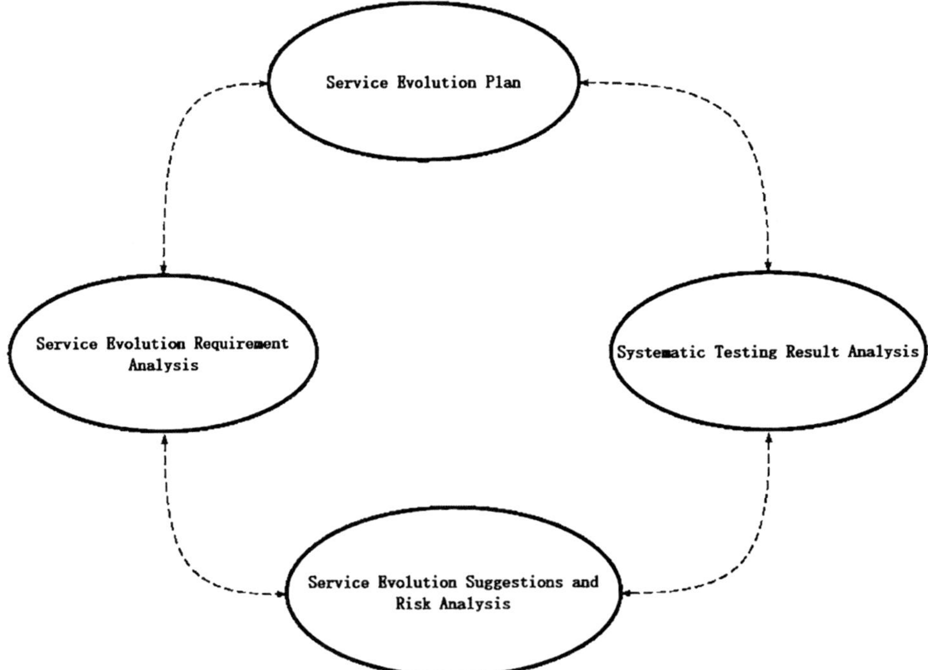

Figure 21. The patient care SaaS inventory evolution

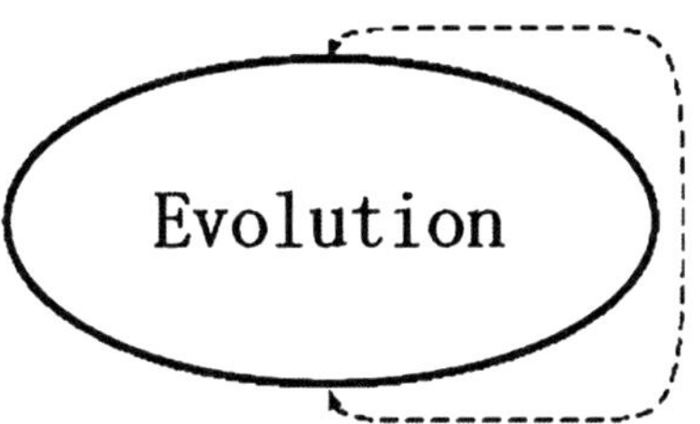

a cloud will participate in the evolution process seamlessly. The process style will be like wiki or web 2.0 styles, that is, a fluid approach with the role of user and developer integrated under the coordination of cloud manager. II) Dynamic. The whole evolution process will happen at run time with little disruption to its service. Iii) Deep and

Figure 22. The approach framework for Cloud Service evolution

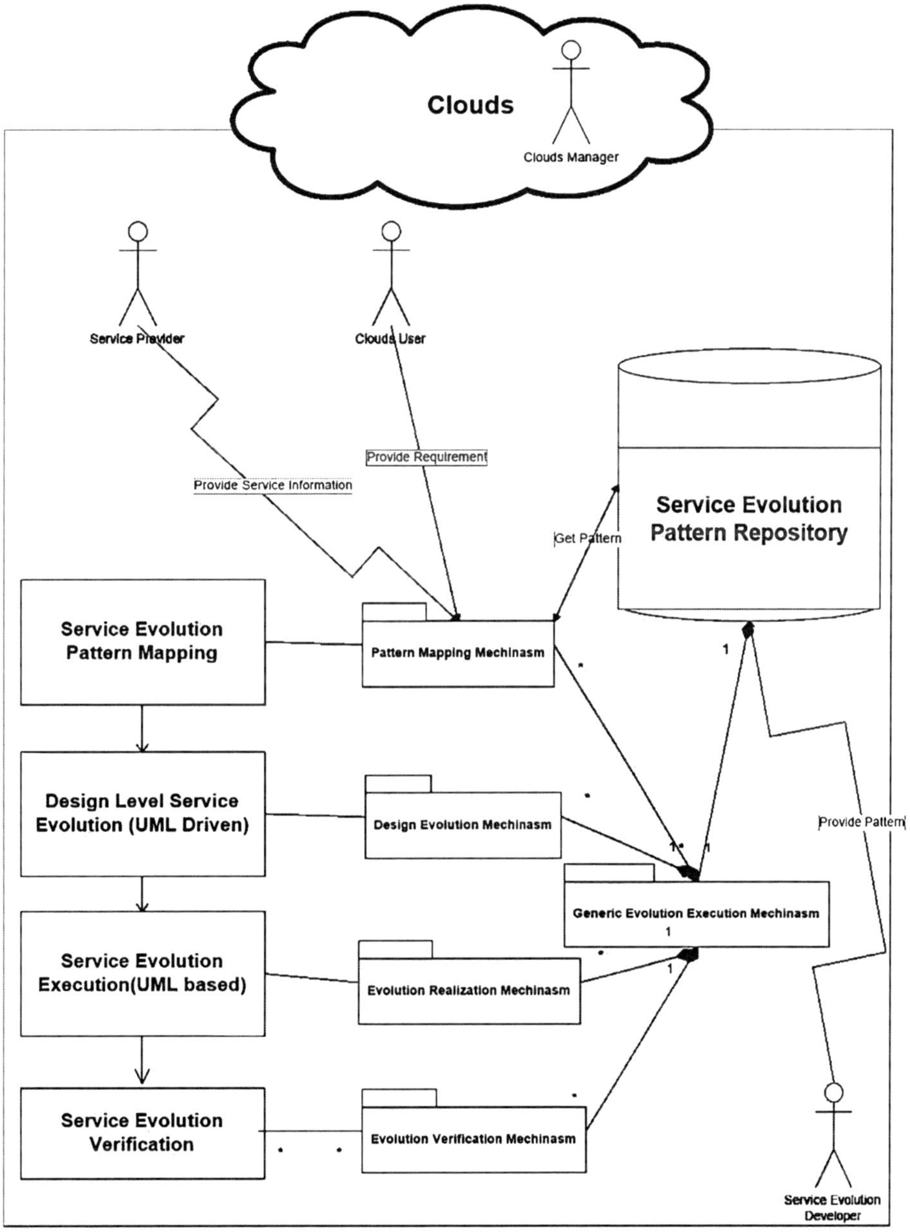

Flexible. The function, QoS and interface of SaaS will be able to be changed at a rather large scale and deep level.

Currently, we've come up with the following ideas to implement the above goals. These ideas or mechanisms are original from us.

- **Stakeholder Interaction Framework:** This will be a process and platform to support the seamless interaction between all stakeholders in clouds regarding service evolution. The interaction will be in an iterative (spiral) manner to allow the refinement and correction of evolution.
- **Evolution Patterns:** Taxonomy of typical evolution of services in clouds will be first generalized. For each type of the evolution, patterns will be developed to implement it, including the process, guideline and possible mechanism.
- **Evolution Enabling Mechanism:** To achieve dynamic and deep evolution, we need to develop appropriate methods or tools to carry out the actually evolution, e.g., via update, replacement, deletion or insertion at multiple structural levels.

The whole process will be based on a Model-Driven Architecture. The process will be driven by the Evolution Execution Mechanism automatically. The execution mechanism will be based on the MDA models In the MDA-based evolution framework, the first step is pattern mapping. The mapping will be based on the requirement proposed by the service user and the service provided by the service provider. The developer will choose a suitable pattern from the pattern repository to evolve the existing service. The pattern problem specification will help the developer to find the appropriate pattern. After the pattern has been selected, the evolution execution mechanism will start the next step which is to carry out the required evolution by updating the UML design diagrams of the services semi-automatically. The

third step is evolution realization, i.e., to propagate the changes in the service UML diagrams to service implementation in BPEL so as to realize the service evolution using BPEL mechanism.

Figure 23. The structure of a service evolution pattern

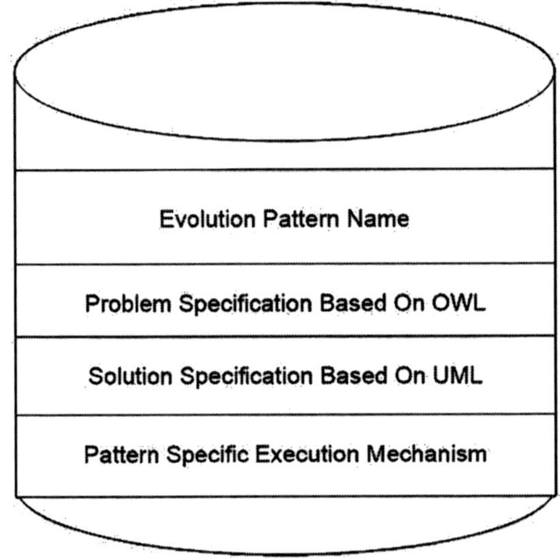

Figure 24. Taxonomy of service evolution patterns

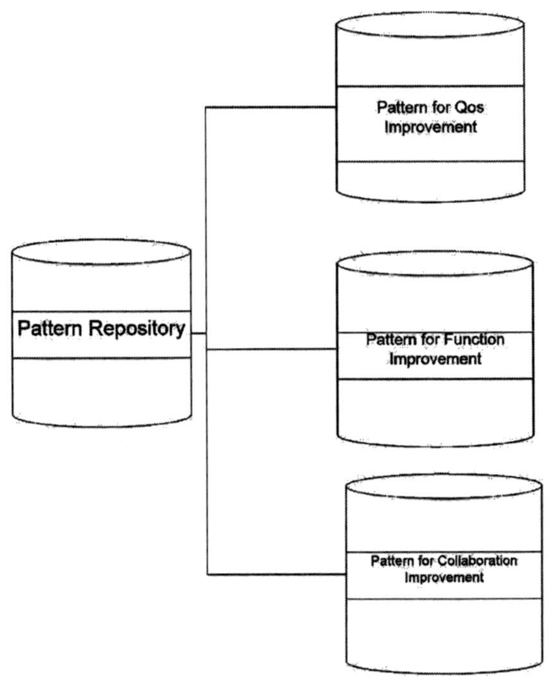

After evolution realization, the evolved services will be verified by using formal methods and software testing methods. The evolution execution mechanism will include the generic evolution execution mechanism, which is shared among all evolution patterns, and the pattern-specific evolution execution mechanism, which is defined and associated with the related pattern(s).

Evolution Pattern Structure and Taxonomy

Inside a pattern, the structure will be comprised by Pattern Name, Problem Specification, Solution Specification and Pattern Specific Evolution Mechanism. Our approach will use OWL to describe the pattern problem, and UML to describe the pattern solution. To find the appropriate pattern to a specific evolution requirement, the pattern name can give the developers a thematic idea of the pattern's purposes, and the OWL problem description can make the machine to find the specific pattern automatically. The UML model can be converted into code automatically based on the pattern evolution execution mechanism. The specific pattern execution mechanism is particularly for the related pattern execution, it will work with the generic execution mechanism together to drive the whole process.

We envision that the evolution patterns will be classified into three types: Pattern for QoS (Quality of Service) Improvement, Pattern for Function Improvement and Pattern for Collaboration Improvement, all based on the real requirements of Clouds service users. QoS, function and collaboration are the three main problems that people will face in the clouds service evolution, these patterns will enhance the service functionality and usability for specific users in their specific domain area. The evolution will make people take advantages of services in clouds as much as possible. For example, the main feature of the clouds is its collaboration environment. Services running inside the clouds should provide such ability to the users and developers and even the clouds manager in order to maximize this advantage of the clouds. QoS and functionality is the common and important feature of services, they will affect the usability mostly, so that the improving of the QoS and functionality for service is necessary.

REFERENCES

Ankolekar, A., Burstein, M., & Hobbs, J. R. (2002). DAML-S: Web service description for the semantic web. In *Proceedings of ISWC 2002* (LNCS), (vol. 2342, pp. 348-363). Berlin: Springer.

Ardagna, D., & Pernici, B. (2007). Adaptive service composition in flexible processes. *IEEE Transactions on Software Engineering, 33*(6).

Baresi, L., & Guinea, S. (2005). Towards dynamic monitoring of WS-BPEL process. In *Proceedings of ICSOC 2005* (LNCS), (vol. 3826, pp. 269-282). Berlin: Springer.

Bass, L., Clements, P., & Kazman, R. (2003). Software architecture in practice (2nd ed.). Academic Press.

Buyya, R., Yeo, C. S., & Venugopal, S. (2008). Market-oriented cloud computing: Vision, hype, and reality for delivering IT services as computing utilities. In *Proceedings of the 10th IEEE International Conference on High Performance Computing and Communications.* IEEE.

Buyya, R., Yeo, C. S., Venugopal, S., Rroberg, J., & Brandic, I. (2009). Cloud computing and emerging IT platforms: Vision, hype, and reality for delivering computing as the 5th utility. *Future Generation Computer Systems, 25*(6), 599–616. doi:10.1016/j.future.2008.12.001

Charfi, A., & Mezini, M. (2004). Aspect-oriented web service composition with AO4BPEL. In *Proceedings of ECOWS 2004* (LNCS), (vol. 3250, pp. 168-182). Berlin: Springer.

Chen, G., & Kotz, D. (2001). *A survey of context-aware mobile computing research.* Dartmouth Computer Science Technical Report TR 2000-381.

Chung, L., & Subramanian, N. (2001). Process-oriented metrics for software architcture adaptability. In *Proceedings of Fifth IEEE International Symposium.* IEEE.

Cinneide, M., & Nixon, P. (2001). Automated software evolution towards design patterns. In *Proceedings of the 4th International Workshop on Principles of Software Evolution.* Academic Press.

Costa, A., Franca, P., & Filho, P. C. L. (2001). Two-level network design with intermediate facilities: An application to electrical distribution systems. *Omega, 39*(1), 3–13. doi:10.1016/j.omega.2010.01.005

Decker, G., Kopp, O., Leymann, F., & Weske, M. (2007), BPEL4Chor: Extending BPEL for modelling choreographies. In *Proceedings of 2007 IEEE International Conference on Web Services.* IEEE. doi:10.1109/ICWS.2007.59

Dey, A. K., & Abowd, G. D. (1999). Towards a better understanding of context and context-awareness. In *Proceedings of the 1st International Symposium on Handheld and Ubiquitous Computing.* Academic Press.

Emmerich, W., Butchart, B., & Chen, L. (2006). Grid service orchestration using the business process execution language (BPEL). *Journal of Grid Computing, 3,* 283-304. DOI:10.1007/s10723-005-9015-3

Fitscapes, F. (2004). Network. *Distributed Computing.*

Foster, H., Uchitel, S., Magee, J., & Kramer, J. (2003), Model-based verification of web service compositions. In *Proceedings of the 18th IEEE International Conference on Automated Software Engineering* (ASE 03). IEEE. doi:10.1109/ASE.2003.1240303

Foster, I., Zhao, Y., Raicu, I., & Lu, S. (2009). Cloud computing and grid computing 360-degree compared. In *Proceedings of Grid Computing Environments Workshop.* Academic Press.

Garlan, D., & Schmerl, B. (2009). A tool for defining and planning architecture evolution. IEEE.

Gibbins, N., Harris, S., & Shadbolt, N. (2003). Agent-based semantic web services. In *Proceedings of the 12th International Conference on World Wide Web.* Academic Press.

Jaroucheh, Z., Liu, X., & Smith, S. (2010), A MDD-based generic framework for context-aware deeply adaptive service-based processes. In *Proceedings of 8th IEEE International Conference on Web Services.* IEEE. doi:10.1109/ICWS.2010.16

John, D. (2001). Model-driven architecture: Vision, standards, and emerging technologies. In *Proceedings of Workshop on Metamodeling and Adaptive Object Models.* Academic Press.

Karanam, M., & Akepogu, A. (2009). Model-driven software evolution: The multiple views. In *Proceedings of the International Multi Conference of Engineering and Computer Scientists.* Academic Press.

Koch, S. (2005). Evolution of open source software systems-A large-scale investigation. In *Proceedings of the First International Conference on Open Source Systems Genova.* Academic Press.

Lee, G. M., & Crespi, N. (2010). Shaping future service environments with the cloud and internet of things: Networking challenges and service evolution, leveraging applications of formal methods, verification, and validation. *Lecture Notes in Computer Science,* 6415.

Leitner, P. (2009). Efficient dynamic web service invocation. *IEEE Internet Computing, 13*(3), 72–80. doi:10.1109/MIC.2009.57

Linthicum, D. (2009). *Cloud computing and SOA convergence in your enterprise –A step-by-step guide*. Academic Press.

Liu, X., Feng, Y., & Kerridge, J. (2008a). Generative aspect-oriented component adaptation. *IET Software, 2*(2).

Liu, X., Feng, Y., & Kerridge, J. (2008b). Automated responsive web services evolution through generative aspect-oriented component adaptation. *International Journal of Computer Applications in Technology, 31*(1/2).

Lucchi, R., & Mazzara, M. (2007). A pi-calculus based semantics for WS-BPEL. *Journal of Logic and Algebraic Programming,* 96-118.

Michel, R. V., Clemens, C., & Reussner, R. S. (Eds.). (2008). Component-based software engineering. In *Proceedings of 11th International Symposium*. CBSE.

Omasreiter, H., Metzker, E., & Chrysler, D. (2004). A context-driven use case creation process for specifying automotive driver assistance systems. In *Proceedings of the 12th IEEE International Requirements Engineering Conference (RE 04). IEEE*. doi:10.1109/ICRE.2004.1335692

Oreizy, P. (1998). Decentralized software evolution. In *Proceedings of the International Conference on the Principles of Software Evolution (IWPSE 1)*. Academic Press.

Paolucci, M., Kawamura, T., Terry, R. P., & Sycara, K. (2002). Semantic matching of web services capabilities. In *Proceedings of ISWC 2002* (LNCS), (vol. 2342, pp. 333-347). Berlin: Springer.

Pearson, S., Shen, Y., & Mowbray, M. (2009). A Privacy manager for cloud computing, cloud computing. *Lecture Notes in Computer Science,* 5931.

Pillai, P., Huang, H., & Kang, G. S. (2003). Energy-aware quality of service adaption. *ADA462108*.

Preuveneers, D., & Berbers, Y. (2005). Automated context-driven composition of pervasive services to alleviate non-functional concerns. *International Journal of Computing & Information Sciences, 3*(2).

Qian, Y., Zhang, S., & Qi, Z. (2008). Mining change patterns in aspectj software evolution. In *Proceedings of International Conference on Computer Science and Software Engineering*. Academic Press. doi:10.1109/CSSE.2008.802

Qu, Y. C., Dumas, M., Breutel, S., & Hofstede, A. T. (2006). Translating standard process models to BPEL. In *Proceedings of CAiSE'06* (LNCS), (vol. 4001, pp. 417-432). Berlin: Springer.

Rajan, H., & Hosamani, M. (2009). Tisa: Toward trustworthy services in a service-oriented architecture. *IEEE Transactions on Services Computing, 1*(4).

Rosenthal, A., Mork, P., Li, M. H., Stanford, J., Koester, D., & Reynolds, P. (2010). Cloud computing: A new business paradigm for biomedical information sharing. *Journal of Biomedical Informatics, 43*(2), 342–353. doi:10.1016/j.jbi.2009.08.014 PMID:19715773

Schilit, B., Adams, N., & Want, R. (1994). Context-aware computing applications - Mobile computing systems and applications. In Proceedings of WMCSA'94. Academic Press.

Shaw, M., & Garlan, D. (2001). *Software architecture – Perspective on an emerging discipline*. Prentice Hall, Pearson Education.

Sindhgatta, R., Nanjangud, C., & Sengupta, B. (2010). Software evolution in agile development: A case Study. In *Proceedings of the ACM International Conference Companion on Object Oriented Programming Systems Languages and Applications Companion. Academic Press*. doi:10.1145/1869542.1869560

Sultan, N. (2010). Cloud computing for education: A new dawn? *International Journal of Information Management, 30*(2), 109–116. doi:10.1016/j.ijinfomgt.2009.09.004

Takabi, H., Joshi, J. B. D., & Ahn, G. (2010). Security and privacy challenges in cloud computing environments. *IEEE Security and Privacy, 8*(6), 24–31. doi:10.1109/MSP.2010.186

Tourwe, T. (2003). *Automated support for framework-based software evolution.* (PhD Dissertation). Programming Technology Laboratory, Vrije University, Brussels, Belgium.

Walkerdine, J., Hutchinson, J., Sawyer, P., Dobson, G., & Oniti, V. (2008). A faceted approach to service specification, Q A76 *Computer software,* ID code 1858.

Wang, Z., & Chalmers, K. (2013). Evolution feature oriented model driven product line engineering approach for synergistic and dynamic service evolution in Clouds:AO4BPEL3.0 proposal. In *Proceedings of International Conference on Information Society (i-Society 2013).* Toronto, Canada: IEEE.

Wang, Z., & Chalmers, K. (2013). Evolution feature oriented model driven product line engineering approach for synergistic and dynamic service evolution in clouds: Four kinds of schema. In *Proceedings of the 4th International Conference on Ambient Systems, Networks and Technologies.* Halifax, Canada: Procedia Computer Science.

Wang, Z., & Chalmers, K. (2013). Evolution feature oriented model driven product line engineering approach for synergistic and dynamic service evolution in clouds: Pattern data structure. In *Proceedings of the 7th International Conference on Complex, Intelligent, and Software Intensive Systeme (CISIS 2013).* IEEE Computational Intelligence Society.

Wang, Z., Chalmers, K., & Cheng, G. (2013). Evolution feature oriented model driven product line engineering approach for synergistic and dynamic service evolution in clouds. *Journal of Industrial and Intelligent Information, 1*(1).

Wang, Z., Chalmers, K., & Kennedy, J. (2014). *An approach to synergistic and dynamic service evolution in clouds.* Inderscience Publishers.

Wang, Z., Chalmers, K., & Liu, X. (2014). Evolution pattern verification for services evolution in clouds with model driven architecture. International Journal for e-Learning Security, 3(3/4).

Wang, Z., Liu, X., Chalmers, K., & Cheng, G. (2012). Evolution pattern for service evolution in clouds. In *Proceedings of the 7th International Conference for Internet Technology and Secured Transactions* (ICITST-2012). London, UK: IEEE.

White, S.A. (2005, March). Using BPMN to model a BPEL process. *BP Trends.*

Yu, B. G., & Wang, X. Z. (2007). *Design and implementation of transaction process system for SOA, VOL 24 NO 11.* Application Research of Computers.

KEY TERMS AND DEFINITIONS

Aspect Generation: Aspect generation is using the model based product line engineering method for aspect code generation.

Aspect Repository: Aspect Repository is used to store the reusable aspect for service evolution.

Aspect Weaving: Aspect weaving is the process of weaving the aspect into the service logic in SaaS.

BEPL: Business Process Execution Language.

Business Process Execution Language: The business process execution language is the service logic execution description language that specific the service logic execution sequence and it needs BPEL engine to execute.

Clouds: Clouds mean several clouds working together by collaboration through the service contained by each cloud.

Dynamic: The dynamic evolution of the service means the changing of the service interface, the changing of the service underlying logic, the changing of the service architecture, the changing of the service orchestration or even the changing of the component that constitute the service are all happened seamlessly based on the AO4PEL3.0 platform we have without shut down the current BEPL process.

Evolution Feature: Evolution Feature is the feature for describing the evolution pattern initial model design.

Evolution Mechanism: Evolution mechanism includes evolution aspect generation and evolution aspect execution.

Evolution Pattern: Evolution pattern is the solution that for solving specific kind of evolution problem.

Evolution Requirement: Evolution requirement is proposed by the user as the demands for service evolution.

Evolution Verification: Evolution verification includes service verification and evolution requirement realization verification.

Evolution: Evolution for the service in clouds is specifically means the changing of the service interface, the changing of the service underlying logic, the changing of the service architecture, the changing of the service orchestration or even the changing of the component that constitute the service.

Fault Handling: Fault handling for service is the evolution process that enhance the service fault handing ability.

Intercepter: Intercepter is used to intercept the message sending between component or service logic in SaaS.

Inventory Application: Inventory Application is the SaaS application that implemented based on Service Inventory.

MDA: Model Driven Architecture.

Message: Message is a data structure for exchanging information between components and service logic.

Model Driven Architecture: Model Driven Architecture is the architecture to implement the software system based on modeling from platform independent to platform dependent.

Requirement Analysis: Requirement analysis is an essential process in Software Engineering for getting the right software requirement information from user.

SaaS: Software as Service.

Security Enhancement: Security enhancement is the evolution process that can enhance the software system's security ability.

Service Bottleneck: Service bottleneck is the limitation of accessing to some services in some overloading period.

Service Façade: Service Façade is the wrapper for service in order to hidden the inside details of the service.

Service Inventory: Service Inventory is the gathering of the related services that belongs to specific enterprise or organization.

Service Reusability: Service reusability is the ability that the service can be reused.

Service Reuse: Service reuse is to reuse the service logic that is reusable in order to enhance the software development efficiency.

Service Usability: Service usability is the level of using the service by people in maximum in every circumstance.

Service Virtualization: Service virtualization is the virtualization for some service to enhance its accessing ability during overloading time.

Service: Service in service-oriented architecture (SOA) and clouds is means software logic. Service in clouds can contain a single software component or many services orchestrated by BPEL engine.

Synergistic: The synergistic evolution process means the evolution of the service happened synergistically based on people involving to define what kind of evolution they need, we introduce evolution feature to solve such problem and how to specifically define the evolution pattern based on people involving, we introduce model-driven product line engineering to solve such problem.

Web Service: Web service is create based on the component technology and deployed to the web for open accessing by soap messaging.

Wrapper: Sometimes called Adapter which used for making the various types component can be compatible with each other.

This work was previously published in Advanced Technological Solutions for E-Health and Dementia Patient Monitoring edited by Fatos Xhafa, Philip Moore, and George Tadros, pages 153-182 copyright year 2015 by Medical Information Science Reference (an imprint of IGI Global).

Chapter 81
Analysis and Linkage of Data from Patient–Controlled Self–Monitoring Devices and Personal Health Records

Chris Paton
University of Oxford, UK

ABSTRACT

This chapter outlines the recent advances in self-tracking technology both for wellness and healthcare purposes. It addresses one of the key challenges in mobile health: how to link the data from self-tracking devices with data in clinical data systems, such as Personal Health Records and Electronic Health Records systems. This chapter also discusses advances in visualisation and analysis for personally controlled data from self-tracking and PHR systems.

INTRODUCTION

In recent years, a large number of personal self-tracking devices have emerged onto the consumer marketplace (Swan, 2009). Self-tracking devices cover a wide range but include devices that measure activity using accelerometers to disposable stick-on patches that measure ECG readings. The vast majority of these devices are used for the purposes of monitoring exercise for fitness and weight-loss, but a significant minority is used for monitoring a range of health conditions including diabetes (Gross, Levin, Mulvihill, Richardson, & Davidson, 1984), COPD (Koff, Jones, Cashman, Voelkel, & Vandivier, 2009), heart failure (Klersy, De Silvestri, Gabutti, Regoli, & Auricchio, 2009) and Parkinson's disease (Little, McSharry, Hunter, Spielman, & Ramig, 2009), to choose a few examples.

In this chapter, we discuss the current landscape of self-tracking devices and examine how the data collected from such devices could be integrated into the clinical health record of the patient or consumer thereby making the data more useful for management of chronic conditions and maintaining good health.

DOI: 10.4018/978-1-4666-8756-1.ch081

Self-Tracking for Wellness

By far the most prevalent group of self-trackers are the fitness fanatics, dieters and "worried well". Arguably, this is also the group where self-tracking can have the largest impact on the health of the individuals and the state of the healthcare system. The personal health benefits of keeping fit and active have long been established (Franco et al., 2005). These include a lower risk of cardiovascular disease (Thompson et al., 2003), cancer (Thune & Furberg, 2001) and diabetes (Manson et al., 1991). From wider societal point of view, by remaining fitter for longer healthy individuals present a lower burden on healthcare services, take less sick-days (Proper, Van den Heuvel, De Vroome, Hildebrandt, & Van der Beek, 2006) and are able to take up caring and support roles longer into their retirement than individuals who take less exercise.

Evidence is emerging that self-tracking offers an increased incentive to keep fit and healthy over not self-tracking by increasing motivation through a process of feedback and a range of gaming effects (Swan, 2009). It will always be difficult to determine a clear link between increased take up of self-tracking technology for health and fitness and the general trend to increased exercise and health-consciousness among affluent consumers. However, recent behaviour change models may be able to demonstrate why this type of technology is enabling people to lead healthier lives. The Fogg behaviour model (Fogg, 2009) outlines a combination of three factors that influence whether or not an individual is likely to change behaviour: motivation, ability and triggers.

Self-tracking equipment has effects in all three of these domains:

Motivation

Many self-tracking tools have a "gamification" (McCallum, 2012) element built into them that can motivate users to compete both with themselves and other users through social networking platforms. For example, the Nike+ Fuelband® will display "points" on the LCD display mounted on the wristband that users can earn through increasing activity levels.

GPS tracker users can upload their GPS data from recent runs and share them with the community of users at Runkeeper.com. This could prove to be a powerful source of motivation as they become part of a community that congratulates and challenges each other to run further and faster.

Ability

Adopting a healthy lifestyle is a difficult challenge for most people. Certain types of self-tracking technology can make this transition easier by offering simple tools that replace the more difficult to maintain paper based systems of recording weights or activity levels. As discussed later in this chapter, the integration of data from self-tracking devices with clinical IT systems may be able to make the transition easier through advice from healthcare professionals on easier and more effective ways to maintain health and fitness that may not have been previously identified by patients.

Triggers

The Fogg model identifies triggers as a key to behaviour change (Fogg, 2009). Even if an individual has a high level of motivation and user-friendly tools that make the behaviour change easy to do, they still require a well-timed trigger to initiative the change. By using reminders and alerts, an ecosystem of technology that uses self-tracking devices, smartphone applications and web-based portals, individuals will be able to create triggers for exercise and activity that fit in with their daily regimens.

Self-Tracking for Long Term Conditions

Many of the positive behaviour changes established for currently healthy self-trackers also apply for patients with long-term conditions. There is increasing evidence that adoption of a healthy diet and exercise regime can help alleviate symptoms in a wide variety of long-term conditions from heart failure to diabetes (Stewart et al., 1994).

However, patients with long-term conditions may also gain additional benefits from self-tracking such as better management and adherence to medications (Smith et al., 2006) and informed decision making by their healthcare professionals who may have access to more accurate and more highly granular data. A short vignette outlines some of these benefits:

Mrs X is a patient with hypertension who is often nervous when her doctor takes her blood pressure. Over the past six months, she has been using a bluetooth home blood pressure monitor that connects wirelessly to her phone. She pulls out her phone and taps on the blood pressure app that shows the doctor her readings since her last visit. Even though her blood pressure was recorded as high by the doctor, the fact that most of her home recordings were within an acceptable range reassures the doctor that he doesn't need to prescribe any new medications or increase her dosage of medications.

Remote monitoring for patients with long-term conditions has a long and venerable history (Picot, 1998). Many patients with diabetes have long been adjusting their medication doses based on readings from home blood glucose monitors (Kovatchev, Cox, Gonder-Frederick, & Clarke, 2002), patients with COPD often alter their daily dose of steroids depending on readings from a home spirometer or peak flow meter (Khdour et al., 2011) and patients with heart failure often use daily weight readings to adjust the level of diuretics they require to keep their fluid levels in check (Klersy et al., 2009).

With more modern tools, these patients and more are now using a range of portable and connected electronic devices to make taking these measures less burdensome and allowing more rapid use of the data by health professionals. In-

stead of needing to bring in a long list of recordings on a piece of paper, the doctor can often view from her office the current readings of patients who are monitoring them through a web-based portal.

SELF-TRACKING TECHNOLOGY

Self-tracking technology is rapidly advancing and a variety of different types of sensor can be integrated in a number of configurations. In this section, we outline some of the commonly used sensors by health-trackers although there are many more highly specific sensors becoming available for certain diseases and conditions.

Self-Tracking Using Built in Smartphone Sensors

Probably the most accessible item of self-tracking hardware is the one a significant proportion of people already own: the smartphone.

Since the introduction of the iPhone in 2007, the smartphone sector has accelerated rapidly with fierce and growing competition between the Apple iOS operating system and the Google-backed Android Open Source platform. Data on smartphone uptake has shown that the majority of phones now being sold are Smartphones, with Android at more the 80% market share (but with Apple taking the lion's share of the profits).

GPS

Most smartphones now include the Global Positioning System (GPS) method of tracking location. Although primarily used for driving directions, GPS can also be harnessed for self-tracking for health and wellness purposes. For example, using the RunKeeper app, a wellness enthusiast can generate maps of runs completed with timings. These can also be shared with other users of RunKeeper on their website.

The GPS sensor can also be used in a number of long-term conditions. For patients suffering from dementia, the GPS sensor on their phone could be used to alert carers if they have wandered off and may need assistance (Bail, 2003). The GPS sensor could also be used to determine whether or not patients are becoming less active and more housebound - this could be an indication of a general deterioration in physical or mental health.

Accelerometer

As well as tracking location through GPS, smartphones are also equipped with an accelerometer that measures the acceleration of the devices across multiple axes of movement. By combining this data with computer algorithms, it is possible to detect the number of steps a person makes during a day, transforming the phone into a pedometer.

This can be used by runners, but also by people with long term conditions such as heart failure who want to maintain a reasonable level of activity but are not wanting to track a pre-determined route.

The accelerometer function can also be used to power sleep-tracking applications. If the smartphone is placed on the bed, the accelerometer can detect movement and hence calculate periods of deep sleep, light-sleep or wakefulness during the night.

Camera

The smartphone camera has a number of applications for self-tracking from the relatively basic snapping of photos of food to keep a food diary to the relatively advanced photoplethysmography applications that use a smartphone camera to determine a patient's pulse rate by the changes in colour caused by tiny blood vessels in their face.

One example is the Foodswitch application that uses the smartphone's camera to scan barcodes in supermarkets to help individual choose healthier meal options (Armstrong, 2012).

Microphone

The smartphone's microphone can also be used as a sensor, picking up ambient sounds to track activities such as mealtimes, exercise or bodily functions. Sonouroflow uses the smartphone's microphone to listen to micturition noises to diagnose prostatic hypertrophy (Zvarova et al., 2011), for example. With improving machine learning algorithms, it is anticipated that the microphone will be able to interpret more activities of daily living and begin to pick up other diagnostic indicators such as heart sounds and breath sounds (Comtois, Salisbury, & Sun, 2012).

Peripheral and Independent Self-Tracking Devices

A number of home monitoring devices and pieces of self-tracking equipment can now be linked via bluetooth to a smartphone (Bluetooth, 2007). This enables users of the devices to use the smartphone to store their readings and view their data. Data collected in this way also offers the opportunity to be linked to electronic health records (described later in this chapter).

Health and Fitness Devices

These types of devices are normally targeted at well individuals looking to increase their fitness and general level of health.

Some of the most commonly used pieces of self-tracking equipment are activity trackers that often take the form of a wristband, pendant or bracelet. These devices usually contain an accelerometer which can be used to track steps and other forms of activity such as time spent in various stages of sleep. By linking with a smartphone via bluetooth, data collected by these devices are immediately viewable and can be edited, annotated or stored by users.

The number of devices classified as 'wearable technology' is rapidly increasing and there are now a number of manufacturers of items of clothing that contain sensors that can be linked to a smartphone. These so called "smartclothes" can detect heart rate, breathing rate and activity when worn as a bra, vest or t-shirt. Socks have been developed that can track activity and numerous other smartclothes are under development with more advanced medical applications. Even diapers are now available as 'smartdiapers' that electronically record an infants bowel and urinary functions (Yambem, Yapici, & Zou, 2008).

Devices for Patients with Medical Conditions

Home monitoring equipment, such as a home blood pressure monitor or weighing scales, have been used by patients to track their health for many years. These devices used to require patients to record their readings in a journal that they could then take with them to their healthcare provider to get advice on managing their conditions.

More recently, however, it has become possible to link such devices with smartphones and tablet PCs to enable the automatic recording of readings and provide feedback to patients when they review their data.

Devices such as implantable cardioverter-defibrillators (ICDs) often contain transmitters that enable the collection of data from the devices. Home monitoring equipment is available that enables patients to transmit the data from their implanted devices on a continuous or intermittent basis.

DATA LINKAGE

Most self-tracking and self-monitoring equipment is designed to be used as a stand-alone device or in a relatively closed ecosystem. For self-tracking bands and pendants, this usually involves the device, and smartphone app and sometimes a website, where data from the smartphone is uploaded into the "cloud" for viewing on the site.

Personal Health Records and Patient Portals

There have been several attempts over recent years of better integrating home monitoring devices used by patients with long-term conditions to clinical IT systems. Some of these show significant promise and appear to be growing in popularity. These systems are often described as Personal Health Records. As well as uploading data, individuals have been encouraged to add descriptive information about their health status and updates on their symptoms or subjective assessment of the health state.

Some of the more high profile PHR endeavors include:

HealthVault

HealthVault (www.healthvault.com) made available a proprietary standard that allowed device manufacturers to allow their users to upload data from their devices to their computers and on, through a internet connection, to the HealthVault website.

Dossia

Dossia (www.dossia.com) is a PHR platform that uses Open Source software to integrate data from a wide variety of healthcare systems with the aim of providing patients with a view of their data, even if it is stored in different organisation's systems.

Google Health

Google Health was a web-based portal that aimed to give patients a place to manually enter details about their health status and to access to health records stored in providers systems that had partnered with Google.

In addition to specific PHR platforms such as those described above many electronic health record vendors and healthcare providers are offering a portal service to patients. These "patient portals" may prove easier to implement and adopt as they are often included as standard in many new EHR installations and, particularly in the UK, the government mandates seem more directed towards providing a view into the patients data rather than a method of contributing data to the system.

Standards for Data Linkage

A wide range of standards has been developed in the healthcare sector of a period of many years. Theses standards were initially developed as messaging protocols to allow medical information to be securely transferred from one system to another. For example, if a hospital laboratory wanted to send their results from their computer system to the system used to administer patients they could format the message in a standardised format that could be read by the other system. Over time, these standards have evolved to include storage as well as messaging and common language or terminology structures have been developed.

HL7 is the most dominant standards set in use in medical informatics today although there are many others with various degrees of overlapping and extended functionality including OpenEHR, IHE, DICOM and CEN. In its latest incarnation (Version 3), HL7 offers an XML based protocol linked to a reference information model (RIM) and common terminology descriptions (using SNOMED-CT) to ensure that medical information conveyed in HL7 messages adhere to a common structure. This means that, for example, a Blood Pressure reading (or any other measurement or term) is recognised as a well-defined concept in other systems that are connecting using HL7 messaging or storage. These allow "semantic interoperability" where the different systems share an understanding of the meaning of the data in the medical context.

Non-Standard Meta-Data

Although many medical systems are adherent to standards like HL7, many home-based monitoring devices and almost all self-tracking devices are not compliant. However, it is not necessary for systems to adhere to the standards as long as appropriate meta-data are attached to data. This is because data can easily be translated using an integration engine such as Mirth from one structure to another as long as the data structures are adherent to a meta-data format that means that mapping can take place.

It is often argued that a lack of health IT standards it the reason why patient-held information is not integrated into clinical systems, but as long as the data are described in meta-data, it should not be an impediment to integration.

DATA ANALYSIS

As these data are collected and integrated there is a danger that both patients and clinicians will become overloaded with the information generated.

Data Visualisation

Instead of presenting data as long lists or tables, it is often more useful for both patients and doctors to present data in the form of charts and diagrams. There has been good progress on data-visualisation by self-tracking equipment providers and PHR providers.

Algorithms

If the data is especially complicated and difficult to understand, it is often useful to reduce the data down using algorithms to a score or summary of the activity or health state. For fitness users, the Nike + Fuelband generates a score rather than the number of steps or GPS route a person has taken. This score is calculated by means of a proprietary algorithm that the manufacturers feel represents a "good" or "bad" level of activity. For patients with long term conditions, there are a number of well established risk scoring systems in the medical literature that can not only summarise complex data but that can be predictive for future events such as risk of heart attack, stroke or hospital admission.

Decision Support Systems

As algorithms become more advanced it may be possible to further reduce the need to present the data to patients and clinicians. What is really needed by users are appropriate alerts and messages that convey the information about the current health state of an individual and trends that may indicate a need for action or intervention. This means that instead of presenting data, either as a chart or table of numbers, it may be preferable to provide alerts and suggestions for altering current treatments, dosages or activities.

For example, if a patient with heart failure begins to become fluid overloaded due to a decrease in the heart function, it may be preferable to simply suggest an increase in dose of medication to the patient while the trend could be presented to the clinician as alert in case a more drastic change in management is required.

One interesting possibility for decision support is the generation of interventions based on "all the data" mapped to health outcomes. The deterioration of a patient is often the result of a multitude of factors some of which may be measured and some of which will not be. With appropriate machine learning technology, it may be possible to data-mine a population of patients to work out correlations between patterns across a range of data inputs (wearable sensors, clinical data form the EHR, demographic data, genomic data, etc.) that do not currently fit our medical model of diagnoses and treating disease. If certain patterns are highly correlated with certain outcomes, it may be possible to intervene with treatment at an earlier stage in a disease process to reduce negative outcomes for patients by spotting the development of these patterns in real time.

DISCUSSION

Two major developments have presented the potential for a merging of personally collected health and lifestyle data and clinical data collected by healthcare professionals:

Wearable Technology

Following Moore's Law, microprocessors are getting smaller and cheaper at an exponential rate. The technology that enables the collection and wireless transmission of data from biometric sensors is now of a small enough size and costs that devices can be manufactured that can fit comfortably into a wristband or wearable pendant. These tiny sensors can be linked to smartphones and tablet computers to enable transmission of the data to the cloud for further review and analysis.

Electronic Health Records

Countries around the world have now adopted Electronic Health Records in their national hospital systems and individual doctors and clinicians use Electronic Medical Records for managing their patients and record keeping. These systems are now becoming increasingly interconnected and many large-scale data aggregation projects are now in motion.

In the US, the HITECH Act (Blumenthal, 2010), part of the Obama stimulus package, has given doctors and hospitals access to over $20 billion to enable them to purchase and install electronic health records systems. As part of the conditions of these grants, these hospitals have to open up their systems for access by patients and be able to share their records with the government and other healthcare providers. This data sharing has promoted the adoption of terminology and interoperability standards such as Health Level 7 and SNOMED-CT.

In the UK, the NHS has been digitising hospital records systems for the last 10 years and is now in the process of creating new data extraction services to pull data from GP systems (Health and Social Care Information Centre, 2013). They have also created a mandate to allow patients access to their electronic health records and have a number of projects that utilise health IT standards to enabling better access to services and transparency of data.

As these two technology trends proceed, it will become inevitable that the demand for data integration will increase. The standards and tools discussed in the previous section will be important for allowing this to happen but a number of socio-political issues will also need to be addressed including data security and privacy and how to better provide personalised services to patients based on their longitudinal readings and lifestyle choices.

CONCLUSION

The rapid growth in wearable technology and the use of electronic clinical systems offers a significant opportunity to provide personalised care to more patients based on data they are collecting about themselves. Whether individuals are simply seeking to prevent the possible onset of future healthcare problems through lifestyle change or if they are trying to mitigate the symptoms of a long term condition such as heart failure or COPD, the linkage of personally generated data with data collected and stored by the healthcare system has the potential to improve clinical decision making and empower patients to make more informed decisions about their treatment or lifestyle options.

REFERENCES

Armstrong, R. M. (2012). App. review-Food-Switch. *The Medical Journal of Australia, 196*(3), 207. doi:10.5694/mja12.10203

Bail, K. D. (2003). Electronic tagging of people with dementia: Devices may be preferable to locked doors. *BMJ, 326*(7383), 281. doi:10.1136/bmj.326.7383.281 PMID:12560288

Bluetooth, S. I. G. (2007). *Specification of the Bluetooth system.* Core Version 1.1. 1 February 22, 2001.

Blumenthal, D. (2010). Launching HITECH. *The New England Journal of Medicine, 362*(5), 382–385. doi:10.1056/NEJMp0912825 PMID:20042745

Comtois, G., Salisbury, J. I., & Sun, Y. (2012). A smartphone-based platform for analyzing physiological audio signals. In *Proceedings of Bioengineering Conference (NEBEC), 2012 38th Annual Northeast* (pp. 69–70). IEEE. doi:10.1109/NEBC.2012.6206966

Fogg, B. J. (2009). A behavior model for persuasive design. In *Proceedings of the 4th International Conference on Persuasive Technology.* ACM.

Franco, O. H., de Laet, C., Peeters, A., Jonker, J., Mackenbach, J., & Nusselder, W. (2005). Effects of physical activity on life expectancy with cardiovascular disease. *Archives of Internal Medicine, 165*(20), 2355–2360. doi:10.1001/archinte.165.20.2355 PMID:16287764

Gross, A. M., Levin, R. B., Mulvihill, M., Richardson, P., & Davidson, P. C. (1984). Blood glucose discrimination training with insulin-dependent diabetics: A clinical note. *Biofeedback and Self-Regulation, 9*(1), 49–54. doi:10.1007/BF00998845 PMID:6487674

Health and Social Care Information Centre. 1 Trevelyan Square. (2013, September 26). *Care. data. standard*. Retrieved April 10, 2014, from http://www.hscic.gov.uk/article/3525/Caredata

Khdour, M. R., Agus, A. M., Kidney, J. C., Smyth, B. M., Elnay, J. C., & Crealey, G. E. (2011). Cost-utility analysis of a pharmacy-led self-management programme for patients with COPD. *International Journal of Clinical Pharmacology, Therapy and Toxicology, 33*(4), 665–673. PMID:21643784

Klersy, C., De Silvestri, A., Gabutti, G., Regoli, F., & Auricchio, A. (2009). A meta-analysis of remote monitoring of heart failure patients. *Journal of the American College of Cardiology, 54*(18), 1683–1694. doi:10.1016/j.jacc.2009.08.017 PMID:19850208

Koff, P. B., Jones, R. H., Cashman, J. M., Voelkel, N. F., & Vandivier, R. W. (2009). Proactive integrated care improves quality of life in patients with COPD. *The European Respiratory Journal, 33*(5), 1031–1038. doi:10.1183/09031936.00063108 PMID:19129289

Kovatchev, B. P., Cox, D. J., Gonder-Frederick, L., & Clarke, W. L. (2002). Methods for quantifying self-monitoring blood glucose profiles exemplified by an examination of blood glucose patterns in patients with type 1 and type 2 diabetes. *Diabetes Technology & Therapeutics, 4*(3), 295–303. doi:10.1089/152091502760098438 PMID:12165168

Little, M. A., McSharry, P. E., Hunter, E. J., Spielman, J., & Ramig, L. O. (2009). Suitability of dysphonia measurements for telemonitoring of Parkinson's disease. *IEEE Transactions on Bio-Medical Engineering, 56*(4), 1015–1022. doi:10.1109/TBME.2008.2005954 PMID:21399744

Manson, J. E., Stampfer, M. J., Colditz, G. A., Willett, W. C., Rosner, B., & Hennekens, C. H. et al. (1991). Physical activity and incidence of non-insulin-dependent diabetes mellitus in women. *Lancet, 338*(8770), 774–778. doi:10.1016/0140-6736(91)90664-B PMID:1681160

McCallum, S. (2012). Gamification and serious games for personalized health. *Studies in Health Technology and Informatics, 177*, 85–96. PMID:22942036

Picot, J. (1998). Telemedicine and Telehealth in Canada: Forty Years of Change in the Use of Information and Communications Technologies in a Publicly Administered Health Care System. *Telemedicine Journal, 4*(3), 199–205. doi:10.1089/tmj.1.1998.4.199 PMID:9831745

Proper, K. I., Van den Heuvel, S. G., De Vroome, E. M., Hildebrandt, V. H., & Van der Beek, A. J. (2006). Dose–response relation between physical activity and sick leave. *British Journal of Sports Medicine, 40*(2), 173–178. doi:10.1136/bjsm.2005.022327 PMID:16432007

Smith, C. E., Dauz, E. R., Clements, F., Puno, F. N., Cook, D., Doolittle, G., & Leeds, W. (2006). Telehealth services to improve nonadherence: A placebo-controlled study. *Telemedicine Journal and e-Health, 12*(3), 289–296. doi:10.1089/tmj.2006.12.289 PMID:16796496

Stewart, A. L., Hays, R. D., Wells, K. B., Rogers, W. H., Spritzer, K. L., & Greenfield, S. (1994). Long-term functioning and well-being outcomes associated with physical activity and exercise in patients with chronic conditions in the medical outcomes study. *Journal of Clinical Epidemiology, 47*(7), 719–730. doi:10.1016/0895-4356(94)90169-4 PMID:7722585

Swan, M. (2009). Emerging patient-driven health care models: An examination of health social networks, consumer personalized medicine and quantified self-tracking. *International Journal of Environmental Research and Public Health*, *6*(2), 492–525. doi:10.3390/ijerph6020492 PMID:19440396

Thompson, P. D., Buchner, D., Piña, I. L., Balady, G. J., Williams, M. A., & Marcus, B. H. et al. (2003). Exercise and physical activity in the prevention and treatment of atherosclerotic cardiovascular disease a statement from the Council on Clinical Cardiology (Subcommittee on Exercise, Rehabilitation, and Prevention) and the Council on Nutrition, Physical Activity, and Metabolism (Subcommittee on Physical Activity). *Circulation*, *107*(24), 3109–3116. doi:10.1161/01.CIR.0000075572.40158.77 PMID:12821592

Thune, I., & Furberg, A.-S. (2001). Physical activity and cancer risk: dose-response and cancer, all sites and site-specific. *Medicine and Science in Sports and Exercise*, *33*(6 Suppl), S530–50, discussion S609–10.

Yambem, L., Yapici, M. K., & Zou, J. (2008). A new wireless sensor system for smart diapers. *IEEE Sensors Journal*, *8*(3), 238–239. doi:10.1109/JSEN.2008.917122

Zvarova, K., Ursiny, M., Giebink, T., Liang, K., Blaivas, J. G., & Zvara, P. (2011). Recording urinary flow and lower urinary tract symptoms using sonouroflowmetry. *The Canadian Journal of Urology*, *18*(3), 5689–5694. PMID:21703041

KEY TERMS AND DEFINITIONS

Electronic Health Records (EHR): Used by clinicians to store data and information about patients.

Personal Health Records (PHR): Used by patients to record their health information online.

Self-Tracking: Measuring subjective and objective measurements about oneself to keep track of changes over time.

Chapter 82
System Upgrade and Integration at a Medium–Sized Dental Clinic

Eun G. Park
McGill University, Canada

Benjamin Paris
McGill University, Canada

ABSTRACT

The implementation of electronic health records systems (EHRS) has a major impact on both clinical staff and physicians. However, it is difficult for small and medium sized clinics to adopt EHRS. Without proper mechanisms and methodologies in place, the transition is often slowed down for several reasons. In order to identify what issues and challenges are involved in transitions, this study was conducted to 1) investigate the current issues and perspectives of employees regarding a system upgrade, database integration and managerial efficiency in order to streamline daily business operations at a medium-sized dental clinic, and 2) suggest the best strategy to solve the identified problems and challenges. Interviews were conducted with administrative staff members, a dentist, a dental resident and the director of the clinic. Interviews were transcribed and grouped into two major categories: managerial efficiency and employees' responses toward system upgrade and integration.

1. INTRODUCTION

As information management and technology have recently improved primary health care, hospitals and medical professionals have expressed a significant interest in adopting electronic health records systems (EHRS) as a reform in the health care sector. Electronic health records (EHR) are defined as electronic records of patients' medical information that are created and managed through a system at hospitals, clinics and physicians' of-fices, health care centers and other institutions in the health care sector (Healthcare Information and Management Systems Society, n.d.). Some examples of this type of information include patient demographics, progress notes, medications, medical history, immunisations, laboratory data and radiology reports (Yoon-Flannery, 2008). EHRS refers to a system which contains, manages, organizes, and uses EHR in the course of medical treatment at hospitals and clinics in the healthcare industry. Some examples of EHRS include VistA

DOI: 10.4018/978-1-4666-8756-1.ch082

(Veterans Health Information Systems and Technology Architecture), VisitA Imaging, Meditech, Kaiser Permanente HealthConnect®, etc. EHRS can support several clinical and administrative functions.

With this major trend in the health care sector, most studies have focused on EHRS implementation issues at large hospitals, where sufficient funding, resources, and personnel are within internal capacities. There are only a few studies that deal with small or medium-sized hospitals and clinics, which seem to be insufficient in most of those factors (Shih et al., 2011; Rao et al., 2011; Carayon, et al., 2009). For example, Rao's study (2011) indicates that providers of small-sized clinics tend to have lower levels of EHR adoption and use these systems less frequently. One of the most significant factors for this is financial barriers, which seem to be a critical factor in the spread of HER systems. Nevertheless, two interesting studies address the advantages of adopting EHRS at small sized providers. Caranyan et al.'s study (2009) illustrates that the work of clinical and office staff has been significantly changed because of decreased time spent distributing charts and on transcription and administrative tasks. In addition, implementing an HERS system and a software upgrade to embed a clinical decision support system can improve comprehensive quality at small primary care practices (Shih et al., 2011).

Therefore, we have conducted a study at a medium-sized dental clinic to assess the feasibility and pre-implementation perspectives of employees regarding a system upgrade, database integration and managerial efficiency in order to streamline daily business operations. The objectives of the study include: 1) investigating the perspectives of employees toward system integration and the current management practices at the dental clinic, and 2) suggesting an implementation strategy to respond to the identified issues and streamline daily business operations at the dental clinic.

Following the introduction, Section 2 reviews literature on relevant topics and Section 3 explains the background of the selected clinic as a case study. Section 4 describes the findings of this study and Section 5 discusses important and relevant issues drawn from the findings and suggests a managerial and implementation strategy for the dental clinic.

2. LITERATURE REVIEW

With technological improvements, information portability and strict legal compliance from the health sector industry in Canada and the United States, many hospitals expressed a significant interest in adopting either partial or full EHRS as a part of health care reforms in the 2000s. Governments began to implement strategies and allocate funds to facilitate the transition from paper records to a digital environment. In Canada, the government has reserved an 800 million dollar Primary Health Care (PHC) Transition Fund to accelerate and facilitate the renewal of its health care system. Among Health Canada's PHC reforms, one of the primary objectives is to create viable Information Management & Technology initiatives and guidelines to assist provincial governments, hospitals, and physicians to meet this challenge (Health Canada, 2007; see details at http://www.healthcanada.ca). In the United States, in 2009 the Obama administration launched the Health Information Technology for Economic and Clinical Health Act (HITECH Act) and provided an assistance package to help hospitals and clinic centers buy EHRS and work with other medical centers to create interoperable records. This act aimed to rigorously adopt EHRS and improve the quality of the health care system as a critical national goal (Blumenthal, 2010). As this stimulus package has allocated 10 billion dollars yearly until the year 2014, the rate of adoption of health information technology has increased to 55% from 45% in 2009 (Yahoo Finance, 2009). Therefore, we expect that information management enabling technology such as EHRS will become more prevalent in hospitals in both North American countries.

EHRS plays a significant role in improving the quality of healthcare in many ways and providing many advantages to clinics and hospitals, as several researchers support this (Boyle, et al. 2010, Friedberg, 2009, Shih, et al. 2011). For example, if a patient's information and data are stored and integrated into one integrated electronic system, the risk of losing vital information and having incomplete patient portfolios would be significantly reduced (Shih, et al. 2011, Dayhoff et al. 1999). In addition, once a patient's information is registered in EHRS, all of the other procedures can be automated, including scheduling, prescription, documenting, billing, as well as the coordination of doctors, pharmacies, patients, etc. In addition, Meidani et al,'s study addresses that as EHR becomes the operating core of the organization, "its adaptation involves the design, delivery and use of the software system in the organization" (2012, 1229). Most of all, EHRS can make contributions to implementing and improving quality in entire hospitals and clinics. Therefore, this has recently become a pressing issue for medical practices in hospitals (Handel & Hackman, 2010, Meidani et al., 2012).

Particularly in small and medium sized hospitals and clinics, the adoption of EHRS has a more prominent impact on the administration and health care provisions. The automated procedures drawn from the implementation of EHRS may make many of the functions and workflow performed by staff unified and streamlined and eliminate the need for some staff members and the administrative tasks of support staff. If the implemented systems were interoperable and integrated to share information, an EHRS would allow doctors to share information easily between two practitioners using one standard technology.

The implementation of an EHRS allows staff members and physicians to spend more time communicating and interacting with patients during a visit (Carayon et al., 2009). It would increase safety through evidence-based decision support, quality management, and outcomes reporting (Health Canada, 2007). With tools for consultation, doctors may reach solutions more effectively than working in isolation. Tamariz et al.'s study indicates that electronic records could be shared among physicians in collaborative environments to make the communication of expertise possible through "teleconsultation," and physicians could also learn about medical procedures used by practitioners from different regions (2009, 448). EHRS can track unprecedented amounts of clinical data to support the research. For instance, clinics and small hospitals can conduct longitudinal comparisons on what treatments have worked in the past.

Regardless of a lot of the advantages, in reality, it is not a simple task to adopt an EHRS in small and medium sized clinics. Rao et al.'s study demonstrates that physicians in small practices have lower levels of EHR adoption than large hospitals and that they were less likely to use these systems (2011). In addition, even among small clinic providers that had adopted EHRS, "there was still a gap in the use of system functions, assuming that the gaps are not just about adoption alone" (Rao, 2011, 271). Regarding the reasons for this, several studies explain that small provider-owned practices have insufficient support staff, substantial financial burden, a risk to the viability of the practice, and scarce resources for improving the delivery of preventive care (Shih et al., 2011; Holanda et al., 2012). It is true that implementing a new information management system is one of the bigger challenges for organizations of any size to overcome. Small clinics and hospitals may have more of an incentive to move towards an EHRS and enable a mass improvement in the delivery of health care. However, small and medium sized clinics are compounded by several difficulties, such as lack of support, slow processing, lack of resources, lack of personnel, lack of training, and lack of integration between the EMR and their workflow (Holanda et al., 2012; Top & Gider, 2012; Carayon et al., 2009). In particular, employees need to take collective responsibility for managing the clinics' information. There are no trained experts to provide guidance and the necessary support throughout the implementation process. When this task is assigned to each employee alongside his or her tasks, it often results in a hindrance to an organization's development (Dawson et al., 2004, 113). Without proper mechanisms and methodologies in place, the EHRS has actually increased the workload of support staff only, while physicians using EHRS do not experience an increase in workload (Carayon et al., 2009, 8).

Therefore, considering that the implementation of EHRS is important at small and medium-sized clinics, this study aims to examine the current issues and challenges during the implementation procedures at a selected real site and suggest feasible solutions that correspond to the issues raised.

3. METHODS

In order to identify which issues are involved in transitions at a medium-sized clinic, the following site was selected as a case study for closer examination.

3.1. Background: Setting of the Clinic

This clinic is a medium-sized, university affiliated Dental Health Clinic (DHC) which is located in Quebec, Canada. It consists of five major divisions: the Student Teaching Clinic, Summer Clinic, Satellite Clinic, Outreach Clinic and Undergraduate Clinic. Currently, the DHC utilizes the main system ABELDent, five databases per clinic and X-rays and radiographic image databases to fulfill each of the major dental clinic divisions. ABELDent is a software application provider. The relationship between the software company and the DHC is well established. Currently the DHC uses Sidexis for X-rays (a digital X-ray tool). Each database in each division is functionally identical but not linked. These systems are mainly used to document administrative, financial, and some medical details for patients in each clinic. This DHC currently uses paper charts to record most of the medical information for each patient. Various forms exist in paper format, such as patient information forms, treatment plans, appointment scheduling with medical students, medical history and consent forms, treatment write-ups, and "chits," respectively. The current situation of the clinic is typical compared to other medium-sized clinics, which have common characteristics.

The existing databases are structured in a decentralized manner, which may cause procedures to be duplicated unnecessarily across the five divisions. If patients have visited the clinic multiple times, each division's database generates its own unique identifier so the same patient may have several different numbers assigned to him or her. It is difficult to track patients who may utilize different divisions at the clinic and assess the financial information of patients who have visited multiple times. This has resulted in the loss of the staff's time and efficiency.

Under the present conditions, the clinic's management team is considering integrating multiple databases into a central database and upgrading ABELDent into a Picture Archiving and Communication System (PACS). In order to successfully perform this integration, we conducted an assessment study to determine the challenges and barriers of proceeding with a system upgrade and database integration. In order to collect the perspectives of employees at the clinic, this study has adopted an interview methodology and examined the system and databases.

3.2. Unstructured Interviews

Prior agreement had been made with the director of the DHCs regarding the day and time of the research team's presence. Then, during the summer of 2009, the research team interviewed five administrative staff members, one dentist, one dental resident and the director of the clinic, totaling 8 participants. The interviews were conducted with unstructured questions about how participants would think and feel regarding the following three topics: 1) current management, 2) current systems and databases, and 3) system integration and upgrade at the clinics (e.g. 1) what do you think of current management? Please feel free to share your opinion on current management, 2) what do you think of the current systems and databases? Please feel free to share your opinion on the current systems and databases, and 3) what do you think of system integration and upgrade? Please feel free to share your opinion on system integration and upgrade). Participants were, on an individual basis, asked to openly and freely share their perspectives on those topics, respectively. Interviews were voluntary based. Each interview lasted approximately thirty minutes to one hour. With the permission of participants, the interviews were recorded.

3.3. Examination of the System and Databases

The research team examined the existing systems and databases directly through a phone interview with the system application ABELDent. The team was permitted to speak with a representative of the company that provided the database for the clinic. This interview enabled the collection of technical information about the main system and a discussion about the feasibility of potential changes and upgrades.

3.4. Qualitative Analysis

The research team transcribed the recorded voices of all interviews and their reliability was double-checked by another research assistant. The answers from participants were grouped into two major themes: 1) managerial efficiency and 2) employees' responses toward system upgrade and integration. The former theme identifies six major issues, including a top-down management approach, the lack of communication between management and employees, dissatisfaction with the current division of tasks, inefficient operational processes, a shortage of staff, and a lack of skills to use the current system. The second theme, the employees' perspectives toward system integration and upgrades, was grouped into positive and negative perspectives. The positive responses from employees toward system integration and upgrade include: the resolution of problems caused by decentralized databases, a reduction in process time, and the elimination of operational mistakes. Employees also have negative views with regards to overburdened workloads, a fear of change, dissatisfaction with the current system, and fear of the new system.

4. FINDINGS

The two major themes that are identified by our research team are demonstrated with important issues in each theme as the following. See the summary of two themes and details in Table 1.

4.1. Overall Managerial Efficiency

- *Top-down Management Approach*: The research team observed that strategic decision-making is mainly left to the director of DHC. The "top down" approach (i.e.

Table 1. Summary of themes and issues

Themes		
Overall Managerial Efficiency	*Employees' Responses Toward System Integration and Upgrade*	
	Positive Responses	*Negative Responses*
• Top-down management approach (director, 5 staff members)* • Lack of communication between management and employees (director, dentist, 5 staff members) • Dissatisfaction with the current division of tasks (5 staff members) • Inefficient operational processes (3 staff members) • A shortage of staff (5 staff members) • Lack of skills for the current system (dentist, dental resident, 5 staff members, and students)	• The resolution of problems caused by decentralized databases (dentist, dental resident, 5 staff members) • A reduction in process time (5 staff members) • The elimination of operational mistakes (5 staff members)	• Overburdened workloads (5 staff members) • Fear of change (dentist, dental resident, 5 staff members) • Dissatisfaction with the current system (5 staff members) • Fear of a new system (3 staff members)

*Each issue is added with the participants in () who expressed the issue.

where one executive and decision maker makes a decision alone) is disseminated under the executive's authority down to the lower levels in the hierarchy, who are, to some extent, bound by the decision. In this case, there was no indication that staff members were actively engaged in the decision-making process and no open venues or tools existed to allow staff members to express their work concerns or identify issues to management.

- ***Lack of Communication between Management and Employees***: Employees felt that there was a lack of connection between management and staff. Interestingly, the management often did not understand the day-to-day concerns of the staff. It was often observed that the organizational culture did not support communication with staff members, bringing about resistance and mistrust toward management decisions. The team thinks that this is reflective of the top-down management approach, as previously mentioned. For example, employees were not aware of the management's strategic business projects and objectives. Employees were not aware of where to find system update notes. Management and staff

who are responsible for installing updates failed to communicate to employees where to find information about the updates.

- ***Dissatisfaction with the Current Division of Tasks***: At the time, each staff member was responsible for various information management tasks as well as their activities in each division. However, the division of these responsibilities created a work environment in which most staff members engaged in similar and repetitive tasks every day. For example, there was an employee whose primary task was to schedule appointments, resulting in employee stagnation along with replacement issues. Staff members believed that roles could be split in different ways to prevent repetition and burnout.

- ***Inefficient Operational Processes***: Three staff members believed that the process used to screen patients was inefficient. For example, sometimes they had to complete a long set of questions in order to guide a patient. In addition, the system they currently used to keep track of patient X-rays seemed inefficient and sometimes led to lost radiographic images or incomplete patient records. Many radiographers forgot to use the sticker system devised to ensure that patient X-rays match with the actual file, resulting in X-rays mismatched with patient charts or lost X-rays.

- *A Shortage of Staff*: The five staff members believed that they were overworked and lacked sufficient staff to efficiently accomplish their day-to-day tasks at the DHC. A new technical process was perceived as having the potential to cause more work for them, resulting in strong opposition and work-related stress.

- *Lack of Skills for the Current System*: It was observed that not all staff members seemed to understand the functionality of ABELDent and there were no formalized training or shared documents in the system. In general, most staff members and students do not use ABELDent as intended, or the system is not user friendly and lacks functionality. For example, staff members mentioned using workarounds to perform simple tasks such as creating a new appointment. When students did not know which treatment codes to record in ABELDent, incorrect and incomplete electrical patient records resulted. In addition, the current system does not allow users (including staff and students) to perform functions that they want to do, such as copying and pasting an entire field screen. It is difficult to edit patient information after it has been saved on the system. Financial data is time-consuming to adjust, causing staff members to spend an inappropriate amount of time fixing simple problems. Furthermore, staff members complained that ABELDent is a slow system that tends to experience slow-downs and random crashes. In addition, all of the participants including staff members, one dentist, and one dental resident expressed the need for more computers at the clinic. Staff members mentioned that at the mo-

ment, students do not have enough computers to support a paperless environment.

- *Employees' Responses Toward System Integration and Upgrade*: Employees demonstrated positive and negative responses toward system integration for the following reasons.

4.2. Positive Responses

- *The Resolution of Problems Caused By Decentralized Databases*: Since the current system and databases may create duplicated copies of records in different ways, the integration of the system into a central database could potentially save significant time and effort, such as locating and tracking a patient's records on appointment history, financial payments, multiple medical charts and treatment plans. It could also eliminate the potential duplication of procedures (e.g. X-rays could be requested if the information was not transferred from one clinic to another).

- *A Reduction in Process Time*: Current inefficient procedures used to screen patients could be solved. Merging the databases will reduce the amount of time spent on the phone with patients collecting information for appointments.

- *The Elimination of Operational Mistakes*: Some business processes are inefficient as a result of incomplete patient records, the loss of radiographic images, X-rays mismatched with patient charts, etc. All staff members interviewed believe that merging systems and using an entirely digital platform can resolve these problems.

4.3. Negative Responses

- *Overburdened Workloads*: Regardless of the advantages, the five staff members are very resistant to the integration of databases. More specifically, staff members indicated that they could not reason or fathom the need to merge the main system and databases at the time. They do not understand the benefits of digital working environments. A major part of the overall resistance has to do with the fact that the DHC is understaffed. This issue is also coupled with a belief that a merger of the databases will increase their workload, either as a result of a physical merger or the process of learning a new system. These may require them to perform beyond their capabilities. Staff members express dismay with merging the databases, as they feel they will bear the brunt of the workload associated with the integration process and the merging process, which may by extension create additional disruptions to staff and their daily functions. While this is a misconception, it stems both out of a lack of understanding the technology and a lack of communicating management strategies and organizational objectives between the managers or the director and the immediate support staff.

- *Fear of Change*: All of the staff members, one dentist, and one dental resident interviewed are somewhat resistant toward integration, which comes from a fear of operational change. They are concerned about the impact that change would have on their individual work. Employees, for the most part, lack the strategic vision to foresee the benefits of merging the databases and going entirely digital with the clinic records.
- *Dissatisfaction with the Current System*: In spite of some shortcomings and the unfriendly functionality of the current system, employees seem to be satisfied with it. No staff member has ever worked with another medical record system, so they are unable to make fair assessments and comparisons with other medical record systems.

- *Fear of a New System*: With a centralized database, the staff fears that there will be an increased number of mistakes because more people will be working on one database and the mistakes could also potentially have a larger impact on their work. They also expressed concern that an integrated database would cause significant slowdowns, and two staff members expressed distaste towards the idea of students accessing certain records or hacking into the system.

5. DISCUSSION

This study examined employees' perspectives and current managerial issues related to the current management and system as well as system integration and upgrade at a medium sized dental clinic. The study also identified a number of challenges and barriers. Considering the overall responses from employees, there are more negative attitudes than positive ones regarding a system merge and upgrade. Most of all, there are major managerial and communication issues that are barriers between management, especially the director of DHC and staff members, in the clinic. In addition, employees know that a system upgrade would bring some benefits and conveniences to the clinic. However, the atmosphere of the dental clinic is characterized by employees who tend to be more hesitant toward system integration, rather than employees who are actively willing to support it.

Although there is often the need for new information management and system integration at small and medium sized hospitals and some benefits can be gained from this, system upgrade in the clinic involves managing employees' resistance to change (Caldeira, et al. 2012). There is also a lack of corresponding resources or expertise to develop and implement policies and procedures. In addition, if the management team and the director focus more on the technological aspects and do not seriously consider employees' perspectives, the implementation of EHRS will result in failure and an oversight of the human impact on the workforce. In light of this result, the findings of this study are in agreement with those of Holanda et al.'s study (2012). We see this study is meaningful by indentifying why small and medium sized clinics have not adopted EHRs and what kinds of barriers there are to new adoptions or benefits to be gained from EHRS. The result of this study could be compared with a case of large sized hospitals. The result of this study sheds light on the state of EHRS adoption to improve patient treatment in small and medium sized clinics and describes the challenges for policymakers who help these providers implement EHRS (Rao, 2011).

Most of all, what we learned from this study is that the technology implementation process is not treated as a technological concern, but is likely to affect all aspects of the job and change work processes (Carayan et al., 2009, 3). In addition, some studies acknowledge that a key element when implementing any EHRS is user acceptance (Johnston & Bowen, 2005). In our diagnosis of the clinic, we point out that the cooperation and collaboration of the staff during any new system implementation should be key, rather than simply imposing upgraded tools upon employees. This approach could minimize the risk of having employees who refuse to adopt new systems and processes. If the desired solution is ultimately to integrate the clinical databases, concerns about whether the staff will receive the change favorably remain. In this situation, the decision about how to implement a merge is difficult.

Therefore, we suggest that technological implementations should be handled as a change management project rather than solely a technological upgrade. Meidani et al.'s study supports this by addressing "the recent theories of EHR success go far beyond technical rationales and focus on organizational and managerial factors in quality improvement" (2012, 1229). If employees establish the need for new systems and create

a sense of voluntary or subjective change from their agreement from the beginning, there will be a positive learning curve for the new EHRS. Careful planning regarding behavior and cultural change is a critical factor in system upgrades and merges because the implementation of new system can transform effect on the way an organization undertakes tasks and the organizational culture (Jones, 2012). The process of change should be gradual and as much training as possible should be provided. To reduce the fears and resistance to change on the part of staff, the management team needs to communicate the organization's strategic direction on a regular basis.

Based on the findings, the research team has prioritized a positive transition with minimal disruption and provided as much information as possible during meetings prior to the merger process. To respond to the identified issues, the following recommendations were made to the clinic.

- **To solve managerial and communication issues:**
  - Educate staff on merging processes through communication. Management should host a series of meetings with staff to explain the proposed merger and the reasons behind it. Management should allow staff members to share their responses and reservations toward the integration, which will lessen any resentment and fear about a top-down decision as well as enable the staff to feel as though they have some input in the decision.
  - Considering the disconnect between employees and management, create a cohesive organizational culture and host open discussions with employees about work-related issues.
  - Make all documents pertaining to vision, objectives, and goals accessible via a website or in print. To address

the dissatisfaction with the division of tasks, balance and redistribute work tasks to prevent employee burnout.

- **To effectively merge the systems and databases**
  - Allow the ABELDent company to lead the merger of databases. The technical database merging process should be outsourced to ABELDent service experts to process and explain technical and administrative procedures in detail, since there is already a well-established relationship between the clinic and the company. This service might incur a negotiated fee.
  - Offer workshops and training sessions to staff conducted by the database company so that the staff can learn how to efficiently and rapidly perform the technical functions of the software. Allow staff members to provide interactive feedback. Highlight the potential positives of the centralized database, such as reduced time for locating and tracking client appointments.
  - After implementation, develop additional internal training sessions about system functions or refresher courses on the impact of hardware, software and networks on daily operations. If possible, create an internal wiki or web page about the functions of ABELDent and FAQs about new systems.
  - Prioritize the merge order step by step: a priority would be to integrate the Summer Clinic database with the Undergraduate Teaching Clinic database and the Satellite clinic. The next priority would be the integration of the Outreach and Student Health databases.
  - Clearly explain to staff that this database merge will be performed on evenings or weekends to minimize disruption. Performing the merge during a relatively less busy period (e.g. after work hours or on weekends) will not add significantly more work for staff.

If the suggested implementation strategy is adopted, merging the databases will streamline operations. In our study, cost issues were not considered because the clinic had allocated funds for the initial installation and implementation at the time this study was conducted. If initial capital expenses are necessary, maintenance costs are expected to decrease over time. Operating expenses need to be appropriately estimated and more computers and technical support must be provided. System migration requires adequate levels of technical equipment, support and training. Patient privacy and security vulnerability issues will be considered at a later time.

Our study has limitations since our findings were collected from one dental school-affiliated clinic as a case study. The results of this study cannot be generalized. We did not assess the actual process of using the EHR by dentists and all administrative staff members. The interview did not assess the views of other personnel, such as nurses, assistants, patients or dental students. Further data collection is necessary in a separate study prior to EHR implementation. Other opinions would enrich an understanding of the real impact of EHR on everyday work and the quality of care. This study was conducted during the planning and early implementation phases. Additional monitoring of practice performance prior to system upgrade and implementation is also beneficial to understanding whether any change is sustainable. Since continuous monitoring and evaluation of the process are essential (Holanda et al., 2012), further study should be concentrated on the measures of process of EHRS use (e.g. usability of the systems, outcomes in patient care, etc.). We hope that the actual implementation of EHRS should integrate all aspects - including health record management, workflow, collaboration and innovation, user governance and participation - which are all intertwined like a chain to improve the quality of health care services (Meidani et al., 2012, 1230).

6. CONCLUSION

EHR has been considered as a key strategy to implementing quality improvements in health care. The primary purposes of this study were to investigate the feasibility of a database merger at a medium sized clinic as well as the general operations in the clinic, and provide the clinic with managerial and implementation suggestions. We found that by purchasing EHRS technology only without an organization-wide understanding and commitment to properly operating the EHRS and without a comprehensive needs analysis and input by stakeholders, small and medium sized hospitals and clinics may find themselves sacrificing employee time and effort during its implementation. It is essential to emphasize that none of the changes mentioned in this study can be achieved efficiently without the input and participation from clinic employees: any implemented changes should be done with the compliance and collaboration of the staff, while ensuring that the appropriate change management procedures are in place. The research team believes that with internal motivation and a degree of cultural acceptance from employees, system upgrade initiatives will have more opportunities to succeed in small and medium sized hospitals.

ACKNOWLEDGMENT

The authors gratefully acknowledge the help of Maimi Niina and Constantina Liatsopoulos in collecting and analyzing data.

REFERENCES

ABELDent. Retrieved May 30, 2013 from http://www.abeldent.com

Blumenthal, D. (2010). Launching HITECH. *The New England Journal of Medicine*, *362*(5), 382–385. doi:10.1056/NEJMp0912825 PMID:20042745

Boyle, R., Solberg, L., & Fiore, M. (2010). Electronic medical records to increase the clinical treatment of tobacco dependence: A systematic review. *American Journal of Preventive Medicine*, *39*(6S16), S77–S82. doi:10.1016/j.amepre.2010.08.014 PMID:21074681

Caldeira, M., Serrano, A., Quaresma, R., Pedron, C., & Romao, M. (2012). Information and communication technology adoption for business benefits: A case analysis of an integrated paperless system. *International Journal of Information Management*, *32*(2), 196–202. doi:10.1016/j.ijinfomgt.2011.12.005

Carayon, P., Smith, P., Hundt, A. S., Kuruchittham, V., & Li, Q. (2009). Implementation of an electronic health records system in a small clinic: The viewpoint of clinic staff'. *Behaviour & Information Technology*, *28*(1), 5–20. doi:10.1080/01449290701628178

Dawson, E., Dodd, R., Roberts, J., & Wakeling, C. (2004). Issues and challenges for records management in the charity and voluntary sector. *Records Management Journal, 14*(3), 111–115. doi:10.1108/09565690410566765

Dayhoff, R., Kuzmak, P., Kirin, G., & Frank, S. (1999). Providing a complete online multimedia patient record. In N. Losenzi (Ed.), American Medical Information Association Annual Symposium 1999: Transforming health care through informatics (pp.241-245). Washington, D.C.: American Medical Information Association. Retrieved May 30, 2013 from http://www.pubmedcentral.nih.gov/picrender.fcgi?artid=2232533&blobtype=pdf

Friedberg, M., Coltin, K., Safran, D., Dresser, M., Zaslavsky, A., & Schneider, E. (2009). Associations between structural capabilities of primary care practices and performance on selected quality measures. *Annals of Internal Medicine, 151*(7), 456–463. doi:10.7326/0003-4819-151-7-200910060-00006 PMID:19805769

Handel, D., & Hackman, J. (2010). Implementing electronic health records in the emergency department. *Emergency Medicine Journal, 38*(2), 257–263. doi:10.1016/j.jemermed.2008.01.020 PMID:18790591

Health Canada. (2007). *Information management and technology: synthesis series on sharing insights.* Retrieved May 30, 2013 from http://www.hc-sc.gc.ca/hcs-sss/alt_formats/hpb-dgps/pdf/prim/2006-synth-tech-eng.pdf

Healthcare Information and Management Systems Society. HER Electronic Health Records. Retrieved May 30, 2013 from http://www.himss.org/ASP/topics_ehr.asp

Holanda, A., do Carmo e Sá, H. L., Vieira, A. P. G. F., & Catrib, A. M. F. (2012). Use and satisfaction with electronic health record by primary care physicians in a health district in Brazil. *Journal of Medical Systems, 36*(5), 3141–3149. doi:10.1007/s10916-011-9801-3 PMID:22072279

Johnston, G., & Bowen, D. (2005). The benefits of electronic records management systems. *Records Management Journal, 15*(3), 420–432. doi:10.1108/09565690510632319

Jones, S. (2012). eGovernment Document Management System: A case of risk and reward. *International Journal of Information Management, 32*(4), 396–400. doi:10.1016/j.ijinfomgt.2012.04.002

Kaiser Permanente HealthConnect®. Retrieved May 30, 2013 from http://xnet.kp.org/newscenter/aboutkp/healthconnect

Meditech. Retrieved May 30, 2013 from http://home.meditech.com

Meidani, Z., Sadoughi, F., Maleki, M., Tofighi, S., & Marani, A. (2012). Organization's quality maturity as a vehicle for EHR success. *Journal of Medical Systems, 36*(3), 1229–1234. doi:10.1007/s10916-010-9584-y PMID:20878212

Rao, S., DesRoches, C., Donelan, K., Campbell, E., Miralles, P., & Jha, A. (2011). Electronic health records in small physician practices: Availability, use, and perceived benefits. *Journal of the American Medical Informatics Association, 18*(3), 271–275. doi:10.1136/amiajnl-2010-000010 PMID:21486885

Shih, S., McCullough, C., Wang, J., Singer, J., & Parsons, A. (2011). Health information systems in small practices improving the delivery of clinical preventive dervices. *American Journal of Preventive Medicine, 41*(6), 603–609. doi:10.1016/j.amepre.2011.07.024 PMID:22099237

Tamariz, F., Merrell, R., Popescu, I., Onisor, D., Flerov, Y., & Boanca, C. et al. (2009). Design and implementation of a web-based system for intraoperative consultation. *World Journal of Surgery*, *33*(3), 1–7. doi:10.1007/s00268-008-9858-4 PMID:19123027

Top, M., & Gider, O. (2012). Nurses' views on electronic medical records (EMR) in Turkey: An analysis according to use, quality and user satisfaction. *Journal of Medical Systems*, *36*(3), 1979–1988. doi:10.1007/s10916-011-9657-6 PMID:21302133

Vist, A. Retrieved May 30, 2013 from http://worldvista.org

Vist, A. Imaging. Retrieved May 30, 2013 from http://www.vistaimaging.com

Yahoo Finance News. (2009). Hospital Information Technology Adoption Rates Going from 10% Today to 55% by 2014 According to US Government, Peak Growth Year to be 2011 According to Industry Experts. Retrieved August 31, 2011 from http://finance.yahoo.com/news/Hospital-Information-twst-3763690005.html?x=0&.v=2

Yoon-Flannery, K., Zandieh S., Kuperman, G., Langsam, D., Hyman, D. & Kaushal, R. (2008). Qualitative analysis of an electronic health record (EHR) implementation in an academic ambulatory setting. *Informatics Primary Care,* 16(4), 277-284.

This work was previously published in the International Journal of Privacy and Health Information Management (IJPHIM), 2(1); edited by Muaz A. Niazi, pages 51-64 copyright year 2014 by IGI Publishing (an imprint of IGI Global).

Chapter 83

Home Telecare, Medical Implant, and Mobile Technology:
Evolutions in Geriatric Care

Vishaya Naidoo
York University, Canada

Yedishtra Naidoo
Wayne State University, USA

ABSTRACT

With a rapidly expanding global aging population, alternatives must be developed to minimize the inevitable increase in acute and long-term care admissions to the health care system. This chapter explores the use of home telecare as an alternative medical approach to managing this growing trend, while also providing superior care to geriatric patients. To address some of the emergent disadvantages of home telecare concerning usability, self-management, and confinement to the home, the use of a cardiac implant in conjunction with a mobile device–to assist in the management of chronic heart failure in seniors–is proposed as a promising technological solution to overcoming these limitations. Ultimately, it seems that the growth of home telecare, as well as the great potential to enhance its services with the use of mobile wireless technology, stands to drastically improve clinical decision-making and management of health services in the future.

INTRODUCTION

We are living in an era when the world's aging population is rapidly expanding. In the year 2000, 600 million people were aged 60 and over, with this number projected to increase to 1.2 billion in 2025 and 2 billion by the year 2050 (WHO, 2006).

At this rate of growth, the inevitable increase in acute and long-term care admissions is a significant concern for policymakers, managers and providers of health care. Concerns arise from the increased economic cost, as well as the potentially lower standard of care that is likely to result from a higher volume of patients seeking treatment in

DOI: 10.4018/978-1-4666-8756-1.ch083

an over-burdened system. Currently, international trends indicate that health care needs increase as people become older, and that the number of people requiring *daily* health care over the age of 85 is now four times more than those aged 65 to 75 (Botsis et al., 2008). One proposed solution to managing this problem is home telecare – a sub-specialty within the larger field of telemedicine. This involves a shift in care with the use of new and emergent information technology in the home, utilizing an array of hardware, software and network services (Roback & Herzog, 2003). With this system, patients can be monitored, consult with their physicians, and receive care without physically leaving their private homes; thereby allowing them to maintain their independence, more conveniently and efficiently manage chronic conditions, and ultimately reduce health care costs to the system (Hébert et al., 2006; Koch, 2006).

In this chapter, we examine the growing arena of home telecare and assess its potential to enhance treatment and clinical decision-making in geriatric medicine. Following a review of important facets of home telecare, as well as a discussion of the advantages of this medical technology for policymakers and patients, we then outline the challenges that arise with this system, proposing the use of an implantable device–under the skin–as a means through which to increase convenience and overcome user-related challenges for seniors with chronic Heart Failure (HF). The use of a cardiac implant in conjunction with mobile wireless technology is a potentially promising solution that addresses some of the emergent challenges of home telecare concerning usability, self-management, and confinement to the home. This proposed technology would allow seniors in chronic HF, and under the monitoring of a home telecare system, to leave their home while maintaining a similarly comprehensive level of medical monitoring and management for their condition. Ultimately, it seems that the growth of home telecare, as well as the great potential to enhance its services with the use of mobile wireless technology, stands to drastically improve clinical decision-making and management of health services in the future.

BACKGROUND

Telemedicine refers to the delivery of medical care–and the sharing of health knowledge–from a distance with the use of telecommunication devices, the Internet, and various monitoring technologies (Allen & March, 2002; Hersh et al., 2002). Home telecare operates on the same premise, allowing health care practitioners to manage and treat patients in their homes from a remote location (Celler et al., 2003; Coughlin et al., 2006). Services encompass a wide array of technologies, including "virtual visiting, reminder systems, home security, and social alarm systems," all of which support the larger goal of home telecare: to manage the care of geriatric patients where they live, and avoid lengthy stays in hospitals or nursing homes (Magnusson, 2004, pp. 224-225). It is a method of health care delivery that addresses many of the existing gaps and weaknesses in the current primary health care system, by providing a higher level of monitoring and medical consultation for patients in their everyday lives. The services provided by this branch of telemedicine are meant to increase convenience for patients, their families, and practitioners, where a higher level of patient autonomy and independence is supported, while also enhancing clinical management and decision-making.

Much of the strength in this system lies in the ability to extensively record and monitor patient data electronically. Clayton and Hripcsak (1995) suggest that the availability of patient information in an electronic format has been one of the most valuable and widely used Decision Support Systems (DSS) in health care. With patient information stored and tracked through home-based DSS, clinicians can potentially make more informed decisions with convenient access to entire patient histories and vital statistics (Cardozo & Steinberg, 2010). Clinicians rely upon timely access to test results and patient records in order to manage care and make efficient treatment decisions. The rapid or real-time transmission of accurate and organized data provided by the monitoring tools of home telecare technologies serve to facilitate this process (Klonoff & True, 2009). Devices are currently in existence to track a number of patient vitals and biostatistics over a period of time, including basic clinical measurements such as temperature, weight, blood pressure, and lung function (Magrabi et al., 2001; Rahimpour et al., 2008). Falas et al. (2003) suggest that providing real-time access to this information allows physicians to rank cases in terms of medical priority, as well as electronically manage how they are handled. This level of monitoring is of particular value to older adults with chronic conditions, who may otherwise find it difficult to physically visit their general practitioner for consultation and treatment of minor symptoms. With this technology, the physical barriers to accessing care are eliminated because minor concerns or changes in vital signs can be dealt with quickly and remotely.

Thornett (2001) indicates that computer-based access to individual patient data can also assist with diagnosis and enhance clinical decision-making through the vast amounts of information that modern practice databases can potentially hold. This allows aging patients to receive more carefully monitored care than if they were to rely upon less-frequent in-person physician visits. Home telecare technologies are used to manage such symptoms as "chronic heart failure, asthma, diabetes, and hypertension" (Celler et al., 2003, p. 242). One of the technological applications used with this form of case management is the video-phone system, allowing nurses and physicians the opportunity to speak directly with and see patients via video monitoring technology, while also wirelessly gathering and assessing data on their vital signs from health monitoring equipment (p. 242).

With this more accessible format to gather and display patient information, a clinician may then also more easily consult electronic decision support materials and evidence – using the Internet or some other form of health information database – to assist in treatment plans and diagnosis.

In addition to videophone technology, and the increased level of decision support that comes with real-time access to patient history and information, another prominent facet of home telecare is teleconsulting. Here, general practitioners can remotely consult with specialists when managing a particular case, thereby interacting with a panel of "experts" when treating a patient (Vitacca et al., 2006). Given that distance is not a barrier with telemedical technology, the geographic location of the consulting panel can potentially include a wide array of international experts. This aspect of telemedicine enables the globalization of medical practice and group decision-making – an important transition in an era when information sharing is becoming increasingly ubiquitous. Here, patients may be treated from a far larger pool of knowledge than they would otherwise receive from traditional care in a physician's office. Instead of one clinician assessing and making decisions about a complex case, there is now the potential to rely upon multiple experts in the delivery of care.

BENEFITS AND CHALLENGES OF HOME TELECARE

Strengths of Home Telecare for Policymakers and Patients

With new home telecare technologies–and access to a more extensive pool of medical expertise–there are several noteworthy aspects of home telecare that are superior to methods of traditional medicine for both policymakers and patients. The first is the reduced economic cost to the health care system itself. This can be seen with less outpatient visits, as well as a reduction in hospital inpatient stays and fewer admissions to nursing homes (Magnusson et al., 2004). Though the initial implementation costs associated with home telecare equipment may be high, it is likely to become lower with the widespread adoption and greater prevalence of such technologies – particularly with the resultant competitive pricing and lowered cost of goods that comes in any rapidly growing market of this nature (Dansky et al., 2001). The benefit of a lesser financial burden to the health care system is particularly important in a time when the scarcity of health care resources is becoming an increasing concern as society's largest age cohort enters the later stages of life. Health care provision has transformed through free market enterprise, to become an increasingly commodified entity, where resources are scarce and care may be compromised (Bambra, et al., 2005; Kearns & Barnett, 1999). As a result, the system is faced with the prospect of being unable to accommodate the needs of all patients equally. The increased use of new information technologies to minimize costs by providing care in the home therefore offers an economic benefit that will enable a greater number of older adults in the growing senior population to efficiently receive treatment and care.

The use of in-home technologies that monitor vital signs and symptoms also benefit patients by allowing individuals to maintain their independence and remain active members of their community. The movement of forcing seniors into a nursing home or other form of long term care facility can be a difficult experience, sometimes fostering a degree of physical, emotional, and/or intellectual decline. When older adults remain in their homes, rather than moving to an institutional environment, they are able to enjoy an overall better quality of life and continue to benefit from enriched social networks (Hébert et al., 2001).

Another important benefit of home telecare technologies is the ability of policymakers to better support patients in rural and other underserved regions (Magnusson et al., 2004). For example, with the use of home telecare technologies, older

adults in northern Aboriginal communities of Canada – where the shortage of physicians is a significant concern – may benefit from the medical expertise of physicians that are remotely located in more populated urban centers. Due to a significant shortage of physicians and specialists in rural areas of Canada, for example, many do not receive medical attention (Dove, 2009). Members of vulnerable groups who require specialized services–particularly women, older adults, and racialized individuals–are at an even greater risk of experiencing compromised care. The use of home telecare technologies has the potential to allow governments to cater to the health care needs of even their most geographically underserved populations.

Finally, home telecare–as with many other branches of telemedicine–allows for greater opportunity to facilitate group clinical decision-making and the sharing of knowledge between clinicians. Quintero et al. (2001) refer to this as "collaborative medical reasoning," where physicians can draw upon knowledge produced in group meetings comprised of both experts and novices (p. 4). This exchange of information ultimately allows for more informed decisions that draw upon a large knowledge base to aid in making treatment and care decisions. With the expertise of more health care professionals, a reduction in medical errors is likely to be realized in treatment and diagnosis. From an international perspective, there is also the added benefit of forging strong partnerships and connections amongst those in the global medical community, while also providing the best possible care from an expansive medical pool of expertise.

Challenges of Home Telecare

Despite the aforementioned benefits of home telecare technologies, prominent research questions, perspectives, as well as concerns emerge with regards to self-management, the changing role of the health care professional, and usability for patients – particularly older adults. The new role of both the patient and the clinician in managing and making decisions about care is an important perspective for consideration. With the growth of home telecare mechanisms and technologies comes a greater emphasis on self-management by the patient and a potentially lesser role for health care professionals. Celler et al. (2003) explore this shift, describing a patient-managed system:

A patient-managed Home Telecare System with integrated clinical signs monitoring, automated scheduling and medication reminders, as well as access to health education and daily logs, is presented as an example of information and communication technology use for chronic disease self-management (p. 242).

This trend is motivated by the economic goals of the home telecare effort, where an important aim is to alleviate cost to the health care system by shifting the responsibility away from the hospital or primary care facility, toward technological solutions to assist in clinical decisions. The de-personalization of medical care, and potential reduction of human contact in clinical care, is one prominent dilemma that has yet to be reconciled (Percival & Hanson, 2006). One aspect of home telecare, for example, is that of "self-assessed patient health status," which essentially monitors and assesses one's health status through electronic questionnaires and provides health information to the patient electronically (Magrabi et al., 2001). A central question that emerges with this increased role of the patient in managing his or her own health is how this will impact both patient care and clinical decision-making at large.

Questions around usability also emerge as a related challenge in discussions about home telecare. Botsis et al. (2008) write of the importance of usability, given that patients and their families are likely to be directly utilizing these technologies in their homes and the design of the information system must be such that it is useable for clinicians *and* their patients. This may be particularly difficult given that geriatric patients are less likely to be technologically inclined and are also more likely to be distrustful of newer methods of care than their younger counterparts (Rahimpour et al., 2008). This concern will only grow as information technology and the field of telemedicine continues to advance. Adaptability, usability, and accessibility are therefore important perspectives of consideration with home telecare for older adults.

Older adults also express reservations about the loss of autonomy and privacy that arises with the self-management and monitoring tools utilized by home telecare systems (Percival & Hanson, 2006). Given that many of these patients are older in age, some prefer human interaction with their health care providers and might be hesitant toward the shifting reliance on technology to assist clinicians with making decisions concerning their care and treatment. Use of computers and the Internet tend to be under-utilized amongst seniors (Kaufman et al., 2003; Magnusson et al., 2004). Given that home telecare is geared mainly toward the aged, accessibility and the use of adaptive technology to make these mechanisms as user-friendly as possible are crucial to the full implementation of the system.

There is also concern with home telecare and the scope of medical conditions that can be effectively managed and monitored with its services. While home telecare efforts have been found to be feasible and effective for monitoring and treating chronic conditions, it is difficult to sustain with more life-threatening and serious conditions given the physical distance between the physician and the patient (Botsis et al., 2008). Such cases potentially require immediate in-person response and action from a treating physician.

Furthermore, technological difficulties from misuse or mis-handling of equipment, faulty devices, or other malfunctioning errors can be frustrating for both providers and patients, making the monitoring process more complex (Roback & Herzog, 2003). Examples include devices that may require manual data entry–such as one's blood pressure level–allowing for the input of potentially incorrect or missing information, depending on who is operating the device and how well-trained or skilled they are in such mechanisms. In the event of technical or human error, there are a number of problems that can result, not the least of which is compromised care or increased risk that can be fatal for the patient.

Finally, given that home telecare is a fairly new field involving a number of technological advancements that could completely alter the way we interact with health care providers, a number of change management challenges are also involved in its implementation and in how the scheme would "operate, define, deliver, and manage care at home and throughout the health care system" (Coughlin et al., 2006, p. 206). With the increased number of actors involved in this transition, for example, significant integration efforts make it difficult to co-ordinate and operationalize a system that is completely aligned with a telemedical effort. This creates not only a potentially difficult transition for those working within the system, but also for patients themselves. In the subsequent section, we propose the use of a medical implant device to address some of these challenges involved with geriatric home telecare for health policymakers, clinical decision-makers and patients.

Mergence of Medical Implant and Mobile Wireless Technology

As has emerged throughout this discussion, usability, accessibility and efficiency are significant areas of concern for home telecare technology in geriatric medicine. One technology that has the potential to address these challenges, and assist physician decision-making in remote patient care, is the implantation of a device–under the skin–that can be used as a tool to monitor physiological statistics and wirelessly transmit real-time patient data. Such technologies currently exist in some forms to assist physicians in monitoring, treating,

and diagnosing conditions related to "heart disease, gastrointestinal tract, neurological disorders, cancer detection, handicap rehabilitation, and general health monitor[ing]" (Zhen et al., 2009, p. 23). Yet, one aspect of this technology that does not emerge in the literature is the potential use of such implants for older patients with chronic Heart Failure (HF).

Chronic HF is a condition that affects an increasing number of older adults each year, impacting more than 350,000 Canadians (Godfrey et al., 2007; Liu et al., 2001). With the rapidly growing aging population, the number of cases is projected to increase in the coming years. Currently, in order to properly manage a chronic condition like HF frequent hospitalization or cardiac monitoring is required (Abraham et al., 2011). Hospitalization rates for this particular condition are therefore high and on the rise, posing some concern over the increased cost of caring for this influx of patients. In treating this condition, the Canadian health care system must sustain a cost of over $1 billion per year for inpatient hospital care (Godfrey et al., 2007). A mechanism for constant monitoring of this condition outside of a health care facility therefore stands to dramatically decrease cost to the primary health care system.

While a home telecare system provides one such solution, it is likely to involve confinement to the home, making it difficult for patients to sustain a high level of social activity and engagement in the community – an integral part of life for older adults who are particularly vulnerable to social isolation. Therefore, the use of an implantable monitoring device for chronic HF would allow those in the vulnerable senior population to more easily leave the home telecare environment, knowing that their condition is still being closely monitored. This also eases the concerns of caregivers who may otherwise have reservations about accompanying these individuals outside of the home and away from monitoring equipment.

To address this need, we propose the merging of two existing technologies with seemingly compatible properties. This proposed amalgamation would allow patient data collected through a specific type of body implant–known as Micro Electro-Mechanical Systems (MEMS)–to be transmitted to a mobile device that the patient carries on their person, allowing for clinical management and decision-making by the patient or caregiver in addition to the remotely located physician. Currently, MEMS transmit detailed health information to the remote physician via the Internet, but not to the patient. Before discussing the proposed use of these technologies together, it is important to first establish how they each separately operate.

First, MEMS are miniature electronic implantable devices that monitor and transmit hemodynamic information directly from a body implant to a secure Website (Botsis et al., 2008). With regards to chronic HF, data recorded by these implants currently include pulmonary artery pressures, systolic and diastolic pressures, heart rate and cardiac output. The purpose of such monitoring is to reduce the number of hospitalizations due to the worsening of chronic HF in patients. Heart failure is broadly defined as the inability of the heart to output sufficient blood to meet the metabolic demands of the body (Borlaug et al., 2006). While it may have numerous causes, it is most commonly due to coronary artery disease and hypertension. Clinical signs and symptoms of the condition include shortness of breath, fatigue, dizziness, and cough. Patients experiencing these symptoms commonly present to emergency departments to alleviate their clinical symptoms. The worsening of chronic HF leads to increased emergency department visits and higher instances of inpatient hospitalization. If a treating physician could monitor blood pressure levels remotely and adjust medications as necessary, however, hospitalization could be prevented, improving the lifestyle of patients and ultimately reducing health-care costs to the system.

CardioMEMS–the company that produces this particular implant–utilizes this technology to monitor symptoms of HF in patients by inserting the implant directly into one of the ventricles of the heart (Raskovic et al., 2004). Transmission occurs when the patient is lying down on a pillow with a built-in antenna. From here, the device records the hemodynamic data previously mentioned, and transmits it via a telephone line to a private Internet database system, allowing remote and real-time access to the information through a secure Web-based server (Abraham et al., 2011). At present, the MEMS device data transmits exclusively to a private Website which can only be accessed by healthcare professionals. Through access to the database, physicians can adjust blood pressure medication dosage or recommend hospitalization, if necessary. After a pressure reading is taken, the patient may then be advised to adjust their medication dosage fairly quickly if a change in levels is detected.

The secure online medical database available to the physician while tracking vital signs in this way greatly assists clinicians in the clinical decision-making process by allowing easy and electronic access to patient histories, teleconsultation with other physicians, as well as access to various health databases and resources to assist in diagnosis. The capability of remote real-time monitoring is a potentially more efficient and direct method that is comparable to patients with diabetes who are similarly given blood glucose monitoring and subsequent prescription medication adjustments. The benefit of this technology for patients is that it allows physicians to frequently monitor cardiac data in a way that many other current non-invasive methods of management for chronic HF cannot (Abraham, et al., 2011). Implant technology is effective for management of this particular condition because if caught early, HF can be efficiently observed before clinical signs and systems manifest themselves, requiring the patient to be hospitalized. This is where mobile device transfer to a portable unit on the patient's person would be the next logical step in utilization of the MEMS device.

The second existing technology that we are suggesting should be adapted for more efficient results with MEMS in the treatment of HF is a mobile device that wirelessly records and processes information directly from the body implant. This device does so in close proximity to the patient – as they would be expected to carry this on their person. Milenković et al. (2006) describe such a system where a personal server application is run on a mobile device and wirelessly linked to medical body sensors, providing feedback through a "user friendly and intuitive graphical or audio user interface," thereby providing an interface custom to the user as well as an interface distinct to the medical server (p. 2523).

The combined use of both of these technologies, as illustrated in Figure 1, involves the short distance transmission of data from the implant to a mobile device, as well as the long distance transmission of patient data to a remotely located physician. In essence, the patient or caregiver is alerted to real time changes in their condition– through the mobile device–and provided with appropriate health information and feedback in instances where symptoms do not necessarily require emergency treatment and can be self-managed. Hospitalization rates can in turn also

Figure 1. Flow of data in telecare system utilizing a body implant in conjunction with a mobile device

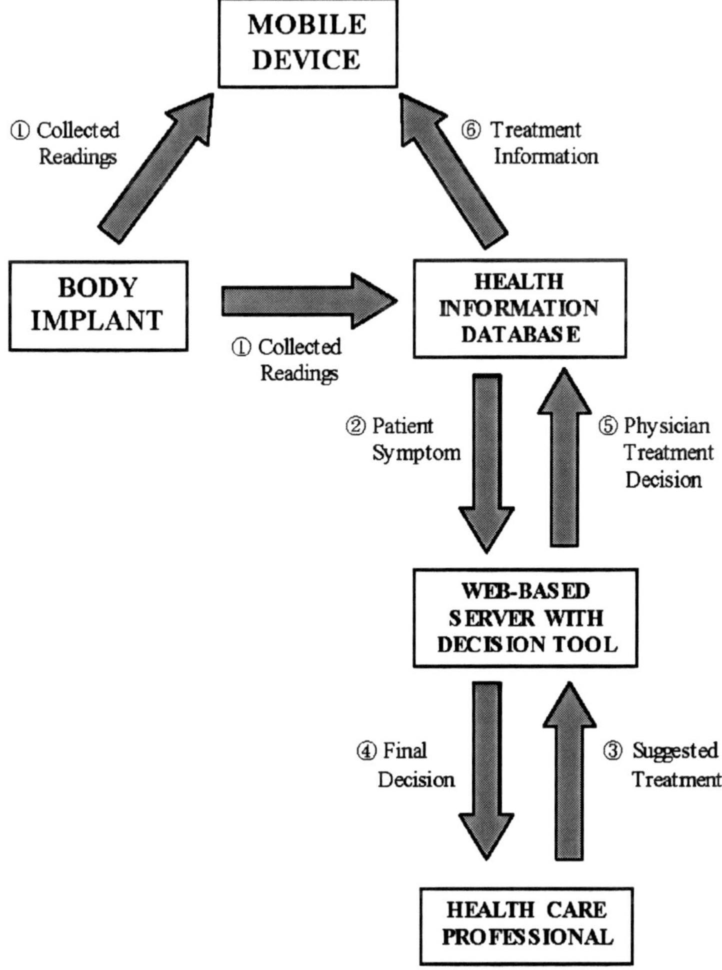

be reduced by optimization of blood pressure symptoms that may lead to the exacerbation of chronic HF (Abraham et al., 2011).

The value of the combined use of these technologies is that the patient can more easily move to a different location or travel without the fear of losing data, and the physician can better assess their condition by monitoring cardiac output during normal daily activities – as opposed to doing so when the patient is bed-ridden or immobile (Tan et al., 2009). Efficiency of monitoring also increases with the use of a mobile device in conjunction with a body monitoring implant such as MEMS by "increasing the amount of data obtained, and streamlining its storage and processing" for faster results (p. 260). Using the example of blood pressure levels, Figure 2 illustrates the efficient use of a Web-based decision support tool in providing accurate diagnosis and treatment. With the combined use of these technologies, and the element of self-care management that it allows, the task of clinical decision-making now has the potential to extend beyond the sole practitioner, to encompass a medical community of both physicians and patients.

Benefits of an Implant

There are several practical applications for this proposed use of MEMS with a mobile device in the monitoring of HF. Firstly, disease management and care are not compromised for aging patients if they leave the confines of their home. Therefore, they are not restricted to one location and can enjoy a more enhanced social life with family and friends – something that is of particular importance to older adults who are already at greater risk of isolation.

Second, the regular and consistent monitoring of HF symptoms provided by the technology allows patients or caregivers the opportunity to more efficiently manage treatment regimes. Users can be trained to use the health tools provided by the mobile device application that would be designed with a simple and highly usable interface. Of course–as established earlier–usability is always a concern when dealing with technology and older adults, but the advent of touch screen devices and large icons with minimalist displays could minimize these limitations. For example, including warning mechanisms for symptoms associated

Figure 2. Web-based server with decision support system for monitoring blood pressure

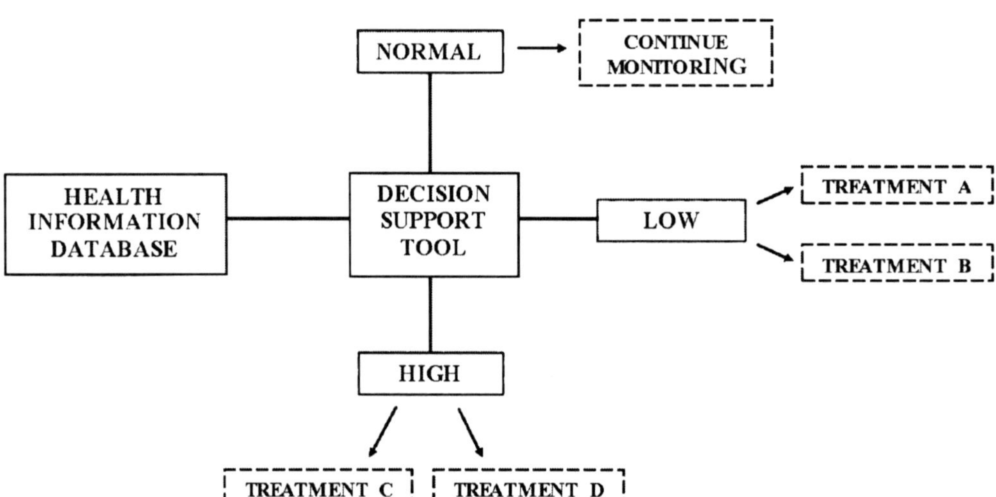

with chronic HF could alert healthcare professionals and patients to the need for more urgent intervention via the emergency department. In less serious instances, patients with blood pressure readings that are either too high or low may also benefit from real-time or immediate adjustment of medication dosages via the mobile device. These elements serve the important goal of alleviating the burden on the health care system by shifting care toward self-management whenever possible.

Another important benefit with this proposed technology concerns medication compliance. One major cause for the worsening of chronic HF in older adults is failing to adhere to medication regimens assigned by a physician. Much of this is due to poor follow up with primary care practitioners, which can result in the worsening of this condition (Schiff et al., 2003). Convenient access to care, self-monitoring and reinforcement are all factors, which have been shown to improve compliance with medication regimes because patients are not required to make multiple visits to their physician for treatment (Haynes et al., 2008). Although further research is needed to explore the extent to which the use of a body implant device with mobile wireless technology would achieve this, it is likely to result in better compliance and in turn, reduced hospitalizations.

Finally, the mobile device also has the potential to facilitate communication with a physician via instant messaging, or make use of videophone technologies that would allow live consultation with a health care professional directly on the screen of the device. Of course, one potential limitation of this is the availability of health care professionals, which may become problematic if the widespread use of this technology involves long wait times for consultation. Ultimately, the goal is a shift towards self-management, where the physician is not over-burdened with treatment decisions if a case can be efficiently managed remotely by a patient or caregiver using assistive tools and devices.

FUTURE RESEARCH DIRECTIONS

There is little doubt that as the aging population continues to grow, policymakers, managers and patients must adapt to the changing landscape of health care delivery. As has been discussed throughout this chapter, the increased use of information technologies and home telecare services are an important avenue through which to meet the needs of aging patients; while also lessening the reliance on what are becoming more limited resources of the primary health care system. With this drastic transition, there are a number of important considerations and difficulties that will require extensive research and effort going forward. As home telecare efforts expand, policymakers will be faced with the ethical questions that will inevitably arise as medicine is delivered at a distance (Botsis & Hartvigsen, 2008). The line between patient- and physician- managed care becomes blurred as the two can now function in entirely different geographic locations during consultation and treatment. The legal aspects of telemedicine also emerge as an immense concern in the future, particularly where medical malpractice policies and technological malfunction and errors are concerned. Additionally, Botsis and Hartvigsen (2008) discuss that while cost savings to the system may be high with these new technologies, a number of countries are not equipped to provide reliable and consistent methods of reimbursement to patients for the purchase of home telecare equipment. Given that older adults are likely to experience greater levels of poverty than their younger counterparts; proper government assistance programs must also be explored and implemented by policymakers.

In addition to these policy considerations, managers of care must also be mindful of the complexities involved in the testing, research and development of new telecare technologies, each of which is likely to involve a number of different dimensions. In order to properly test and determine the efficacy of adapting a technology such as the MEMS cardiac implant for use with a mobile device, for example, a number of actors would need to be involved. First, as a primary corporate actor, the CardioMEMS company would need to invest in research and development to adapt the MEMS implant for use with a mobile device. Once a prototype version of the device is developed and ready for testing, a willing health care facility or hospital must be selected to test the product, in conjunction with a leading academic research team to conduct the study. Here, a lead physician is needed to manage a clinical trial involving an appropriately selected group of geriatric participants with chronic HF. In the trial phase of the study, a team of experts in information technology would also be required to facilitate and guide the creation, implementation and maintenance of the software tools and health information database to be accessed by patients on the mobile device, as well as by physicians at a distance. Such a process is likely to take time and involve a number of patient safety considerations from both managers and health care providers.

Finally, future research and effort must also be concentrated on the increasing trend of self-care amongst patients and caregivers who are required to take a more prominent role in the delivery of telecare – alongside physicians. User-friendly technology is critical in this endeavour. Patients, along with policymakers and managers will need to adapt to constant changes in the rapidly changing and evolving sphere of information technology and health. In this effort, more comprehensive studies and literature on the efficacy and efficiency of home telecare will be needed as new avenues–including the adaptation of mobile wireless technology in this field–emerge.

CONCLUSION

In this chapter, we have explored the use of home telecare technology as a promising application for enhanced clinical decision-making in geriatric medicine. With the growing aging population, telemedicine is likely to become a very attractive option to increase efficiency in health care management. Throughout this analysis, several challenges arise in the areas of usability, privacy, patient autonomy, self-management and group clinical decision-making. To address some of these concerns, particularly with self-management and usability, we suggest the use of the MEMS cardiac implant in conjunction with a mobile device to assist in more efficient clinical decision-making for physicians, as well as an improved standard of care for patients and caregivers. Ultimately, it seems certain that home telecare is an expanding field that is sure to be met with significant innovation in the coming years. Going forward, despite the immense promise for clinical management that stands to result from the use of these new methods, the inevitable dramatic shift in the way that medicine is delivered must be handled carefully so that patient care remains as a fundamental priority.

REFERENCES

Abraham, W. T., Adamson, P. B., Bourge, R. C., Aaron, M. F., Costanzo, M. R., & Stevenson, L. W. et al. (2011). Wireless pulmonary artery haemodynamic monitoring in chronic heart failure: A randomised control trial. *Lancet, 377*(9766), 658–666. doi:10.1016/S0140-6736(11)60101-3 PMID:21315441

Abraham, W. T., Adamson, P. B., Hasan, A., Bourge, R. C., Pamboukian, S. V., Aaron, M. F., & Raval, N. Y. (2011). Safety and accuracy of a wireless pulmonary artery pressure monitoring system in patients with heart failure. *American Heart Journal, 161*(3), 558–566. doi:10.1016/j.ahj.2010.10.041 PMID:21392612

Allen, A., & March, A. (2002). Telemedicine at the community cancer center. *Oncology Issues, 17*(1), 18–24.

Bambra, C., Fox, D., & Scott-Samuel, A. (2005). Towards a politics of health. *Health Promotion International, 20*(2), 187–193. doi:10.1093/heapro/dah608 PMID:15722364

Borlaug, B. A., Melenovsky, V., Russell, S. D., Kessler, K., Pacak, K., Becker, L. C., & Kass, D. A. (2006). Impaired chronotropic and vasodilator reserves limit exercise capacity in patients with heart failure and a preserved ejection fraction. *Circulation, 114*(20), 2138–2147. doi:10.1161/CIRCULATIONAHA.106.632745 PMID:17088459

Botsis, T., Demiris, G., Pedersen, S., & Hartvigsen, G. (2008). Home telecare technologies for the elderly. *Journal of Telemedicine and Telecare, 14,* 333–337. doi:10.1258/jtt.2008.007002 PMID:18852311

Botsis, T., & Hartvigsen, G. (2008). Current status and future perspectives in telecare for elderly people suffering from chronic diseases. *Journal of Telemedicine and Telecare, 14,* 195–203. doi:10.1258/jtt.2008.070905 PMID:18534954

Cardozo, L., & Steinberg, J. (2010). Telemedicine for recently discharged older patients. *Telemedicine and e-Health, 16*(1), 49-55.

Celler, B. G., Lovell, N. H., & Basilakis, J. (2003). Using information technology to improve the management of chronic disease. *The Medical Journal of Australia, 179*(5), 242–246. PMID:12924970

Clayton, P. D., & Hripcsak, G. (1995). Decision support in healthcare. *International Journal of Bio-Medical Computing, 39*(1), 59–66. doi:10.1016/0020-7101(94)01080-K PMID:7601543

Coughlin, J. F., Pope, J. E., & Leedle, B. R. (2006). Old age, new technology, and future innovations in disease management and home health care. *Home Health Care Management & Practice, 18*(3), 196–207. doi:10.1177/1084822305281955

Dansky, K. H., Palmer, L., Shea, D., & Bowles, K. H. (2001). Cost analysis of telehomecare. *Telemedicine Journal and e-Health, 7*(3), 225–232. doi:10.1089/153056201316970920 PMID:11564358

Dove, N. (2009). Can international medical graduates help solve Canada's shortage of rural physicians? *Canadian Journal of Rural Medicine, 14*(3), 120–123. PMID:19594998

Falas, T., Papadopoulos, G., & Stafylopatis, A. (2003). A review of decision support systems in telecare. *Journal of Medical Systems, 27*(4), 347–356. doi:10.1023/A:1023705320471 PMID:12846466

Godfrey, C. M., Harrison, M. B., Friedberg, E., Medves, J. M., & Tranmer, J. E. (2007). The symptom of pain in individuals recently hospitalized for heart failure. *The Journal of Cardiovascular Nursing, 22*(5), 368–374. PMID:17724418

Haynes, R. B., Ackloo, E., Sahota, N., McDonald, H. P., & Yao, X. (2008). Interventions for enhancing medication adherence [review]. *Cochrane Database of Systematic Reviews, 2*(2), 1–127.

Hébert, M. A., Korabek, B., & Scott, R. E. (2006). Moving research into practice: A decision framework for integrating home telehealth into chronic illness care. *International Journal of Medical Informatics, 75,* 786–794. doi:10.1016/j.ijmedinf.2006.05.041 PMID:16872892

Hébert, R., Dubios, M., Wolfson, C., Chambers, L., & Cohen, C. (2001). Factors associated with long-term institutionalization of older people with dementia: Data from the Canadian study of health and aging. *Journal of Gerontology, 56*(11), 693–699.

Hersh, W., Helfand, M., Wallace, J., Kraemer, D., Patterson, P., Shapiro, S., & Greenlick, M. (2002). A systematic review of the efficacy of telemedicine for making diagnostic and management decisions. *Journal of Telemedicine and Telecare*, *8*, 197–209. doi:10.1258/135763302320272167 PMID:12217102

Kaufman, D. R., Patel, V. L., Hilliman, C., Morin, P. C., Pevzner, J., Weinstock, R. S., & Starren, J. (2003). Usability in the real world: Assessing medical information technologies in patients' homes. *Journal of Biomedical Informatics*, *36*(1-2), 45–60. doi:10.1016/S1532-0464(03)00056-X PMID:14552846

Kearns, R. A., & Barnett, J. R. (1999). Auckland's starship enterprise: Placing metaphor in a children's hospital. In A. Williams (Ed.), *Therapeutic landscapes: The dynamic between place and wellness* (pp. 169–200). Lanham, MD: University Press of America Inc.

Klonoff, D. C., & True, M. W. (2009). The missing element of telemedicine for diabetes: Decision support software. *Journal of Diabetes Science and Technology*, *3*(5), 996–1001. PMID:20144411

Koch, S. (2006). Home telehealth–Current state and future trends. *International Journal of Medical Informatics*, *75*(8), 565–576. doi:10.1016/j.ijmedinf.2005.09.002 PMID:16298545

Liu, P., Arnold, M., Belenkie, I., Howlett, J., Huckell, V., & Ignazewski, A. et al. (2001). The 2001 Canadian cardiovascular society consensus guideline update for the management and prevention of heart failure. *The Canadian Journal of Cardiology*, *17*(Suppl E), 5E–25E. PMID:11773943

Magnusson, L., Hanson, E., & Borg, M. (2004). A literature review study of information and communication technology as a support for frail older people living at home and their family carers. *Technology and Disability*, *16*(4), 223–235.

Magrabi, F., Lovell, N. H., Huynh, K., & Celler, B. G. (2001). *Home telecare: System architecture to support chronic disease management.* Paper presented at the 23rd Annual International Conference of the IEEE Engineering in Medicine and Biology Society. Istanbul, Turkey.

Milenković, A., Otto, C., & Jovanov, E. (2006). Wireless sensor network for personal health monitoring: Issues and implementation. *Computer Communications*, *29*, 2521–2533. doi:10.1016/j.comcom.2006.02.011

Percival, J., & Hanson, J. (2006). Big brother or brave new world? Telecare and its implications for older people's independence and social inclusion. *Critical Social Policy*, *26*(4), 888–909. doi:10.1177/0261018306068480

Quintero, J., Abraham, M., Aguilera, A., Villegas, H., Montilla, G., & Solaiman, B. (2001, October). *Collaborative medical reasoning in telemedicine.* Paper presented at the 23rd Annual International Conference of the IEEE Engineering in Medicine and Biology Society. Istanbul, Turkey.

Rahimpour, M., Lovell, N. H., Celler, B. G., & McCormick, J. (2008). Patients' perceptions of a home telecare system. *International Journal of Medical Informatics*, *77*, 486–498. doi:10.1016/j.ijmedinf.2007.10.006 PMID:18023610

Raskovic, D., Martin, T., & Jovanov, E. (2004). Medical monitoring applications for wearable computing. *The Computer Journal*, *47*(4), 495–504. doi:10.1093/comjnl/47.4.495

Roback, K., & Herzog, A. (2003). Home informatics in healthcare: Assessment guidelines to keep up quality of care and avoid adverse effects. *Technology and Health Care*, *11*, 195–206. PMID:12775936

Schiff, G. D., Fung, S., Speroff, T., & McNutt, R. A. (2003). Decompensated heart failure: Symptoms, patterns of onset, and contributing factors. *The American Journal of Medicine*, *114*(8), 625–630. doi:10.1016/S0002-9343(03)00132-3 PMID:12798449

Tan, R., McClure, T., Lin, C. K., Jea, D., Dabiri, F., & Massey, T. et al. (2009). Development of a fully implantable wireless pressure monitoring system. *Biomedical Microdevices*, *11*, 259–264. doi:10.1007/s10544-008-9232-1 PMID:18836836

Thornett, A. M. (2001). Computer decision support systems in general practice. *International Journal of Information Management*, *21*, 39–47. doi:10.1016/S0268-4012(00)00049-9

Vitacca, M., Assoni, G., Pizzocaro, P., Guerra, A., Marchina, L., & Scalvini, S. et al. (2006). A pilot study of nurse-led, home monitoring for patients with chronic respiratory failure and with mechanical ventilation assistance. *Journal of Telemedicine and Telecare*, *12*(7), 337–342. doi:10.1258/135763306778682404 PMID:17059649

World Health Organization. (2006). *Active aging – A policy framework*. Retrieved September 3, 2012, from http://whqlibdoc.who.int/hq/2002/who_nmh_nph_02.8.pdf

Zhen, B., Li, H., & Kohno, R. (2009). Networking issues in medical implant communications. *International Journal of Multimedia and Ubiquitous Engineering*, *4*(1), 23–37.

ADDITIONAL READING

Amala, L., Turner, T., Gretton, M., Baksh, A., & Cleland, J. (2003). A systemic review of telemonitoring for the management of heart failure. *European Journal of Heart Failure*, *5*(5), 583–590. doi:10.1016/S1388-9842(03)00160-0 PMID:14607195

Audebert, H. J., Boy, S., Jankovits, R., Pilz, P., Klucken, J., Fehm, N. P., & Schenkel, J. (2008). Is mobile teleconsulting equivalent to hospital-based telestroke services? *Stroke*, *39*(12), 3427–3430. doi:10.1161/STROKEAHA.108.520478 PMID:18787198

Barlow, J., Bayer, S., Curry, R., Hendy, J., & McMahon, L. (2010). From care closer to home to care in the home: The potential impact of telecare on the healthcare built environment. In M. Kagioglou & P. Tzortzopoulos (Eds.), *Improving healthcare through built environment infrastructure* (pp. 131–150). Malden, MA: Blackwell Publishing Ltd. doi:10.1002/9781444319675.ch9

Barlow, J., Singh, D., Bayer, S., & Curry, R. (2007). A systemic review of the benefits of home telecare for frail elderly people and those with long-term conditions. *Journal of Telemedicine and Telecare*, *13*(4), 172–179. doi:10.1258/135763307780908058 PMID:17565772

Bates, D. W., & Bitton, A. (2010). The future of health information technology in the patient-centered medical home. *Health Affairs*, *29*(4), 614–621. doi:10.1377/hlthaff.2010.0007 PMID:20368590

Bellazzi, R., Montani, S., Riva, A., & Stefanelli, M. (2001). Web-based telemedicine systems for home-care: Technical issues and experiences. *Computer Methods and Programs in Biomedicine, 64*(3), 175–187. doi:10.1016/S0169-2607(00)00137-1 PMID:11226615

Bertera, E. M., Tran, B. Q., Wuertz, E. M., & Bonner, A. (2007). A study of the receptivity to telecare technology in a community-based elderly minority population. *Journal of Telemedicine and Telecare, 13*(7), 327–332. doi:10.1258/135763307782215325 PMID:17958932

Cartwright, L. (2000). Reach out and heal someone: Telemedicine and the globalization of health care. *Health, 4*(3), 347–377.

Coleman, E. A. (2003). Falling through the cracks: Challenges and opportunities for improving transitional care for persons with continuous complex care needs. *Journal of the American Geriatrics Society, 51*(4), 549–555. doi:10.1046/j.1532-5415.2003.51185.x PMID:12657078

Freedman, V. A., & Martin, L. G. (1998). Understanding trends in function among older Americans. *American Journal of Public Health, 88*(10), 1457–1462. doi:10.2105/AJPH.88.10.1457 PMID:9772844

Hersh, W. R., Hickam, D. H., Severance, S. M., Dana, T. L., Krages, K. P., & Helfand, M. (2006). Diagnosis, access and outcomes: Update of a systematic review of telemedicine services. *Journal of Telemedicine and Telecare, 12*(Suppl. 2), 3–31. doi:10.1258/135763306778393117 PMID:16884561

Jerant, A. F., Azari, R., & Nesbitt, T. S. (2001). Reducing the costs of frequent hospital admissions for congestive heart failure: A randomized trial of a home telecare intervention. *Medical Care, 39*(11), 1234–1245. doi:10.1097/00005650-200111000-00010 PMID:11606877

Koch, S. (2006). Meeting the challenges – The role of medical informatics in an ageing society. *Studies in Health Technology and Informatics, 124*, 25–31. PMID:17108500

Koch, S., & Hägglund, M. (2009). Health informatics and the delivery of care to older people. *Maturitas, 63*(3), 195–199. doi:10.1016/j.maturitas.2009.03.023 PMID:19487092

Lehoux, P., Sicotte, C., Denis, J., Berg, M., & Lacroix, A. (2002). The theory of use behind telemedicine: How compatible with physicians' clinical routines? *Social Science & Medicine, 54*(6), 889–904. doi:10.1016/S0277-9536(01)00063-6 PMID:11996023

Liddy, C., Dusseault, J. J., Dahrouge, S., Hogg, W., Lemelin, J., & Humber, J. (2008). Telehomecare for patients with multiple chronic illnesses. *Canadian Family Physician Medecin de Famille Canadien, 54*(1), 58–65. PMID:18208957

Mann, W. C., Marchant, T., Tomita, M., Fraas, L., & Stanton, K. (2002). Elder acceptance of health monitoring devices in the home. *Care Management Journals, 3*(2), 91–98. PMID:12455220

McColl, M. A., Jarzynowska, A., & Shortt, S. E. D. (2010). Unmet health care needs of people with disabilities: Population level evidence. *Disability & Society, 25*(2), 205–218. doi:10.1080/09687590903537406

Meredith, S., Feldman, P. H., Frey, D., Hall, K., Arnold, K., Brown, N. J., & Ray, W. A. (2001). Possible medication errors in home healthcare patients. *Journal of the American Geriatrics Society, 49*(6), 719–724. doi:10.1046/j.1532-5415.2001.49147.x PMID:11454109

Nebeker, J. R., Hurdle, J. F., & Bair, B. D. (2003). Future history: Medical informatics in geriatrics. *Journal of Gerontology, 58*(9), 820–825.

Rialle, V., Duchêne, F., Noury, N., Bajolle, L., Demongeot, J. Health 'smart' home: Information technology for patients at home. *Telemedicine and e-Health, 8*(4), 395-409.

Rialle, V., Lamy, J., Noury, N., & Bajolle, L. (2003). Telemonitoring of patients at home: A software agent approach. *Computer Methods and Programs in Biomedicine, 72*(3), 257–268. doi:10.1016/S0169-2607(02)00161-X PMID:14554139

Vitacca, M., Scalvini, S., Spanevello, A., & Balbi, B. (2006). Telemedicine and home care: Controversies and opportunities. *Breathe, 3*(2), 149–158.

Wyatt, S., Henwood, F., Hart, A., & Platzer, H. (2004). Extending patient's world: The internet, health information and everyday life. *Sciences Sociales et Sante, 22*(1), 45–68. doi:10.3406/sosan.2004.1608

Xiao, Y., & Chen, H. (2008). *Mobile telemedicine: A computing and networking perspective.* Boca Raton, FL: Auerbach Publications.

KEY TERMS AND DEFINITIONS

Decision Support System: An electronic system that stores data and assists in decision making. In a clinical context, it can be used to store detailed patient data and vital statistics that can then be accessed and used by clinicians to assist in treatment decisions.

Home Telecare: A subspecialty within the larger field of telemedicine that involves clinical monitoring and the collection of patient data–with the use of information technologies–in a private home.

Medical Implant Device: A device placed under the skin that both records and transmits data to a sensor or other device located outside of the body.

Mobile Device: A handheld device with a display screen that can be used as a communicative tool to convey information to a user.

Self-Management: In clinical practice, a process by which a patient takes responsibility in managing their own care.

Telemedicine: Medicine performed at a distance using telecommunications technology. This branch of medicine allows for the exchange of clinical information and provision of care by physicians and other medical professionals from a remote location.

Usability: The extent to which a technology is user friendly and accessible to a patient who may lack technological expertise.

Chapter 84
Tracking Future Path of Consumers' Empowerment in E-Health

Muhammad Anshari
Universiti Brunei Darussalam, Brunei

Mohammad Nabil Almunawar
Universiti Brunei Darussalam, Brunei

ABSTRACT

Developments in ICT have created a new generation of networking technology that affects all areas, including healthcare. The use of ICT in healthcare organizations, for example in health information systems (HIS), has developed the same way as the wider landscape, and includes the use of Internet-based technology. The adoption of social network features as the 'front end' of electronic health (e-health) systems is believed to boost sharing between consumers, leading to greater satisfaction. E-health is likely to become more consumer-centric, accommodating consumers' participation in the healthcare process, including decision-making. The government of Taiwan has successfully implemented a National Health Insurance (NHI) system as the foundation for e-health. Improvements in technology may drive changing consumer behavior concerning healthcare services. This paper addresses some important concepts, milestones, challenges, and future direction of consumer empowerment in Taiwan, and proposes that empowerment will be personal, social, and medical.

INTRODUCTION

Information and communications technology (ICT) now permeates almost all facets of life, including healthcare. ICT is able to improve consistency, accuracy, and efficiency of processes and detailed clinical information flow (Conrick, 2006).

Healthcare organizations, with their requirements for knowledge and an educated workforce, are considered likely to be rapid adopters of ICT (Erl, 2005), but in practice, many healthcare providers are slow to adopt it, and healthcare as a whole is one of the sectors that invests least in it (CSC, 1999; E-Health Ontario, 2009).

DOI: 10.4018/978-1-4666-8756-1.ch084

A health information system (HIS) processes data, and provide information and knowledge in healthcare environments to support high-quality and efficient patient care (Haux et al., 2006. An HIS can be successfully adopted when it integrates people, processes (procedures), strategies (effective implementation), and technologies appropriately to support operations and management, and deliver essential information to improve the quality of healthcare (Almunawar & Anshari, 2014). The HIS has evolved through several stages that have been primarily influenced by the advancement of ICT.

There are several other technologies closely related to HIS. *Health information technology* (HIT) is computer hardware and software that deals with the storage, retrieval, sharing, and use of healthcare information, data, and knowledge for communication and decisions (Goldschmidt, 2005). *Health informatics* is concerned with the cognitive, information-processing, and communication tasks of medical practice, education and research, using information science and technology to support those tasks. Health informatics tools include computers, clinical guidelines, formal medical terminologies, and information and communication systems. The emphasis is on clinical and biomedical applications with the added possibility of integrating clinical components together or with administrative health information systems (Conrick, 2006).

Electronic health (e-health) has been described as the single most important revolution in healthcare since the advent of modern medicine, vaccines, or public health measures such as sanitation and clean water (Silber, 2003). Electronic health records (EHRs) reside at the centre of any health information system. An EHR is an individual patient's medical record in a digital format. EHRs are the building blocks of an HIS that substitutes for the traditional paper record. An EHR system (EHR-S) coordinates the storage and retrieval of individual records with the aid of computers. EHRs are usually accessed via computer, often

through a network, enabling telemedicine. This enables the remote practice of medicine through the exchange of clinical information where patients and providers are geographically separated (Gustafson et al., 1993).

Consumer empowerment in healthcare is a feature of e-health deployment. Empowerment can be considered as a new paradigm in healthcare scenarios, allowing patients to make their own health-related decisions (Anshari & Almunawar, 2012). Consumer empowerment can be supported by allowing customers to control the process of their interactions with their healthcare providers, such as in accessing online services, booking online consultations, and paying online. Empowerment allows patients and their families to access their medical records online, which helps to create individual awareness of health.

In Taiwan, an e-health system called the National Health Insurance (NHI) system has achieved availability, accessibility, and utilization by providers, as shown by the high percentage of online claims and digital records (Chunhuei, Lee & Schoon, 2012). Its low administrative costs, 1.51% of its total expenditure for 2009 (BNHI, 2010), are strong evidence of its high impact.

This paper reviews literature on the healthcare system in Taiwan, identifies the current state of knowledge about e-health systems, and discusses emerging trends and their effect on consumer participation and empowerment. In Section 2, we discuss the background to the study. In Section 3, we focus on some challenges in the recent development of e-health. Future trends in e-health are discussed in Section 4, and Section 5 is the conclusion.

BACKGROUND

In their early stages, in the 1960s, HIS were primarily used for financial accounting of medical transactions and computerized medical record-keeping (Haux, 2006). By the mid-1970s, most

Table 1. HIS by Industry Phase in United States (Bourke, 1994)

Industry phase	Data	Technology
1945–1965 Govt. sponsored growth	Manual	Almost no IT
1965–1973 Medicare introduced	Accounting	Mainframes, stand-alone. No standard
1973–1983 Disenchantment on many fronts	Utilization data, profitability reporting	Minicomputers, PC, DBMS on mainframe
1983–1991 Diagnosis-related groups (DRGs) introduced	Data collection dictated by external organizations	PC networks, PC database
1991–2000 Prospect of national health care	Product line, Market segment, Demographic segment	PC networks and database, AI, data exchange

hospitals used computers for business purposes. Since then, healthcare organizations have become more computerized and their operations significantly dependent on information systems (Haux, 2006). HIS have helped healthcare professionals to improve their efficiency and effectiveness in providing healthcare services. With their ability to record and locate important information quickly, they have become standard in many healthcare organizations.

Haux (2006) categorized the milestones of HIS into several stages. First, there was a shift from paper- to computer-based processing and storage, as well as the increased amount of data in healthcare settings. Second, the focus moved from institution-centered departmental systems toward regional and global HIS. Third, patients and health consumers became HIS users, as well as healthcare professionals and administrators. Fourth, HIS data was used for healthcare planning and clinical and epidemiological research, as well as patient care and administrative purposes. Fifth, there was a shift from technical HIS problems to those of change management and strategic information management. Sixth, the data changed from alpha numeric to images, and to the molecular level. Seventh, there was a steady increase in inclusion of new technologies such as ubiquitous computing environments and sensor-based technologies for health monitoring.

Bourke (1994) summarized HIS phases in the United States (Table 1). From the late 1980s, technology was developed to deliver more tailored services and products at lower prices. During this period, healthcare organizations shifted toward integrated care systems. The introduction of the personal computer (PC) during the 1980s and 1990s, later supported by Local Area Networks (LAN), made the use of HIS widespread. HIS vendors began to reengineer their products and collaborated with others to make the systems more open. Database management systems (DBMS), equipped with query languages, enabled other vendors to access the databases. Query language has mediated interoperability and heterogeneous databases across HIS providers.

A trend toward open systems and objective technologies emerged during the 1990s (Kuhn & Giuse, 2001), probably influenced by the increase in the connectivity of networks and the ability of database management systems to multitask across networks and databases. Networking technologies and database management systems were able to incorporate better healthcare services, increasing response times and making it easier to meet the increasing demands for system integration. The use of broader technologies including expert systems, voice recognition, electronic imaging, and voice synthesis were also introduced during the 1990s. Later, the merger of healthcare organizations and stakeholders into large integrated healthcare networks has been described as a dominant trend (Smith, 1997).

The current status of HIS varies around the world. In 2009, 193 countries were members of the World Health Organization and 114 of them participated in the global survey on e-health (WHO, 2011). Most developed countries have fully utilized HIS, because they have the necessary resources, expertise, and capital. In developing countries, HIS are yet not fully utilized. Most countries are seeing the slow adoption of EHRs as part of e-health systems. These systems move patient information from paper to electronic file formats so they can be easily and effectively managed. The trend toward clinical computing and a patient-centered computer-based record was, however, seen worldwide by the 1980s (Ball, Peterson & Douglas, 1999).

Deployment of HIS has changed business processes for healthcare organizations. The earlier HIS, mainly designed to support administrative functions, have evolved into systems focused on clinical and patient records, and are more open in a technological as well as an organizational sense. People tend to know more about their condition, and actively participate in health promotion, prevention, and care, as they exercise the rights that have become a standard guide in the development of HIS. The trend is therefore toward more involvement of patients or citizens in receiving information, decision-making, and responsibility for their own health. In the next section, we discuss the concept of e-health, and its advantages, including cost efficiency, effectiveness, and improvements in the quality of healthcare.

E-Health

This section sets out some important features of e-health and its related technologies, especially Internet-based technology and social networks. E-health is an intersection between healthcare systems, users/people (healthcare staff and patients),

and information technology, aiming to deliver better healthcare services for the community (Low & Anshari, 2013). The nature of healthcare services, which are highly influenced by economic, social, political, and technological factors, has changed over time, and this includes e-health adoption. E-health embraces home-based, mobile, and more personalized patient-centric services, which often enable active participation of patients and their families (Nugent et al., 2007). E-health can remove time and distance barriers from the flow of health information and ensure that collective knowledge is brought to bear effectively on health problems throughout the world (Kwankam, 2004). For instance, online consultations can reach consumers (patients) who cannot physically be present for a consultation. Physicians can provide consultations over the Internet without meeting their patients in person. E-health also allows doctors and other healthcare professionals to connect with their patients online (Marchibroda, 2009).

Many statistics are available to illustrate the pervasiveness, effects, and advantages of e-health. For example, the European e-health industry leads in emerging fields such as personalized health systems, medical equipment and several sectors of integrated e-health solutions. The focus is on two main areas, telemedicine/homecare and clinical information systems in primary healthcare.

Among the countries that have implemented e-health systems are Canada, Singapore, and Australia. Canada established e-health Ontario in March 2009, with targeted strategies to improve diabetes management, medication management and waiting times. One service offered is e-prescribing, under the medication management stream. This authorizes and transmits prescriptions from physicians and other prescribers to pharmacists and other dispensers. It prevents medication errors due to illegible prescribing and reduces fraud. "Participating prescribers and pharmacies at both sites will continue electronically prescribing until a provincial Medication Management System is in place" (e-Health Ontario, 2009).

Australia is progressively adopting e-health as part of the Government's national health reform agenda, designed to provide better health services and outcomes for all Australians. This approach is similar to other international e-health initiatives such as those in Canada, the United States, United Kingdom, Hong Kong, Singapore, Denmark, and Germany. In July 2012, Australians started to have access to Personally Controlled Electronic Health Records (PCEHR), helping to improve access to health information held in dispersed records across the country. For the first time, all Australians who chose to participate could see their health information when and where they needed it, and share this information with trusted healthcare providers (ehealthinfo, 2012).

The Internet has changed the way that consumers engage with health information (Powell, Darvell & Gray, 2003). It allows consumers to share their opinions on the products and services that they buy, and these opinions are often more useful to others than information from providers. This triggered a significant change in how organizations treat consumers. They started to engage with their consumers, by listening to their concerns or even involving them in improving the quality of products and services. The Internet has become a popular channel to deliver information, including for healthcare. Its use as an e-health platform has increased significantly, as browsers offer a dynamic and interactive user interface (Anshari, et al., 2012).

The feasibility of building web interfaces for clinical information systems was shown in 1996 (Sittig, Kuperman & Teich, 1996), and reports of other successful projects followed. WebCIS is an example of implementation of a web server on top of clinical information system architecture, with a central data repository (Hripcsak, Cimino & Sengupta, 1999). The Internet is popular and holds great promise of being able to reach consumers (patients) anytime, anywhere. E-health using web-based systems may fill information needs and empower consumers by making accessible high-quality healthcare information and services.

Taiwan's Context

Taiwan embarked on healthcare reform in the 1980s, after two decades of economic growth (Reid, 2008a). The government of Taiwan formed the National Health Insurance (NHI) system on March 1st 1995, providing universal health insurance coverage (Chunhuei et al., 2012). The model has many similarities to Medicare in the United States. Working citizens and their employers both pay premiums, and others pay a flat rate, which the government subsidizes. Poorer and older people are fully subsidized (Reid, 2008b). NHI is compulsory for all Taiwanese and foreign nationals holding residency permits, and its membership covers 99.6% of the population. It is administered by the NHI bureau under the Department of Health (DoH), providing guaranteed access for all through premium subsidies and installment plans (Chan, 2012).

Under this scheme, citizens are able to choose healthcare centers and physicians. NHI covers comprehensive benefits including exemptions of co-payment for child delivery, preventive health services, medical services in remote areas, low-income households, older people, and catastrophic diseases such as cancer, chronic mental illness, hemodialysis and congenital illness, covering most illnesses with medical expenses too high for an average family to afford. Most preventive services are free, including annual checkups and maternal and child care. Regular office visits have co-payments as low as US $5 per visit. Co-payments are fixed and do not depend on income (Lu & Hsiao, 2003).

In 1985, the DoH initiated an infrastructure project to be completed by 2000, for a 15-year, three-phase project to build capacity for better distribution of medical resources in 17 regions and 63 sub-regions. Phases one and two (1985–1995) developed primary and secondary care by encouraging private investment in rural and mountain areas. Phase three (1996–2000) covered rehabilitation, long-term care, psychiatric care, and quality assurance (see Table 2).

Table 2. Capacity building (DoH, 2011a)

	Project Goals	**Health Status**
Physicians	13.3 / 10,000 patients	15 / 10,000 patients
Hospital beds	35 / 10,000 patients	56.8 / 10,000 patients
Psychiatric care	10 / 10,000 patients	6.7 / 10,000 patients
Nursing homes	35.2 / 10,000 patients	507 / 14,094 patients

Most healthcare providers in Taiwan are private. Of the 508 hospitals in Taiwan in 2010, 82 (16.1%) of them were state-owned and 426 (83.9%) were privately-owned (Chunhuei et al., 2012). These hospitals provided 68.61 beds per 10,000 population (DoH, 2011a). State hospitals tend to be large general hospitals and although they make up only 16.1% of total hospitals, they provide 33.79% of total hospital beds (BNHI, 2011a).

Chan (2012) mentioned that the challenges faced by the government in delivering healthcare services include that healthcare expenditure accounts for only 6.7% of Taiwan's gross domestic product. This is lower than many other members of the Organisation for Economic Co-operation and Development. Another problem is that Taiwan needs more doctors. Residents in mountain areas and offshore islands rely heavily on local health stations. Since 1979, the government has sent mobile medical teams to remote villages on a regular basis. In 1995, a boat was built for mobile medical treatment. In 1996, a helicopter-landing pad was provided in some remote areas to improve local emergency care.

E-Health in Taiwan

In 2008, realizing the advantages of ICT in healthcare, the Taiwanese government included telecare as a development project in the emerging service industry (Huang, 2013). Taiwan aims to create outstanding e-health services and deliver high quality medical care. In 2009, Taiwan introduced computerized medical records and a central database network that links government administrative agencies, physicians and patients under strict conditions of privacy. The system expected to connect all healthcare centers by 2016. It also includes electronic kiosks in many of Taiwan's hospitals, enabling patients to make an appointment with a doctor or review their medical records by using an identification card. Medical staff in mobile clinics in rural areas are equipped with laptops attached to the NHI data center (Chan, 2012).

The system now includes online data exchange among all databases, search functions for important medical orders in various medical institutions via the Internet, broadband networks for NHI, electronic patient records and medical information standards. Other major healthcare information applications are being developed. Taiwan began implementing its health information network in the 1980s and continues to invest in HIT. It acknowledges that HIT not only helps to provide efficient and safe medical care but will also play a significant role in sustaining the national health system (DoH, 2011b).

Currently, all hospitals and most clinics are connected to the Bureau of National Health Insurance through a virtual private network (VPN) for e-claim purposes. Taiwan also developed digital accreditation procedures, and set up a system of cross-branch operations at one counter, voice service systems, and an NHI card. All residents use health smart cards that contain limited EHRs. There is a low doctor-to-population ratio resulting in too many patients depending on too few doctors. Patients visit the doctor frequently, causing doctors to limit visits to about 2–5 minutes per patient (Gunde, 2004).

Milestones in HIS Development

Since starting to implement NHI, the BNHI has been very aggressive in adopting various HIT (Chunhuei et al., 2012). In 1990, the government of Taiwan invested in IT infrastructure to support an information network backbone to connect the DoH, regional information centers, and BNHI. The network was also intended to support telemedicine centers to facilitate collaboration with several university hospitals (Li, 2007).

Table 3 shows the milestones in HIS implementation in Taiwan. During its early development, HIT was used to support basic public health administration, hospital regulation, and cancer registries. Later in 1999, the government launched Phase II of its health information network plan, which included VPN connections and placed emphasis on privacy and security, EHRs, a health insurance smart card, and access to information for health professionals (Li, 2007).

The BNHI has established very accessible and user-friendly websites for beneficiaries to access their entire medical care utilization information, stored as an electronic record (Chunhuei et al., 2012). Information is also available for beneficiaries dealing with disputes. Besides serving beneficiaries, the BNHI website provides comprehensive information for employers, including an online application to enroll their new employees into NHI (BNHI, 2011b).

The DoH provides a free interactive online education program called Formosa e-Medical School (DoH, 2011b). This offers full-length courses of online learning for the general population. The website also provides extensive online medical consultations, including pharmaceutical, nutritional, and health promotion consultations. It also contains online self-assessments for various health status measurements (DoH, 2011b).

Through BNHI in 2001, the Taiwan government introduced a smart ID card system to store patient information and speed up the administration process. This ID card serves multiple functions:

1. Personal basic information (such as name, photo identification, ID number, birth date, and sex);
2. Health insurance information (such as most recent utilization code number, cumulative medical care utilization, cumulative medical care costs, cumulative cost sharing, insurance tax, and preventive care);
3. Medical information (such as major diagnoses, prescriptions, and allergies to pharmaceuticals and biological products); and
4. Health administration information that includes vaccinations and organ donation information.

All information on the ID card is encrypted, and only BNHI-issued card readers can read and retrieve information (Chunhuei et al., 2012). For

Table 3. HIS adoption in Taiwan (Li, 2007)

Year	Adoption
1989	Government-initiated decision to establish a National Health Information Network (HIN)
1991–1993	Pilot HIN tested in Hsinchu medical care region
1994–1996	HIN plan extended to other regions in Taiwan
1999	Phase II of HIN began with focus on bandwidth and VPN upgrades, local resources analysis, and web-based application and standards development.
2001	BNHI introduced smart cards

healthcare providers, the smart card system changed the business process. Healthcare providers upload electronic records daily to BNHI, and on every sixth patient visit, card information is uploaded online for data analysis, audit, and authentication. The system also accelerates the reimbursement process (Smart Card Alliance, 2005).

The smart card replaced paper-based patient ID to improve efficiency and effectiveness, and reduce fraud. This system contributes to a reduction of duplications in diagnostic procedures and laboratory tests, and duplications or contraindications of prescription drugs. Because Taiwan's residents have complete freedom to seek healthcare from any contracted providers, from private clinics to teaching hospitals' outpatient departments, there was significant duplication of diagnostic procedures and laboratory tests before this system was implemented (Chunhuei et al., 2012).

The development of e-health in Taiwan began under the National Information Infrastructure (NII) initiative. Major progress made under the umbrella of the NII includes distance education, tele-consultation, video-on-demand, and the existence of an electronic library. Taiwan used e-health for learning to distribute medical resources and support medical staff in rural areas (Wang, 2008). E-health in learning is needed in rural areas because medical resources are poorly distributed, the quality of consultation and referral needed improvement, peer communication among healthcare providers was difficult, there was a need to provide continuing medical education online, and it was hard to provide services for older people, disabled people, and those with terminal illnesses (Chen, 2006).

Taiwan's health system now incorporates reports to medical facility and patient records from the national medical image exchange centre, and issuing of health smart cards. Efforts have been made to establish medical kiosks and telehealth services for remote areas. Patient privacy is guaranteed using dedicated smart card readers activated by special issue staff cards. Every hospital in

Taiwan now offers patients a range of self-service options, including registration, payments and in some cases, access to health records (Hou, 2011).

Challenges

Consumer expectations of healthcare services are high, which creates serious challenges for healthcare providers worldwide (Anshari et al., 2013a). Healthcare providers have to make an exceptional impression on consumers, and need health information for decision-making and medical issues (Warner & Procaccino, 2004). The critical issue in healthcare information systems is not merely technology but also people. Technology is the enabler, not the driver (Ball et al, 1999).

Taiwan's NHI system has moved further in providing a good quality service. NHI ensures that each consumer receives the same service at any healthcare provider across the country, which is efficient, affordable, and higher quality. The best practice in developing e-health, however, is to promote patient empowerment by ensuring that channels for e-communications and information exchanges are in place (Alpay et al., 2010). There are three challenges NHI systems face in managing consumer empowerment, and ensuring that e-health can be facilitated to manage empowerment and participation in NHI systems.

First, *patient self-empowerment* is when the patient is personally empowered, as an individual, to access personalized e-health systems (interface), to enable them to update, record, or just view their personal information (personal account details including password, ID, phone number, email, address, and other contact details) or daily life activities (for example, eating and sleeping habits, and exercise). Consumers are empowered to customize those services, within certain limits set out in rules and regulations.

Interaction between consumers (patients) is a form of social empowerment, where patients' participation in social networks can be accommodated by e-health systems as part of the healthcare process, to enable them to share and discuss information with other patients who have similar conditions. This type of interaction is often unstructured, which can provide new insights for people involved in the management of healthcare and chronic conditions. Finally, *consumer–healthcare provider interaction* is a form of medical empowerment where consumers can interact with medical staff online within the e-health system, for a consultation (telehealth). Those three interactions need to be considered in e-health systems.

Future Directions

The vision of a paperless NHI system is delineated as the embodiment and foundation of future e-health systems, with the hope that it will make delivery of healthcare more reliable, effective, and efficient. Paper-based systems in healthcare business processes are perceived as inefficient, more expensive, and lower quality.

The trend in e-health is a shift from institution to consumer-centered care, emphasizing the continuity of care in prevention, care, and rehabilitation. This vision can be achieved through shared care, which builds on e-health networks and services, linking hospitals, laboratories, pharmacies, primary care, consumers, and social centers, and provides individuals with a "virtual healthcare center" and a single point of entry. This implies provision of health services using innovative services such as personal health monitoring, support systems, and user-friendly information systems that support health education and awareness (Iakovidis, 1998). The use of the Internet and applications is vital as it can help to improve the quality of healthcare provision.

Figure 1 shows consumer empowerment in e-health, so that healthcare providers can extend existing services to be more consumer-centric. We propose that consumer empowerment must be personal, social, and medical. Personal empowerment is self-participation and direct interaction with the e-health system. Social empowerment is consumers connecting with others in the e-health system. Medical empowerment is the ability of consumers to connect and interact with online healthcare staff (Almunawar, Wint, Low, & Anshari, 2012). Empowerment in e-health needs to consider people, process, strategies, and technologies. People are the actors in the systems, using them directly or indirectly. The process describes standard operating procedures in implementing the systems. The

Figure 1. Consumer empowerment in e-health

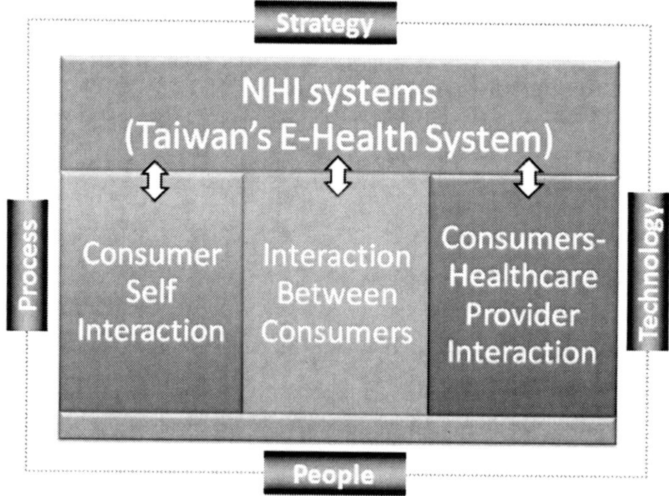

strategy is how to effectively and efficiently deliver the service. It is important to consider the organization's choice of service productivity level as a strategic decision variable to be optimized. Finally, technologies are the appropriate means for system interface, such as mobile or Internet technology, which support operations, management, and delivering essential information.

Personal Empowerment

Empowerment is an important feature in e-health services. Enabling patients to generate their own personal health records can improve both health literacy and customer satisfaction (Anshari et al, 2012). Consumers can produce electronic health record content that may help healthcare staff make a diagnosis. This is the opposite of a conventional e-health system, where consumers cannot generate content. Future e-health systems should help healthcare providers by empowering their customers.

Social empowerment

Embedding social networks into e-health systems is challenging but may be beneficial for consumers. The recent development of social networking services such as Facebook, Twitter, Myspace, Friendster, and LinkedIn has facilitated peer-to-peer collaboration, participation, and networking (Anshari & Almunawar, 2012). These tools have made it possible to extend e-health services by enabling consumers, their families, and the wider community to participate more actively in health promotion, interaction, conversation, and education through social networking. Using social networks in e-health could provide a new means to build relationships between patients and healthcare organizations. It could also be important in encouraging patients to share their experiences and related information to achieve better health outcomes. The use of such tools, particularly in healthcare, has not, however, been

widely discussed. The main advantages are the linkages among people, ideas, processes, systems, content and other organizational activities (Askool & Nakata, 2010). Social networks may affect healthcare business processes, especially those relating to interactions between patients, because they offer a new way to engage, manage and maintain relationships.

Medical Empowerment

E-health initiatives are designed to move from paper-based to paperless business, particularly with the implementation and integration of digitalized medical record systems. At this level, the empowerment is very limited from the patient's perspective, because only healthcare providers have access to the EHR. Medical empowerment requires the patient to be able to access their EHR, as has now begun in Australia (Pearce & Bainbridge, 2014).

In contrast, many healthcare providers prevent patients from accessing their EMRs prior to a consultation, so that they cannot see their medical history. This may imply that whenever a patient needs to consult a different healthcare provider, they will need to go through a redundant diagnosis process. Similarly, whenever a patient visits another doctor, the patient will have to explain their symptoms and problems all over again. The aim of e-health should be to educate patients (Eysenbach, 2001) about their health status, condition, and history. Therefore, medical empowerment is pivotal to improve patient literacy and education.,

Scope of Context in Taiwan

Embedding empowerment into e-health is primarily designed to promote consumer participation in three dimensions of health services, personal, social, and medical. Figure 2 shows how additional value will be generated by involving consumers, healthcare providers, medical staff, and the wider community through an inclusive system design.

It is particularly useful for illustrating the system boundaries and the relationships among the key entities of the system.

The NHI at the center of the diagram indicates that influencing those dimensions is the primary goal of the system. Naming the other important entities connected to the system indicates that value is added to the system by involving and integrating these elements. The bidirectional arrows show that all of the components and entities in the system interoperate. The dotted arrow shows that the system is founded on a set of fundamental principles. Finally, each of the major components of the system contributes to its goals.

CONCLUSION

The adoption of NHI systems has made it possible to have interoperable input, accessed from multiple locations, with the ability to process different types of data across systems. Through information exchange and interoperability, healthcare profession-als have access to a longitudinal medical record. This interoperability is a fundamental requirement for the healthcare system to derive the societal benefits promised (Brailer, 2005). Technological advancement also, however, drives consumer demands for more personalized healthcare services, often involving social networking (Anshari et al, 2013a). Internet technologies facilitate processing, storage, retrieval, and dissemination of data and information remotely anytime and anywhere. This has dramatically changed the ways in which healthcare organizations operate. Consumer demands have changed, as consumers have been empowered by the availability of information (Almunawar & Anshari, 2011). Social networking tools have also enabled consumers to access information from other users, and not just providers, on products and services. Healthcare providers may therefore consider consumer empowerment to be adaptive and changing. We propose the adoption of three dimensions of consumer empowerment (personal, social, and medical) in e-health, to give an alternative direction for the NHI system in Taiwan.

Figure 2. Generating value by involving parties through an inclusive system design

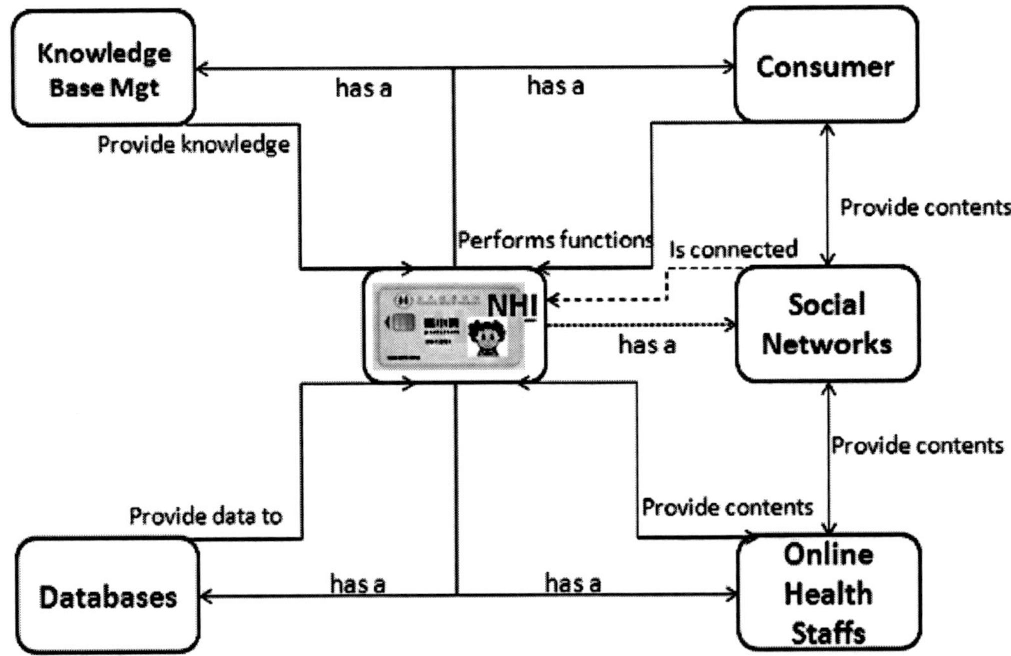

ACKNOWLEDGMENT

The authors are grateful for support from the Taiwan Fellowship program 2014.

REFERENCES

Almunawar, M. N., & Anshari, M. (2011). Improving customer service in healthcare with CRM 2.0. *Global Science and Technology Forum (GSTF). Business Review (Federal Reserve Bank of Philadelphia), 1*(2), 228–234.

Almunawar, M. N., & Anshari, M. (2014). Empowering customers in electronic health (e–health) through social customer relationship management. International Journal of Electronic Customer Relationship Management. *InderScience, 8*(1), 87–100.

Almunawar, M. N., Wint, Z., Low, K. C. P., & Anshari, M. (2012). Customer's Expectation of E-Health Systems in Brunei. *Journal of Health Care Finance. Aspen Publishers, 38*(4), 36–49.

Alpay, L. L., Henkemans, O. B., Otten, W., Röve-kamp, T. A. J. M., & Dumay, A. C. M. (2010). E-health applications and services for patient empowerment: Directions for best practices in The Netherlands. *Telemedicine Journal and e-Health, 16*(7), 787–791. doi:10.1089/tmj.2009.0156 PMID:20815745

Anshari, M., & Almunawar, M. N. (2012). Framework of social customer relationship management in e-health services. *Journal of Health Management, 2012*, 1–14. doi:10.5171/2012.766268

Anshari, M., Almunawar, M. N., Low, P. K. C., & Al-Mudimigh, A. S. (2013). Empowering Clients Through E-Health in Healthcare Services: Case Brunei [Baywood Publishing Co., Inc.]. *International Quarterly of Community Health Education, 33*(2), 191–221. PMID:23661419

Anshari, M., Almunawar, M. N., Low, P. K. C., & Wint, Z. (2012). Customer empowerment in healthcare organisations through crm 2.0: Survey results from Brunei tracking a future path in e-health research. *ASEAS – Austrian. Journal of Southeast Asian Studies, 5*(1), 139–151.

Anshari, M., Almunawar, M. N., Low, P. K. C., Wint, Z., & Younis, M. Z. (2013). Adopting customers' empowerment and social networks to encourage participations in e-health services'. *Journal of Health Care Finance. Aspen Publishers, 40*(2), 17–41. PMID:24551960

Askool, S. S., & Nakata, K. (2010). Scoping study to identify factors influencing the acceptance of social CRM. *Proceedings of the 2010 IEEE ICMIT*, 1055-1060. doi:10.1109/ICMIT.2010.5492888

Ball, M. J., Peterson, H., & Douglas, J. V. (1999). The computerized patient record: a global view. *MD Computing: computers in medical practice, 16*(5), 40-46.

Bourke, M. K. (1994). *Strategy and architecture of health care information systems*. New York: Springer-Verlag. doi:10.1007/978-1-4757-2338-0

Brailer, D. (2005). Interoperability: the key to the future health care system. *Health Affairs – Web Exclusive*, W5-19-W5-21.

Bureau of National Health Insurance (BNHI). (2010). *Financial status of BNHI, 1996–2009, Table 8*. Taipei: Bureau of National Health Insurance, Department of Health.

Bureau of National Health Insurance (BNHI). (2011a). *National health insurance annual statistical report 2010*. Taipei: Bureau of National Health Insurance, Department of Health.

Bureau of National Health Insurance (BNHI). (2011b). Home website. Retrieved 15 October 2011 from http://www.nhi.gov.tw/

Chan, R. (2012). US scholar praises Taiwan health care system. Retrieved 15 June 2015 from http://taiwantoday.tw/ct.asp?xItem=194109&ctNode=413

Chen, H. (2006). Telemedicine & e-Health in Taiwan. Internet2 Spring Meeting International Task Force Panel Session, Arlington, USA.

Chunhuei, C., Lee, J.-L., & Schoon, R. (2012). Assessing health information technology in a national health care system: An example from Taiwan. *Advances in Healthcare Management, 12*, 75–109. PMID:22894046

Conrick, M. (2006). *Health informatics: Transforming healthcare with technology*. Thomson Social Science Press.

CSC. (1999). Critical Issue of Information Systems Management. 1999 CSC, El Segundo.

Department of Health (DoH). (2011a). Taiwan health statistics 2010. Retrieved from http://www.doh.gov.tw/CHT2006/DM/DM2_2.aspx?now_fod_list_no=11926&class_no=440&level_no=4 on October 22, 2011.

Department of Health (DoH). (2011b). Online medical consultation website. Retrieved from http://sp1.cto.doh.gov.tw/doctor/Question.php?PHPSESSID=a0dde120efcd979b34834d5c178ebade on October 22, 2011.

E-Health Ontario. (2009). ePrescribing. Retrieved from http://www.ehealthontario.on.ca/programs/ePrescribing.asp on 1 March 2011. ehealthinfo, (2012). About the PCEHR system. Retrieved from http://www.ehealthinfo.gov.au. on 15 June 2015

Erl, T. (2005). *Service-oriented architecture: Concepts, technology, and design*. Prentice Hall.

Eysenbach, G. (2001). What is e-health? *Journal of Medical Internet Research, 3*(2), e20. doi:10.2196/jmir.3.2.e20 PMID:11720962

Goldschmidt, P. G. (2005). HIT and MIS: Implications of health information technology and medical information systems. *Communications of the ACM, 48*(10), 69-74.Gunde, Richard.(2004). "Healthcare in Taiwan: Opportunities and Success." UCLAInternational Institute. Retrieved 2015 From http://www.international.ucla.edu/article.asp?parentid=15333

Gustafson, D., Wise, M., McTavish, F., Taylor, J. O., Wolberg, W., Stewart, J., & Bosworth, K. et al. (1993). Developing and pilot evaluation of a computer-based support system for women with breast cancer. *Journal of Psychosocial Oncology, 11*(4), 69–93. doi:10.1300/J077V11N04_05

Haux, R. (2006). Health information systems – past, present, future. *International Journal of Medical Informatics, 75*(3-4), 268–281. doi:10.1016/j.ijmedinf.2005.08.002 PMID:16169771

Hou, E. (2011). DOH minister highlights Taiwan's e-health services. Retrieved from http://www.taiwantoday.tw/ct.asp?xItem=164387&ctNode=445 on 15 June 2015.

Hripcsak, G., Cimino, J. J., & Sengupta, S. (1999). WebCIS: large scale deployment of a Web-based clinical information system. In N. M. Lorenzi (ed). *Proceedings of the AMIA Symposium* (p.804-808). American Medical Informatics Association.

Huang, J. C. (2013). Innovative healthcare delivery system–a questionnaire survey to evaluate the influence of behavioral factors on individuals' acceptance of telecare. *Computers in Biology and Medicine, 43*(4), 281–286. doi:10.1016/j.compbiomed.2012.12.011 PMID:23375377

Iakovidis, I. (1998). Towards personal health record: Current situation, obstacles and trends in implementation of electronic healthcare record in Europe. *International Journal of Medical Informatics, 52*(1), 105–115. doi:10.1016/S1386-5056(98)00129-4 PMID:9848407

Kuhn, K. A., & Giuse, D. A. (2001). From hospital information systems to health information systems; problems, challenges, perspectives. *Methods of Information in Medicine, 40*(4), 275–287. PMID:11552339

Kwankam, S. (2004). What e-Health can offer. *Bulletin of the World Health Organization, 82*(10), 800–802. PMID:15643805

Li, Y. (2007). Taiwan HIT Case Study. Retrieved from http://www.pacifichealthsummit.org/downloads/hitcasestudies/economy/taiwanhit.pdf on 15 June 2015.

Low, K. C. P., & Anshari, M. (2013). Incorporating social customer relationship management in negotiation. International Journal of Electronic Customer Relationship Management. *Inder-Science, 7*(3), 239–252.

Lu, J. F. R., & Hsiao, W. C. (2003). Does universal health insurance make health care unaffordable? Lessons from Taiwan. *Health Affairs, 22*(3), 77–88. doi:10.1377/hlthaff.22.3.77 PMID:12757274

Marchibroda, J. M. (2009). eHealth, and communication: putting the consumer first. Paper presented at the IOM (Institute of Medicine) Health Literacy Workshop Summary. Washington, DC: The National Academies Press.

Nugent, C., Finlay, D., Davies, R., Mulvenna, M., Wallace, J., Paggetti, C., & Black, N. et al. (2007). The next generation of mobile medication management solutions. *International Journal of Electronic Healthcare, 3*(1), 7–31. doi:10.1504/IJEH.2007.011478 PMID:18048259

Pearce, C., & Bainbridge, M. (2014). A personally controlled electronic health record for Australia. *Journal of the American Medical Informatics Association, 21*(4), 707–713. doi:10.1136/amiajnl-2013-002068 PMID:24650635

Powell, J. A., Darvell, M., & Gray, J. A. (2003). The doctor, the patient and the world-wide web: How the internet is changing health care. *Journal of the Royal Society of Medicine, 96*(2), 74–76. doi:10.1258/jrsm.96.2.74 PMID:12562977

Reid, T. R. (2008a). "FRONTLINE: Sick Around the World". Public Broadcasting Service. Retrieved from http://www.pbs.org/wgbh/pages/frontline/sickaroundtheworld/ on 15 June 2015.

Reid, T. R. (2008b). Taiwan takes fast track to universal health care. Retrieved from http://www.npr.org/templates/story/story.php?storyId=89651916 on 15 June 2015.

Silber, D. (2003). The case for eHealth. Paper presented at the European Commission's first high-level conference on eHealth, May 22/23 2003. European Institute of Public Administration.

Sittig, D. F., Kuperman, G. J., & Teich, J. M. (1996). WWW-based interfaces to clinical information systems: the state of the art. In J. J. Cimino (ed). *Proceedings of the AMIA Annual Fall Symposium*, 694-698.

Smart Card Alliance. (2005). The Taiwan health care smart card project. Retrieved from http://www.smartcardalliance.org/resources/pdf/Taiwan_Health_Card_Profile.pdf on 15 June 2015.

Smith, R. (1997). The future of healthcare systems. *British Medical Journal, 314*(7093), 1495–1496. doi:10.1136/bmj.314.7093.1495 PMID:9183186

Warner, D., & Procaccino, J. D. (2004). Toward wellness: Women seeking health information. *Journal of the American Society for Information Science and Technology, 55*(8), 709–730. doi:10.1002/asi.20016

World Health Organization. (2011). Publications. Retrieved from http://www.who.int/goe/publications/en/ on 4 March 2011. [1]

This work was previously published in the International Journal of E-Health and Medical Communications (IJEHMC), 6(3); edited by Joel J.P.C. Rodrigues, pages 63-76 copyright year 2015 by IGI Publishing (an imprint of IGI Global).

Chapter 85
Information Systems in Healthcare with a Special Focus on Developing Countries

Ahed Abugabah
American University in the Emirates, UAE

Osama Afarraj
King Saud University, Saudi Arabia

Louis Sansogni
Griffith University, Australia

ABSTRACT

Information Systems offer tremendous opportunities to improve healthcare services. Thus far, they have a proven track record as a way to improve the quality of services, and work processes effectiveness. However, Health Information Systems can be inappropriately specified, having functional errors, being unreliable, and not user friendly. Such breakdowns may affect working processes and decisions of healthcare providers, resulting in potential harm to patients. This chapter will elaborate a number of important issues/problems related to Information Systems in healthcare with the aim of providing a deeper contextual insight into their application in healthcare and offer advice on the factors that should be considered when designing and evaluating them. The chapter aims at providing a literature review of Information Systems in healthcare and highlight the challenges Information Systems face in this domain by providing a significant review of Information System theory in healthcare.

INTRODUCTION

A host of academic articles and agency reports have argued that information and communication technologies (ICT) can make considerable contributions to improving healthcare in developing countries. However, development practitioners have learned from bitter experience that 'technological fixes' often deliver far less than promised when confronted with the chaotic and sometimes corrupt health systems in many countries. Generally speaking, healthcare systems are at risk due to

DOI: 10.4018/978-1-4666-8756-1.ch085

increasing demand, spiralling costs, inconsistent and poor quality of care, and inefficient, poorly coordinated care processes (Llucha, 2011). In response, governments are developing various strategies, one of which consists of heavy investments in information systems in healthcare as the use of information systems in the healthcare domain has been proven as a way to improve the quality of services, and work process and effectiveness (Johnson, Johnson and Zhangal, 2005; Easona and Waterson, 2013; Waterson, 2014). For example, the recent health reform in the USA includes plans to spend $18.9 billion to promote Healthcare Information Systems (HISs) and provide incentives for information systems adoption by healthcare organizations (Llucha, 2011).

The global shift in orientation and health strategy from curative to preventive care and from centralized to decentralized health care, has necessitated the need for comprehensive and efficient health information systems. This led to a communication revolution brewing in the modern healthcare system fuelled by the growth of powerful new health information technologies that hold tremendous promise for enhancing the delivery of healthcare and the promotion of health. As a result, an ongoing research activity has been witnessed recently investigating different aspects of healthcare informatics and making significant progress toward understanding the information Technology (IT) phenomena in healthcare(Lopez and Blobel, 2009; Ludwick and Doucette, 2009; Martikainen et al., 2011). Despite the successes of health informatics research, numerous challenges to developing, implementing, and evaluating HISs still remain (Chiasson et al., 2007, Easona and Waterson, 2013).

While it is evident that information systems offer tremendous opportunities to improve healthcare services by for example reducing clinical medication and diagnostic errors, supporting healthcare professionals in providing timely, up-to-

date patient information, increasing the efficiency of care and improving the quality of patient care (Ammenwerth et al., 2004). However, hazards also remain associated with information systems in health care. HISs can be inappropriately specified, having functional errors, be unreliable, user-unfriendly. Such breakdowns may affect working process and decisions of healthcareproviders and results in harm for the patients (Lapointe, Mignerat and Vedel, 2011; Chiasson & Davidson, 2004).

This chapter will elaborate a number of important issues/problems related to information systems in healthcare in developing countries with the aim of providing more insight to better understand information systems in healthcare and provide some recommendations about the factors that should be considered when design and evaluate information systems in healthcare especially in developing countries. The chapter aims at providing a literature review of the Information Systems (IS) in healthcare and highlight the challenges of IS in healthcare, by providing an up to date literature review of the IS theory in health care. A significant part of this chapter will be covering the main challenges of information systems in health care.

Literature Review

This section presents a selective literature review focusing on different aspects of IS in healthcare in general, followed by a discussion to the main lessons learned from the literature and the most important issues related to IS and Healthcare Information Systems (HIS) in different settings in the healthcare domain with a special focus on developing countries. The literature review covered in this section was organized and categorised according to the main factors and issues investigated in the studies to help better understand HIS from different perspectives as explained below:

Historical View

The historical view of HIS started a few decades ago. The actual use of Information technology in healthcare has existed for about three decades, and has gained widespread usage (Ammenwerth et al., 2004). There were many attempts made in discussing different issues of health information and health information systems in healthcare, the focus of these attempts was on the tremendous shift from paper-based processing and storage to computer-based processing and storage. In general, in the 1960s as medical informatics was mostly focused on small (functionally limited) applications in special departments of hospitals. Consequently, there was limited research in that field due to the simple of application of information systems at that time. In additions, earlier efforts could not be implemented successfully due to lack of software and hardware techniques (Haux, 2006), and the lack of wide knowledge in this field. A gradual change occurred highlighting the move from electronic data processing to health informatics from the nature of papers that were presented at World Congresses Medical Informatics in 1974 in Stockholm, as cited in (Hovenga et al, 1998).

However, serious efforts and research started later in 1970s (Haux, 2006). Starting with Martin and Norman 25 years ago (1970) predicted that the computer promised revolutionary changes in medicine, as cited in (Hovenga et al., 2010). Some contributions to the same topic have been made; it may be permitted to use some of the earlier ideas. Most of these efforts lack methodological development as well as software and hardware techniques.

In 1974 year, the year of publication of the first article to evaluate the effect of IT in healthcare organizations was conducted by De Dombal et al, (1974) to evaluate the impacts of Clinical Decision Support System (CDSS) on clinician performance. They carried out many trials and stated that the clinician's diagnostic performance improved significantly during the period of the trial. Although the article was important as an early start, it did not identify any factors that probably affect healthcare services. But at least it opened the path for more critical thinking about HIS applications and healthcare services.

In 1984, Peter Reichertz gave a lecture on the past, present and future of health information systems. The lecturer tried to collect all previous HIS work to build on a new orientation in the field and open the gate for more research. He mentioned the importance of Health information systems by explaining the future of these applications. Since then, there has been a tremendous progress in health informatics (Haux, 2006). This progress, leading to aging societies, is of influence to the organization of healthcare and to the future development of its information systems. Two decades later, referring to Peter Reichertz' lecture, considering HIS, Haux, (2006) introduced two important questions: which discusses the development in HIS from the past until today and the consequences for HIS in the future?

Although Reichertz' lecture was simple, it was one of the most serious and important works at the time. In additions, this view necessitated the need for reorganizing healthcare in an aging society, as last consequence the need for research around HIS is seen.

After that date many research has been carried out about the critical role information technology plays in healthcare organizations, and will continue to play, in the reduction of medical errors, as well as its impact on improving the quality of medical care (Moore and Berner, 2004). According to Ammenwerth et al (2003) information technology offers tremendous opportunities to reduce clinical errors such as, medication and, diagnostic errors, and also support healthcare professionals to increase the efficiency of healthcare and to improve the quality of patient care.

Noticeably, in 1990 the evolution of the IT in healthcare took a place and received attention from researchers. However, most of these studies are evaluation studies, they tried to evaluate HISs from different perspectives and examine the successes of and opportunities for using advanced information systems (Bates and Gawande, 2003), and/ or examine the user acceptance of new technology (Pai and Huange, 2011, Yi et al., 2006; Schaper and Pervan, 2007).

Van der Loo et al., (1995) conducted a literature review to classify evaluation studies of information systems in health care. Seventy-six studies published between 1974 and 1995 were included in the study. Many different performance measures or success factors were applied in the included studies. The study found that the evaluation methods and effect measures depended on the characteristics of the information system under evaluation. Some important variables that were mentioned in their study are costs, changes in time spent by healthcare personnel, changes in care process, database usage, performance of the system and user, and job satisfaction. Researchers also suggested some approaches to evaluating information technology in healthcare (i.e. Yusof et al, 2008). However, these approaches concerned assessment of technical, sociological, and organizational impact and did not specify an appropriate frameworks and factors that should be taken into consideration when evaluate HIS impacts in organizations (Rippen et al., 2012)

RE-STRUCTURING THE RESEARCH ON HIS

Studies on HIS research focused on a different type of information systems or different aspects of the systems, some of them tried to investigate how technologies can improve medical practice and patient care. Although these studies provided useful explanation about some important issues relevant to HIS, but they did provide a clear framework to further investigate HIS and even did not provide clear measurements of HIS evaluation and outcomes in healthcare. Furthermore, majority of the studies used clinical data and patient outcomes

(feedback) to measure practitioner performance and healthcare services (Ludwick and Doucette, 2009).

Consequently, and due to the limited research in this field and the rapid growing of information technologies, some researchers have tried recently to re-structure the research in this filed to improve the quality of research, formalize a more incorporated framework which might be used to evaluate HIS in health organizations, give directions and maps for new and future researches in this filed and to identify what has been done and what has not been done yet. For example, Yusof et al, (2008, 2008a) attempted to show how a framework could be derived for HIS evaluation that incorporates comprehensive dimensions and measures of HIS and provides a technological, human and organizational fit. The researchers tried to identify a more comprehensive model from the existing studies to evaluate HIS. Although their study has brought valuable contributions, however, they did not specify the critical dimensions that could affect the outcomes of the systems and/or their study was restricted only to shape a framework to evaluate the system itself and implementation aspects rather that system impacts on the organizations and services provided (Rippen et al., 2012). The study explained indicated that human, organizational and technical elements should have a mutual alignment or 'fit' in order to ensure successful HIS implementation. It is crucial that HIS fit organizational aspects as well as align with work routines, management assumptions, and patient care philosophies and users' needs as the introduction of a system affects different dimensions of fit in complex ways (Yusof et al., 2008a; Lee et al., 2008).

Another recent view was conducted by Ammenwerth and Keizer, (2005) supporting the need for more studies in HIS field in general and emphasizes the need for more structured, well-defined and clear methodology, reliable data and well-descried studies.

Overall, these studies proved the importance of HIS to the quality of the services provided proved that the use of modern information and communication technology offers tremendous opportunities to improve health care. However, they showed that there are also hazards associated with information technology in health care.

Evaluating the quality of service, quality impacts, value, effects and impacts of information systems and applications in healthcare environment is still required in many aspects. For example, Ammenwerth et al., (2004) investigated many aspects in their study related to HIS and its impacts in healthcare organizations. The study concluded several important contributions including the need for a good framework to evaluate the HIS impacts in health organizations. It stated that the contributions of HIS still need more research empirically to explain the payoff of HIS application in these organizations.

Furthermore, the call for shifting the focus into user needs and perspectives has been emphasised nowadays by academic and partitioner community. For example, De Rouck, Jacobs and Leys, (2008) emphasised the need to shift the concentration into user perspectives.

Although the progress in HIS is increasingly growing, limitation of research on user requirements and needs, and other aspects of HIS at the user level seems to be a major limitation in this area. Previous studies depended on case studies, which make the generalizability of these studies very low, although some studies tried to build a framework to evaluation (Lee et al., 2008). Kaplan (2001) reviewed CDSS's literature with a focus on evaluation, indicating general consensus that CDSSs are thought to have the potential to improve care. Evidence is more equivocal for guidelines and for systems to aid physicians with diagnosis. There is also general consensus that a variety of systems are little used despite demonstrated or potential benefits. The results indicate that there is a lack of information useful for understanding why CDSSs may or may not be effective.

Yusof et al, (2008) presented an overview of evaluation in health informatics and information systems. They evaluated HIS to assess the extent to which HIS are fulfilling their objectives in supporting healthcare outcomes. They found that the potential of HIS to improve performance of clinicians is often thwarted by the users' reluctance to accept and adopt it. Therefore, the usefulness of HIS depends largely on users and their evaluation of the systems. They stated that a HIS evaluation should be comprehensive and with specific measures that would incorporate technological, human and organizational issues to facilitate HIS evaluation. In Table 1, we listed some selective and high contributing evaluation studies in HIS.

HEALTH INFORMATICS IN DEVELOPING COUNTRIES

The apparent need for the adoption of Health Information Systems (HISs) and the positive impact that these systems can have on the quality, effectiveness and efficiency of care services have been analysed and depicted over the years in the health informatics literature studies (Mukred, Singh & Safie, 2013). In many European nations, as well as other countries around the world, there is a growing awareness that strategic investments in innovative clinical information system as well as other types of (HISs) can yield significant improvement for an entire healthcare system (Kitsiou et al., 2010).

Recent studies related to IT projects and investments stated that more than 40% of ICT developments in various sectors including the health sector have failed or been abandoned and one of the major factors leading to the failure is the inadequate understanding of the sociotechnical aspects of ICT (Kijsanayotin et al., 2009). More specifically, the knowledge of how people who work in the health sector accept and use health ICT, their basic ICT knowledge and acceptance, and use will enable more efficient implementation

Table 1. Selective evaluation studies in HIS

De Dombal et al, (1974)	Clinical decision support systems impact on the clinician performance, and the clinician's diagnostic performance improved markedly.
Reichertz (1984)	The lecturer tried to collect all previous HIS works to build a new orientation in this field and open the gate for more research and study.He mentioned the important of Health information systems by explaining the future of these applications.
Gremy and Degoulet, (1993)	Human factors are very critical when study HIS. Human interaction must be involved when investigating HIS
Johnston et al, (1994)	Some CDSSs can improve physician performance. Studies are needed to assess effects on cost and patient outcomes.
Hunt et al, (1998)	The CDSSs can enhance clinical performance, patient outcomes and other aspects of medical care.
Berner et al, (1999)	Physicians' performed better on the easier cases and on the cases for which QMR could provide higher-quality information.
Kaplan, (2001)	There is little research involves field tests and almost none take place in actual and there is little explicit theory that informs many evaluations, the need to broaden evaluation through a variety of methods and approaches that investigate many important aspects in healthcareinformation systems.
Van der Meijden et al. (2003)	IS success model is applicable in the evaluation of HIS. More studies of patient care information systems can be performed to address factors that contribute to systems' success and failures.
Ammenwerth et al, (2004)	The contributions and the foundations of good HIS still ambiguous and also HIS Research in health information is still at its infancy. That is, apparently it is desirable to have a broadly accepted, detail evaluation framework that could guide researcher to undertake evaluation studies and formulate relevant questions, to find adequate methods and tools, and to apply them in a sensible way.
Ammenwerth & Keizer, (2005)	The continuous and dominant number of non-RCT studies reflects the various approaches applicable to evaluate IT systems in health care. Despite the increasing discussion on evidence-based health informatics, the quality of published evaluation studies on IT interventions in healthcareis still insufficient in some aspects.
Haux, (2006).	Comparing the world in 1984 and in 2004.the study concluded that many questions still unsolved, development and investigation of methods for modelling and evaluating health information systems as well as studying HIS properties through evaluation studies still also needed and investigating several aspects for the various users of health information systems.
Despont-Gros et al, (2005)	The study led to the identification of eight key variables, among which satisfaction, acceptance, and success were found to be the most referenced. And the study model links the dimensions in traditional clinical information systems evaluation and the dimensions from the human–computer interaction (HCI) perspective
Yusof et al., (2008a).	Evaluation is complex; it is easy to measure many things but not necessarily the right ones. Nevertheless, it is possible to consider, a HIS evaluation framework with more comprehensive and specific measures that would incorporate technological, human and organizational issues to facilitate HIS evaluation.
De Rouck, Jacobs and Leys, (2008)	The research confirms that systematic approaches are needed to understand and systematically assess user needs and expectations, to design electronic health applications.
Yusof et al., (2008).	Comprehensive, specific evaluation factors, dimensions and measures in the new framework (HOT-fit) are applicable in HIS evaluation. The use of such a framework is argued to be useful not only for comprehensive evaluation of the particular system under investigation, but potentially also for any Health Information System in general. The need for comprehensive framework has been stated.

of HIS in health sector. Overall, research in this particular area reported different factors beyond the noteworthy failure of IT projects in health sector, taking into account the difference exist in developing countries.

Recently, HISs in developing countries have gained more attention as more efforts made by governments, international agencies, nongovernmental organizations, donors and other development partners seek to improve healthcare (Nyella,

2009). Early computer-supported health information systems were primarily intended to support healthcare professionals, mainly physicians, as well as administrative staff in hospitals. Later, there was also a focus on nurses. For the last few years, the focus has shifted to support patients and their relatives often denoted as health consumers (Mukred, Singh & Safie, 2013).

In developing countries, it is important to adopt a holistic approach to cultivate a more mature Information Culture in healthcare systems to increase the adoption level of the technological innovation. This means that to adopt such a holistic approach, it is necessary to build conditions and capacities for interpreting, evaluating and utilizing information resources (Zheng, 2005). For example, prior to creating electronic medical records systems for a developing country, it must be noted that each nation would most probably have different requirements that need to be satisfied. Therefore, undertaking research in these countries will demand proper consultation concerning the laws and regulations of the country (Mukred, Singh & Safie, 2013).

Krickeberg (2007) provided a framework for HIS in developing countries highlighting most important principles and issues related to success HIS in developing countries. The design or reform of a HIS should be based upon an understanding of six principle objectives or applications of the system including planning and managing the health system, publishing health-related information, epidemic surveillance, supporting daily clinical work, obtaining information for local use and conducting studies. With these functions in mind, some structural principles necessary for this process have been identified such as logical and transparent structure flexibility, coordination minimal flow of information and autonomy regarding information. Although these principles may appear in part fairly theoretical and technical, they are intimately tied to the daily practice of the system. Observing them will motivate and enlighten the health workers handling the

system, increase its reliability, enlarge its scope, improve its usefulness on all levels, and reduce costs (Krickeberg, 2007).

Research on HIS adoption and implementation in developing countries clearly documents a number of benefits of Health Information Technology (HIT). However, it also identified a various types of barriers to the widespread adoption of these systems such as for example, physician acceptance, security, authentication concerns and improper primary focus on technology. Researchers in different countries reported many factors in addition to the aforementioned ones that affect HIS in developing countries. Some of these factors relate to IT aspects and technical issues, while others relate to human and usability aspects as discussed in details below:

Aldosari (2014) studied the implementation of electronic health records in Saudi Arabia. The study indicated that adoption rates compare favorably with those reported from other countries and other districts in Saudi Arabia, but wide variations exist among hospitals in the levels of adoption of individual items. General weaknesses in the implementation phase concern the legacy of paper data systems, including document scanning and data conversion; in the maintenance phase concern updating/maintaining software; and in the improvement phase concern the communication and exchange of health information. In addition, in developing countries for implementation, there is a cluster of low preparation/action regarding scanning strategy, management of old paper records, and converting data and issues of compatibility. Therefore, further research is needed on the determinants of adoption by incorporating a more widespread sample and cross-country evaluation will help gain more insights about the adoption and implementation issues of HIS in developing countries.

Yusof et al. (2008) in two different studies mentioned that adoption factors of HISs of the specific users in a particular setting have influenced the adoption negatively. These factors include system usefulness, technical support, response time, ease of use, user perception and user IT background and knowledge. On the other hand, the studies showed some other factors that contribute significantly to the positive adoption of HIS including information relevancy, user attitude, leadership, medical sponsorship, organizational readiness.

Littlejohns et al. (2003) reported the reasons for failure of a large computerized HIS project in developing countries like South Africa resulted from a lack of users' understanding of reasons for the new system and the underestimation of the complexity of the healthcare system. The lack of acceptance is a fundamental barrier to the implementation of HISs (Croll, 2009). The same researcher argued that there are many reasons for the lack of acceptance or actual resistance to HISs, such as unwillingness of stakeholders to learn new routines, lack of ICT training as major barriers to the acceptance and implementation of HISs and lack of insight into the benefits and lack of concern about the sheer magnitude of the change caused by HIS (Croll, 2009). Young (1984) identified the nature of the doctor's work, his attitudes, interests and enthusiasms to be the major reasons for the non-acceptance of computer systems. Thus, Agrawal (2011) argued that physicians may be more reticent to adopt PHRs than other health professionals.

Yusof et al. (2008) stated that having the right user attitude and skills base together with good leadership, ICT-friendly environment and good communication have positive influence on the system adoption. In addition, Mosse (2004) stated that HISs emphasize aspects of humans, technologies, organizational procedures and their inter-linkages. Individual, organizational, technological and external environmental factors were identified as factors that impede or facilitate e-health adoption (Baroud, 2008). Croll (2009) identified some barriers facing HISs, which include factors such as system failure, cost, fears about confidentiality, security and privacy, inefficiency, poorer quality of healthcare, the change in the work process,

complexity of healthcare and lack of acceptance by clinicians. Croll (2009) added that usability is important to the adoption of health information systems. Lack of awareness, information sharing and accessing information are among the barriers to acceptance of ICT. Kushniruk and Borycki (2008) argued that lack of ease of use of HISs has been a major impediment to the adoption of such systems

Ludwick and Doucette (2009) studied health information systems implementation in seven countries and reviewed the literature of HIS in significant number of databases, journal websites, from grey sources, medical colleges and professional associations as well as a number of government databases. The study showed that systems' graphical user interface design quality, feature functionality, project management, procurement and users' previous experience affect implementation outcomes. Implementers had concerns about factors such as privacy, patient safety, provider/patient relations, staff anxiety, time factors, quality of care, finances, efficiency, and liability. The study also highlighted some important issues such as the quality of the implementation process as important as the quality of the system being implemented. In addition to the important of health system usability, computer skills and the system's fit within the organizational culture and processes as significant factors in implementation success.

LESSONS LEARNED FROM DEVELOPING COUNTRIES

There is a growing consensus that the impact of ICT on health systems will be substantial or even revolutionary in developing countries. However, there is much less agreement as to the likely nature of that impact. Lessons that could be learned from HIS in developing countries vary. The implementation and the influencing factors that affect the success and the benefits of the system in such countries are relatively different from those exist in other countries. However, there is an acceptable level of agreement among prior studies that investigated HIS in developing countries where HIS provide important benefits for healthcare, including positive effects on outcomes such as the efficiency of care, the effectiveness of care, the reduction of error rates, and the reduction of healthcare costs. Such systems will be particularly important in helping relieve overburdened health systems in the face of aging populations and dramatic increases in the prevalence of chronic conditions. For example, Electronic Health Records Systems (EHR) should enable new interfaces to be established between healthcare and research environments, leading to improvements in the scope and efficiency of research and the integration of new scientific evidence into practice.

Recent studies reported that most HIS systems designed to produce management information have an inherent deficiency. This is compounded by the fact that in most developing countries' situation management decisions are not based on information and, therefore, a need for a long-term investment in training and changing the processes in such situations for HIS needs to be used. Furthermore, studies reported that both complexity and context of internal and external environment are key to sustainability of computerized HIS in developing countries. HIS systems that are aligned to the technical environment of the context (country) and those that can be localized will be sustainable, as long as their product has currency to the users (Jayasuriya, 2014).

DISCUSSION AND FUTURE DIRECTION

Previous studies in HIS could be divided into many streams where each stream focuses on a specific part of health informatics. In general, they concentrate on evaluating HIS and investigating factors that affecting on the adopting HIS in general, in addition to user acceptance of HIS and implementation issues. These studies also evaluated the external environment in which HIS is operating and how so far new application will operate in healthcare organizations besides the costs of implementing new systems. On the other hand, some of these studies focused on the critical success factors of clinical IT systems, IT as changer of healthcare delivery, What is 'good practice of information management and technology' in healthcare and IT as an enabler of re-engineering of healthcare delivery processes (Brender et al, 2000).

Another stream of previous studies has concentrated on system use and user satisfaction of HIS, these studies tested the extent of user satisfaction with various systems (Pai and Huang, 2011), reporting in many cases a relevant degree of satisfaction about HIS in different health organizations and strong intention to continue using the particular system by medical staff which seems to be perceived favourably by physicians, with user satisfaction being mainly positive. Similarly, patient satisfaction has been analysed by previous studies, examining the impacts of implementing HIS on patient care. Positive impacts and reasonable satisfaction have been confirmed in most of these studies.

A recent review of HIS reported many problems in health organizations in general including data collection and processing, and weak use of information, poor quality and efficiency and application problems related to the functionality, and reliability of the system (Maenpaa et al., 2009). Ammenwerth and Keizer, (2005) investigated designs and study methods used in research evaluating IT in healthcare and indicated that evaluation studies on HIS in healthcare still has to be improved in some aspects. This poses a problem as evaluation research form the basis of any further analysis about the effects and quality of IT in health organizations.

Despite the proliferation of IS in health care, usefulness has been limited to date and technologies have not had the wide impact predicted (Gawande and Bates, 2000). However, few systems have been evaluated with respect to the impact of these systems on clinical performance and patient outcomes. Factors included in these studies were limited and many critical factors were excluded in the investigation. This limited our awareness of important factors that might contribute to success and failure of the HIS and/or the benefits of the systems gained by organizations. Therefore, researchers should take into account that not only IT factors when evaluating HIS but also other relevant factors such as human factors, usage and usefulness of HIS, user factors, the consistency between IT and actual needs, and the outputs of these factors (Ammenwerth et al, 2003). Thus, to be able to evaluate the impacts of HIS the interaction between all above factors should be analysed.

In general, information system research is very rich in many industries for example banking and manufacturing. However, its application in the health sector is still in its infancy, studies are limited in their focus because they often rely on descriptive information (Schaper and Pervan, 2007). In other words, research in health information systems is still very poor, this area needs more empirical and analytical research, little is known about IT and health organizations but much is still unknown about the benefits of these systems to organizational outcomes, performance, strategy and employees performance (Saitwal et al., 2010). In conclusion, early efforts addressing evaluation methods and their applications have been published in 1990s to guide researchers and practitioners in evaluating IT healthcare applications (Yusof et al., 2008).

Previous evaluation studies dealt with two distinct trends of HIS: The first one considers human and organizational issues, while the other is concerned with the approach that has employed to study HIS. Methods complement each other in that they evaluate different aspects of HIS and they can be improved upon. Additionally, most of these studies are case studies, they focus on specific aspects in healthcare information systems specially

implementation and installation issues; thus, there is limited knowledge in this field regarding several important factors which have essential influences on HIS user and its outcomes. Moreover, previous studies in HIS have limitation in the approaches that were used to study HIS, these approaches are based on very tight perspective ranging from for example technical, sociological, economic, human and organizational. In addition, they did not evaluate the potential effects of the system itself from a technological perspective as well as a user perspective. Such evaluation can lead to several outcomes for instant determine characteristics of IS in healthcare organizations in general and improve clinical performance, and potentially help improve the quality of care (Yusof et al., 2008).

Some of the typical problems that have been noted by many researchers are insufficient description or lack of control in these studies, use of inadequate designs besides limited power of studies and inadequate methods or inconsistent results of studies (Ammenwerth and Keizer, 2005). Furthermore, these studies are theoretical studies rather than empirical, and if they are empirical they depended on case study methodology and very narrow view. In a similar vein, Ammenwerth et al, (2004) discussed that the problem of inadequate and incomplete reporting of IT evaluation studies to improve standards and the significant of these studies. Therefore, studying HIS still needs more development in regard to methodology, data sufficient, framework and aspects that should be taken into account when analysing these complex applications especially at that time while HIS and medical technology is growing rapidly. Moreover, the evaluation of IT in previous studies gives the impression that it is insufficient especially with regard to a clear description of the IT system and to the methods used to capture and analyse data (Heeks, 2005). In addition, a major weakness in the prior research in this area that is most evaluation studies have been limited to technical performance or sometimes cost-effectiveness assessments and they have not taken a broader view in evaluation even though some authors go as far as to plea for controlled clinical trials of information systems in healthcare in the 'real world' as an approach to evaluate the impact of information systems in healthcare practice.

In summary, prior research that evaluated HIS has measured many aspects but not necessarily the right aspects. Therefore, a wider and more comprehensive framework that captures more relevant and essential variables, and meets the evaluation needs in this sector is highly desirable.

Before discussing the importance of Internet for accessing healthcare information, there are some issues that must be addressed by the different nations particularly the developing ones for example, poor Internet skills, lack appropriate tools and /computer systems/utilities to access the relevant information and lack of adoption of appropriate hardware and software, which are crucial for successful implementation of HIS in developing countries (Qureshi et al., 2014)

HIS adoption by healthcare professionals has shown to be a challenging endeavour due to a variety of barriers. Multidisciplinary approaches can enlighten and assist in HIS implementation (Peleg et al., 2009). Some of the barriers to successful HIS implementations can be approached from an organisational management perspective, while others most importantly from a users perspective. This section highlights some important issues that were commonly reported in the literature to be critical success factors to HIS implementations. These factors contribute significantly to the potential outcomes of successful and ideal HIS.

The ideal HIS provides real time access to a patient's medical history and health information, and accessibility to data that are not easily found within the patient chart. This improves the quality of patient care through improved patient records. Ensure that patient data are accurate and allow healthcare professionals to more easily and more quickly track the quality of patient care provided through the use of automated summary reports.

However, in many cases this does not come through all the time. Healthcare organizations report many difficulties everyday related to systems success and outcomes gained after and during the implementation of HIS projects.

There is generally no one reason for difficulties and failures in implementing HIS. In the IS literature and HIS literature researchers reported over thirty factors beyond a system failure ranging from systems and technology factors to human and behavior factors. Furthermore, while certain factors appear to be major contributors to the failure of many HIS, there are no data to measure the relative importance of each potential cause of failure. A common approach used in most studies conducted to evaluate success and failure HIS projects and explore the barriers to successful HIS implementation, is the analysis of critical factors to the successful HIS which offer general guidelines for implementation. The ideal HIS, however, does not yet exist. Furthermore, what is ideal within one healthcare setting may not be deemed so in another, and what is considered to be ideal may change over time. At least, these studies provided a common guidance to healthcare organizations and systems designers to avoid what might be applicable in their own situations to increase the probability of success implementation and minimize the probability of success. Based on the literature review the following factors deemed to be some of the most critical barriers to successful implementation of HIS is discussed below:

Work Redesign

Implementing a new system in any work environment requires some work redesign and process reengineering. In healthcare the situation might even requires more changes, as the environment of healthcare is complex and multifaceted. This necessitates a certain degree of redesigning the way the office works. This will lead to more system usage and

SYSTEM INTEGRATION

System integration is a main component of HIS and one of the HIS packages core capabilities. This capability is important as it impacts on the level of system usability. System integration is also designing the system for various types of users from different educational backgrounds. This enhances the ability of users to rely on these systems for all tasks in different functional areas and increases the usefulness of the systems

HIS must support the integration of functions, divisions of organizations in terms of information exchange and flow, and the integration of core business process (Kim and Chang, 2007).

Integration implies also that all relevant data for a particular bounded and closed set of business processes is processed in the same software application. Updates in one application or component are reflected throughout the whole business process logic, with no complex external interfacing. Information and data are stored one time in the main database, which enable users to share all information and data instantaneously that are supported and enabled by the system. In healthcare, unfortunately, as noted by many researchers integration was described as difficult due to the already demanding pace and responsibilities at the clinical setting. In effect, the benefits of a HIS, or its usability, must outweigh the costs associated with its implementation.

User Training and Systems Usage

User training is a very important factor, as users need to adequately learn how to use the new system and maximize the benefits of the use. Some authors identified the training and competences of healthcare professionals as the end-users operating a specific application as key factors in HIS adoption. In many cases, system use does not reflect the level of utilization. Some researchers described that as main obstacle to HIS successful implementation; regardless of the savings in time, reduction in errors, and improved patient care that can result (Mostashari, Tripathi and Kendall, 2009).

In healthcare many studies reported lack of sufficient training provided to users and/or lack of planned training before and during implementation stage. This led to lower system usage and utilization, and unrecognized benefits of the HIS implementation specially when it comes to cost benefits analysis comparing the countless hours of implementation and huge investments made in adopting and implementing HIS (Beuscart-Zéphir et al., 1997; Blobel and Roger-France, 2001).

Teamwork and Cooperation

A substantial number of studies in HIS research identified the current structure of healthcare organizational systems as a barrier of HIS success and argue that the current structure does not encourage teamwork involving different tiers of the healthcare organizational system, as mentioned in Lluch, (2011), others pointed out that team-based care strategies are needed, but missing for successful implementations of HIS (Mostashari, Tripathi and Kendall, 2009).

Cultural Change

Face-to-face interaction versus new ways of working is another major concern for HIS success. Healthcare delivery has traditionally been associated with face-to-face interaction between the patient and the health- care professionals. In many cases researchers highlight the fact that clinicians have expressed fears that the increasing use of HIS solutions will lead to the depersonalization of healthcare hence the need for cultural change.

Complexity and Multidimensionality

When understanding HIS as part of the information system of an organization, evaluation should not concentrate only on hardware and software, but on the information processing, i.e. usability and on the interaction between HIS and users in a particular environment. Thus, evaluation requires not only an understanding of computer technology, but also of the social and behavioral aspects that affect and are affected by the technology. The success of IT depends on several factors such as how IT matches with clinical workflow, on the quality of information it offers, on training and support, and on the depth of usage (Blobel and Roger-France, 2001). Therefore, evaluating HIS in any healthcare organization is a multidimensional and complex process that requires a broader view of many factors and aspects including the users, process and technology (Verhoeven et al., 2009).

Despite their promise, implementing HIS has proved to be difficult. In this chapter, based on a selective review of evaluation studies of HIS, some barriers and challenges to HIS adoption and successful implementation in general and in developing countries in particular have been identified. We suggest that several additional empirical studies need to assess future areas of HIS deployment and data sharing that lead to more realized benefits and successful HIS implementation in developing countries. There is a need for further research providing evidence of cost-effectiveness of HIS and information regarding organizational structure and change, work design, liability issues, end-users competences and skills, and work process issues involved in realizing the benefits gained from HIS.

Majority of the healthcare organizations in developing countries possess huge information but lack the capability to manage and analyze the information by using IT applications for decision-making. Therefore the users of such applications must be properly trained for the success of HIS. These application were described by may researchers as beneficial for healthcare sectors in developing states to effectively plan, control, and communicate health related information. It must be noted that healthcare related information systems and hardware are now easily available with affordable cost round the world. However successful adoption of these systems depends on the infrastructural arrangements, the willingness and interest of healthcare professionals about the usage of the system applications.

In summary, HIS is a multifaceted complex discipline. The complexity of the field and the barriers related to HIS research such as methodology, multidisciplinary and costs, have been already discussed in previous studies and confirmed in meta-analysis research (Ammenwerth et al., 2003). The lack of required considerations of design principles centred in human factors makes them very difficult to learn and use, and this difficulty leads to strong resistance by users, in some cases it leads to abandoning the HIS altogether or increasing "human error" resulting from an incorrect usage (Zhang et al., 2002). One plausibly solution is successful design and development of HIS that can increase efficiency and productivity and simultaneously, can help to decrease medical errors as well as to reduce support and training cost. These facts accentuate the need for a rigorous and deliberate consideration of above-mentioned requirements when design, develop and implement HISs. Therefore, a more inclusive framework in the retrospective investigation of the previous IS design approaches and models seems necessary to better understand and design a healthcare information system. Such an effective consideration and identification of the user requirements can guide HIS decision-making related to system development and implementation and have the potential to avert system failure and thus save human and financial investments (Curriea, 2005).

In this chapter, we elaborated a number of important problems to some more detail. Other researchers might find further evaluation problems, or may structure them differently. As many others authors pointed out, the necessity for a more incorporative framework to facilitate evaluation studies of HIS may be useful to address more issues and help searchers to better understand HIS in different settings.

REFERENCES

Aldosari, B. (2014). Rates, levels, and determinants of electronic health record system adoption: A study of hospitals in Riyadh, Saudi Arabia. *International Journal of Medical Informatics, 83*(5), 330–342. doi:10.1016/j.ijmedinf.2014.01.006 PMID:24560609

Ammenwerth, E., & De Keizer, N. (2005). An inventory of evaluation studies of information technology in health care: Trends in evaluation research 1982-2002. *Methods of Information in Medicine, 44*(1), 44–56. PMID:15778794

Ammenwerth, E., Gaber, S., Herrmann, G., Burkle, T., & Konig, J. (2003). Evaluation of health information systems – problems and challenges. *International Journal of Medical Informatics, 71*(2-3), 125–135. doi:10.1016/S1386-5056(03)00131-X PMID:14519405

Ammenwerth, E., Nyknen, P., Rigby, M., & de Keizer, N. (2004). Clinical decision support systems: Need for evidence, need for evaluation. *Artificial Intelligence in Medicine, 59*(1), 1–3. doi:10.1016/j.artmed.2013.05.001 PMID:23810731

Andersson, A., Hallberg, N., & Timpka, T. (2003). A model for interpreting work and information management in process-oriented healthcare organisations. *International Journal of Medical Informatics, 72*(1), 47–56. doi:10.1016/j.ijmedinf.2003.09.001 PMID:14644306

Baroud, R. M. (2008). *How ready are the stakeholders in the Palestinian healthcare system in the Gaza Strip to adopt e-Health?* (1st ed.). Ottawa: Library and Archives.

Bates, D. W., & Gawande, A. A. (2003). Improving safety with information technology. *The New England Journal of Medicine, 25*(19), 2526–2534. doi:10.1056/NEJMsa020847 PMID:12815139

Berner, E., Richard, E., Maisiak, S., Cobbs, G., & Taunton, D. (1999). Effects of a decision support system on physicians' diagnostic performance. *Journal of the American Medical Informatics Association, 6*(5), 420–427. doi:10.1136/jamia.1999.0060420 PMID:10495101

Beuscart-Zéphir, M., Brender, J., Beuscart, R., & Depriester, I. (1997). Cognitive evaluation: How to assess the usability of information technology in healthcare. *Computer Methods and Programs in Biomedicine, 54*(1-2), 19–28. doi:10.1016/S0169-2607(97)00030-8 PMID:9290916

Beuscart-Zéphir, M., Pelayoa, S., & Bernonvillea, S. (2010). Example of a human factors engineering approach to a medication administration work system: Potential impact on patient safety. *International Journal of Medical Informatics, 79*(4), E43–E57. doi:10.1016/j.ijmedinf.2009.07.002 PMID:19740700

Blobel, B., & Roger-France, F. (2001). A systematic approach for analysis and design of secure health information systems. *International Journal of Medical Informatics, 62*(3), 51–78. doi:10.1016/S1386-5056(01)00147-2 PMID:11340006

Chiasson, M., Reddy, M., Kaplan, B., & Davidson, E. (2007). Expanding multi-disciplinary approaches to healthcare information technologies: What does information systems offer medical informatics? *International Journal of Medical Informatics, 76*(S1), S89–S97. doi:10.1016/j.ijmedinf.2006.05.010 PMID:16769245

Chiasson, M. W., & Davidson, E. (2004). Pushing the contextual envelope: Developing and diffusing IS theory for health information systems research. *Information and Organization, 14*(3), 155–188. doi:10.1016/j.infoandorg.2004.02.001

Croll, J. (2009). *The impact of usability on clinician acceptance of a health information system* (Ph.D. thesis). Brisbane: Queensland University of Technology.

Curriea, L. (2005). Evaluation frameworks for nursing informatics. *International Journal of Medical Informatics, 74*(11-12), 908–916. doi:10.1016/j.ijmedinf.2005.07.007 PMID:16099711

De Dombal, F., Leaper, D., Horrocks, J., Staniland, J., & McCann, A. (1971). Human and computer-aided diagnosis of abdominal pain: Further report with emphasis on performance of clinicians. *British Medical Journal, 2*(1), 376–380. PMID:4594585

De Rouck, S., Jacobs, A., & Leys, M. (2008). A methodology for shifting the focus of e-health support design onto user needs: A case in the homecare field. *International Journal of Medical Informatics, 77*(9), 589–601. doi:10.1016/j.ijmedinf.2007.11.004 PMID:18248846

Easona, K., & Waterson, P. (2013). The implications of e-health system delivery strategies for integrated healthcare: Lessons from England. *International Journal of Medical Informatics, 82*(5), E96–E106. doi:10.1016/j.ijmedinf.2012.11.004 PMID:23266062

Grémy, F., & Degoulet, P. (1993). Assessment of health information technology: Which questions for which systems? Proposal for a taxonomy. *Medical Informatics, 18*(3), 185–193. doi:10.3109/14639239309025309 PMID:8289530

Haux, R. (2006). Health information systems, past, present, future. *International Journal of Medical Informatics, 75*(3), 268–281. doi:10.1016/j.ijmedinf.2005.08.002 PMID:16169771

Heeks, R. (2006). Health information systems: Failure, success, and improvisation. *International Journal of Medical Informatics, 75*(2), 125–137. doi:10.1016/j.ijmedinf.2005.07.024 PMID:16112893

Hovenga, E. (1998). Health and medical informatics education for nurses and health service managers. *International Journal of Medical Informatics, 50*(1-3), 21–29. doi:10.1016/S1386-5056(98)00047-1 PMID:9726489

Hovenga, E., Kidd, M. R., Garde, S., & Cossio, H. (2010). *Health informatics: An overview (Studies in health technology and informatics)*. Amsterdam: IOS Press.

Hunt, D., Haynes, B., Hanna, S., & Smith, K. (1998). Effects of computer-based clinical decision support systems on physician performance and patient outcomes: A systematic review. *Journal of the American Medical Association, 21*(15), 1339–1346. doi:10.1001/jama.280.15.1339 PMID:9794315

Jayasuriya, R. (2014). *Sustainability of computerized health information system implementation in developing countries: A meta-analysis of evidence*. University of Wollongong. Australia: School of Health Sciences.

Johnson, C., Johnson, T., & Zhang, J. (2005). A user-centered framework for redesigning healthcare interfaces. *Journal of Biomedical Informatics, 38*(1), 75–87. doi:10.1016/j.jbi.2004.11.005 PMID:15694887

Jydstrup, A., & Gross, M. (1966). Cost of information handling in hospitals. *Health Services Research, 1*(3), 235–271. PMID:5971636

Kaplan, B. (2001). Evaluating informatics applications – some alternative approaches: Theory, social interactionism, and call for methodological pluralism. *International Journal of Medical Informatics, 64*(1), 39–56. doi:10.1016/S1386-5056(01)00184-8 PMID:11673101

Kijsanayotin, B., Pannarunothai, S., & Speedie, S. M. (2009). Factors influencing health information technology adoption in Thailand's community health centers: Applying the UTAUT model. *International Journal of Medical Informatics*, *78*(6), 404–416. doi:10.1016/j.ijmedinf.2008.12.005 PMID:19196548

Kim, D., & Chang, H. (2007). Key functional characteristics in designing and operating health information websites for user satisfaction: An application of the extended technology acceptance model. *International Journal of Medical Informatics*, *76*(11-12), 790–800. doi:10.1016/j. ijmedinf.2006.09.001 PMID:17049917

Krickeberg, K. (2007). Principles of health information systems in developing countries. *Health Information Management Journal*, *36*(3), 1833–3575. PMID:18195412

Kushniruk, A. W., & Borycki, E. M. (2008). *Human, social, and organizational aspects of health information systems* (1st ed.). Hershey, PA: IDEA Group. doi:10.4018/978-1-59904-792-8

Lapointe, L., Mignerat, M., & Vedel, I. (2011). The IT productivity paradox in health: A stakeholder's perspective. *International Journal of Medical Informatics*, *80*(2), 102–115. doi:10.1016/j.ijmedinf.2010.11.004 PMID:21147023

Lee, T., Mills, M., Bausell, B., & Lu, M. (2008). Two-stage evaluation of the impact of a nursing in- formation system in Taiwan. *International Journal of Medical Informatics*, *77*(1), 698–707. doi:10.1016/j.ijmedinf.2008.03.004 PMID:18457988

Lluch, M. (2011). Healthcare professionals' organizational barriers to health information technologies – A literature review. *International Journal of Medical Informatics*, *80*(12), 849–862. doi:10.1016/j.ijmedinf.2011.09.005 PMID:22000677

Lopez, D., & Blobel, B. (2009). A development framework for semantically interoperable health information systems. *International Journal of Medical Informatics*, *78*(2), 83–103. doi:10.1016/j. ijmedinf.2008.05.009 PMID:18621574

Lucas, H. (2008). Information and communications technology for future health systems in developing countries. *Social Science & Medicine*, *66*(10), 2122–2132. doi:10.1016/j. socscimed.2008.01.033 PMID:18343005

Ludwick, D., & Doucette, J. (2009). Adopting electronic medical records in primary care: Lessons learned from health information systems implementation experience in seven countries. *International Journal of Medical Informatics*, *78*(1), 22–31. doi:10.1016/j.ijmedinf.2008.06.005 PMID:18644745

Maenpaa, T., Suominen, T., Asikainen, P., Maass, M., & Rostila, I. (2009). The outcomes of regional healthcare information systems in health care: A review of the research literature. *International Journal of Medical Informatics*, *78*(11), 757–771. doi:10.1016/j.ijmedinf.2009.07.001 PMID:19656719

Martikainen, S., Viitanen, J., Korpela, M., & Lääveri, T. (2011). Physicians' experiences of participation in healthcare IT development in Finland: Willing but not able. *International Journal of Medical Informatics*, *81*(2), 98–113. doi:10.1016/j. ijmedinf.2011.08.014 PMID:21956004

Moore, R. A., & Berner, E. S. (2004). Assessing graduate programs for healthcare information management/technology (HIM/T) executives. *International Journal of Medical Informatics*, *73*(2), 195–203. doi:10.1016/j.ijmedinf.2003.12.002 PMID:15063380

Mosse, E. L. (2004). *Understanding the introduction of computer-based health information systems in developing countries: Counter networks, communication practices and social identity – A case study from Mozambique* (Doctoral dissertation). Oslo: University of Oslo.

Mostashari, F., Tripathi, M., & Kendall, M. (2009). A tale of two large community electronic health record extension projects. *Health Affairs*, *28*(2), 345–356. doi:10.1377/hlthaff.28.2.345 PMID:19275989

Mukred, A., Singh, D., & Safie, N. (2013). A review on the impact of information culture on the adoption of health information systems in developing countries. *Journal of Computer Science*, *9*(1), 128–138. doi:10.3844/jcssp.2013.128.138

Nyella, E. (2009). Challenges in health information systems integration: Zanzibar experience. *Proceedings of the International Conference on Information and Communication Technologies and Development*, April 17-19. Doha: IEEE Xplore Press. doi:10.1109/ICTD.2009.5426679

Pai, F.-Y., & Huang, K.-I. (2011). Applying the technology acceptance model to the introduction of healthcare information systems. *Technological Forecasting and Social Change*, *78*(4), 650–660. doi:10.1016/j.techfore.2010.11.007

Peleg, M., Shachak, A., Wang, D., & Karnieli, E. (2009). Using multi-perspective methodologies to study users' interactions with the prototype front end of a guideline-based decision support system for diabetic foot care. *International Journal of Medical Informatics*, *78*(7), 482–493. doi:10.1016/j.ijmedinf.2009.02.008 PMID:19328739

Qureshi, A., Bahadar, S.,..... (2014). *Infrastructural barriers to e-Health implementation in developing countries* (Doctoral dissertation). Available from ProQuest Dissertations and Theses database.

Reichertz, P. L. (1984). Hospital information systems – past, present, future. *Medical Informatics Europe, Fifth Congress of the European Federation for Medical Informatics, Brussels*, September 10-13.

Rippen, H., Pan, E., Russell, C., Byrne, C., & Swift, E. (2012). Organizational framework for health information technology. *International Journal of Medical Informatics*, *82*(4), E1–E13. doi:10.1016/j.ijmedinf.2012.01.012 PMID:22377094

Saitwal, H., Feng, X., Walji, M., Patel, V., & Zhang, J. (2010). Assessing performance of an electronic health record (EHR) using cognitive task analysis. *International Journal of Medical Informatics*, *79*(7), 501–506. doi:10.1016/j.ijmedinf.2010.04.001 PMID:20452274

Schaper, L. K., & Pervan, G. P. (2007). ICT and OTs: A model of information and communication technology acceptance and utilisation by occupational therapists. *International Journal of Medical Informatics*, *76*(1), S212–S221. doi:10.1016/j.ijmedinf.2006.05.028 PMID:16828335

Seffah, A., Gulliksen, J., & Desmarais, M. (2005). An introduction to human-centered software engineering: Integrating usability in the development process. In A. Seffah, J. Gulliksen, & M. Desmarais (Eds.), *Human-centered software engineering – Integrating usability in the software development lifecycle* (pp. 3–14). Netherlands: Springer. doi:10.1007/1-4020-4113-6_1

Teixeira, L., Ferreira, C., & Santos, B. S. (2010). User-centered requirements engineering in health information systems: A study in the hemophilia field. *Computer Methods and Programs in Biomedicine*, *106*(3), 160–174. doi:10.1016/j.cmpb.2010.10.007 PMID:21075471

Tsiknakis, M., & Kouroubali, A. (2009). Organizational factors affecting successful adoption of innovative eHealth services: A case study employing the FITT framework. *International Journal of Medical Informatics, 78*(1), 39–52. doi:10.1016/j.ijmedinf.2008.07.001 PMID:18723389

Van der Loo, R. P., Van Gennip, E. M., Bakker, A. R., Hasman, A., & Rutten, F. F. (1995). Evaluation of automated information systems in health care: An approach to classifying evaluative studies. *Computer Methods and Programs in Biomedicine, 1*(2), 45–52. doi:10.1016/0169-2607(95)01659-H PMID:8846711

Van der Meijden, M. J., Tange, H. J., Troost, J., & Hasman, A. (2003). Determinants of success of inpatient clinical information systems: A literature review. *Journal of the American Medical Informatics Association, 10*(3), 235–243. doi:10.1197/jamia.M1094 PMID:12626373

Verhoeven, F., Steehoudera, M., Hendrix, R., & Van Gemert-Pijnena, J. (2009). Factors affecting healthcare workers' adoption of a website with infection control guidelines. *International Journal of Medical Informatics, 78*(10), 663–678. doi:10.1016/j.ijmedinf.2009.06.001 PMID:19577956

Waterson, P. (2014). Health information technology and sociotechnical systems: A progress report on recent developments within the UK National Health Service (NHS). *Applied Ergonomics, 45*(2), 150–161. doi:10.1016/j.apergo.2013.07.004 PMID:23895916

Yi, M. Y., Jackson, J. D., Park, J. S., & Probst, J. C. (2006). Understanding information technology acceptance by individual professionals: Toward an integrative view. *Information & Management, 43*(3), 350–363. doi:10.1016/j.im.2005.08.006

Young, D. (1984). What makes doctors use computers? *Journal of the Royal Society of Medicine, 77*, 663–667. PMID:6481741

Yu, P., Li, H., & Gagnon, M. P. (2009). Health IT acceptance factors in long-term care facilities: A cross-sectional survey. *International Journal of Medical Informatics, 78*(4), 219–229. doi:10.1016/j.ijmedinf.2008.07.006 PMID:18768345

Yusof, M. M., Kuljis, J., Papazafeiropoulou, A., & Stergioulas, L. K. (2008). An evaluation framework for health information systems: Human, organization, and technology-fit factors (HOT-fit). *International Journal of Medical Informatics, 77*(6), 386–398. doi:10.1016/j.ijmedinf.2007.08.011 PMID:17964851

Zhang, J. (2005). Human-centered computing in health information systems – Part 1: Analysis and design. *Journal of Biomedical Informatics, 38*(1), 1–3. doi:10.1016/j.jbi.2004.12.002 PMID:15694880

Zhang, J., Patel, V., Johnson, K., & Smith, J. (2002). Designing human-centered distributed information systems. *IEEE Intelligent Systems, 17*(5), 42–47. doi:10.1109/MIS.2002.1039831

KEY TERMS AND DEFINITIONS

Developing Countries: A nation with an underdeveloped industrial base, a moderate to low HDI index, and a relatively low standard of living.

Evaluation Framework: A set of processes for evaluating the benefits derived from the implementation of Information Systems in Healthcare. Increasing the understanding of the goals and objectives and articulating the internal and external elements that affect the implementation.

Health Informatics: The study of information processing as it relates to health care provision.

Healthcare Information Systems: The integration of business, financial, and clinical data into an effective database for the purpose of streamlining the management and delivery of healthcare.

Healthcare Services: A range of practices designed for the prevention, diagnosis, treatment, of maladies as they relate human beings.

Information Culture: Activities and behaviours associated with knowledge, communication, information, and data that play a major role in the success the organisation.

Information Systems: A composite technology used to store, process, and interpret information.

This work was previously published in Transforming Public Health in Developing Nations edited by Mohamud Sheikh, Aziza Mahamoud, and Mowafa Househ, pages 309-327 copyright year 2015 by Information Science Reference (an imprint of IGI Global).

Chapter 86
Mobile Technologies in the Emergency Department:
Towards a Model for Guiding Future Research

Judith W. Dexheimer
Cincinnati Children's Medical Center, USA

Elizabeth Borycki
University of Victoria, Canada

ABSTRACT

Hand-held and mobile technology is steadily expanding in popularity throughout the world. Mobile technologies (e.g. mobile phones, tablets, and smart phones) are increasingly being used in Emergency Departments (ED) around the world. As part of this international trend towards introducing mobile technologies into the ED, health professionals (e.g. physicians, nurses) are now being afforded opportunities to access patient information and decision supports anywhere and anytime in the ED. In this chapter, the authors present a model that describes the current state of the research involving mobile device use in the ED, and they identify key future directions where mobile technology use is concerned.

INTRODUCTION

Mobile technologies are increasingly being used in regional health authorities, health care systems, hospitals, and clinics throughout the world. Mobile technologies have afforded healthcare providers (e.g. physicians, nurses, therapists) the ability and opportunity to access patient information anytime and almost anywhere in and outside of health care organizations (i.e. in the hospital and in the community). This rapid access to patient information has made mobile technologies a valuable tool and provided health professionals with an aid in supporting patient care related decision making. When first implemented in health care organizations, mobile technologies provided limited access to health information on the World Wide Web. They were a significant contrast to desktop computers that provided access to electronic health records in hospitals. Electronic health records (EHRs) were

DOI: 10.4018/978-1-4666-8756-1.ch086

accessed via desktop computers that were located in specific areas of the health care organization (e.g. at the nursing station, at the end of a hallway). Desktop computers could not be easily moved from one location to another. With the development of varying types of mobile technologies, EHRs and their components including provider order entry, medication administration systems, laboratory information systems, and others can now be accessed anytime and anywhere.

There is a need to understand how these technologies are being used in EDs. Therefore, the researchers will present the findings of a scoping review addressing the current literature focusing on the use of mobile devices in the ED environment. In this chapter, we outline the current state of the research in using mobile devices and identify future research directions. We will also present a model. We will begin by providing background information about the ED, EHRs and Decision Support Systems (DSS) followed by information about mobile device technologies and software use in the ED.

BACKGROUND

The Emergency Department

The emergency department (ED) see patients needing critical or urgent care. Visits range from life-threatening to minor and non-acute complaints. From 1996-2006, ED visits increased by 3% annually (Pitts, Niska, Xu, & Burt, 2008) and utilization rate increased by 18% (Pitts, et al., 2008). The majority of visits occur in community EDs. A dedicated ED includes access to a wide-variety of specialists. The ED plays an important role in addressing, treating, and stabilizing life-threatening conditions. To address the unique needs of providing patient care there is a need to identify technologies that would best support health professional work in these settings. These technologies include EHRs, DSS and mobile technologies.

Electronic Health Records and Decision Support Systems

Approximately 55% of hospitals have a comprehensive HER (Jamoom et al., 2012); 46% of EDs have EHRs (Geisler, Schuur, & Pallin, 2010) 34.3% have Computerized Provider Order Entry and 26.7% have clinical guideline support (Nakamura, Ferris, DesRoches, & Jha, 2010). Children's hospitals have a smaller rate of EHR implementation with approximately 2.8% of children's hospitals have a comprehensive EHR with 17.9% having some form of basic system (Nakamura, et al., 2010). However, EHRs are increasingly implemented in hospitals, with the adoption of EHRs doubling over the last two years (U.S. Department of Health & Human Services (HHS), 2011). EHRs are replacing paper-based processes and records. Computer-based decision support is provided to healthcare providers to support clinical decision making and standardize care. Decision support systems are integrated with EHRs to guide treatment decisions and to aid the decision-making process at the point of care. Decision support can be delivered in a variety of ways, such as suggesting medications, medication warnings, providing guideline recommendations, alerting about abnormal values, and many other suggestions.

Fifty-five percent of U.S. healthcare institutions have EHRs (Jamoom, et al., 2012); decision support is frequently part of implementation and is defined as "any program designed to help health-care professionals make clinical decisions (Musen, Shakar, & Shortliffe, 2006)." It can cover many aspects of care including patient-specific recommendations (Slagle et al., 2010), information management (Chute, Beck, Fisk, & Mohr, 2010), and guideline compliance (Bell et al., 2010). The framework for decision support (Miller, Waitman, Chen, & Rosenbloom, 2005) outlines the types of support and the options for ideal workflow integration. Decision support should be provided at the right place, to the right person, at the right time, and these ideas should be incorporated into the design (Sirajuddin et al., 2009). CDS should improve performance so that the computer is a tool not a hindrance (Friedman, 2009). Design elements of effective decision support have been reported in the literature (Garg et al., 2005; Kawamoto, Houlihan, Balas, & Lobach, 2005; Sittig et al., 2008). Three key axes to consider in the design and implementation of decision support are: the role, when to intervene, and the method of intervention (Miller, et al., 2005). CDS is frequently built on evidence-based guidelines that represent the expert consensus on the ideal ways to manage patients and decrease variation in practice (Bakken, Cimino, & Hripcsak, 2004). Such systems have demonstrated positive effects on patient outcomes (Dexter, Perkins, Maharry, Jones, & McDonald, 2004). However, barriers exist that limit the implementation and integration of these into clinical practice and one of these is accessibility.

Mobile devices can help overcome the accessibility issue. These devices are already integrated into health care facilities for general use by health professionals to input, access and review patient information, or even as a source of information. They have provided health professionals with ubiquitous access to DSS which can be used during care.

Mobile Devices and Software in the ED

Ideally, access to the EHR and DSS via mobile technologies such as a tablet and the Smartphone can influence how a healthcare provider delivers patient care. Through mobile technologies, providers have the ability to access EHR data and decision supports in real time and virtually anywhere. This is vital in the ED, a location where having instantaneous access to information can be critical for patients with life threatening injuries or illnesses. Therefore, the ED context is ideal for mobile device use. In the ED, patients are treated by a variety of providers who move from one location to another. Over the past several years emergency departments (ED) have increasingly become more computerized with desktop computers, laptops, hand-held tablets, smartphones, and other portable devices.

The ED is conducive to the use of mobile devices as healthcare providers move constantly from room to room to treat patients. The episodic nature of the care visits lends itself to studying a clinician workflow or presentation of a disease instead of the chronic disease model, which is more patient-oriented. As part of this trend towards computerization of EDs, we have seen the introduction of mobile devices (e.g. tablets) as a way of providing health care professionals (e.g. physicians, nurses) with access to patient information and decision supports in the ED in real-time, anywhere and anyplace. In the next section of this book chapter the researchers will outline the findings of our scoping review.

METHODS AND PROCEDURES

Scoping Review of the Literature

The researchers conducted a scoping review to assess the state of mobile technology use in the ED. They systematically assessed the body of literature at the intersection of mobile devices and use of these technologies in the ED. Key studies were identified. Following this the studies were reviewed for key themes and findings. The researchers' inclusion criteria were broad as this area of research is only beginning to emerge (Arksey & O'Malley, 2005; Landa et al., 2011). The researchers reviewed studies that: (a) examined mobile devices such as wireless mobile computers, mobile work stations, personal digital assistants (PDAs), mobile handheld computers, tablets and smart phones, and (b) evaluated a software and mobile hardware intervention in the ED. Studies were excluded if they did not involve humans, focused on software design alone, lacked an evaluation component, studied a clinician or patient educational intervention only, took place outside of the ED or were a case report, abstract, survey, editorial, letter to the editor, or non-English language report. Articles were excluded when their focus was upon the use of a mobile device for only image-display purposes such as radiology report reading. Do you need to discuss the dates of the searches?

We searched the major electronic databases PUBMED® (MEDLINE®) ("PUBMED,"), OVID CINAHL® ("CINAHL®,"), ISI Web of Science™ ("ISI Web of Knowledge,"), and EMBASE ® ("EMBASE ®,"). Searches were performed from the databases' inception through July 18, 2012. In all databases, searched terms were classified as keywords. In PUBMED, search terms were defined as keywords and Medical Subject Headings (MeSH®) where appropriate. We based the search strategy on including emergency medicine facility, mobile devices, and medical informatics. Search terms included the following:

'emergency medicine' and any combination of the terms 'tablet computer,' 'phone,' 'medical informatics,' 'mobile,' 'tablet,' 'iPad,' or 'PDA' and relevant plurals.

A sample query is shown below:

(emergency medicine OR emergency services, hospital) AND (tablet computer OR phone OR medical informatics OR mobile OR tablet OR iPad OR PDA).

After completion of the first search, we performed an additional MeSH term search to be more inclusive. The results were included in the title and abstract review:

(medical informatics AND emergency medicine AND computers, handheld).

The two authors reviewed the titles and abstracts of all articles identified through the keyword searches. Disagreements between the authors were resolved through consensus. Articles meeting inclusion criteria were pulled for review. We removed any identified duplicate manuscripts describing the same study as another included manuscript. Duplicate results were removed. Included manuscripts were reviewed by both authors to ensure meeting inclusion criteria and references were examined for any missed manuscripts. Additional disagreements were resolved through consensus.

RESULTS

The literature search produced 6,672 articles, after exclusions, 38 articles were selected for inclusion. Of these, 28 articles were excluded for not meeting the inclusion criteria. Ten articles were included in the analysis. Several themes emerged from our reviews of the articles (see Figure 1).

Much of the research has focused on physician and nurse's use of mobile technologies in ED settings. Nurses were the focus of the research when a triage system was used. Alternatively, physician users were studied for all other types of systems. Physicians and nurses are not the only users of technology in a busy ED. Every person who has patient contact potentially uses technology from registration, to treatment, to discharge. In pediatric EDs, child-life specialists may use mobile technology to help entertain children during their visit. Additional research assistants are increasingly able to use mobile technology to screen patients, perform surveys, and collect basic research-related information on patients. We focused on physician and nurses as the users of the technology since they are most likely to use the tablet for situations that would benefit from decision support.

As physicians and nurses were the users of the mobile technology in conjunction with the software tools much of the research focused on how physician and nurse work was affected by the introduction of an intervention (i.e. mobile device + a software tool) in the ED. We focused on mobile technology providing some form of decision support for providers. By limiting to decision support, the total number of studies was reduced, however given the large range of uses

Figure 1. Overview of key themes emerging from the scoping review

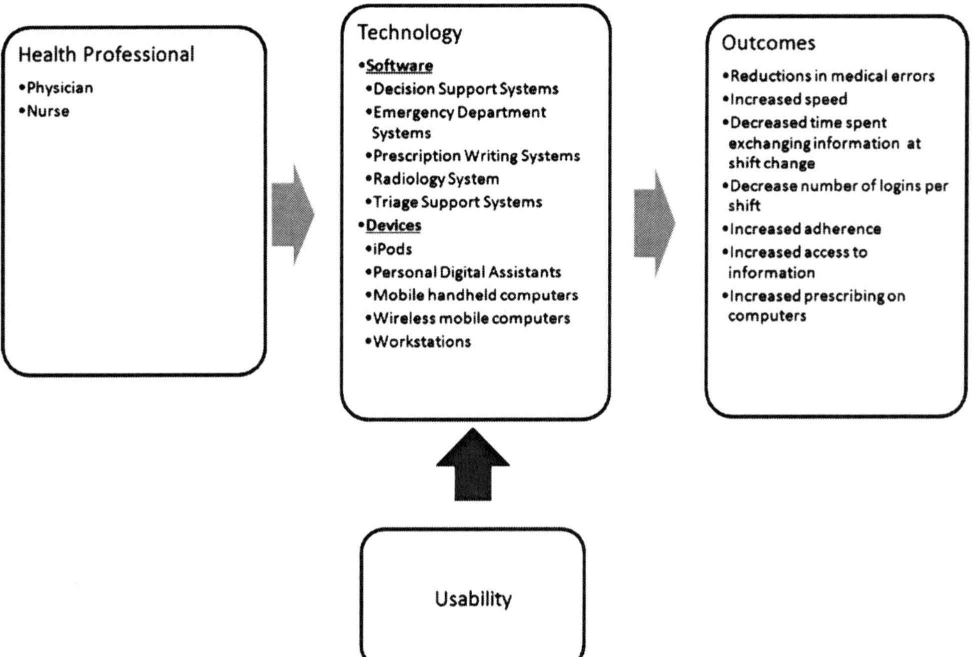

for mobile technologies from telephone calls to games, we wanted to focus on an area that had the potential to show direct clinical benefit (e.g. decision-making support).

As patients move through the ED during a visit, physicians or nurses lead their care predominantly in different areas and stages. In Figure 2, we present a simplified view of a patient's movement through the ED from arrival to discharge. In this figure, we have labeled where the nurse or physician is the predominant decision-maker. In a typical ED, the nurse would perform triage. This flow suggests the basic stages where mobile technology could be employed. Each of these steps is more complicated than it appears. A patient room may be changed during treatment, and there are other

providers who participate in patient care who aren't mentioned. Mobile devices, however, can be employed at any of these steps to provide additional information, improve team communication, or provide decision support.

Mobile Devices

Mobile devices were treated as the primary intervention in all of the studies. Here, the researchers attempted to evaluate the impacts of introducing these mobile technologies upon nurse and physician work in the ED setting. Several differing types of mobile devices were studied by the researchers. Our findings identified that a range mobile devices were studied by researchers. The devices included

Figure 2. Simplified view of patient movement through an Emergency Department

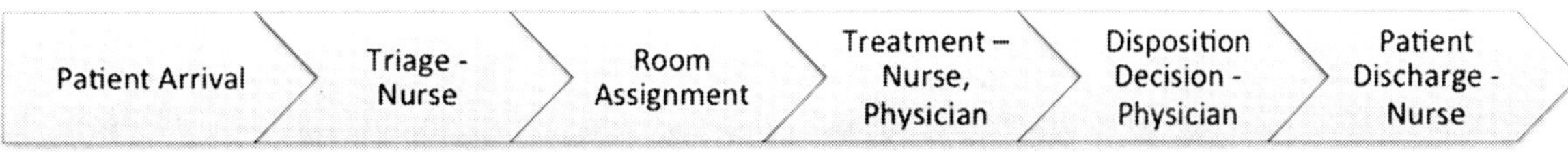

iPods, Personal Digital Assistants (PDAs), Mobile Handheld computers, wireless mobile computers and mobile workstations. Only one study examined the implementation of a Smartphone, the current dominant technology in the global consumer market. The majority of the devices were studied were personal digital assistants (PDAs) (n=6) (See Figure 1). PDAs differ in terms of shape and size and have limited ability to run complex software applications.

Software Tools

The published articles we reviewed in this work documented that there were a range of software tools that were used in conjunction with mobile technologies in the ED setting. These tools included software that would allow health professionals to triage patients (i.e. a triage support system used by nurses), review patient data (i.e. radiology system software, emergency department system), write prescriptions (i.e. prescription writing software) and view information/guidelines (i.e. videos, guidelines) (See Figure). No one type of software tool predominated in the studies. Each study represented an evaluation of one type of software tool with no other study evaluating the same or a similar software tools; for example, there was only one study that focused on the use of prescription writing software use in the ED. Instead a range of differing types of software were studied in conjunction with the above outlined mobile technologies. As a result, we found it difficult to make recommendations about the use of any particular software tool or type of software (e.g. prescription writing system or triage tool) for use in ED settings. According to the literature, differing types of software tools enable users to perform differing actions. As mentioned earlier in this scoping review, there were single study descriptions and evaluations of single software tools. Therefore, it was not possible to make comparisons across studies for an individual type

of software or software tool (e.g. all prescription writing systems used on a PDA). More research is needed on specific types of software that are used in the ED and there is also a need for several studies using the same software tool as such research would also provide additional insights as to the utility of the tool in differing ED settings (e.g. adult and pediatric contexts).

As well, little information was provided about the software tools themselves. For example, the publications provided limited information to the reader about the features and functions of each of the software tools. Therefore, it was difficult for the readers to determine what features and functions should be present in ED software tools and if the tools themselves were fully effective in supporting ED work and workflows. We find it difficult to recommend that specific features and functions be present in specific software tools such as triage systems because of a lack of information about software features and functions.

Usability and Workflow of Software Tools and Mobile Devices

Research has found that the usability and workflows emerging from mobile devices and software tools can influence their use. In this scoping review, only one study examined the usability of the software tools that were deployed in the ED. In this study, the investigator attempted to evaluate users perceived usability of the software tool. The focus of this research was a triage support system used in conjunction with a PDA. The researchers surveyed the study participants about their perceived ease of use of the system. Research from the usability literature suggests surveys of users perceived usability of a technology often do not provide detailed information that could be used to rectify specific usability problems and that further usability testing involving real users in laboratory and naturalistic contexts would need to be conducted to fully understand how a technology's features and functions support or detract from work in ED contexts (Kushniruk & Patel, 2004). None of the studies looked specifically at the effects of providing software tools via a mobile device upon workflow. Recent publications suggest there is a need to fully understand the impacts of these technologies upon workflow as some software/device configurations may introduce new types of workflow that are more cumbersome and may not fully support work in specific health care contexts such as an emergency departments (Borycki, Kushniruk, Kuwata, & Watanabe, 2009; Kushniruk, Borycki, Kuwata, & Kannry, 2006).

Usability and workflow are increasingly being recognized in the health informatics literature as important aspects of evaluating mobile technology and software configurations prior to implementation in real-world settings (Kushniruk, Triola, Borycki, Stein, & Kannry, 2005). Poor usability and workflow have been implicated in reducing adoption rates among users (Kushniruk, Patel, & Cimino, 1997), introducing inefficiencies in the process of using the technology (Borycki, et al., 2009; Kushniruk, et al., 2006) and introducing new types of errors into clinical settings - technology-induced errors (Kushniruk, et al., 2005). Technology induced errors are "medical errors that arise from the: design and development of a technology; implementation and customization of a technology; and interactions between the operation of a new technology and the new work processes that arise from the technology's use. (Borycki & Kushniruk, 2008)" As well, usability and workflow can have a significant impact on study outcomes. This is especially the case when the focus of these studies is to assess whether the mobile device and software tools when combined have an effect upon the ability of users to effectively and efficiently use the technologies to conduct their work (Borycki, et al., 2009; Kushniruk, et al., 2006). More research will be needed to identify the best mobile device and software tool combination for use by specific ED users and in differing ED contexts. As well, research is needed to determine the types of devices that will be needed in the ED and the features and functions that are needed for specific types of software used in the ED.

Outcomes

In our work, we found no one particular outcome of introducing a mobile device and software tool combination was studied, although several key themes emerged where outcomes were concerned. Much of the research focused upon how the software/mobile device combinations could reduce the amount of time spent undertaking specific ED activities as well as how these software/mobile device combinations could improve the quality of patient care that was provided. In terms of improving efficiency of work, the focus of this research was upon time spent performing activities (increasing the speed associated with performing tasks or decreasing the amount of time spend performing specific activities). Alternatively, other studies described how the mobile technology/software tool combination would improve access to patient information, improve adherence to guidelines and reduce medical error rates – all key indicators of improved healthcare quality. No one particular measure of efficiency or quality was used by the researchers. As a result it was difficult to compare across studies in terms of mobile device/software tool device combinations or their impacts on efficiency or quality of healthcare. Health informatics researchers need to identify key outcomes variables that should be used across studies so that there is an opportunity to make comparisons between mobile devices, software tools and mobile technology/device combinations. As well, there is a need to identify other potentially relevant outcome measures from the ED literature that can be used to compare mobile device/software tool measures to other types of interventions implemented in an ED setting such as the introduction of new paper based protocols to assess clinical and patient care impacts of the technologies across studies and interventions.

FUTURE TRENDS AND RESEARCH

Mobile devices are increasingly permeating work and home life. Mobile devices are in no way limited to providing decision support. Many studies used the mobile devices to view radiology images in the ED (http://www.ncbi.nlm.nih.gov/pubmed/23893749, http://www.ncbi.nlm.nih.gov/pubmed/23413062). This is an apt use for the devices but was not included in our research question. Before choosing a methodology, this would certainly bear examining and discovering. This did not provide any direct decision support help or advice but acted as an image-viewer only.

There were fewer studies of mobile devices in the ED than expected. With the great demand for mobile devices and the many options of downloadable applications, we expected more research on how well these systems performed during clinical care. We suggest more research to examine how much these systems do improve either care or clinician satisfaction. We understand that this is a rapidly moving field but mobile technology does have the potential to improve care if implemented and used properly.

CONCLUSION

In summary, ten studies were identified in our scoping review of the literature. Research examining the effects of introducing mobile devices and their associated software tools is in its infancy. To date few studies have focused upon any one type of mobile software tool in evaluating its interface design or workflow and its impact on health care outcomes in terms of efficiency and ability to improve the quality of care in the ED. Alternatively, although there are more studies specifically looking at the introduction of the PDA in the ED setting, the PDA itself has become obsolete as a

technology that can be used in the ED. More recently, Smartphones have become popular among healthcare consumers and health professionals. Health professionals are increasingly demanding that the technology be used in ED settings. Yet, few studies have specifically explored the impact of the device upon health professionals working in the ED. There is a great deal of variability in the types of outcomes variables that were measured. There is a need to identify key indicators of mobile device/software tool quality that can be used to evaluate the impacts of introducing these technologies across differing types of hardware and software. Lastly, there is a need to conduct usability and workflow studies involving software and mobile devices used in the ED. Such work is necessary as there is little known about the qualitative impacts of the software features and functions as well as workflows emerging from the use of software and mobile devices on the quality of patient care, health professional work and medical error rates.

REFERENCES

Arksey, H., & O'Malley, L. (2005). Scoping Studies: Towards a Methodological Framework. *International Journal of Social Research Methodology*, 8(1), 19–32. doi:10.1080/1364557032000119616

Bakken, S., Cimino, J. J., & Hripcsak, G. (2004). Promoting patient safety and enabling evidence-based practice through informatics. *Medical Care*, 42(2Suppl), II49–II56. PMID:14734942

Bell, L. M., Grundmeier, R., Localio, R., Zorc, J., Fiks, A. G., Zhang, X., & Guevara, J. P. (2010). Electronic health record-based decision support to improve asthma care: A cluster-randomized trial. *Pediatrics*, 125(4), e770–e777. doi:10.1542/peds.2009-1385 PMID:20231191

Borycki, E., & Kushniruk, A. (2008). Where do technology-induced errors come from? Towards a model for conceptualizing and diagnosing errors caused by technology. In A. W. Kushniruk & E. Borycki (Eds.), *Human, social, and organizational aspects of health information systems* (pp. 148–166). Hershey, PA: Information Science Reference. doi:10.4018/978-1-59904-792-8.ch009

Borycki, E., Kushniruk, A., Kuwata, S., & Watanabe, A. (2009). Simulations to assess medication administration systems. In B. Staudinger, V. Höss, & H. Ostermann (Eds.), *Nursing and clinical informatics: Socio-technical approaches* (pp. 144–159). Hershey, PA: Information Science Reference. doi:10.4018/978-1-60566-234-3.ch010

Chute, C. G., Beck, S. A., Fisk, T. B., & Mohr, D. N. (2010). The Enterprise Data Trust at Mayo Clinic: A semantically integrated warehouse of biomedical data. *Journal of the American Medical Informatics Association, 17*(2), 131–135. doi:10.1136/jamia.2009.002691 PMID:20190054

CINAHL®. (n.d.). Retrieved 1 August 2012, from http://web.ebscohost.com/ehost/search/selectdb?sid=a54fae89-7491-46d4-953c-958345858902%40sessionmgr4&vid=1&hid=28

Dexter, P. R., Perkins, S. M., Maharry, K. S., Jones, K., & McDonald, C. J. (2004). Inpatient computer-based standing orders vs physician reminders to increase influenza and pneumococcal vaccination rates: A randomized trial. *Journal of the American Medical Association, 292*(19), 2366–2371. doi:10.1001/jama.292.19.2366 PMID:15547164

EMBASE ®. (n.d.). Retrieved 6 November 2012, from http://www.embase.com/

Friedman, C. P. (2009). A fundamental theorem of biomedical informatics. *Journal of the American Medical Informatics Association, 16*(2), 169–170. doi:10.1197/jamia.M3092 PMID:19074294

Garg, A. X., Adhikari, N. K., McDonald, H., Rosas-Arellano, M. P., Devereaux, P. J., Beyene, J., & Haynes, R. B. (2005). Effects of computerized clinical decision support systems on practitioner performance and patient outcomes: A systematic review. *Journal of the American Medical Association, 293*(10), 1223–1238. doi:10.1001/jama.293.10.1223 PMID:15755945

Geisler, B. P., Schuur, J. D., & Pallin, D. J. (2010). Estimates of electronic medical records in U.S. Emergency departments. *PLoS ONE, 5*(2), e9274. doi:10.1371/journal.pone.0009274 PMID:20174660

ISI Web of Knowledge. (n.d.). Retrieved 1 August 2012, from http://apps.webofknowledge.com/UA_GeneralSearch_input.do?product=UA&search_mode=GeneralSearch&SID=2DPDdNGBCKHI7NPmmI5&preferencesSaved=

Jamoom, E., Beatty, P., Bercovitz, A., Woodwell, D., Palso, K., & Rechtsteiner, E. (2012). Physician adoption of electronic health record systems: United States, 2011. *NCHS Data Brief,* (98), 1-8.

Kawamoto, K., Houlihan, C. A., Balas, E. A., & Lobach, D. F. (2005). Improving clinical practice using clinical decision support systems: A systematic review of trials to identify features critical to success. *British Medical Journal, 330*(7494), 765. doi:10.1136/bmj.38398.500764.8F PMID:15767266

Kushniruk, A., Borycki, E., Kuwata, S., & Kannry, J. (2006). Predicting changes in workflow resulting from healthcare information systems: Ensuring the safety of healthcare. *Healthcare Quarterly, 9,* 114–118. doi:10.12927/hcq..18469 PMID:17087179

Kushniruk, A. W., & Patel, V. L. (2004). Cognitive and usability engineering methods for the evaluation of clinical information systems. *Journal of Biomedical Informatics, 37*(1), 56–76. doi:10.1016/j.jbi.2004.01.003 PMID:15016386

Kushniruk, A. W., Patel, V. L., & Cimino, J. J. (1997). *Usability testing in medical informatics: Cognitive approaches to evaluation of information systems and user interfaces.* Paper presented at the AMIA Annual Symposium: American Medical Informatics Association. Retrieved from http://www.ncbi.nlm.nih.gov/pubmed/9357620

Kushniruk, A. W., Triola, M. M., Borycki, E. M., Stein, B., & Kannry, J. L. (2005). Technology induced error and usability: The relationship between usability problems and prescription errors when using a handheld application. *International Journal of Medical Informatics, 74*(7-8), 519–526. doi:10.1016/j.ijmedinf.2005.01.003 PMID:16043081

Landa, A. H., Szabo, I., Le Brun, L., Owen, I., Fletcher, G., & Hill, M. (2011). An Evidence-Based Approach to Scoping Reviews. *Electronic Journal of Information Systems Evaluation, 14*(1), 46–52.

Miller, R. A., Waitman, L. R., Chen, S., & Rosenbloom, S. T. (2005). The anatomy of decision support during inpatient care provider order entry (CPOE), empirical observations from a decade of CPOE experience at Vanderbilt. *Journal of Biomedical Informatics, 38*(6), 469–485. doi:10.1016/j.jbi.2005.08.009 PMID:16290243

Musen, M. A., Shakar, Y., & Shortliffe, E. H. (2006). Clinical Decision-Support Systems. In E. H. Shortliffe & J. J. Cimino (Eds.), *Biomedical informatics: Computer applications in health care and biomedicine* (3rd ed., pp. 698–736). New York: Springer. doi:10.1007/0-387-36278-9_20

Nakamura, M. M., Ferris, T. G., DesRoches, C. M., & Jha, A. K. (2010). Electronic health record adoption by children's hospitals in the United States. *Archives of Pediatrics & Adolescent Medicine, 164*(12), 1145–1151. doi:10.1001/archpediatrics.2010.234 PMID:21135344

Pitts, S. R., Niska, R. W., Xu, J., & Burt, C. W. (2008). National Hospital Ambulatory Medical Care Survey: 2006 emergency department summary. *National Health Statistics Reports,* (7), 1-38.

PUBMED. (n.d.). Retrieved 1 August 2012, from http://www.ncbi.nlm.nih.gov/pubmed/

Sirajuddin, A. M., Osheroff, J. A., Sittig, D. F., Chuo, J., Velasco, F., & Collins, D. A. (2009). Implementation pearls from a new guidebook on improving medication use and outcomes with clinical decision support: Effective CDS is essential for addressing healthcare performance improvement imperatives. *Journal of Healthcare Information Management, 23*(4), 38–45. PMID:19894486

Sittig, D. F., Wright, A., Osheroff, J. A., Middleton, B., Teich, J. M., Ash, J. S., & Bates, D. W. (2008). Grand challenges in clinical decision support. *Journal of Biomedical Informatics, 41*(2), 387–392. doi:10.1016/j.jbi.2007.09.003 PMID:18029232

Slagle, J. M., Gordon, J. S., Harris, C. E., Davison, C. L., Culpepper, D. K., Scott, P., & Johnson, K. B. (2010). MyMediHealth - Designing a next generation system for child-centered medication management. *Journal of Biomedical Informatics, 43*(5Suppl), S27–S31. doi:10.1016/j.jbi.2010.06.006 PMID:20937481

U.S. Department of Health & Human Services (HHS). (2011). *We Can't Wait: Obama Administration takes new steps to encourage doctors and hospitals to use health information technology to lower costs, improve quality, create jobs.* Retrieved November 4, 2013, from http://www.hhs.gov/news/press/2011pres/11/20111130a.html

KEY TERMS AND DEFINITIONS

Decision Support or Clinical Decision Support: Using a system (computerized or paper-based) to help healthcare providers make care and treatment decisions.

Human Factors: A multidisciplinary field that studies the design of equipment and how it relates to a user's physical space and cognitive ability.

Medical Informatics: The field of study that broadly addresses information and computer science in healthcare.

Prospective Study: A type of analytic study that is designed to identify if there is a relationship between a condition and a selected characteristic that is shared by members of a particular group.

Scoping Review: A review that gathers information in the literature and presents a mapping of the results.

Usability: the study of the ease of use of a user interface typically in a computerized system. It evaluates the system's learnability, efficiency, memorability, errors, and user satisfaction.

User Interface Design: Aspects of a health information system which are seen by human users.

User-Centered Design: An approach to the development of products, devices, or systems to be used to complete tasks efficiently, effectively, safely and satisfactorily by their intended users.

Workflow: The the tasks and steps in a procedure that people and organizations undertake as part of a health care or business process.

This work was previously published in Social Media and Mobile Technologies for Healthcare edited by Mowafa Househ, Elizabeth Borycki, and Andre Kushniruk, pages 48-58 copyright year 2014 by Medical Information Science Reference (an imprint of IGI Global).

Chapter 87

Cloud–Based Healthcare Systems:
Emerging Technologies and Open Research Issues

Ahmed Shawish
Ain Shams University, Egypt

Maria Salama
British University in Egypt, Egypt

ABSTRACT

Healthcare is one of the most important sectors in all countries and significantly affects the economy. As such, the sector consumes an average of 9.5% of the gross domestic product across the most developed countries; they should invoke smart healthcare systems to efficiently utilize available resources, vastly handle spontaneous emergencies, and professionally manage the population health records. With the rise of the Cloud and Mobile Computing, a vast variety of added values have been introduced to software and IT infrastructure. This chapter provides a comprehensive review on the new Cloud-based and mobile-based applications that have been developed in the healthcare field. Cloud's availability, scalability, and storage capabilities, in addition to the Mobile's portability, wide coverage, and accessibility features, contributed to the fulfillment of healthcare requirements. The chapter shows how Cloud and Mobile opened a new environment for innovative services in the healthcare field and discusses the open research issues.

1. INTRODUCTION

Healthcare provision varies around the world; almost all wealthy nations provide universal healthcare. Health provision is challenging due to the costs required, as well as various social, cultural, political and economic conditions. However, many nations around the world spend considerable resources trying to provide it. Based on the 2012 statistics mentioned in (Organization of economics co-operation and development, 2013), most of the developed countries consumed an average of 9.5%

DOI: 10.4018/978-1-4666-8756-1.ch087

of their gross domestic product. For example, The United States (17.6%), Netherlands (12%), France and Germany (11.6%) were the top four spenders in this sector. One of the most critical disease and daily consume a lot of healthcare resources is the diabetes.

Efficient healthcare systems are hence critically important and need to be smartly incorporated. Such systems should fulfill a list of urgent requirements. They should efficiently utilize and allocate the available health resource; i.e., equipments and medications. They also have to be fast enough to effectively cope with spontaneous emergency calls and cases handling. In addition, they should be more flexible to move toward the patients as well as being able to explore critical probes and provide a pro-active model for healthcare crisis management. However, these requirements are not yet totally achieved through the classical healthcare systems that depend on the old technologies.

With the rise of new technologies like Cloud and Mobile Computing, new solutions have been introduced in healthcare field. The smart mobile is emerged as a fast, portable, widely available and efficient connection channel with the patients. Through such channel, data can be vastly acquired from the field with very low expenses. Guiding instructions as well can be also delivered to the patients anywhere and anytime. Developed smart medical mobile applications have hosted and helped patients to fully mange their daily treatment process. The Cloud, on the other hand, has incorporated to accommodate the healthcare system due to its broadly availability, scalability, and storage capability that makes it possible to acquire real updated data and feedbacks from both patients and healthcare managers.

This chapter provides a comprehensive review on the new Cloud-based and Mobile-based applications that have been developed in the healthcare field. Solutions related to Hospital Management System, Emergency Healthcare Systems, Healthcare Records Systems, Social Healthcare Systems, and Medical Imaging systems are addressed and

discussed in details; in terms of their features, functionalities and architecture. As illustrated and discussed along the chapter, these solutions have proven to fulfill the critical healthcare requirements and also Cloud and Mobile have opened a new environment for innovation in the healthcare field. The chapter also covers and discusses the hot research points that need to be addressed in this area.

The rest of this chapter is organized as follows. Section 1, introduces the background on the Cloud-based and mobile-based solutions in the healthcare field. In section 2, cloud-based and mobile-based healthcare systems are presented, and we illustrate their functionalities, features and architectures, along with discussions about their open research points. Finally, the road ahead is discussed in section 3 and the chapter is concluded in section 4.

2. BACKGROUND

This section provides a comprehensive background on the Cloud-based and mobile-based solutions in the healthcare field.

2.1 Cloud Computing and Healthcare

Healthcare and medical services consist of general and emergency medical services. General medical services involve provision of hospital numbers for appointments whereas emergency medical services consist of various pre and in-hospital activities. These activities are performed by various individuals (administrative, hospital staff and paramedical). These individuals differ on grounds of knowledge, experience and status. These activities are interconnected to provide services in case of emergency. Thus, during the process of development of this project, an essential emphasis has to be made over individual and combined processes.

According to the National Institute of Standards and Technology (NIST), Cloud computing is a pay per use model for enabling convenient, on demand network access to a shared pool of configurable computing resources (e.g., networks, servers, storage, applications, and services) that can be rapidly provisioned and released with minimal management effort or service provider interaction (Mell & Grance, 2009).

A cloud provides sharing of data and reducing the amount of local storages required. The advantages of using cloud computing can be mentioned as:

- **Reduced Cost:** Cloud technology is paid incrementally, saving organizations money.
- **Increased Storage:** Organizations can store more data than on private computer systems.
- **Highly Automated:** No need to worry about keeping software up to date.

- **Flexibility:** Cloud computing offers much more flexibility than past computing methods.
- **More Mobility:** Users can access information wherever they are.
- **Allows Shifting Focus:** No need to worry about constant server updates.

Given the characteristics of Cloud Computing and its service models, thus improves the ability of accessing the information by the users being able to rapidly and inexpensively re-provision technological infrastructure resources. Device and location independence enable users to access systems using a web browser regardless of their location or the device they are using. Multi-tenancy enables sharing of resources and costs across a large pool of users thus allowing for centralization of infrastructure in locations with lower costs. Reliability improves through the use of multiple redundant sites, which makes Cloud

Figure 1. Benefits of emerging cloud computing into healthcare

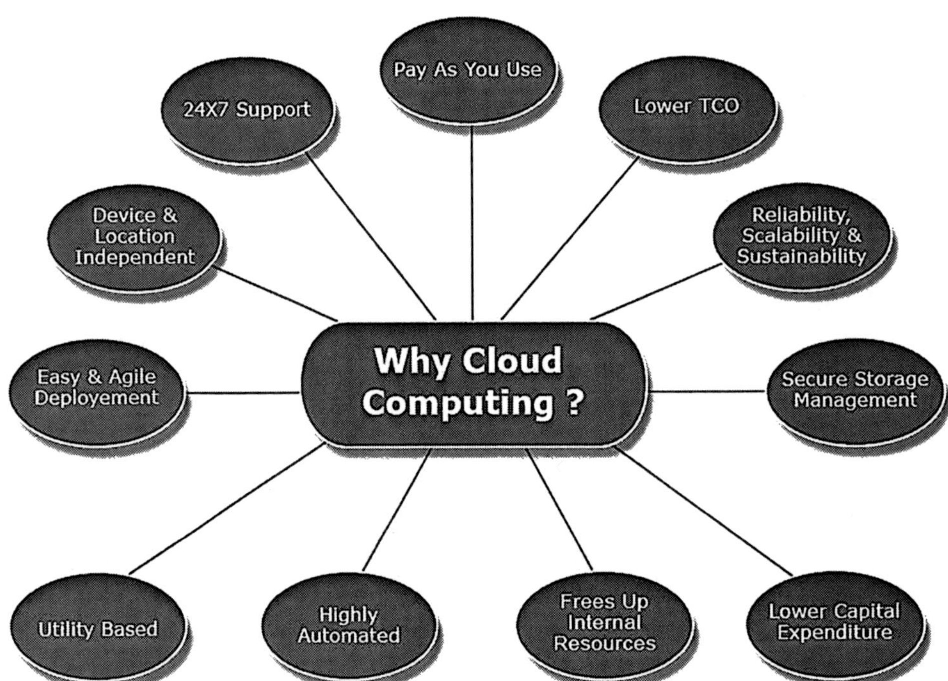

Computing suitable for business continuity and disaster recovery. Security typically improves due to centralization of data and increased security-focused resources. Sustainability comes about through improved resource utilization, more efficient systems.

2.2 Mobile Cloud Computing and Healthcare

Mobile Cloud Computing is a type of cloud computing in which some of the devices that are used for providing the services, are mobiles. Mobile devices have many constraints imposed upon them because of the desirability of smaller sizes, lower weights, longer battery life and other features. These constraints cause inflexibility in hardware and software development for these devices. Cloud computing can be used to allow the mobile devices to avoid these constraints by making the resource intensive tasks and complex functions to be performed on desktop systems and having the end results sent to the device (Doukas, Pliakas, & Maglogiannis, 2010). This enables the Mobile Cloud Computing to be a very efficient and effective way to develop robust applications in the healthcare sector. The end user will benefit, as they can share resources and applications without high capital expenditure on hardware and software resources. The end users can easily run the applications from the mobile without any costly hardware to run applications as the operations are run within the cloud.

Mobile Cloud Computing (MCC) is gradually becoming a promising technology, which provides a flexible stack of massive computing, storage, and software services in a scalable and virtualized manner at low cost (X. Wang et al., 2013). The integration of WBANs and MCC is expected to facilitate the development of cost-effective, scalable, and data-driven pervasive healthcare systems, which must be able to realize long-term health monitoring and data analysis of patients in different environments (Wan, et al., 2013).

The purpose of applying MCC in medical applications is to minimize the limitations of traditional medical treatment (e.g., small physical storage, security and privacy, and medical errors (Kohn, Corrigan, & Donaldson, 1999), (Kopec, Kabir, Reinharth, & Rothschild, 2003)). Mobile healthcare (m-healthcare) provides mobile users with convenient helps to access resources (e.g., patient health records) easily and quickly. Besides, m-healthcare offers hospitals and healthcare organizations a variety of on-demand services on clouds rather than owning standalone applications on local servers. There are a few schemes of MCC applications in healthcare. For example, five main mobile healthcare applications in the pervasive environment were presented (Varshney, 2007):

- Comprehensive health monitoring services enable patients to be monitored at anytime and anywhere through broadband wireless communications.
- Intelligent emergency management system can manage and coordinate the fleet of emergency vehicles effectively and in time when receiving calls from accidents or incidents.
- Health-aware mobile devices detect pulse-rate, blood pressure, and level of alcohol to alert healthcare emergency system.
- Pervasive access to healthcare information allows patients or healthcare providers to access the current and past medical information.
- Pervasive lifestyle incentive management can be used to pay healthcare expenses and manage other related charges automatically.

3. HEALTHCARE CLOUD-BASED SYSTEMS

In this section, the cloud-based and mobile-based healthcare systems are presented. These solutions

Figure 2. Emergence of mobile cloud computing into healthcare

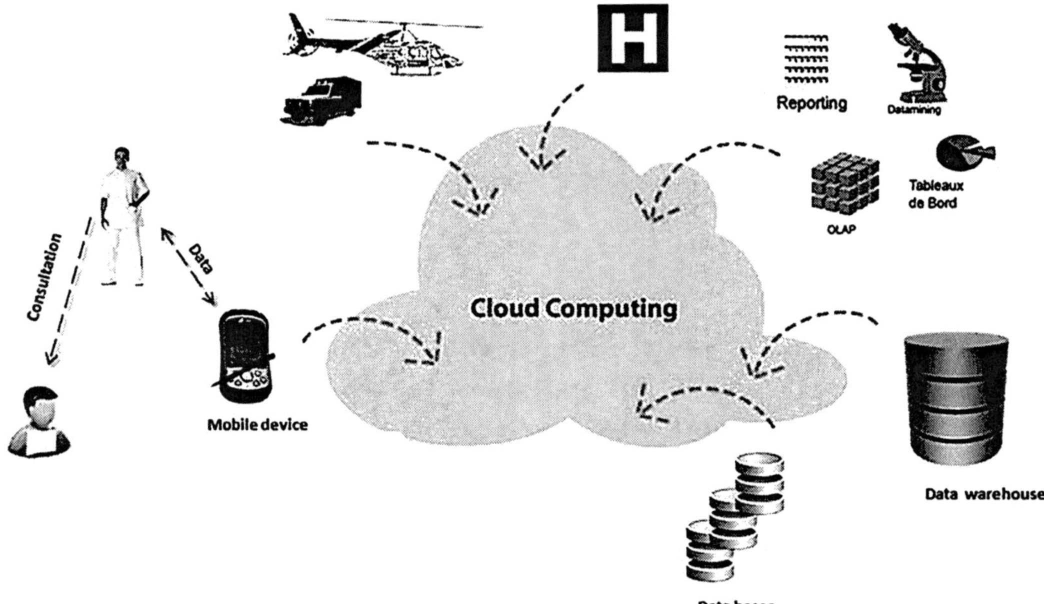

are categorized into Hospital Management System, Emergency Healthcare Systems, Healthcare Records Systems, Social Healthcare Systems, and Medical Imaging systems.

3.1 Hospital Management System

Many studies have demonstrated that there is a very limited access to patient-related information in hospital system which is available, during decision-making and the communication among patient observation team members are usual causes of medical errors in healthcare. Thus, there is a need for the pervasive and ubiquitous access to healthcare data is considered to be most essential for the proper diagnosis and treatment procedure for the patient. Cloud Computing is a model for enabling convenient, on-demand network access to a shared group of configurable computing resources (e.g., networks, servers, storage, applications, and services) that can be rapidly provisioned and released with minimal management effort or service provider interaction. This cloud model promotes availability and is composed of five essential characteristics, three service models, and four deployment models (Vinutha, Raju, & Siddappa, 2012).

The major characteristics of Cloud Computing can be summarized into the following:

1. **On-Demand Self-Service:** A consumer can unilaterally obtain access to computing capabilities, such as server computing time and/or network storage, as needed automatically without requiring human interaction with each service's provider;
2. **Broad Network Access:** Resources are available over the network and accessed through standard mechanisms that promote use by heterogeneous thin or thick client platforms;
3. **Resource Pooling:** The provider's computing resources are pooled to serve multiple consumers using a multi-tenant model, with different physical and virtual resources dynamically assigned and reassigned according to consumer demand. Examples of resources include storage, processing, memory, network bandwidth, and virtual machines;

4. **Rapid Elasticity:** Resources can be rapidly and elastically provisioned, in some cases automatically, to quickly scale out and rapidly released to quickly scale.

Given the characteristics of Cloud Computing and the flexibility of the services that can be developed, a major benefit is the agility that improves with users being able to rapidly and inexpensively re-provision technological infrastructure resources. Device and location independence enable users to access systems using a web browser regardless of their location or the device used. Multi-tenancy enables sharing of resources and costs across a large pool of users thus allowing for centralization of infrastructure in locations with lower costs. Reliability improves through the use of multiple redundant sites, which makes Cloud Computing suitable for business continuity and disaster recovery. Security typically improves due to centralization of data and increased security-focused resources. Sustainability comes about through improved resource utilization, more efficient systems. A number of Cloud Computing platforms are already available for pervasive management of user data, either free; e.g., iCloud, Box, Mozy and DropBox; or commercial; e.g., GoGrid and Amazon AWS. The majority of them however, do not provide to developers, the ability to create their own applications and incorporate Cloud Computing functionality, apart from Amazon AWS (Vinutha, Raju, & Siddappa, 2012).

3.1.1 Electronic Hospital Management System

The prevalent functionality of the application is to provide medical experts and patients with a mobile user interface for managing healthcare information more securely. The latter interprets into storing, querying and retrieving patient health records and patient-related medical data. The data may reside at a distributed Cloud Storage facility, initially uploaded/stored by medical personnel through a Hospital Information System (HIS). In order to be interoperable with a variety of Cloud Computing infrastructures, the communication and data exchange has to be performed through non-proprietary, open and interoperable communication standards. Electronic hospital management utilizing Web Services connectivity and Android OS supports the following functionality: Seamless connection to Cloud Computing storage: The main application allows users to retrieve, modify and upload medical content (medical images, patient health records and biosignals) utilizing Web Services and the Representational State Transfer (REST) API. The content resides remotely into the distributed storage elements but access is presented to the user as the resources are located locally in the device. Patient Health Record Management: Information regarding patient's status, related bio-signals and image content can be displayed and managed through the application's interface. Image viewing support: The Digital Imaging and Communications in Medicine (DICOM) medical image protocol is supported, while the JPEG2000 standard has been implemented to support loss and lossless compression, progressing coding and Region of Interest (ROI) coding. The progressive coding allows the user to decode large image files at different resolution levels optimizing network resources and allowing image acquisition even in cases network availability is limited. The code for performing wavelet decoding on mobile devices in has been modified to support the JPEG2000 standard on the Android platform. Image annotation is also supported, using the multi-touch functions of the Android OS. Proper user authentication and data encryption: User is authenticated at the Cloud Computing Service with SHA1hashing for message authentication and Secure Sockets Layer (SSL) for encrypted data communication (Vinutha, Raju, & Siddappa, 2012).

Figure 3 illustrates the system architecture for developing and deploying the electronic hospital management system application that utilize Cloud Computing and the VPN connection. The

Figure 3. Electronic hospital management system architecture

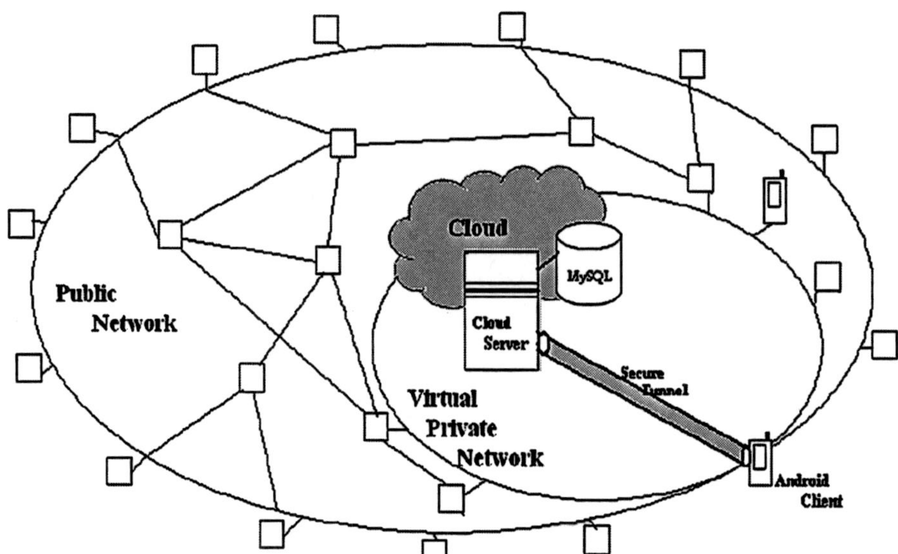

main components of a Cloud Computing Service usually are the platform front-end interface that communicates directly with users and allows the management of the storage content. The interface can be a web client or a standalone application.

The Cloud Storage Facilities manages the physical infrastructure (e.g., storage elements) and is also responsible for performing maintaining operations (e.g., backing up data) The Cloud Platform interface is also connected to the Cloud Service module, which handles and queues user requests. Finally, the Cloud Infrastructure module manages user account, accessibility and billing issues. Electronic hospital management system has been developed based on Google's Android mobile Operating System (OS) (Hung, Shih, Shieh, Lee, & Huang, 2011) using the appropriate Software Development Kit (SDK). Android is a mobile operating system running on the Linux kernel. Several mobile device vendors already support it. The platform is adaptable to larger and traditional smart phone layouts and supports a variety of connectivity technologies (CDMA, EV-DO, UMTS, Bluetooth, and Wi-Fi). It supports a great variety of audio, video and still image format, making it

suitable for displaying medical content. Finally, it supports native multi-touch technology, which allows better manipulation of medical images and generally increases the application's usability. The Cloud Service client running on Android OS consists of several modules. The Patient Health Record application acquires and displays patient records stored into the cloud. Data in Cloud are seamlessly stored and presented to the user as if they reside locally. This means that the Cloud repository is presented as a virtual folder and does not provide the features of a database scheme. In order to provide the user with data querying functionality, medical records and related data are stored into a SQLite file. SQLite is the database platform supported by Android. The file resides into a specific location at the Cloud and is retrieved on the device every time user needs to query data. The query is performed locally and the actual location of the data in the cloud is revealed to the applications. The database file is updated and uploaded into the Cloud every time user modifies data, respectively (Vinutha, Raju, & Siddappa, 2012).

3.2 Emergency Healthcare Systems

Emergency healthcare, divided as pre-hospital and in-hospital emergency care, involves a range of interdependent and distributed activities that can be interconnected to form emergency healthcare processes (Poulymenopoulou, Malamateniou, & Vassilacopoulos, 2003). These processes are executed within and between the ambulance services and hospitals Emergency Departments (EDs). ED physicians need the richest possible picture of the emergency case condition and health status. Hence, it is important to provide to authorize emergency healthcare participants readily access to both pre-hospital emergency case data and selected portions of past medical data (e.g., patient allergies and chronic diseases) of the patients by accessing their Personal Health Record (PHR).

3.2.1 Emergency Medical Systems (EMS) and PHR-Based EMS

Emergency Medical Systems (EMS) are among the most crucial ones as they involve a variety of activities which are performed from the time of a call to an ambulance service till the time of patient's discharge from the emergency department of a hospital and are closely interrelated so that collaboration and coordination becomes a vital issue for patients and for emergency healthcare service performance (Wooten, Klink, Sinek, Bai, & Shar, 2012).

EMS is an emergency medical system that accesses personal health records of patients and helps provide timely care. There are three groups of users in the EMS:

1. Ambulance Paramedics who have access to read and write data regarding paramedic activities performed at an incident site;
2. Emergency department physicians who have access to their respective authorized portions of medical data and can use the data to evaluate medical history, patient allergies and other critical health factors;
3. Nurses who can access their authorized portion of the data and provide the required medication to the patients.

EMS mainly consists of three components, Personal Health Record (PHR) platform, EMS application and a Portal to access the former. The PHR platform is composed of a user interface and medical record repository. The user interface allows patients to access their own medical history data and authorized healthcare professionals to access appropriate parts of the data. While the EMS application stores emergency medical information along with application software. The application software includes a number of web services that are only accessible by authorized personnel in the ambulance and the emergency department. Authorized healthcare professionals can interact with PHR and EMS via mobile phones and personal digital assistants, thus providing timely assistance to patients. This process gets initialized when a telephone operator receives an emergency call and records the patient's demographic and emergency medical information. After that, a physician who requests past medical data of the current patient is given access using a web service invocation. This service takes the doctor's role and the patient's name as input and searches the patient's PHR to retrieve authorized portions of medical data. The case data collected by both the ambulance service personnel and the personnel in the emergency department is captured in two separate XML documents. These XML documents are generated automatically upon ambulance arrival at the emergency department of a hospital and also when the patient is discharged from the emergency department.

EMS uses a private cloud to store data. In particular, PHR data is stored on multiple data centers on the cloud. It helps facilitate a timely access of relevant information by authorized people in case of emergencies (Koufi, Malamateniou, &

Vassilacopoulos, 2010). It was developed as a web application using Apache/Tomcat. Its prototype has been implemented on a laboratory cloud computing infrastructure. As of today, usability of the system has not been evaluated (Wooten, Klink, Sinek, Bai, & Shar, 2012).

3.2.2 Cloud-Based Information Support for Emergency Healthcare

Combining cloud computing with Service-Oriented Architectures (SOA) presents a new way for Service-Oriented Integration (SOI) of existing healthcare systems and for developing distributed applications within and between healthcare organizations (Zhou, et al., 2010). Through emergency healthcare process automation, ambulance service and hospital EDs can automate their operations by making information available where and when needed and by providing an infrastructure for the integration of pre-hospital and in-hospital emergency medical care.

At each healthcare organization (e.g. hospitals and ambulance services) there exists an information system. Figure 4 illustrates the information support for emergency healthcare system architecture.

On Amazon EC2 virtual images there exists a SOA platform that consists of a database server,

a business process server that hosts the BPEL processes and an application server that hosts the web services (Poulymenopoulou, Malamateniou, & Vassilacopoulos, 2003). In addition, on Amazon EC2 virtual images a global security server has been installed to enforce the global security policy. Patient data created in the form of XML Clinical Document Architecture (CDA) based documents are stored in and retrieved from the cloud servers with the use of Amazon S3 service and are made available to appropriate authorized recipients through messages sent by the Amazon SQS service.

During pre-hospital emergency healthcare delivery, emergency case data is stored in the ambulance service database servers. Upon ambulance arrival at the ED, a BPEL process is automatically triggered to call web and cloud services that retrieve pre-hospital emergency case data from ambulance service database servers and, optionally, designated portions of medical data from the patient's PHR, transform this data into a CDA document which is stored in the cloud servers and send this document to the ED where it is made readily available to authorized users. In this way, it is assured that timely and accurate patient information is made available at the point of care when needed (e.g. on a tablet pc or mobile phone).

Figure 4. Information support for emergency healthcare system architecture

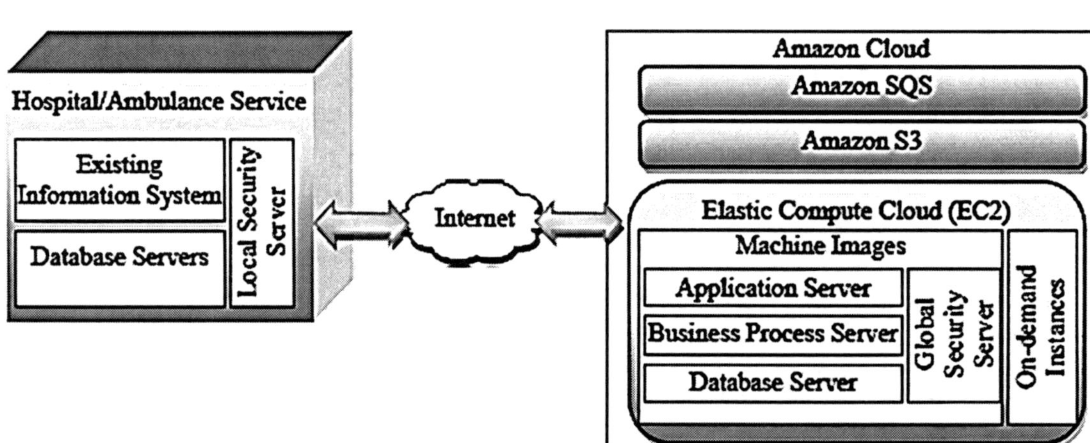

3.2.3 Discussion

Cloud-based services can prove important in emergency care delivery since they can enable easy and immediate access to patient data from anywhere and via almost any device.

3.3 Healthcare Records Systems

Using Cloud Computing, electronic health information is accessed by all the participants of healthcare system such as patients, healthcare providers, healthcare payer using open source cloud which acts as a server that faces several challenges, like data storage and management (e.g., physical storage issues, availability and maintenance), interoperability and availability of heterogeneous resources, security and privacy (e.g., permission control, data anonymity, etc.), unified and ubiquitous access.

On the other hand, mobile applications are used as a client to focus towards achieving two specific goals: the availability of e-health applications and medical information anywhere and anytime and the invisibility of computing. Mobile applications basically support electronic billing and EHR activities of patient and their medical history which can be accessed individually by patient, healthcare provider, healthcare payer by authenticating themselves with the cloud server.

3.3.1 Health Cloud eXchange (HCX)

HCX is a distributed web interactive system that provides a private cloud-based data sharing service allowing dynamic discovery of various health records and related healthcare services. In particular, HCX allows sharing health records between different EHR systems. It automatically adapts to changes in the cloud (Mohammed, Servos, & Fiaidhi, 2010).

With the maturity of Web Services and Enterprise Service Oriented Architectures (SOA), new delivery and Web interaction models are now demonstrating how services can be traded outside traditional ownership and provisioning boundaries. The value of SOA comes from having an architecture that readily accommodates change. The more the business changes, the more SOA pays for itself. However, the initial build-out of SOA, prior to business change or service sharing, is cost-ineffective. By incorporating cloud computing in SOA, the time to value is shortened because you leverage 'other people's work' as well as saving on infrastructure cost by leveraging on demand cloud based infrastructure services. HCX is a distributed web interactive system for sharing health records on the cloud using distributed OSGi services and consumers. This system allows for different health record and related healthcare services to be dynamically discovered and interactively used by client programs running within a federated private cloud (Mohammed, Servos, & Fiaidhi, 2010).

3.3.2 Healthbook

The development of HealthBook provides ease of access to patient's data in case of emergency by any responsible authority. These authorities have access to patient's medical information like previous medical histories, blood group, allergies, uploaded blood and electrocardiogram reports. The patient is initially required to access the web application to register for the service of HealthBook and then use the mobile application made available over his/her mobile device and enter all the required details about the type of service needed (Ujjwal, Manglani, Akarte, & Jain, 2012).

The architecture of the HealthBook system is shown in Figure 5. The system consists of three operating systems namely OS1, OS2 and OS3. Database is distributed on all these OS. The node controller represents the main user namely patient. It is the cloud deployment platform. The node controller comprises of the BPEL engine which has the designed BPEL rules and checks the queries accordingly and processes the output

Figure 5. HealthBook architecture

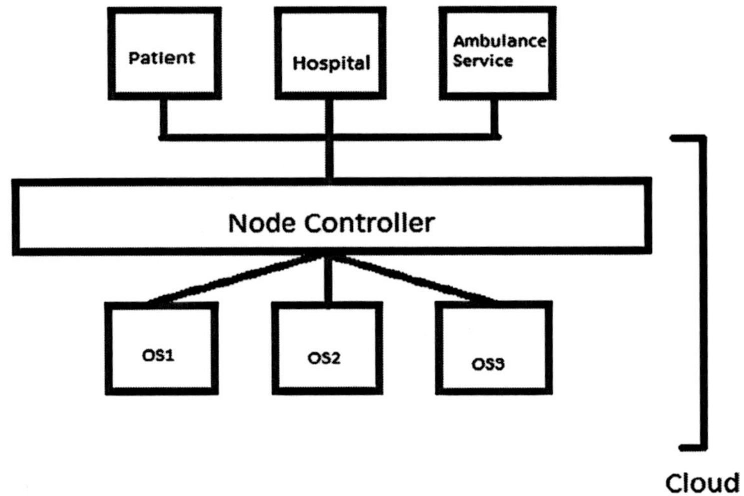

and makes it available over the user's device. The node controller and the database servers are located over the cloud. The user fires a query to the node controller according to the services he/she demands. The node controller which consists of the BPEL engine processes this query using the information stored in the database. The node controller has a complete access to the database servers OS1, OS2 and OS3 (Ujjwal, Manglani, Akarte, & Jain, 2012).

The HealthBook consists of various BPEL-orchestrated services which are usually called by the patient or the ambulance operator or the hospital authority. The entire process begins after a call is made by the patient to the ambulance service. Appropriate web services are used for various services requested. Likewise, if an ambulance operator or hospital doctor requests for previous medical history of the patient then in that case an appropriate web service is invoked. Case history collected by the ambulance service doctor and the hospital doctor form two separate XML documents. These XML documents are automatically generated as the ambulance reaches the hospital and when the patient is discharged, respectively. The applications for HealthBook are licensed for use and these are provided only

upon registration to the service. The application software for PHR and HealthBook component are comprised of various web services which are deployed using BPEL rules. Users can interact with the application either by using desktops or mobile devices.

The HealthBook consists of various BPEL-orchestrated services which are usually called by the patient or the ambulance operator or the hospital authority. The entire process begins after a call is made by the patient to the ambulance service. Appropriate web services are used for various services requested. Likewise, if an ambulance operator or hospital doctor requests for previous medical history of the patient then in that case an appropriate web service is invoked. Case history collected by the ambulance service doctor and the hospital doctor form two separate XML documents. These XML documents are automatically generated as the ambulance reaches the hospital and when the patient is discharged, respectively. The applications for HealthBook are licensed for use and these are provided only upon registration to the service. The application software for PHR and HealthBook component are comprised of various web services which are deployed using BPEL rules. Users can interact with the application either by using desktops or mobile devices (Ujjwal, Manglani, Akarte, & Jain, 2012).

The architecture can be broadly termed consisting of following components:

- **PHR Application:** Responsible for centrally locating the patient information as well as giving the patient privileges to view his/her profile anytime with an access to edit it. Thus, the PHR application consists of a data repository to store the data globally and not locally. The PHR application also consists of a user application which enables user and ambulance or hospital authority to access the patient's information.
- **HealthBook Application:** Stores the hospital and ambulance data which consists of the phone numbers and addresses. This also consists of various BPEL –orchestrated web services. Registered patients only can use these services.
- **Graphical User Interface:** Provides front-end to the services provided by the processes. Users interact with the GUI to access PHR and HealthBook Application. The size of the GUI is flexible so that it can be easily accessed over any device. This property enables the efficient use of GUI in case of emergency when the application has to be accessed through a mobile device.

3.3.3 E-Healthcare Billing and Record Management Information System (MedBook)

Electronic Health Records (EHR) and Electronic Medical Billing (EMB) have been proposed as a mechanism which reduces healthcare disparities and ensures adequate privacy and security. One potential solution for addressing all aforementioned issues is the introduction of Cloud Computing concept in electronic healthcare systems. This mechanism pursued the idea of using open-source public cloud computing Technologies and mobile

plus cloud paradigm to build an affordable, secure and scalable platform that supports billing as well as EHR operations. A platform called *MedBook* has been proposed (Vanitha, Narasimha Murthy, & Chaitra, 2013). MedBook is a cloud solution that provides patients, healthcare professionals/ providers and healthcare payers a platform for exchange of electronic information about billing activities, benefit inquiries and EHR operations such as insert delete and update record using open source cloud services and Android operating system (OS).

MedBook is Software–as-a-Service (SaaS) platform built on top of open source public cloud technologies and running on the top of an Infrastructure-as-a Service (IaaS) platform. Generally the server applications are implemented as a collection of web services and web applications using MySQL, Tomcat 6or7 server, Apache web server. All the web services run on virtual machines powered by Windows XP or Ubuntu Linux 10.04.These servers are hosted inside an open source cloud which can be Jelastic, Eucalyptus 2.0, Open Stack and so forth. The client applications are mobile apps run from Google's Android Enabled phones. These client applications are built using Java 1.7 or 1.6 and uses REST based API to interact with MedBook SaaS Infrastructure (Vanitha, Narasimha Murthy, & Chaitra, 2013).

MedBook provides a highly reliable and secure electronic billing and record management system. It also helps reduce the occurrences of medical errors due to incomplete medical information. Privacy of medical information is maintained to prevent unauthorized access and misuse of electronic information. Since the MedBook is Mobile plus cloud paradigm, the various participants such as patients, health care payers, healthcare professional can exchange information regardless of time, location, cost involved in it. Since the system utilizes open source cloud computing technologies, the interaction of healthcare participants with MedBook SaaS application can be done globally which reduce the cost associated in accessing medical information to certain limit. In addition, by integrating and correlating the billing system with EHR, it becomes possible to find that a given procedure was actually performed or the medical history of the patient utilized such procedures.

Figure 6 depicts the MedBook system architecture. MedBook SaaS application serves as an integration point between the various participants in the healthcare delivery system. MedBook architecture basically contains two Modules such as Client Module which uses the Mobile apps such as android enabled phones to interact with MedBook application. Server Module which consists of a series of web services and databases residing inside an IaaS cloud that maintains the information about each patient's EHR (Vanitha, Narasimha Murthy, & Chaitra, 2013).

The MedBook Client applications are mobile apps which uses Android enabled phones that connect with the MedBook SaaS infrastructure by means of REST based API. An android enabled phone is an open source and basically supports large number of applications compared to other Smart phones. Android client application is designed for Patients, Healthcare provider/professional, Healthcare payers to perform billing and EHR activities with MedBook. The MebBook client application is designed for patients, healthcare payers, and healthcare providers/professionals (Vanitha, Narasimha Murthy, & Chaitra, 2013).

MedBook Server Application consists of a series of web services and databases residing inside an IaaS cloud that maintains the information related to each patient's EHR activities. The server module is designed to perform the following activities; service description, submitting Billing Transactions, representing and accessing EHR's (Vanitha, Narasimha Murthy, & Chaitra, 2013).

3.4 Social Healthcare Systems

Health and social care is a vast service sector undergoing rapid change, with new government initiatives giving it a higher profile than ever. Priorities on the

Figure 6. MedBook system architecture

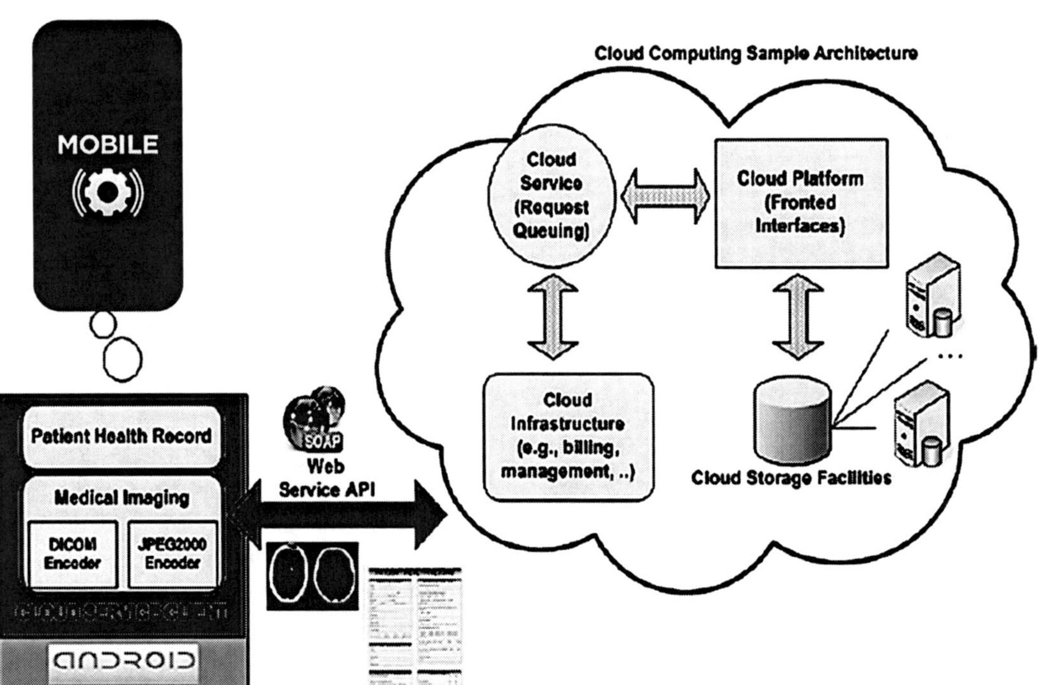

healthcare agenda include being more responsive to patient needs, and preventing illness by promoting a healthy lifestyle. The focus in frontline health and social care is on giving service-users more independence, choice and control.

Some new ideas have been developed in the context of providing healthcare personalized system on hold with the citizen. Ideas; such as kiosks, health cloud and information system for rural areas; are briefed below.

3.4.1 HealthATM Kiosks

HealthATM kiosks are developed for patients to manage their own personal health data. It integrates services from Google's cloud computing environment. It provides timely access to relevant health data to patients and strengthens patients' communication with their care providers (Botts, Thoms, Noamani, & Horan, 2010). Although, it is also a cost effective solution of personal healthcare management; as they makes use of cloud computing architectures, the systems currently cannot be directly handed over to patients; for constant training, outreach, education and collaboration are must.

3.4.2 @HealthCloud

@HealthCloud is a mobile healthcare information management system that is based on cloud computing and Android OS. It enables healthcare data storage, update and retrieval using Amazon Simple Storage Service (S3). It includes a PHR application that acquires and displays patient records stored in the cloud and a medical imaging module to display medical images on the device. It also supports native multi-touch technology which allows better manipulation of medical images and increases the application's usability (Doukas, Pliakas, & Maglogiannis, 2010).

3.4.3 Rural Healthcare Information System Model

Information management in hospitals, dispensaries and healthcare centres particularly in rural areas is a complex task. High quality healthcare depends on extensive and carefully planned information processing. In this context, a cloud based rural healthcare information system model has been introduced (Padhy, Patra, & Chan, 2012). The Cloud-based information system requires creating a secure, state-of-art facility to store the data / information available in different healthcare centres and to provide access to users in a secured manner, as per their roles and privileges. Figure 7 depicts the cloud-based model rural healthcare centre.

The model is composed of:

- **Cloud Control Server:** In a typical cloud, the cloud controller is responsible for managing physical resources, monitoring the physical machines, placing virtual machines, and allocating storage. The controller reacts to new requests or changes in workload by provisioning new virtual machines and allocating physical resources. This server also helps several ways in order to facilitate better control over the network.
- **Authentication Server:** Because in the application and data is hosted outside of the organization in the cloud computing environment, the cloud service provider has to use Authentication and Authorization mechanism. Authentication means that each user has an identity which can be trusted as genuine. This is necessary because some resources may be authorized only to certain users, or certain classes of users.

Figure 7. Architecture of cloud-based model rural healthcare centre

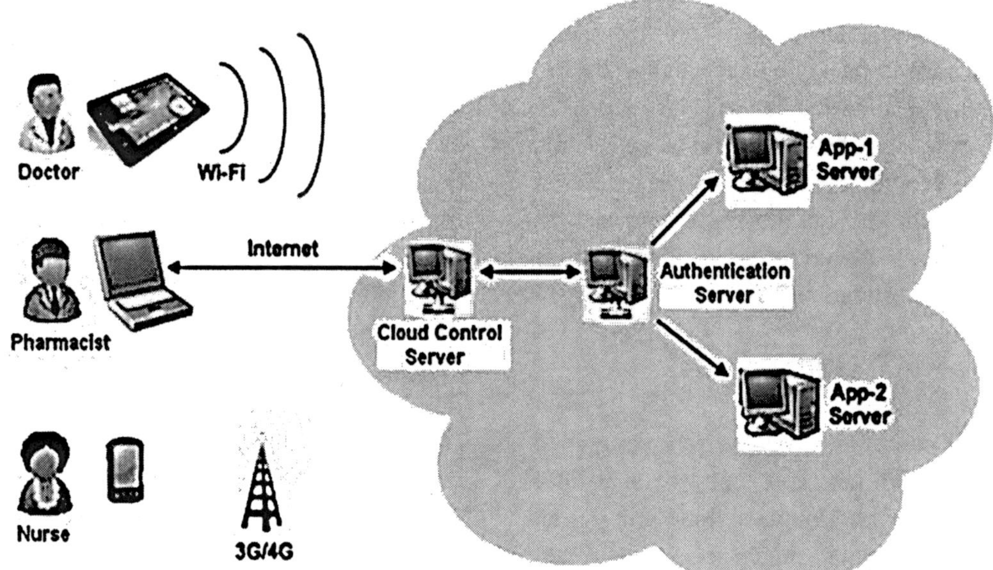

- **Resource Access:** Resource Access means that remote resources can be accessible to Grid users. These resources could mean anything from CPU time to disk storage, to visualization tools and data sets. Everyone should not be able to access all resources.
- **Resource Discovery:** Resource Discovery means that users can access remote resources that they can use.

The connectivity and configuration of the Cloud-based rural healthcare Information system is based on the service provider policy and domain location; i.e. cloud data centre location. Internet is the main communication link between the service provider and the Rural Healthcare centre. Users access cloud computing using networked client devices, such as desktop computers, laptops, tablets and smart phones. Some of these devices - cloud clients - rely on cloud computing for all or a majority of their applications so as to be essentially useless without it. Examples are thin clients and the browser. Many cloud applications do not require specific software on the client and instead use a web browser to interact with the cloud application (Padhy, Patra, & Chan, 2012).

Regarding, the system message flow, a nurse documents a visit of that patient when a patient visits a Rural Healthcare Centre. The Rural Healthcare Centre Information support centre supports an interface that closely used the SOAP protocol for documenting a visit. SOAP is an acronym comprising of the four stages involved; subjective which captures a patient's conditions in her own words, Objective consisting of notes made from measurements, physical examination and tests, Assessment consisting of a summary and differential diagnosis and finally Plan which is the care-provider's recommended course of action that includes prescriptions and referrals. As part of the plan, the care provider also recommends, if she deems necessary, a follow up to be done by the Health Extension Worker. Every visit documented by the nurse goes through an approval by a doctor and, the health care provider can access the history of visits for every patient (Padhy, Patra, & Chan, 2012).

3.4.4 Discussion

Directed to a new area, Cloud Computing would help rural healthcare centres to achieve efficient use of their hardware and software investments and to increase profitability by improving the utilization of resources to the maximum.

3.5 Medical Imaging systems

The Digital Imaging and Communication in Medicine (DICOM) standard, is the de facto format for medical images produced by various modalities. DICOM has become an indispensable component for the integration of digital imaging systems in medicine. DICOM offers solutions for many communication related applications - in a network as well as off-line. The keyword "DICOM" by itself, however, is no guarantee for a "plug and play" integration of all information systems in a hospital. Such a scenario requires a careful combination of all the partial solutions offered by DICOM.

DICOM image analysis and visualization systems have become important tools that can help to diagnose various pathological disorders affecting human beings. Currently, there are numerous systems that allow medical professionals to access DICOM images located on PACS servers (Pasha, et al., 2012), while some even offer collaborative analysis features for image based discussion with their medical peers via computer networks (Drnasin & Grgic, 2010).

Research and development into advanced medical image analysis and visualization mostly focus on creating algorithms to analyze image features, segment specific soft tissues and ultimately identify lesions. Today, pervasive and cloud computing technology is also receiving widespread acceptance in the healthcare industry (Doukas, Pliakas, & Maglogiannis, 2010) (Vlahu-Gjorgievska & Trajkovik, 2011).

Several mobile applications to retrieve and display DICOM images already exist on the market today. Most are only available on the iOS platform with one application utilizing Android (Doukas, Pliakas, & Maglogiannis, 2010).

3.5.1 Android-Based Mobile Medical Image Viewer

The rationale behind the adoption of the Android platform for the mobile system is because Android provides higher flexibility to third parties on development and licensing issues, compared to the closed approach of the iOS platform. In addition, it is supported by a majority of mobile device manufacturers today. This is seen through the formation of the Open Handset Alliance, comprising of 80 pioneering software, hardware, and telecommunication companies committed to promoting open standards in the mobile technology sector. Thus, the large number and variety of devices running on the Android platform will be advantageous for the mobile solution.

Figure 8 shows the complete architectural design of the mobile system. Overall, it has four major components: the Viewer component, the Preference Store component, the Browse and Import component, and the Collaborative Module (Pasha, et al., 2012). For the database, the SQLite relational embedded database is implemented to store data. In addition, a lightweight collaborative server implementation with infrastructure support for the mobile system collaborative annotation feature is designed.

The Viewer component is basically the main component of the mobile system. It links the other components and manages the data flow between the user and the system. Since the system is designed to run on Android-based devices with touch screens, the viewer component also implements the required touch gestures to control the system. Lastly, it also has three sub-components to provide different functionalities (Pasha, et al., 2012).

The first sub-component is the DICOM reader, which implements the needed functionality to read

Figure 8. Mobile medical image viewer and collaborative annotation system architecture

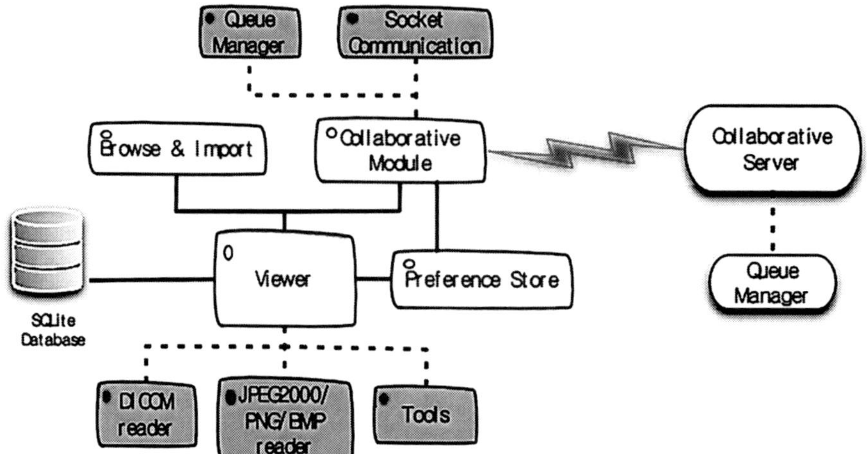

DICOM images and the included metadata. The second sub-component is a conventional image reader that focuses on reading compressed lossless JPEG images. And the last sub-component is the tools module providing the needed tools to highlight regions of interest.

The viewer component is linked with the three other components; the Browse and Import component, the Preference store, and the Collaborative Module component. The Browse and Import component is a module designed to scan the mobile device's local directory for DICOM files. It also implements an import function to import local DICOM files and stores its location and metadata into the SQLite database. The Preference store module basically implements the standard system preference settings for storage in mobile devices.

Next, the Collaborative Module component is the core element of the Android-based mobile medical image viewer and collaborative annotation system. It allows multiple experts from different geographical sites, to confer and annotate images in real time without altering the original data. Medical experts can use this functionality to review the same medical images or radiological reports and conduct discussions in real-time. The Collaborative Module component uses the same drawing tools from the Viewer component's Tools

module. The drawings of rectangles, freehand shapes, arrows, or measurement rulers are overlaid upon the images and subsequently displayed on the display screens of all participants in a discussion session.

The Collaborative Module component also provides an alternative way to import medical images from external sources, rather than local DICOM files which can be accessed via the Browse and Import component itself. It downloads medical images from the collaborative server.

Currently this image download feature is designed to only support the collaborative annotation feature, with a single medical image downloadable per instance. There are two sub-components designed to support the collaboration functionality: the Queue Manager and the Socket Communication. The Queue Manager is designed to handle multi-user annotation by queuing up the process of annotations to avoid loss of information due to multiple users annotating at the same time. The Queue Manager module is also implemented in the Collaborative Server to serve multiple mobile users. Next, the Socket Communication module implements a standard socket based function in Android to connect to a Java socket running on the server side.

To offer seamless collaborative annotation functionality, the Collaborative Module relies upon a stable Client-Server based implementation. For this, two mechanisms were designed in the Queue manager module, namely; the circular token passing mechanism and hash polling mechanism. These two mechanisms are designed to enable multiple users to effectively conduct virtual meetings and annotate images in turn. Annotations are transferred independently of the images and are recombined later to avoid bandwidth issues. To enhance usability and reliability of annotating on relatively small screened mobile devices, an image scaling module was designed for precise annotation. This is to ensure that regardless of the screen size and resolution, annotations drawn will appear in the same precise location and shape for all participants in a session. Via this functionality, users will be able to annotate even a small region of interest within the medical image using only their fingertips. It will also enable the annotation to be shared precisely with other users, regardless of what device they are using.

3.5.2 Medical Image Data Management System

The HMS application is designed to make available the prescriptions and health records, medical image records (like scanned images etc.) of patients, on their Android powered mobile phones. The health records are stored and managed in the cloud OS. The records are transferred from the cloud to the mobile device, where it is displayed. EyeOS is the cloud platform used to build this application. This cloud OS can be easily downloaded for free. Since Android powered mobile devices are available in the market at affordable rates, they can be easily used in such healthcare applications. Several authors have already presented ideas of mobile platforms for information exchange (like text and images) over internet. The MADIP system is a distributed information platform allowing wide-area health information exchange based on mobile agents. But most of them are based on expensive and inflexible communication methods

that require the installation of software and hardware components. These issues are solved using the cloud computing concept, as there is no need for extra storage and computation medium. The information that resides in the cloud is managed by the hospital management staff and the doctors (for uploading prescriptions and medical image records). The Android OS supports the connection to the Cloud OS that allows the patient to retrieve, modify, manage and upload medical images and text data using the internet services and REST API concepts like HTTP URLs. The image support is provided by DICOM protocol and the pixel data of images are compressed by the JPEG standard. The progressive coding allows the user to decode large image files at different resolution levels optimizing network resources and allowing image acquisition even in cases network availability is limited. The code for performing wavelet decoding on mobile devices in has been modified to support the JPEG2000 standard on the Android platform. Image annotation is also supported, using the multi-touch functions of the Android OS (Somasundaram, Gitanjali, Govardhani, Priya, & Sivakumar, 2011). The system architecture of the implementation is shown in Figure 9.

The entire process works as follows:

1. The client at the mobile end opens the cloud application as either patient or doctor and is authenticated by the cloud end.
2. The client enters his/her profile details by registering first, and then logging in. The username is the corresponding 'id' and password is the one set by him/her in the cloud server.
3. Then the Patient id is required to "search" for the records under that id. Then the particulars, diagnosis details and medical images are viewed by selecting the same via the checkbox.
4. When the user requests for an operation in the mobile end, the request is sent via Rest API like HTTP URL to the cloud OS.

Figure 9. Medical image data management system architecture

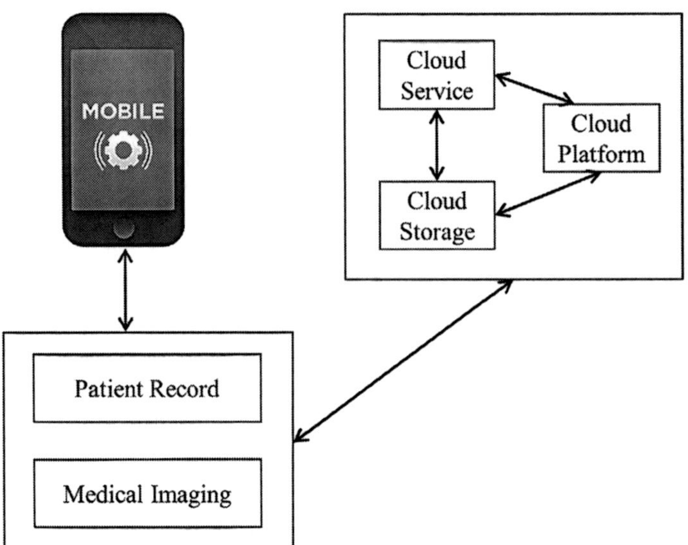

5. The cloud OS responds by sending the requested information by searching in the database and sending them back to client.
6. The mobile application checks whether there are any files that were received and are waiting to be downloaded, and will download them and make them viewable to the client.

3.5.3 Discussion

In summary, different cloud-based medical applications and systems are being investigated. As seen above, some systems are designed to maximize the benefits of treatment, while others to assist patients in managing their own care. Yet, the benefits of mobile and cloud computing are not yet interactively used by governments when implementing their e-health solutions.

The healthcare industry is a prominent user of mobile cloud computing. The industry had developed applications which allow patients and doctors access to information anywhere at any time, the ability to monitor patients remotely and enhance emergency response. Due to the sensitive nature of health information, mobile cloud computing for the healthcare industry faces many challenges such as data storage, heterogeneous resources, and last but not least, security (Ahuja & Rolli, 2012).

Nevertheless, mobile cloud computing is being identified as one of the "key factors contributing to better health care for the society." Mobile cloud computing utilized in fields like the healthcare industry offer improved efficiency and improved quality.

4. OPEN RESEARCH ISSUES

The emergence of cloud computing leads to new developments for diverse application domains. This is particularly true for healthcare with its tremendous importance in today's society, thus making it worth to investigate the relevant perspectives and insights. Healthcare, as with any other service operation, has been impacted by the cloud computing phenomenon with the literature reporting both benefits and challenges of cloud computing in the area. However, despite the significant advantages for the utilization of cloud computing as part of Healthcare IT, security and privacy, reliability, integration and data portability are some of the significant challenges and barriers to implementation that are responsible for its slow adoption.

4.1 Privacy and Security

Healthcare data has stringent requirements for security, confidentiality, availability to authorized users, traceability of access, reversibility of data, and long-term preservation. Hence, cloud vendors need to account for all these while conforming to government and industry regulations. Problems in making IT systems interoperable have delayed cloud computing growth in the health care industry.

Data maintained in a cloud may contain personal, private or confidential information; such as healthcare related information that requires the proper safeguards to prevent disclosure, compromise or misuse. Globally, concerns related to data jurisdiction, security, privacy and compliance are impacting adoption by healthcare organizations.

Data leaving a mobile device onto a commercial 3G or 4G network is typically the responsibility of the network operator to ensure that the data is securely transported. All major domestic carriers have developed encryption measures designed to safeguard data flowing through their cellular networks. Without proper data encryption methods in place, sensitive data may be passed through non-secure networks such as the Internet or transmitted through an open Wi-Fi hot spot.

Medical devices also pose potential privacy risks. As medical devices and sensors become more sophisticated, they may allow for not only external monitoring and data gathering for storage in a Big Data cloud but for their control as well. Improper controls or management of these patient medical devices may compromise patient information, or provide a mechanism for inappropriate access to or tampering of the device itself.

Another critical component is the process of correctly identifying and authenticating users along with a comprehensive authorized privilege and role-based access control. Passwords or other safeguards are necessary to confirm the identity of all those seeking to access information. Currently, varying forms of user authentication and authorization are used to provide access to cloud based capabilities with personal access information required for each system or application. This results in a potential plethora of user accounts, account IDs and passwords, which not only makes it challenging for the user but also reduces privacy and security.

Future Identity Management advances should provide for end-to-end full life-cycle capabilities, including change management, that will not only provide a single point of user authentication / authorization but a single site for user control and access to their related personally identifiable information. Additionally, such a capability should also work across all device types (PCs, cell phone, mobile computing devices and sensors) to provide a unified user-centric secure and private digital identity. Associated with user access is the necessity to track the actions or behaviors of users in audit logs to determine data usage. In order to maintain data confidentiality and data integrity, the appropriate access controls should be in place so no accidental or unauthorized disclosure of data takes place or that data does not get unintentionally or maliciously altered.

4.2 Service Reliability

From an operational standpoint, the reality is that all cloud ecosystems and enterprise infrastructures will have disruptions to some degree at some point in time. Mission critical healthcare applications must meet very high performance, availability and reliability standards. The growing reliance on distributed network-based solutions; such as Service-Oriented Architecture (SOA) web services, Cloud-based service providers and Software as a Service (SaaS) solutions, are only increasing the complexities of managing, securing and maintaining these dynamic environments. These types of services may be hosted by multiple heterogeneous, geographically distributed CSPs or in local on-premise data centers. In order to meet overall mission performance goals, the service capabilities may have their workloads shifted across the cloud ecosystem in order to optimize processing and storage resources.

Disaster recovery is a component of service reliability that focuses on processes and technology for resumption of applications, data, hardware, communications (such as networking), and other IT infrastructure in case of a disaster. The process of devising a disaster recovery plan starts with identifying and prioritizing applications, services and data, and determining for each one the amount of downtime that's acceptable before there is a significant business impact. In general, current cloud Service Level Agreements (SLAs) provide inadequate guarantees in case of a service outage due to a disaster. Most cloud SLAs provide cursory treatment of disaster recovery issues, procedures and processes.

The healthcare industry's dependence on the availability and reliability of information can be a matter of life and death. Performance is another factor that is slowing the pace at which cloud computing is adopted by healthcare organizations. Globally, hospitals, physicians and patients have different types of Internet connections that can impact performance of a healthcare system. For example, many rural healthcare facilities still use modems to connect to the Internet. Uptime and other appropriate service levels should be reviewed and included as part of the service level agreement.

4.3 Integration and Interoperability

A key component to healthcare that transcends the IT domain is the reliable exchange of commonly understood information to facilitate coordinated patient care. Different participants (e.g., surgeons, pediatricians, nurses) in the healthcare ecosystem have different terminologies and requirements. Delivering an end-to-end system that fully integrates all patient information, including emergency and in-patient care, pharmacies, billing, reimbursement and more requires standardization and interoperability. Certain standards are needed to help drive the transfer and storage of data within the cloud through common and unifying components.

Some of the risks associated with migration to the cloud include incompatibilities with the enterprise organization, strategic vision, its business or operational processes, managing a new services-based financial/billing chargeback model, dealing with the lack of transparency of off-loaded data and applications, or leveraging existing system architecture. A typical cloud computing environment consists of disparate components from multiple participants and legacy on-premise data center applications. Ultimately the legacy system infrastructure, business process improvements, financial management, and operations and maintenance; all need to be an integral part of the cloud strategy.

4.4 Data Portability

Another barrier that impacts some healthcare organizations' willingness to adopt cloud computing is the concern regarding the ability to transition to another cloud vendor or back to the healthcare organization without disrupting operations or introducing conflicting claims to the data. With traditional IT, the healthcare organization has physical control of systems, services and data. The concern is that if a provider were to suspend its services or refuse access to data, a healthcare organization may suddenly be unable to service its patients or customers. Or, if the healthcare organization were given notice that the cloud service would be discontinued, the lack of interoperability across cloud systems could make it very challenging to migrate to a new cloud service provider. This risk highlights the need for provider agreements that address termination rights, rights to access and retrieve data at any time, termination assistance in moving to another provider and cure periods to allow breach of contract to be remedied before the provider terminates or suspends services.

5. CONCLUSION

This chapter provided a comprehensive review on the Cloud-based and Mobile-based applications that have been developed in the healthcare field. The review covered different solutions related to Hospital Management, Emergency Healthcare, Healthcare Records, Social Healthcare, and Medical Imaging systems, where each solution was addressed and discussed in terms of its features, functionalities and architecture. The chapter discussed how these solutions fulfilled the healthcare requirements and even provide new services. The chapter illustrated how the emergence of both Cloud and Mobile in the healthcare field have reduce the cost overhead, increase the storage capability, keep high level of automation, provide mobility, and eliminate technical administrative burden. The chapter had discussed some open research issues that need to be addressed in this field.

REFERENCES

Ahuja, S., & Rolli, A. (2012, June). Exploring the convergence of mobile computing with cloud computing. *Journal of Network and Communication Technologies, 1*(1).

Botts, N., Thoms, B., Noamani, A., & Horan, T. (2010). Cloud computing architectures for the underserved: Public health cyberinfrastructures through a network of HealthATMs. In *Proceedings of 43rd Hawaii Int. Conf. on System Sciences (HICSS)* (pp. 1-10). IEEE. doi:10.1109/HICSS.2010.107

Doukas, C., Pliakas, T., & Maglogiannis, I. (2010). Mobile healthcare information management utilizing cloud computing and Android OS. In *Proceedings of 32nd Annual International Conference of the IEEE Engineering in Medicine and Biology Society (EMBC)*. Buenos Aires, Argentina: IEEE.

Drnasin, I., & Grgic, M. (2010). The use of mobile phones in radiology. *ELMAR, 2010*, 17–21.

Hung, S., Shih, C., Shieh, J., Lee, C., & Huang, Y. (2011). An online migration environment for executing mobile applications on the cloud. In *Proceedings of 2011 5th International Conference on Innovative Mobile and Internet Services in Ubiquitous Computing*. Seoul, Korea: Academic Press.

Kohn, L., Corrigan, J., & Donaldson, S. (1999). *To err is human: Building a safer health system.* Washington, DC: National Academy Press.

Kopec, D., Kabir, M., Reinharth, D., & Rothschild, O. (2003, August). Human errors in medical practice: Systematic classification and reduction with automated information systems. *Journal of Medical Systems, 27*(4), 297–313. doi:10.1023/A:1023796918654 PMID:12846462

Koufi, V., Malamateniou, F., & Vassilacopoulos, G. (2010). Ubiquitous access to cloud emergency medical services. In *Proceedings of 10th IEEE Int. Conf. on Information Technology and Applications in Biomedicine (ITAB)* (pp. 1-4). Corfu, Greece: IEEE. doi:10.1109/ITAB.2010.5687702

Mell, P., & Grance, T. (2009). *Draft NIST working definition of cloud computing - v15.* National Institutes of Standard and Technology, Information Technology Laboratory.

Mohammed, S., Servos, D., & Fiaidhi, J. (2010). HCX: A distributed OSGi based web interaction system for sharing health records in the cloud. In *Proceedings of IEEE/WIC/ACM Int. Conf. on Web Intelligence and Intelligent Agent Technology (WI-IAT)* (pp. 102-107). Toronto, Canada: IEEE. doi:10.1109/WI-IAT.2010.26

Organization of Economics Co-Operation and Development. (2013). Retrieved from http://www.oecd.org/

Padhy, R., Patra, M., & Chan, S. (2012). Design and implementation of a cloud based rural healthcare information system mode. *UNIASCIT, 2*(1), 149–157.

Pasha, M., Supramaniam, S., Liang, K., Amran, M., Chandra, B., & Rajeswari, M. (2012, January). An Android-based mobile medical image viewer and collaborative annotation: Development issues and challenges. *International Journal of Digital Content Technology and its Applications, 6*(1).

Poulymenopoulou, M., Malamateniou, F., & Vassilacopoulos, G. (2003). Emergency healthcare process automation using workflow technology and web services. *Med Inform Internet, 28*(3), 195–207. doi:10.1080/14639230310001617841 PMID:14612307

Somasundaram, M., Gitanjali, S., Govardhani, T., Priya, G., & Sivakumar, R. (2011). Medical image data management system in mobile cloud computing environment. In *Proceedings of International Conference on Signal, Image Processing and Applications (ICSIPA 2011)*. Kuala Lumpur, Malaysia: Academic Press.

Ujjwal, A., Manglani, B., Akarte, D., & Jain, A. (2012, March-April). Healthbook – Ubiquitous solution for heath services. *International Journal of Engineering Research and Applications, 2*(2), 965–967.

Vanitha, T., Narasimha Murthy, M., & Chaitra, B. (2013). E-healthcare billing and record management information system using Android with Cloud. *IOSR Journal of Computer Engineering, 11*(4), 13-19.

Varshney, U. (2007, March). Pervasive healthcare and wireless health monitoring. *Journal on Mobile Networks and Applications, 12*(2-3), 113–127. doi:10.1007/s11036-007-0017-1

Vinutha, S., Raju, C., & Siddappa, M. (2012, July). Development of electronic hospital management system utilizing cloud computing and Android OS using VPN connections. *International Journal of Scientific & Technology Research, 1*(6), 59–61.

Vlahu-Gjorgievska, E., & Trajkovik, V. (2011). Personal healthcare system model using collaborative filtering techniques. *Advances in Information Sciences and Service Sciences, 3*(3), 64–74. doi:10.4156/aiss.vol3.issue3.9

Wan, J., Zou, C., Ullah, S., Lai, C., Zhou, M., & Wang, X. (2013, September-October). Cloud-enabled wireless body area networks for pervasive healthcare. *IEEE Transactions on Network, 27*(5).

Wang, X., et al. (2013, February). AMES-cloud: A framework of adaptive mobile video streaming and efficient social video sharing in the clouds. *IEEE Trans. Multimedia, 10*(1109).

Wooten, R., Klink, R., Sinek, F., Bai, Y., & Shar, M. (2012). Design and implementation of a secure healthcare social cloud system. In *Proceedings of 12th IEEE/ACM Int. Symp. Cluster, Cloud and Grid Computing (CCGRID 2012)* (pp. 805-810). Ottawa, Canada: IEEE/ACM. doi:10.1109/CCGrid.2012.131

Zhou, Y., Liu, X., Xue, L., Liang, X., & Liang, S. (2010). Business process centric platform-as-a-service model and technologies for cloud enabled industry solutions. In *Proceedings of 3rd International Conference on Cloud Computing* (pp. 534-537). Miami,FL: Academic Press. doi:10.1109/CLOUD.2010.52

KEY TERMS AND DEFINITIONS

Cloud Computing: A market-oriented distributed computing paradigm consisting of a collection of inter-connected and virtualized computers that are dynamically provisioned and presented as one or more unified computing resources based on service-level agreements established through negotiation between the service provider and consumers.

Cloud: A large pool of easily usable and accessible virtualized resources (such as hardware, development platforms and/or services). These resources can be dynamically reconfigured to optimum resource utilization. This pool of resources is typically exploited by a pay-per-user model in which guarantees are offered by the Infrastructure Provider by means of customized SLA's.

eHealth: A relatively recent term for healthcare practice supported by electronic processes and communication, dating back to at least 1999. Usage of the term varies: some would argue it is interchangeable with health informatics with a broad definition covering electronic/digital processes in health while others use it in the narrower sense of healthcare practice using the Internet.

Emergency Medical Services: A type of emergency service dedicated to providing out-of-hospital acute medical care, transport to definitive care, and other medical transport to patients with illnesses and injuries which prevent the patient from transporting themselves.

Healthcare System: The organization of people, institutions, and resources to deliver health care services to meet the health needs of target populations.

Hospital Information System: A comprehensive, integrated information system designed to manage all the aspects of a hospital operation, such as medical, administrative, financial, legal and the corresponding service processing.

Hybrid Cloud: A Cloud Computing environment in which an organization provides and manages some resources in-house and has others provided externally.

Infrastructure-as-a-Service (IaaS): A provision model in which an organization outsources the equipment used to support operations, including storage, hardware, servers and networking components, where the service provider owns the equipment and is responsible for housing, running and maintaining it and the client typically pays on a per-use basis.

Medical Imaging: The technique and process used to create images of the human body (or parts and function thereof) for clinical purposes (medical procedures seeking to reveal, diagnose, or examine disease) or medical science (including the study of normal anatomy and physiology).

mHealth: A term used for the practice of medicine and public health, supported by mobile devices. The mHealth field has emerged as a sub-segment of eHealth, the use of information and communication technology (ICT); such as computers, mobile phones, communications satellite, patient monitors; for health services and information. mHealth applications include the use of mobile devices in collecting community and clinical health data, delivery of healthcare information to practitioners, researchers, and patients, real-time monitoring of patient vital signs, and direct provision of care (via mobile telemedicine).

Mobile Cloud Computing (MCC): The state-of-the-art mobile distributed computing paradigm comprises three heterogeneous domains of mobile computing, cloud computing, and wireless networks aiming to enhance computational capabilities of resource-constrained mobile devices towards rich user experience.

Private Cloud: A marketing term for a proprietary computing architecture that provides hosted services to a limited number of people behind a firewall.

Public Cloud: One based on the standard Cloud Computing model, in which a service provider makes resources, such as applications and storage, available to the general public over the Internet. Public Cloud services may be free or offered on a pay-per-usage model.

Software-as-a-Service (SaaS): A software distribution model in which applications are hosted by a vendor or service provider and made available to customers over a network, typically the Internet.

This work was previously published in Emerging Research in Cloud Distributed Computing Systems edited by Susmit Bagchi, pages 315-338 copyright year 2015 by Information Science Reference (an imprint of IGI Global).

Chapter 88

Coalitions:
The Future of Healthcare in Public Private Partnerships

Erinn N. Harris
Baltimore City Fire Department, USA

ABSTRACT

Demands in healthcare have placed a strain on healthcare providers trying to provide quality care while maintaining accreditations and planning for the possibility of expansion of resources as well as patients. Public Private Partnerships (PPPs) have been used to help ease this strain and increase the capabilities of healthcare systems all over the country. In an effort to "level the playing field," the federal government has recently decided to mandate the structure of these healthcare PPPs. That is, a new form of these partnerships (i.e. coalitions) has been designated the organizational model that healthcare PPPs must evolve into in order to receive certain types of federal grants. This chapter discusses these coalitions as well as challenges for PPPs that are just now in the process of forming. Also discussed is the increased effort required to form coalitions from PPPs that have already been in existence for any length of time.

INTRODUCTION

Public private partnerships have existed in the United States for hundreds of years (Cellucci, 2010) and have been used for endless types of projects branching from infrastructure to housing to tourism. Another area that has had high use of public private partnerships is healthcare. With the Baby Boomer Generation putting more demand on the healthcare industry in the form of number of physicians, medications and treatments to new healthcare legislation, the price of healthcare is steadily increasing. This cost increase is not only affecting the people requiring these services, but it is also increasing the cost of doing business within the healthcare industry itself. The American Heart Association estimates that by the year 2030, the number of people over the age of 65 will have doubled, increasing the number to more than 70 million Americans. Of all these people, more than one out of every six baby boomers will be managing more than one chronic condition. That is an estimated 37 million Americans. For all populations, the American Heart Association predicts that the number of physician's visits will double by the year 2030. This is slightly over 1.3 trillion visits to a doctor.

DOI: 10.4018/978-1-4666-8756-1.ch088

Hospitals, emergency medical service providers and health departments are all struggling to find funds for continuing to provide the best and latest services as quickly and safely as possible. These costs come from several areas. For patient related costs, there is diagnostic testing such as x-rays, blood work, specimen collection, etc. Treatment costs include not only the people needed for the procedure, but the equipment and supplies also needed. Overhead is included in the form of bed a patient needs (admitted into a specialty area, kept in the ER, bariatric beds) and for how long they need to occupy that space. Not only are there costs of helping to physically repair the patient, but there are mental care issues as well. Was the patient injured in an isolated incident, or do they need to talk to social services? Do they need to enter a detox program for drugs or alcohol? Are there ongoing care issues where the patient would not be able to return home but needs to be evaluated for entry into a rehabilitation facility? While admission into a hospital was mentioned, most if not all of the issues that were listed can be handled within the Emergency Department of a hospital. The Center for Medicare and Medicaid released a statement in the Federal Register in 2002 that at least half of all emergency services go uncompensated.

Patient costs are not the only costs generated by the hospital. There are also the costs of becoming accredited to provide as many services as they are able. The process for becoming recognized as a cardiac catheter center, a primary stroke center, a trauma center, or even a location that pre-hospital services can consult with a physician at is a long one that has many loopholes to jump through. This means that aside from treatments, hospitals for example must also have a required number of training hours, assemble different types of response plans and be integrated with other aspects of the community in which they are located (for example the local health department). All of these things cost money. So the healthcare industry has turned to public private partnerships to try and offset any direct costs they might incur. One can see this in the number of hospital conglomerations that have been increasing in the past 5 years. Take for example MedStar Health in the Baltimore/Washington DC area. It consists of 10 hospitals, and has its own research institute and medical education program through Georgetown University. (MedStar Health, 2014) MedStar Health generates 4.2 billion dollars annually and in 2013 listed a total of 551,292 emergency room visits in their hospitals. It is proving to be much easier to expand and generate money with a group of healthcare entities, who each can focus on a small group of specialties, than a single hospital trying to offer everything itself. While this type of public private partnership has proven to be beneficial, within the past five years there has been an attempt by government agencies to modify these partnerships into a mold so that they are all operating under the same rules and guidelines. MedStar Health is a non-profit organization. (MedStar Health, 2014) While there are certain advantages to being labeled this way and they have listed sizeable yearly revenue, what was not accounted for was how much of the revenue goes into the training, maintenance of current facilities and expansion projects that MedStar is undertaking. Billing for their services alone would not bring in enough to cover all of this organization's expenses. For this reason, most hospitals also need assistance from the government in the form of grants. The main supplier of these grants on the federal level is the Department of Health and Human Services (DHHS). Since there are so many forms hospitals and their partnerships can assume, it is difficult for DHHS to designate appropriate amounts of funds annually so that everyone has what they need. It is for this reason that DHHS is guiding healthcare public private partnerships to reorganize themselves into "coalitions." If public private partnerships would like to receive the same funding they have been getting in the future, or really any type of funding at all, then they need to transform into "coalitions" and operate under certain regulations.

This chapter focuses on what healthcare public private partnerships are being transitioned into, the reasons behind the change, and gives the specific example of how one public private partnership in Baltimore, Maryland is attempting to make this change. Discussed will be the history of how this public private partnership was operating before the change, the mindset of the partnership during the change, and the challenges observed as this partnership attempts to make the necessary changes to stay in existence.

BACKGROUND

Region III Health and Medical Taskforce

In Maryland, the Maryland Institute for Emergency Medical Services Systems (MIEMSS) oversees coordination of statewide emergency medical service assets. (MIEMSS, n.d.) This includes assets such as infrastructure, communications, research, training and oversight needed for all aspects of patients needing emergency healthcare services. In terms of emergency healthcare, this would include everything from pre-hospital care (public and private transport units) through treatment and also incorporates rehabilitation services if necessary. For the state of Maryland alone, there are 631 public transportation units. (MIEMSS, n.d.) This includes ambulances, medic units and ambo buses that are "in-service" and ready to receive 911 calls at any time. There are just over 400 private transport units not including those labeled as neonatal. Forty eight hospitals in the state have emergency departments that can handle calls 24 hours a day. (MIEMSS, n.d.)

MIEMSS is an independent state agency, governed by an 11-member EMS Board appointed by the Governor. (MIEMSS, n.d.) MIEMSS has worked to formalize, through statute and regulation, the administration, regulation and operation of the statewide EMS system. In an attempt to stay within the National incident Management System's definition of span of control, the state has been divided into five regions, each having their own director and chain of command. Baltimore and its surrounding counties comprise Region III. Region III by itself includes 21 hospitals, 7 counties and their respective health departments and emergency medical services. The counties include: Baltimore City, Baltimore County, Harford County, Carroll County, Howard County, Anne Arundel County and Annapolis. Hospitals include:

- Anne Arundel Medical Center
- Baltimore Washington Medical Center
- Bon Secours Hospital
- Carroll Hospital Center
- Franklin Square Hospital
- Good Samaritan Hospital
- Greater Baltimore Medical Center
- Harbor Hospital
- Harford Memorial Hospital
- Howard County General Hospital
- Johns Hopkins Bayview Medical Center
- Johns Hopkins Hospital (Adult ED)
- Johns Hopkins Hospital (Pediatric ED)
- Maryland General Hospital
- Mercy Medical Center
- Mount Washington Pediatric Hospital
- Northwest Hospital
- R Adams Cowley Shock Trauma Center
- Sinai Hospital of Baltimore
- St. Agnes Hospital
- St. Joseph Medical Center
- Union Memorial Hospital
- University of Maryland Medical Center
- Upper Chesapeake Medical Center (MIEMSS, n.d.)

Each region monitors and advocates for their area. In the event of large scale incidents, the officers of the Regional Office would be expected to help coordinate their resources and be the first State representative on scene if needed.

In terms of large scale healthcare related incidents, we have so far covered the local entities that would be covered as well as the state. In terms of federal assistance, one of the representatives that one would expect to see in the case of an incident in the Baltimore/DC area would be a member of the local Urban Area Security Initiative.

The Urban Area Security Initiative (UASI) is formed through the Department of Homeland Security. Its purpose is to address the unique planning, organization, equipment, training, and exercise needs of high-threat, high-density urban areas, and assists them in building an enhanced and sustainable capacity to prevent, protect against, mitigate, respond to, and recover from acts of terrorism. (FEMA, 2014) The concept of the UASI was initially created in 2003 through the Homeland Security Grant Program (HSGP). HSGP gave funds out to locations for preparation for attacks and other hazards. In 2010, the Department of Homeland Security allocated over 500 million dollars to the different UASIs in the nation. (FEMA, 2014) State agencies are the only ones who are allowed to apply for these grants. In the case of the Baltimore UASI group, the Mayor's Office of Emergency Management is the lead agency submitting applications for the program.

In 2010, there were a total of 64 UASI groups in the United States. (FEMA, 2014) By 2013 that number had decreased to 25 areas eligible for funding. "Eligible candidates for the FY 2013 UASI program were determined through an analysis of relative risk of terrorism faced by the 100 most populous metropolitan statistical areas in the United States, in accordance with the 9/11 Act." (FEMA, 2014) Baltimore is the core city of the federally designated Baltimore Urban Area Security Initiative, which is comprised of the cities of Baltimore and Annapolis and the counties of Anne Arundel, Baltimore, Carroll, Harford, and Howard. (MOEM, n.d.) As one can see, the Baltimore UASI and Region III defined by MIEMSS encompass the same stakeholders.

In 2006, the UASI created what was called the Region III Health and Medical Task Force to coordinate regional healthcare resources attached to the UASI. The taskforce was asked to focus on the healthcare projects that were to be funded by UASI grant money. The taskforce included all entities from MIEMSS Region III as well as representation from Baltimore City's Mayor's Office of Emergency Management (MOEM), The Department of Health and Mental Hygiene (DHMH), and Maryland Institute for Emergency Medical Services Systems (MIEMSS). Standing members include representatives from the following hospitals:

- Anne Arundel Medical Center,
- Baltimore Washington Medical Center,
- Bon Secours Baltimore Health System,
- Carroll Hospital Center,
- MedStar Franklin Square Medical Center,
- MedStar Good Samaritan Hospital,
- Greater Baltimore Medical Center,
- MedStar Harbor Hospital,
- Harford Memorial Hospital,
- Johns Hopkins Bayview Medical Center,
- The Johns Hopkins Hospital and Health System,
- Howard County General Hospital,
- Kennedy Krieger Institute,
- Kernan Orthopedics and Rehabilitation Hospital,
- Maryland General Hospital,
- Mercy Medical Center,
- Mt. Washington Pediatric Hospital,
- Northwest Hospital,
- Sinai Hospital,
- St. Agnes Hospital,
- St. Joseph Medical Center,
- Sheppard Pratt Hospital,
- MedStar Union Memorial Hospital,
- University of Maryland Medical Center,
- Upper Chesapeake Medical Center. (MIEMSS, n.d.)

The Taskforce is led by a chairperson that is nominated and elected annually by the group. They also have several subcommittees which are formed to work on individual projects. They meet monthly and the meeting place rotates through the different member's hospitals.

From 2006 to present the Taskforce has used the funding to accomplish several projects. They have created an electronic patient tracking system which can start from the time 911 arrives at the patient's side through to when they are discharged from the hospital. "In addition to family reunification, such a system was also necessary for law enforcement to locate individuals during an investigation and for public health officials to document patients who were in direct contact with an infected individual, as well as track clients and medications at the points of distribution." (Maloney, 2012) This system has been tested in several large events held in the state including Sailabration. This event was held in Baltimore City in 2012 celebrating the 200th anniversary of the War of 1812. "The weeklong event celebrating the bicentennial of the War of 1812 drew more than a million Marylanders from across the state, almost half a million out-of-state tourists and $166 million for the local economy." (WJZ, 2012)

The funds have also been used for surge capacity planning as well as an alternate care site (ACS). There were no standard interagency SOP's within metro Baltimore to pre-identify staff, hospital beds, or other resources that can be deployed following a catastrophic event. The establishment of an alternate care site (ACS) post disaster would be ad hoc and undersupplied. Standard operating procedures were developed so that all partners would be operating under the same system. In addition, common equipment was purchased and partners were all trained to be able to use the same devices so that there would be a more streamlined response in the event of an incident. This location can serve as a medical facility if required, but also acts as a warehouse that can ship out supplies to the hospitals that need them

in the case of a surge event. To date, this capability has not had to be utilized. "Work surrounding the ACS continues. Current objectives include arrangement of pre-designation and pre-approval of the facility as an ACS by the Maryland Office of Health Care Quality, development of MOUs with public and private partners for critical elements of site operation such as security and mortuary services, and development of protocols for triggering direct EMS transport during a public health emergency. DHS grant funds continue to support the development of additional ACS sites, as well as sustainment and environmental maintenance of existing facilities. A loss of funds could result in the loss, or deterioration, of this regional institution that has demonstrated to close a capability gap." (Maloney, 2012)

The taskforce has been able to add two "ambo buses" to their resource list as well as complete several evacuation drills of large hospitals in the region, one of which was Johns Hopkins Hospital. In addition to these completed projects, the taskforce has a list of 30 projects that have been started or are awaiting funds to be able to accomplish. Projects range from training and exercises to planning and policy, response and support and advocacy.

Hospital Preparedness Program

The Region III Health and Medical Taskforce was also put in charge of the spending of Hospital Preparedness Program (HPP) funds. The Hospital Preparedness Program (HPP) is a cooperative agreement program created by the Department of Health and Human Services (HHS). HHS uses this program to distribute funding to the states for hospital preparedness. The national budget allotted for HPP finds in FY12 was just over 315 million dollars. Fiscal year 2013 saw a budget of 331 million dollars which is in direct contrast to the money available under UASI funds. (HHS, 2013) In 2011, Baltimore UASI was granted 7.8 million dollars. For FY12 it was announced that budget cuts were causing grant moneys to be reduced by 40-50% nationally. This corresponded with the 4.1 million dollars granted to the Baltimore UASI in 2012. (Maloney, 2012)

The purpose of the HPP is to use grant funding to increase preparedness for all hazards, to be able to handle increase surge capacity, to be able to track the availability of beds and other resources electronically as well as develop communication systems that are inoperable with other response partners. (HHS, 2009a) It was decided that the states needed to be better aligned with Federal preparedness grant programs, specifically, that the states needed broader, more community based healthcare preparedness approaches including the building and strengthening of healthcare coalitions. (HHS, 2009a) "Partnerships and coalitions unify the management capability of the healthcare system and provide support both when normal day–to-day operations of the health system are distressed, as well as when the system is overwhelmed, and disaster operations become necessary." (HHS, 2009a)

In 2006, HPP was transferred over to the Assistant Secretary for Preparedness and Response (ASPR). ASPR is considered the lead for all matters related to public health and response to public health emergencies. (HHS, 2009a). They serve as the single point of contact for coordination and integration for all public health and medical preparedness programs with medical response programs and activities for the federal government. (HHS, 2009a) Health and Homeland Security is the lead agency for emergency support function 8 (ESF-8) and they use HPP to help grantees address gaps in healthcare preparedness in order to augment damaged or overwhelmed local medical systems in health emergencies. (HHS, 2009a) HHS feels that the best way to achieve these goals is through the formation and the use of coalitions. Coalitions strengthen efforts of the jurisdiction by providing a single functional entity that will unify management capability and provide support. (HHS, 2009a)

While HHS provides the funding and sets the priorities, the funding is not given to the jurisdictions or local medical systems. The money is given to the state who then in turn will distribute it as they see fit. In Maryland, the agency controlling distribution of these funds is the Department of Health and Mental Hygiene (DHMH). DHMD reports their goals as the following:

- Medical surge planning
- Interoperable communications equipment
- Conducting drills and exercises

DEFINING THE NEW PUBLIC PRIVATE PARTNERSHIP

In order to form a coalition, one must understand what constitutes a coalition. ASPR defines coalition as a formal collaboration among healthcare organizations and public and private sector partners that is organized to prepare for and respond to an emergency, mass casualty or catastrophic health event. (ASPR, 2014)

It includes (HHS, 2009a):

- Hospitals,
- Skilled nursing facilities,
- Nursing homes,
- Hospices,
- Community health centers,
- Home care,
- Physician and other ambulatory care providers,
- Specialty services like
- Dialysis centers,
- Poison control centers, and
- Emergency medical services

All of these services under their normal operational guidelines might compete with one another for business. This competition, promotes lack of information sharing, poor resource sharing and lack of common operating procedures and equipment utilized during an incident. By joining all of these entities into a public private partnership, referred to as a coalition, individual capabilities are unified during events when resources are stressed. "To overcome the day-to-day business competition that exists between healthcare organizations, the Coalition must promote open and fair representation for all its members. At the same time, the Coalition must respect the management sovereignty of each organization during incident response and recovery, as well as the inherent governmental authority of Emergency Management, Public Health, Emergency Medical Services, and other relevant public agencies." (HHS, 2009b)

Coalition duties include:

- In order to respond to a disaster:
  - Planning
  - Organizing
  - Equipping
  - Training
- During response:
  - Provide multiagency coordination
  - Advice on decisions made by incident management
  - Information sharing
  - Resource coordination

The measurement criteria for funding were established under two headings: medical surge and continuity of healthcare operations. (ASPR, 2014) Medical surge as defined by the Department of Health and Human Services is "the ability to evaluate and care for a markedly increased volume of patients–one that challenges or exceeds normal operating capacity. The surge requirements may extend beyond direct patient care to include such tasks as extensive laboratory studies or epidemiological investigations." (HHS, 2009a) This would be what healthcare coalitions face during the incident itself or just immediately after. Continuity of healthcare operations would be during the recovery phase of an incident and how these healthcare organizations can maintain

their normal day to day operation in light of events like medical surge. Each of the two categories had seven indicators. The current status of each of these indicators was to be reported by either the awardee (a single healthcare entity) or a healthcare coalition (HCC). In addition to the fourteen indicators, there were also nineteen developmental assessment factors. In the big picture, out of thirty three reporting factors, only three of the indicators were allowed to be reported on by an awardee. The rest were only to be reported on by an HCC. This indicates how little an awardee can accomplish or hope to be given in funding without the backing of a coalition.

As a result of the new demand for healthcare public private partnerships to become "coalitions", several steps have been taken by the Region III Health and Medical Taskforce. They have acknowledged the fact that they need to change their formal structure. They have established a wish list for what they would like to be developed through the transformation to a coalition. Finally, they have hired a company to help the taskforce in their strategic planning efforts. Since hiring this company, there have been two meetings; one in the fall of 2013 and the second in the spring of 2014. The company they have hired and the results of the two meetings will be discussed in the following section.

STRATEGIC PLANNING

The company hired by the Region III Health and Medical Task Force is a nonprofit organization called the National Healthcare Coalition Resource Center (NHCRC). They were established in 2013 after the Inaugural National Healthcare Coalition Preparedness Conference held in November of 2013. (NHCRC, 2013a) The group provides technical assistance to emerging and established coalitions. (NHCRC, 2013a) They were formed by members of three other existing coalitions. The first is the North Virginia Hospital Alliance.

NVHA was formed in October of 2002 and is comprised of 14 hospitals, and 6 free standing emergency departments. (Hanfling, 2013) NVHA was an offshoot of Northern Virginia Emergency Response Coalition (NVERC) because hospitals needed a different approach than the health department, law enforcement, fire department and emergency medical services during an incident. (Hanfling, 2013) NVHA states that they are a planning and response agency with a focus on real time information sharing. (NVHA, 2014)

The second entity of NHCRC is Managed Emergency Surge for Healthcare (MESH) in Indianapolis. They were formed in 2007 and include not just hospitals but healthcare facilities. (MESH, 2010) They state that they provide education and training, healthcare intelligence, preparedness and planning, and policy analysis services to healthcare agencies, government agencies and non-government organizations. (MESH, 2010)

Finally, the third member of NHCRC is the Northwest Healthcare Response Center (NWHRC). They were created in 2012 by a merging of King County and Pierce County Coalitions, both located in Washington State. (NWHRC, 2013) King County alone brought 20+ hospitals and medical group leaders to the NHRCR. (NWHRC, 2013)

Fall 2013

The initial meeting held between the NHCRC and the Region III Health and Medical Taskforce was held in October of 2013. Prior to the meeting through the use of surveys to individual members, NHCRC asked the taskforce what they though the coalition should look like when it was finished. (NHCRC, 2013b) The three to five year goals of the taskforce were found to be:

- Become a fiduciary agent
- Establish a regional emergency equipment and supply inventory plan
- Increase engagement from the non-hospital sector
- Establish response capabilities
- Hire staff

In terms of fiduciary agent, NHCRC recommended the taskforce to look at the following governance models:

- 509(a)3: Supporting Organizations
- 501(c)6: Business League/Trade Organizations
- 501(c)3: Nonprofit
- Private Embed
- Public Embed

In response to the requirement to become a coalition, the taskforce must do more than simply change its name on funding applications. This public private partnership needs to be a formal collaboration between individual healthcare organizations. Part of this would be to draw up a legal and ethical agreement that all individual entities agree upon and that establishes the fact that the coalition can act on behalf of these entities during certain times. What decisions and power of authority the coalition is granted needs to be spelled out as well as when this authority is granted and when the authority comes to an end. Different models exist in the business world and as a group the taskforce needs to decide which model best fits what the coalition wants to become and what the coalition will be doing in the future (planning, response, recovery, information sharing, resource sharing, mutual aid, etc.).

In terms of increasing engagement from the non-hospital sector, the following additional entities were listed by the taskforce:

- Long term care facilities
- Mental health providers
- Federally qualified health centers
- Medical and pharmaceutical suppliers

- Law enforcement agencies
- Faith based organizations
- Funeral and mortuary service providers
- Voluntary Organizations Active in Disasters (VOADs)
- Media
- Transportation Authorities
- Academia
- Utility Providers
- Dialysis Providers
- Private EMS
- Baltimore Metropolitan Council

It was agreed upon that the numbers of members in the coalition needs to increase substantially from what it is today. One problem discussed is the lack of knowledge in the region about the taskforce. While healthcare entities like hospitals are included, the taskforce is not restricted to this type of partner. Other organizations that do not deal directly with healthcare should still be included in this coalition.

Spring 2014

The second meeting held between NHCRC and the taskforce was in May of 2014. This workshop was used for the development of values, creation of a mission statement, a SWOT analysis was performed, a vision statement was created, and goals and objectives were created. Finally, the current project list for the taskforce was examined and projects were prioritized. While nothing was set in stone at this workshop, it enabled NHCRC to gather enough data to then try and create a strategic plan for the taskforce. This plan would be presented and edited/tailored by the taskforce for their new identity as a coalition.

There were approximately 25 people at the second meeting. Together, the entire group created a list of values for the coalition. Values were defined as items or concepts that the coalition as a whole deemed either important for the coalition to have or imperative for the coalition to obtain. The top contenders in a list of about 20 were:

- Collaborative
- Resilient
- Innovative
- Proactive
- Integrated

From there a SWOT analysis was performed on the following five factors that were chosen by NHRCR to be importance for healthcare coalitions to consider:

- External factors
- Local Healthcare Environment
- Operations
- Finances
- Marketing/Public Relations

SWOT is for an assessment of the taskforce to develop a profile for the coalition. It sets a foundation for the strategic plan to be built upon. It analyzes strengths, weaknesses, opportunities and threats. Due to the small amount of time needed to perform a SWOT analysis, it is often used to address issues that have the potential to cause the biggest impact during periods where time is of the essence. (NetMBA, 2010) It also serves as a filter to focus on key issues and should be performed by all stakeholders instead of just one or two members of upper management.

It also is a good visual tool to use when brainstorming in a group. Divide a square into four equal squares. This also produces two columns and two rows, or four quadrants total. The overall analysis is a focus on one element. An example of this would be local healthcare environment. The left column has a heading called 'helpful', or things that can be used to help achieve the objective. The right column is for things that can be considered 'harmful' to achieving the objective. The upper row is reserved for things of an 'internal origin' while the lower row is considered things that are of 'external origin'. The top left quadrant will be strengths of the element you are analyzing. The upper right is for weaknesses. The lower left quadrant is where one would list opportunities, and the lower right quadrant is reserved for threats.

For the first element, local healthcare environment, the taskforce considered strengths to be: wealth of healthcare resources, their relationship with the state, growing focus on meeting standards will entice participation in the taskforce, no geographical challenges, and structure of both private and public healthcare systems in the region. Weaknesses were listed to be: the amount of resources can be overwhelming/difficult to engage. Opportunities were seen in: collaboration with the state, developing governance structure, and an increase in joint planning among the members. Threats were listed as: competition for limited funding, any incident would impact available resources, how decisions were made (political v. analytical), competition in the region, and no response role has been defined for the taskforce. (Taskforce, 2014)

In terms of general environment, internal strengths could be considered to be increased expertise in hospital preparedness, leadership, strong history and relationships between members, the structure of the existing healthcare systems and having the members that currently exist be so involved withint he taskforce. Internal weaknesses were considered to be limited ability to make changes the taskforce recommended within their own organizations, lacking membership of certain healthcare providers within the taskforce and limited engagement with hospital executives. External opportunities were better organization through formation of a coalition, increases engagement of existing members, and increased attention by Center for Medicare and Medicaid (CMS). Although it was noted in the external threats that this increased attention might bring about unfounded mandates. (Taskforce, 2014)

In terms of operations, strengths were considered to be the communications within the taskforce, the level of competency in the healthcare systems, the ability to track patients within the healthcare system, the level of experience within the taskforce. The structure of the healthcare systems was again mentioned in this analysis as a positive. While the expertise was seen as a positive, the lack of experience of the providers during actual disasters was seen as a weakness. The professionals were also seen as having no autonomy or authority to make decisions for their respective healthcare organizations. Potential opportunities were seen as ability to increase coordination with public safety agencies and further development of the existing patient tracking system. There was discussion on choosing an organizational model that would allow for an increase in freedom and less mission creep, improved decision making once a solution has been identified and increasing ability to raise funds to help sustain the coalition. Threats were seen in competition for funding sources that were currently available, the relationship with local and state health departments and new political mandates requiring a shift in priorities. (Taskforce, 2014)

In the financial realm, opportunities definitely outweighed any other category. There was an increase in donors, engagement from hospitals as required by the Joint Commission, addition of smaller facilities to the coalition to fill in existing gaps, improvement of advocacy all around, etc. The only strength recognized was the resilience of the current healthcare system at the current time. Weaknesses were seen with limitation of reimbursement, lack of transparency for funding, and lack of infrastructure for fundraising. Threats financially took the shape of declining federal funding and the desire for healthcare systems to pay into supporting the work performed by the coalition. (Taskforce, 2014)

Finally, in the area of public relations, the only threat mentioned was competition with the North Capitol Region. Weaknesses were several: no formalized committee for this function, state wants all regions to be equal, and counties being based off the actions of other counties instead of their own actions. Strengths lie in the healthcare community's credibility, networking within the community, educational opportunities, forums, and friendly competition. Opportunities were identified as highlighting individual achievements, increasing external communications, engagement of executives during response, enhancing political relationships, and promotion of healthy competition. (Taskforce, 2014)

For the mission and vision statements, the workshop was broken into five smaller groups and each was asked to come up with their own statements for the coalition. These were then reviewed by the whole group. Parts of each were taken and reassembled to form one statement.

The mission statement was described as having to answer four questions:

- What do we do?
- How do we do it?
- For whom do we do it?
- What value are we bringing?

The mission statement needs to be relevant and should be able to identify the group with what it is saying. NHCRC described it as something that will "brand" the coalition. As a potential mission statement, the taskforce created the following:

"To lead, educate, plan and respond for all hazard preparedness though collaboration and integration with all health and medical community stakeholders in order to enhance recovery and resiliency in our communities." (Taskforce, 2014)

It was noted during the workshop that there was some difficulty in groups trying to create a mission statement as several members were still unsure of what it is that a coalition actually does. This lack of information was an area of frustration for the entirety of the workshop. It went beyond people disagreeing on where they should go in the future. There was a basic lack of knowledge into what this transition would cause this group to become. If it would mean that they could no longer work on the same projects, if they would have to do more work, or what would be expected of them from both the state and federal entities

in charge of grant money as well as if there was any hope of achieving different sources of funding were all questions repeatedly asked by different taskforce members. It was also noted that there was no one person standing up to try and answer these questions. While this taskforce has been in existence for years and these people have all worked together on projects, there was still a divided feel among the partners as to their acceptance of these changes. This will be a challenge for this taskforce to overcome in the future. The federal government is requiring the taskforce become a coalition, but that does not mean that the attitude of the individual partners within this public private partnership will suddenly become the same, or that issues these organizations have had with each other in the past will suddenly be forgotten.

The next exercise was to attempt to create a rough version of a vision statement for the coalition. A vision statement was described as something that would describe the "end-state". It is to be what this coalition sees as its perfect world. This statement should be written in clear terms but reference an abstract goal. If one is too succinct about its goal, then it is easily obtained and then the coalition would have nothing further to accomplish (for example, building a structure). However, it needs to be clear enough that people can understand what the coalition wants to accomplish. It should not be more than one or two sentences long. The five groups again created their own statements and then all five were morphed into a rough draft for consideration. The combined vision statement was as follows:

A fully integrated emergency preparedness and response network to support healthcare resilience. (Taskforce, 2014)

In the final part of the brainstorming session, goals and objectives were discussed. Goals were defined as things needed to achieve your vision statement. They should be broad, not specific. It is the objectives that should be specific. They are what are used to reach your goals. It was stated that they needed to be SMART objectives, meaning that they needed to be specific, measurable, attainable, relevant and time bound. Goals and objectives both should reflect back to what is found through a SWOT analysis. Goals for this taskforce were set to five and were determined to be:

1. Determine organizational model for a sustainable coalition
2. Increase community awareness of the coalition
3. Enhance active/engaged coalition membership
4. Enhance coalition programming to demonstrate a return on investment
5. Define the response role of the coalition

From there, each of the five groups were given one of the goals and told to make no more than five SMART objectives to try and achieve their assigned goal. Sample objectives are as follows:

1. Have a complete and approved (by taskforce, DHMD and executives) strategic plan in 8 months
2. By 7/2015 have a subcommittee of public information officers (PIOs) draft a regional public relations campaign for the coalition (to increase internal/healthcare entity awareness of the coalition)
3. Develop an internal marketing subcommittee by 7/15
4. Survey members for training needs within the next year
5. Within the next 18 months, develop and after action report to analyze defects and improve coordination within the coalition

In the last two hours of the workshop, the current list of projects was analyzed and sorted. Projects were categorized as short term or long term. It was looked to see if any of the projects could be removed from the list or if certain things were missing.

Projects were consolidated into categories such as planning and policy, training and exercise, advocacy, etc. Projects ranged from a variety of evacuation preparedness activities to decon/HAZMAT training, to outreach campaigns for the taskforce. Each of the proposed projects was then put into the categories of short term, long term and ongoing.

It was understood that at the conclusion of the workshop, NHCRC would take the information they had gathered and create a strategic plan for the taskforce.

CHALLENGES

While the people within the room seemed to work well together, several challenges were spoken of both as a whole group and in side conversations throughout the room. In general, people are wary of change. The unknown can bring about new rules, new responsibilities and new players into a situation where the existing members have grown comfortable. While change is necessary in both emergency preparedness and healthcare, it is usually met with friction which can sometimes increase to unwillingness. In the creation of timelines, people's unwillingness to change can often prevent deadlines from being met or even assigned, resulting in friction within the group as a whole.

In addition to being cautious about what will change overall with the transition of the taskforce into a coalition, there is the fear that more work will be expected of each and every individual member. There is not a single member of the Region III Health and Medical Taskforce that can say their only job is to help out on the taskforce. Most of the time, emergency planners for a healthcare entity are also healthcare providers or administrative staff already working within that organization, health department, or jurisdiction. It may have been a voluntary decision to take on the added responsibility, or it may have been required of that person due to their training or experience. Regardless, each member has other time restraints in their schedule that would prevent them from assuming additional responsibilities. So how then could it be expected that they do more than they already are?

While it was a common goal that the taskforce as a coalition would like to add response to their capabilities, many people questioned how they could make this possible. In the event of an emergency, as the members do have multiple responsibilities, in the event of an incident they would be expected to stay on location at their organization. How would these people be able to leave and meet the rest of the taskforce to respond on the regional level at the same time?

Another concern was support from the state level. The grant funding from federal levels is given to the state to distribute how they see fit. Maryland has five regions. If the coalition for Region III does not have the same goals or priorities as the state, would their amount of funding be reduced and given elsewhere? If the coalition was focusing on areas that the State did not deem important, would the coalition receive the same amount of funding in future years? Also adding in the fact that the coalition intends to seek additional sources of funding, the State could be seen as seeming resistant to the taskforce changing into a coalition. If other areas of funding were not in the control of the state to distribute, they would not have the control over the activities of the coalition that they might have otherwise. People who have control are reluctant in relinquishing it. This issue was not addressed by any member of the taskforce during the workshop, but talked about among several of the smaller groups. DHMH was part of the workshop, and there were several veiled comments and sideways looks given during certain discussions as the day progressed. Since the workshop was held, DHMH has released how they will be distributing HPP funding next year. In previous years, the amount designated to each region was based on the size of the region, the number of facilities in the region and that region's population. According to a source that does not want to be named, for FY15, the state decided that each region can request up to $150,000. As this is less than it has ever been previously, it is not known whether there will be enough funding for sustainment of the taskforce, let alone development into a coalition. There does not appear to be a direct link between the development of a coalition and decrease in funding. However, the state does need to realize that failure of the taskforce to become a coalition would directly impact any future funding the state receives.

CONCLUSION

In 2006 the Region III Health and Medical Taskforce was created from the Baltimore Urban Awareness Security Initiative and MIEMSS Region III with the purpose of having subject matter experts decide what the best fit was for grant money being received for healthcare emergency preparedness. They created what is essentially a healthcare public private partnership consisting of hospitals, health departments, jurisdictions with emergency medical services, etc. In the time since then, the taskforce has accomplished several high priority projects and has amassed a list of at least 30 more. The issue is that the requirements for continuation of funding are changing.

The Federal Government through the Assistant Secretary for Preparedness and Response representing the Department of Health and Human Services has determined that the most efficient and effective way for the healthcare field to become prepared for emergencies is through the formation of healthcare coalitions. While the obvious answer is to just change the name of the group from taskforce to coalition, the Region III taskforce is taking this change and trying to make the partnership better and more capable in the process. They are analyzing their shortcomings and their gaps like lack of amount of time members are able to spend with this group to looking to increase sources of revenue and trying to plan ways of bridging what they have with where they would like to be.

This is not an easy process. There are many challenges. Trying to make a group of 25+ members agree on a single point on anything is a task in itself. Take into account people's reluctance for change and the extra work it might bring, and people's fear of losing power, progress might be much slower than anticipated. The HPP has already announced selection criteria for grants for the FY15. Coalitions will be the ones receiving the money. It is in the best interest of all parties that coalition development progress so that all may benefit. Coalitions are the model for healthcare public private partnerships to become. The Region III Health and Medical Taskforce acknowledges this fact and is using this opportunity to create a better coalition out of a productive and effective taskforce.

REFERENCES

ASPR. (2014). *HPP cooperative agreement.* Washington, DC: HHS.

Cellucci, T. (2010). *Innovative public private partnerships: A pathway to effectively solving problems.* Washington, DC: Department of Homeland Security.

FEMA. (2014). *FY 2013 homeland security grant program (HSGP).* Retrieved 05 20, 2014, from FEMA: http://www.fema.gov/fy-2013-homeland-security-grant-program-hsgp-0

Hanfling, D. (2013). *Role of regional healthcare coalitions in managing and coordinating disaster reposnse.* Washington, DC: National Academy of Science.

HHS. (2009a). *From hospitals to heralthcare coalitions: Transforming health preparedness and response in our communities.* Wsahington, DC: HHS.

HHS. (2009b). Medical surge capacity and capability: The healthcare coalition in emergency response and recovery. Washington, DC: HHS.

HHS. (2013, July 3). *HHS grants to bolster disaster preparedness for health care, public health.* Retrieved July 15, 2013, from http://www.hhs.gov/news/press/2013pres/07/20130703a.html

MedStar Health. (2014). *About us.* Retrieved 08 14, 2014, from MedStar Health: https://www.medstarhealth.org/Pages/About-Us.aspx

MESH. (2010). *About our coalition.* Retrieved 05 14, 2014, from MESH: www.meshcoalition.org

MIEMSS. (n.d.). *Who we are.* Retrieved 05 14, 2014, from Maryland Institute of Emergency Medical Services Systems: https://www.miemss.org/home/Home/WhoWeAre/tabid/74/Default.aspx

MOEM. (n.d.). *Regional planning.* Retrieved 05 23, 2014, from Mayor's Office of Emergency Management: http://emergency.baltimorecity.gov/Programs/RegionalPlanning.aspx

NetMBA. (2010). *SWOT analysis.* Retrieved 05 24, 2014, from NetMBA Business Knowledge Center: http://www.netmba.com/strategy/swot/

NHCRC. (2013a). *National healthcare coalition resource center.* Retrieved 05 14, 2014, from http://healthcarecoalitions.org/

NHCRC. (2013b). *Region III health and medical taskforce strategic planning workshop october 2013 final report.* Indianapolis, IN: NHCRC.

NHCRC. (2014). *Region III health and medical taskforce startegic plan final report.* Indianapolis, IN: NHCRC.

NVHA. (2014). *About us*. Retrieved May 12, 2014, from http://www.novaha.org/about-us/

NWHRC. (2013). *Who we are*. Retrieved May 13, 2014, from http://www.nwhrn.org/about-the-network/

WJZ. (2012, October 18). *Baltimore's star-spangled sailabration drew big business*. Retrieved May 15, 2014, from http://baltimore.cbslocal.com/2012/10/18/study-baltimore-sailabration-drew-big-business/

KEY TERMS AND DEFINITIONS

Alternate Care Site or Alternate Care Facility (ACF): Is a (physical) location that can be used to provide healthcare in the event of a surge that overwhelms local resources.

Coalition: An alliance of related organizations (in the context of this chapter these are healthcare related organizations) and other individual healthcare assets intended to maximize medical surge capacity and capability (MSCC).

Homeland Security Grant Program (HSGP): Is intended to cover all projects through which the U.S. Department of Homeland Security (DHS) provides funding to local, state, and Federal agencies in support of the National Preparedness Goal, i.e. in support of mitigation, protection, prevention, response and recovery as well as related capabilities.

Hospital Preparedness Program (HPP): Is a program administered by the U.S. Department of Health & Human Services that provides leadership and funding to States, territories, and local jurisdictions intended to enhance public health preparedness.

Maryland Institute for Emergency Medical Services Systems (MIEMSS) Region III: Is a high quality, state-wide, coordinated emergency medical system (EMS) system in the State of Maryland (for more information see: http://www.miemss.org/home/). There are five regions within the MIEMSS each having a Regional EMS Advisory Council. Region III is an area that includes Baltimore City as well as Anne Arundel, Baltimore, Carroll, Harford, and Howard counties.

Medical Surge Capacity and Capability (MSCC): Is a management methodology utilizing the tenets of emergency management and the Incident Command System (ICS) to coordinate between various medical/healthcare organizations and disciplines as well as providing a foundation for integration with other emergency management systems, e.g. fire service, law enforcement, etc. MSCC is a tiered system comprised of: *Tier 1:* Management of Individual Healthcare Assets, e.g. outpatient clinics, private physician offices etc., *Tier 2:* Management of a Healthcare Coalition, *Tier 3:* Jurisdiction Incident Management, i.e. integration across the emergency management systems (healthcare, fire services, law enforcement, etc.) within a jurisdiction, *Tier 4:* Management of State Response, *Tier 5:* Interstate Regional Management Coordination, *Tier 6:* Federal Support to State, Tribal, and Jurisdiction Management.

Office of the Assistant Secretary for Preparedness and Response (ASPR): Is an agency within the U.S. Department of Health & Human Services charged with preventing, preparing for, and responding to the adverse health effects of public health emergencies and disasters in the U.S.

Task Force: Is a work group or team established to work on a single task.

Urban Area Security Initiative (UASI) Program: Is intended to be a conduit for financial assistance to address the unique multi-discipline planning, organization, equipment, training, and exercise needs of high-threat, high-density Urban Areas, and to assist these areas in building and sustaining capabilities to prevent, protect against, mitigate, respond to, and recover from threats or acts of terrorism using the Whole Community approach.

U. S. Department of Health and Human Services (DHHS): Is a U.S. federal agency charged with protecting the health of all Americans and providing essential human services, especially for those who are least able to help themselves.

Work Groups and Teams: A *work group* is a group of 2 or more, working individually to achieve a common goal or goals. This is in contrast to a *team*, which is also a group of 2 or more but who are working together to achieve a common goal or goals. Where the emphasis in work groups is on individual contribution (or work product), the emphasis in teams is on the collective contribution (or work product).

This work was previously published in Emergency Management and Disaster Response Utilizing Public-Private Partnerships edited by Marvine Paula Hamner, S. Shane Stovall, Doaa M. Taha, and Salah C. Brahimi, pages 240-255 copyright year 2015 by Information Science Reference (an imprint of IGI Global).

D

fault handling 1633
febrile neutropenia 1445, 1448, 1452, 1463
future healthcare professionals 49, 56

G

genomics 277, 515, 847, 874, 967, 1209, 1456
geocoding 577, 588, 601
Geographic Information System (GIS) 769-770
Google Map 282, 587, 589, 601, 781, 930-931
Graphical User Interface (GUI) 189, 380, 501, 768, 1695
grounded theory 362, 367
guideline rules 666
gyroscope 941, 943

H

health apps 265, 428
healthcare delivery 25, 34, 50-51, 97, 222, 273, 284, 320, 337, 341, 346, 537, 576, 657, 949, 962, 967, 979, 1001, 1008, 1200, 1280, 1320, 1325, 1551, 1696, 1699, 1726, 1730
healthcare industry 2, 222, 260, 262, 276, 282, 443, 467, 710-711, 1001, 1097-1101, 1103-1104, 1107-1111, 1117, 1120, 1122, 1126, 1131, 1202, 1442-1443, 1466, 1507, 1512, 1515, 1518, 1524-1526, 1645, 1733, 1736, 1738, 1743-1744
Healthcare Information Systems (HIS) 222, 710, 1083-1084, 1325, 1681, 1689, 1697, 1705
healthcare management 1092, 1531, 1545, 1731
healthcare-managers 1549
healthcare monitoring 332, 466, 468, 1039, 1088, 1435
healthcare operations 1321, 1323, 1329, 1749
healthcare providers 149, 151, 157, 266-267, 272, 275, 277-278, 281-282, 287, 299-301, 438, 467-468, 472, 582, 718, 842, 846, 851, 863, 875, 895, 899, 948, 963, 969, 983, 1083, 1122-1123, 1156, 1279-1280, 1290, 1299-1300, 1315, 1321, 1323-1324, 1439, 1507, 1509-1510, 1512, 1515-1516, 1547, 1553, 1640-1641, 1674-1675, 1678-1679, 1681-1684, 1688, 1707-1709, 1717, 1727, 1730, 1743, 1752, 1754
healthcare services 77-81, 85, 94, 105, 277, 319, 321-322, 334, 342, 346, 348, 357, 524, 537-538, 540, 547, 642, 656-657, 695-696, 710, 721, 730, 734, 784-789, 792, 802, 863, 893, 896, 947-949, 961, 965, 967, 971, 975, 1001, 1020, 1087, 1089-1090, 1107, 1200, 1330, 1397, 1403, 1413, 1441, 1492, 1494-1495, 1507, 1552-1553, 1562, 1636, 1674, 1676-1677, 1679, 1681, 1684, 1688-1691, 1706, 1727, 1745

healthcare system 77-78, 156, 261, 273, 277, 301, 336, 581, 637-638, 658, 747, 784, 786-787, 795, 800-801, 1002, 1092, 1101, 1156, 1186-1187, 1312, 1325, 1436, 1494, 1508, 1510, 1553, 1636, 1642, 1675, 1684, 1689, 1692, 1695, 1719, 1726-1727, 1738, 1741, 1748, 1752
health disparities 118, 120-121, 128, 131
Health & Human Services (HHS) 239, 257, 1708, 1757
healthinfo engineering 537-538, 541, 545, 547
health informatics 64, 89, 131, 160, 418, 487-488, 499, 560, 562, 956, 962, 965, 977-978, 1254, 1303, 1675, 1689-1690, 1692, 1696, 1705, 1713, 1741
Health Information Exchange (HIE) 82, 445, 488-489, 491, 509-510, 513-514, 517, 520, 1001, 1008, 1245-1246, 1248-1249, 1251-1254, 1256, 1259, 1735
Health Information System (HIS) 88, 161, 222, 225, 235, 332, 336, 578, 582, 588-589, 596, 1323, 1435, 1490, 1534, 1545, 1675, 1717
Health Information Technology for Economic and Clinical Health (HITECH) Act 1008, 1301, 1432, 1444, 1509, 1646
Health Information Technology (HIT) 2, 50, 60, 64-65, 67, 120, 122, 129-130, 356, 395, 431, 443, 488, 490-491, 502-503, 509, 511-513, 517, 520-521, 523-524, 534, 683, 962-963, 966, 974, 1005, 1008, 1079, 1245-1247, 1251, 1259, 1301, 1320, 1324-1325, 1432, 1442, 1444, 1488-1490, 1509, 1646, 1675, 1694
Health Insurance Portability and Accountability Act (HIPAA) 489, 515, 752, 764, 1006, 1012, 1246, 1301, 1432, 1444, 1518
health monitoring 276, 335, 348, 543, 551-553, 555-557, 559, 576, 584, 586-587, 602-608, 610-611, 613-615, 618, 738, 751, 753, 763, 768, 787, 797, 1020, 1022-1023, 1039, 1088, 1660, 1676, 1682, 1721
health prevention 1156-1158, 1173-1174, 1185
health privacy 419, 1207-1214, 1218-1219
Health Record Trust (HRT) 1436
health services 8, 28, 32, 56, 77-90, 93, 227, 250-251, 319, 321, 348, 351, 537, 578, 582, 584, 619, 623, 637-641, 655-656, 663, 787, 814, 823, 825, 834, 854, 863, 894-895, 961, 969, 1057, 1101, 1143, 1279-1281, 1290, 1395-1396, 1407, 1430, 1507, 1516, 1529, 1540-1541, 1551-1555, 1557-1558, 1560, 1600, 1658-1659, 1678, 1682-1683, 1741
health technologies 79-80, 93, 260, 284, 438, 578, 580-581, 601
Health Technology Competency (HTC) 977, 1000

N

National Electronic-Health Transition Authority (NEHTA) 1444
National Health System (NHS) 376, 637, 1444, 1679
natural disasters 1271, 1273
neonatal health 1141, 1143, 1150
neurosurgery 1338-1340, 1342-1343, 1346-1347
non-adoption 391-392, 395-396, 400-401, 404-405, 407-408
Noncommunicable Chronic Diseases (NCD) 295
noncommunicable diseases 260, 267, 270, 281
norm analysis 26, 33, 35, 38, 41-42, 44, 329, 1059, 1066, 1070

O

ontological approach 445, 458-459
ontological model 32, 450, 578, 582-584, 586, 591-592, 595-597, 601
Operative Role Management (ORM) 1379-1381, 1384, 1388-1389, 1391, 1394
Opportunistic Mobile Networks (OMN) 1045
organizational learning 360-361, 366-367, 1537
organizational semiotics 26, 37, 45, 319-320, 328, 330, 332, 336, 341, 346, 363, 1059

P

palliative care 183-189, 191-196, 199
Parkinson's Disease (PD) 555, 694, 1174, 1635
participative health 1185
participatory mapping 1361, 1365, 1374-1375
pathology services 60-63
pathway knowledge 26, 32, 42, 45
patient monitoring 320-321, 323-324, 331, 336, 346, 469, 472, 475, 483, 551-553, 555-556, 567-570, 605-606, 736, 751-753, 787, 842, 854, 862, 874, 1017, 1019-1022, 1026-1027, 1029-1030, 1033, 1040-1041, 1552, 1606-1607, 1609-1610, 1624, 1626
patient outcomes 19, 25, 823-824, 843, 846, 848-851, 855, 863-864, 874, 903, 1103, 1121, 1187, 1507, 1691, 1697, 1709
patient safety 25-28, 30-35, 45, 63-65, 104, 120, 320-321, 346, 361-362, 365-367, 416, 531, 606, 821-825, 834, 841, 900-901, 903-904, 909, 918, 962, 1001, 1008, 1048-1049, 1062-1063, 1069, 1108, 1119, 1122, 1127, 1186-1187, 1198, 1223-1227, 1230-1232, 1234, 1238, 1244, 1338, 1347, 1398, 1442, 1445-1447, 1449, 1453-1456, 1493, 1510, 1536-1537, 1540, 1546, 1568-1569, 1579, 1593, 1600, 1668, 1695

patient-safety culture 26-27
patient view 1097, 1099, 1104, 1106, 1109, 1111, 1117, 1436
pay-as-you-go 710, 1414, 1427, 1431
pelvic floor muscle training 304, 317
perceived enjoyment 238, 241, 243, 248-249, 251-252, 257
perceived irritation 238, 242, 247, 257
perceived monetary value 238, 241, 248-249, 251, 257
perceived usefulness 49-52, 55-57, 195, 197, 241, 252, 686, 1555, 1557
performance dashboards 1135
perioperative process 1119-1125, 1127-1129, 1131, 1135
Personal Health Records (PHR) 490-491, 500-502, 509, 511-512, 521, 597, 962, 1073, 1079, 1081, 1083-1084, 1087-1088, 1096, 1246-1247, 1253, 1260, 1435, 1438, 1444, 1467, 1725
Personal Health Systems (PHS) 659, 1110, 1396, 1398, 1401, 1404
Personal Identifiable Information (PII) 510, 516, 521
personalized medicine 717, 842, 847, 857-859, 862, 864, 874, 962, 1246-1248, 1251-1252
Personally Controlled Electronic Health Records (PCEHR) 50, 980, 1320-1322, 1324, 1337, 1436, 1444
Personal Medical Device (PMD) 1087-1088, 1096
pervasive healthcare 319-324, 328, 330-332, 334, 337-342, 346, 1721
Pervasive Healthcare Information Provision (PHIP) 319-322, 324, 330-332, 334, 338-342, 346
PGOT framework 1511-1512, 1518, 1524, 1526
pharmaceutical care 1445-1447, 1455-1456, 1463
pharmaceutical protocols 641, 660
pharmaco-cybernetics 1445, 1447, 1449, 1452, 1455-1456, 1463
pharmaco-informatics 1447, 1463
physical therapy 298-299, 301-305, 312, 317
Platform-as-a-Service (PaaS) 563, 576
Platform for Privacy Preferences (P3P) 1442, 1444
political attitudes 822, 1207-1208, 1210-1214, 1218-1219
post-analytical 1223-1226, 1228, 1235, 1244
Post-Traumatic Stress Disorder (PTSD) 512, 1339, 1360, 1437
power outage 877-881, 883, 887-888, 1012
pre-analytical 1223-1226, 1228-1232, 1234-1238, 1244
price premium 846, 874
Principal Component Analysis (PCA) 1449, 1463
privacy rule 515, 1006-1007, 1432-1435, 1439, 1444

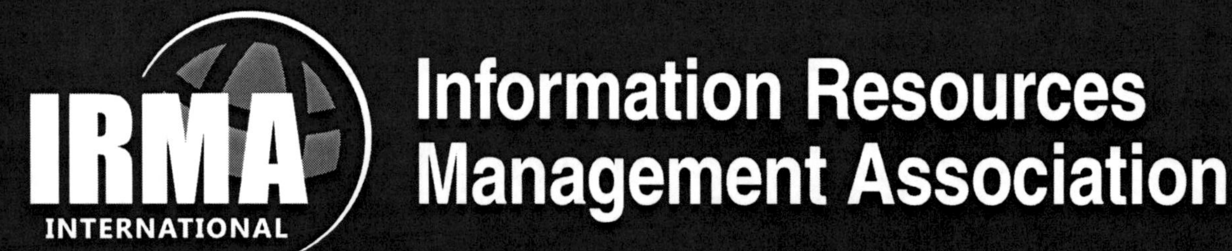

Become an IRMA Member

Members of the **Information Resources Management Association (IRMA)** understand the importance of community within their field of study. The Information Resources Management Association is an ideal venue through which professionals, students, and academicians can convene and share the latest industry innovations and scholarly research that is changing the field of information science and technology. Become a member today and enjoy the benefits of membership as well as the opportunity to collaborate and network with fellow experts in the field.

IRMA Membership Benefits:

- **One FREE Journal Subscription**

- **30% Off Additional Journal Subscriptions**

- **20% Off Book Purchases**

- Updates on the latest events and research on Information Resources Management through the IRMA-L listserv.

- Updates on new open access and downloadable content added to Research IRM.

- A copy of the Information Technology Management Newsletter twice a year.

- A certificate of membership.

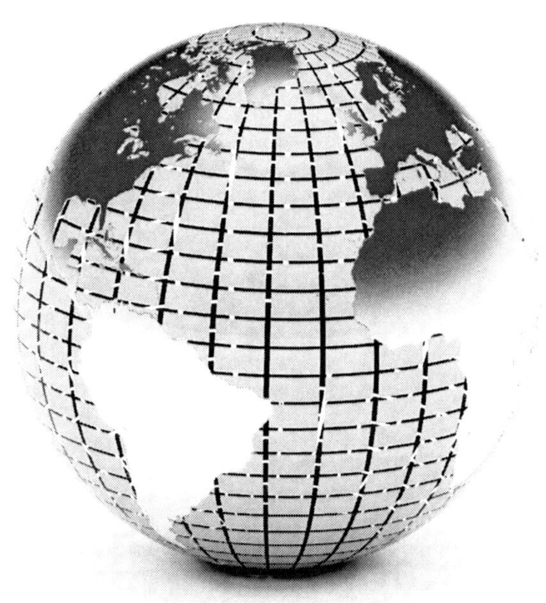

IRMA Membership $195

Scan code to visit irma-international.org and begin by selecting your free journal subscription.

Membership is good for one full year.